Diagnostic Imaging in Head and Neck Cancer

Hiroya Ojiri
Editor

Diagnostic Imaging in Head and Neck Cancer

Springer

Editor
Hiroya Ojiri
Department of Radiology
The Jikei University School of Medicine
Tokyo
Japan

ISBN 978-981-15-3187-3 ISBN 978-981-15-3188-0 (eBook)
https://doi.org/10.1007/978-981-15-3188-0

This Springer imprint is published by the registered company Springer Nature Singapore Pte Ltd.
The registered company address is: 152 Beach Road, #21-01/04 Gateway East, Singapore 189721, Singapore

Preface

Head and neck cancer, the main subject of this textbook, is a heterogeneous disease encompassing epithelial malignancies of the upper aerodigestive tract, including paranasal sinuses, nasal cavity, oral cavity, pharynx and larynx. Worldwide, it represents the 6th most frequent neoplasia (approximately 650,000 new cases diagnosed annually) and accounting for 6% of all cases, and is also responsible for approximately 1–2% of tumor deaths (350,000 deaths per annum worldwide). As a whole, the disease group is associated with different epidemiology, etiology and treatment strategy. Tobacco and alcohol abuse have been major risk factors of head and neck cancer. More recently, high-risk HPV (human papilloma viruses) infection is implicated in the development of oropharyngeal cancer although HPV- related cancer has a distinct clinical entity with a better prognosis. Treatment selection for head and neck cancer is based on the location and stage of the disease. Early-stage diseases are often treated with single modality such as surgery or radiation therapy alone, while advanced tumors are usually treated with multiple modalities, usually including systemic therapy. Organ preservation therapy has been increasingly adopted, without causing significant compromise of locoregional control and survival rate, mainly due to its excellent functional and/or cosmetic outcomes.

Diagnostic imaging, particularly CT and MRI, plays an important role in the diagnosis of head and neck cancers, evaluation of the disease extent (to stage the disease accurately) and post-treatment follow-up. To evaluate images of head and neck cancers adequately, radiologists should thoroughly understand the regional anatomy, both typical and atypical imaging features of the disease, differential diagnosis, patterns of disease spread, treatment complications and patterns of recurrence. Despite the recent progression of the imaging techniques, only a few subspecialized head and neck radiologists can fully meet the needs of referring clinicians.

We have attempted to make diagnostic imaging of head and neck cancers clear and concise in this text by reviewing the recent advances in this field, with an emphasis on practical aspects of the evaluation of such diseases. The authors of each chapter, who are all at the forefront in this field, discussed and summarized the points based on their considerable knowledge and abundant experience. Especially, my mentor and one of my best friends, Tony (Mancuso AA, M.D.), kindly joined us to write an introductory chapter "Perspectives and trends in diagnostic imaging of head and neck cancer". This chapter tells us exactly what I wanted to express in this textbook. I believe that all chapters will bring the readers up to date about head and neck cancer and about the future of this field. This textbook is warmly recommended to radiologists, head and neck surgeons, ENT doctors, and radiation oncologists.

Finally, I would like to express my sincere thanks to all the authors for their tremendous effort in enhancing the value of this textbook. I am very grateful to Ms. Guruprasad Kripa and Ms. Yoko Arai at Springer for promotion of this project and detailed editing of the manuscripts.

Tokyo, Japan — Hiroya Ojiri

Contents

1 Perspectives and Trends in Diagnostic Imaging of Head and Neck Cancer

Anthony A. Mancuso

Abstract

A meaningful and accurate report is the central responsibility of those interpreting imaging studies of patients with head and neck cancer. This chapter will draw on the approximately 80 years of knowledge that has contributed meaningfully to the understanding of the factors that define competent reporting and consultation in head and neck cancer imaging. This begins with a consideration of the fundamental structure and content of consistent and meaningful reports. Next, the chapter will define processes that create a pathway to becoming expert enough to exercise imaging professional behavior that defines an optimal and efficient standard of practice in head and neck cancer imaging. The central theme will continuously reflect how the expectation of such expert practice relates to foundations of knowledge and experience that began in the 1930s and have reached a reasonably defined steady state at this time. Finally, the chapter will summarize suggested improvements in the current state of our imaging techniques that remain primarily of investigational and/or speculative interest. This will include suggestions in the literature, for possible marginal improvements in the data we generate from images and conclusions drawn from that data we provide in reports.

Keywords

Cancer · Spread patterns · Regional adenopathy · Perineural · Post treatment · Imaging · Reporting

A. A. Mancuso (✉)
Department of Diagnostic Radiology, University of Florida College of Medicine and UF Health—Shands Hospital, Gainesville, FL, USA
e-mail: mancua@radiology.ufl.edu

1.1 The Central Task: A Competent Report/Consultation

A meaningful and accurate report is the central responsibility of those interpreting imaging studies of patients with head and neck cancer. This chapter will draw on the approximately 80 years of knowledge that has contributed meaningfully to the understanding of the factors that define competent reporting and consultation in head and neck cancer imaging. This begins with a consideration of the fundamental structure and content of consistent and meaningful reports. Next, the chapter will define processes that create a pathway to becoming expert enough to exercise imaging professional behavior that defines an optimal and efficient standard of practice in head and neck cancer imaging. The central theme will continuously reflect how the expectation of such expert practice relates to foundations of knowledge and experience that began in the 1930s and have reached a reasonably defined steady state at this time.

Finally, the chapter will summarize suggested improvements in the current state of our imaging techniques that remain primarily of investigational and/or speculative interest. This will include suggestions in the literature, for possible marginal improvements in the data we generate from images and conclusions drawn from that data we provide in reports. Pursuing those ends can become a distraction from our central responsibilities to our patients and clinical colleagues, while providing no added value especially with respect to time and effort that might be expended. Implementing some of these suggestions can create real expense in addition to the human capital investment with no return on investment. At its conclusion, this chapter will recommend avoiding some of these specific suggestions that make their way into the literature as part of a standard portfolio of imaging in head and neck cancer.

Patients with head and neck cancer are at high risk for very significant functional and cosmetic deficits because of the nature of this disease and the effects of these therapeutic options. Value-added in our reports is directly linked to

H. Ojiri (ed.), *Diagnostic Imaging in Head and Neck Cancer*, https://doi.org/10.1007/978-981-15-3188-0_1

exploiting our extraordinary imaging tools to produce as accurate an account of the disease extent as possible to limit this morbidity and, in some cases, avoid fruitless attempts at definitive therapy moving the patient to a disease "management" rather than curative strategy.

The suggested basic structure of the diagnostic imaging report differs within four basic clinical situations encountered in a practice of head and neck cancer imaging. However, there is commonality in the report structure and content between those four following clinical settings that follow:

1. **The initial staging and treatment planning study**.

   This requires that diagnostic imaging specialists understand that they do not, themselves, stage cancers although "staging the tumor" often becomes a focus of educational effort in head and neck cancer imaging. It would be unfortunate if patients who are reading their imaging reports, as well as their own medical records, were to become confused by a TNM stage offered by a diagnostic radiologist's report that was different from that offered by the physicians who are actually responsible for officially assigning a stage in the medical record. This can lead to needless time spent on reconciling such recorded disparities.

   Diagnostic radiologists must offer clear and accurate subjective and objective data that contributes to the staging process. A recent and somewhat belated educational effort, sometimes presented as "Contextual Reporting", is a more appropriate educational approach to ensure that report content is complete, consistent, and useful in the staging process [1]. Staging does not dictate specific treatment. Tumor staging does contribute the process of treatment planning since the staging process relies on our reported granularity of extent of primary, regional, and distant disease, which is a real and central determinant of treatment strategy.

   Staging is important for accurate end results reporting, which is a significant responsibility of our clinical colleagues who rely on our data to also execute that responsibility as accurately as possible in keeping with the most current staging guidelines. At times, integration of imaging data into staging systems has created a phenomenon referred to as "stage creep". This has resulted in some degree of over staging some cancers compared to historic baselines. Still it is a system that is essential and requires careful thought as imaging data continues to be integrated with staging criteria.
2. **The search for a clinically occult primary cancer** that might be producing symptoms or signs of disease such as otalgia, metastatic cervical adenopathy, or signs and symptoms related to the Trigeminal or Facial nerve.
3. **Routine surveillance** of the treated patient.
4. **The staging and treatment planning study of the patient with newly discovered recurrent cancer**.

The suggested commonality in these situations and related report structure includes (**terms in bold are suggested sections for creation of a shell for a structured report**):

1. **Evaluation of the primary site:** A clear description of the full extent of the primary tumor. This includes spread within **soft tissues** especially along known pathways in the deeper soft tissue spaces of the head and neck (such as the parapharyngeal pre- and retrostyloid components) and **cartilage** and **bone invasion**, when appropriate, for the given primary site.
2. **Perineural spread:** An accounting of the likely presence and extent of perineural spread of cancer based on pathoanatomic image analysis informed by known tendencies that vary with cancer tissue type and primary site location.
3. **Regional adenopathy:** A full accounting of regional nodal metastatic disease. This should be based on known trends and patterns and must account for **all lymph node groups** including retropharyngeal, retrostyloid, facial, parotid, and posterior neck groups. This assessment should also include the presence and extent of **extranodal extension** including the likelihood of **deep neck fixation and/or involvement of vascular structures** including the jugular vein, especially the carotid artery.
4. **Risk of distant metastases (optional as appropriate):** A suggestion with regard to the necessity of evaluation of distant metastatic disease based on the extent of local regional spread: typically, this is a suggestion for chest CT and possibly FDG-PET imaging.

Such a suggested report structure should remain essentially the same in evaluating a confirmed cancer recurrence. In the other two alternative settings of searching for clinically occult primary tumors and imaging in the surveillance mode for recurrence, the reporting responsibilities shift to primarily expressing a degree of confidence in the presence or absence of disease. The ACR NI-RADS initiative is a useful attempt to standardize the approach to surveillance imaging. In both these alternative clinical scenarios expressing such a degree of confidence, with regard to the presence or absence of tumor, is one of the most difficult tasks in head and neck cancer imaging. In my years of practice, it has come to require the most experience and care in report preparation. Patients are currently reading either the report impression section and/or the full report in the United States. The responsibility of an expert imaging consultant in these clinical scenarios is to create a clear understanding of degree of confidence in the meaning of the imaging findings and to avoid confusing and/or insensitive language or needless equivocation that might provoke unnecessary patient anxiety. That responsibility in reporting must be balanced with an honest assessment of risk so as not to mislead the ordering physician with ambiguous language. Current training programs are only beginning to address these nuances in report creation, at this point, marginally approaching the challenge by encouraging a standard report structure as embodied by concepts of "Contextual Reporting" [1] and the ACR NI-RADS initiative. Such initiatives are only now emerging, almost four decades into the evolution of modern head and neck cancer imaging.

In the post-treatment surveillance scenario, the basic report structure is modified as follows (**terms in bold are suggested sections for creation of a shell for a structured report**):

1. **Expected post-treatment changes:** A succinct discussion of the presence and nature of postoperative and/or postradiation changes. Avoidance of unnecessary and essentially meaningless verbiage is important to keep the "fog" out of these reports. If those post-treatment changes are relatively routine, a summary statement to that effect can be made. This would include such findings as generalized lymphedema affecting the skin, superficial fascia and deeper soft tissue planes and pharyngeal walls, free margin of the epiglottis and aryepiglottic folds. There is no reason to clutter the report by using either a "macro" with sometimes inappropriate, to an individual case, content describing such findings or dictated, variable quality and sometimes confusing syntax to document these routine types of expected post-treatment findings.
2. **Primary Site**
   (a) If there has been reconstructive surgery, what is **the extent of the entire construct** including status of the soft tissue free or otherwise vascularized flap, its vascular pedicle, and the status of any metallic and bony combination component of the construct.
   (b) Changes in the construct or remaining anatomic structures that constitute a definite or suspicious **complication of treatment** such as construct failure, infection, or developing osteonecrosis.
   (c) The presence of any **atypical or worrisome residual focal changes**, including unusually asymmetric or excessive edema, after allowing for asymmetry that may be related to IMRT or other focal treatment planning methodology.
   (d) If there are worrisome or atypical focal changes at the primary site, a **suggestion for short interval follow-up or alternative imaging** follow-up such as with FDG PET (as suggested in ACR NI-RADS guidelines).
   (e) If there is clear evidence of **primary site recurrence,** a report that fully evaluates the extent of disease as presented previously.
3. **Regional Adenopathy:** An assessment of regional adenopathy including possible atypical nodal patterns of spread due to alteration of drainage patterns by therapy.
4. **Risk of Distant Metastases (optional as appropriate):** A suggestion with regard to the necessity of evaluation of distant metastatic disease based on the extent of local regional spread: typically a suggestion for Chest CT and possibly FDG-PET imaging.

In the setting of the search for a clinically occult primary cancer, the task shifts to a statement of confidence in the exclusion or discovery of a malignancy responsible for the suspicious clinical scenario. This includes accounting for variations in normal anatomy such as the superficial asymmetric appearance of pharyngeal lymphoid tissue that might be mistaken for a significant finding. This task requires a significant amount of experience with regard to the range of normal variation of structures in the head and neck region and recognition of early signs of infiltration of deeper tissue space [2]. The latter observation is an essential skill for identifying potentially aggressive and, therefore, malignant pathology. This is a skill set that is not delivered in the context of usual residency and even neuroradiology fellowship training. The fidelity of statements with regard to the presence or absence of significant findings in this particular setting is directly proportional to the experience of the interpreting physician. *An expert imaging consultant must be able to identify negative exams with a very high degree of confidence.*

1.2 Knowledge Base for Progress Toward Becoming an Expert Head and Neck Cancer Imaging Consultant

1.2.1 The Beginnings: Becoming a "Student of the Disease"

To become an expert at interpreting images of patients with head and neck cancer, the interpreting physician must become a student of the natural history of head and neck cancer and how it is altered by therapeutic interventions. The foundational knowledge for this pursuit resides in first understanding evolution of knowledge in the domain of anatomy and pathologic behavior of these malignancies in the untreated state. The important tendencies in this regard are primary site specific with regard to both local and regional lymphadenopathy spread patterns. It is worth a careful review of how such foundational knowledge has come about and contributed to our image interpretive processes over the last 80+ years.

The birth of modern Head and Neck Imaging occurred in the 1970s but the core knowledge for its application came at least three decades before the advanced imaging studies of the modern era were invented and then refined over the next four decade to reach their current state. Compared to the state of the available diagnostic imaging in head and neck cancer early in the 1970s, our current imaging capability to provide useful information is beyond extraordinary. The pre CT/MRI era required that treatment planning rely on the history and physical examination, plain films, contrast studies (such as laryngo-pharyngography), and multidirectional tomography. The ensuing development of imaging modalities beginning with the advent of whole body CT imaging and grey scale ultrasound in the second half of the 1970s is one of the most compelling stories about the impact of a technological improvement in attacking this often devastating disease.

The revolution and rapid evolution of CT, MRI, US, and radionuclide tumor imaging from the late 1970s onward combined with innovative IT advances that were given birth in the early 1990s have made it possible to provide informative images paired with timely reports to all treating practitioners since the late 1990s. With these advances diagnostic radiologists have become ***potential*** providers of valuable, real-time data for medical decision-making in the treatment planning and follow-up care of patients with head and neck cancer. However, the value added by the diagnostic radiologist is directly proportional to a willingness to earn a respected position as part of a multidisciplinary team by becoming *student of this disease* and the information needed by our clinical partners. This requires expert-level training and is a skill set that is not even adequate in a radiology residency training and often does not reach a proficient level of practice in the context of a 1-year neuroradiology fellowship.

While our current advanced imaging tools are powerful, when used with optimal technique, a lack of a fundamental understanding of how this disease grows and spreads at each individual site of origin can limit the optimal acquisition and interpretation of these diagnostic images. This makes it essential for the expert to become fully confident in the practice of imaging that is relevant and shown to contribute to improved outcomes. In treatment planning, such ignorance of fundamental, proven pathoanatomic precepts or reliance on unsubstantiated "new techniques" can lead to poor outcomes. True experts and students of this disease will avoid these pitfalls by studying and understanding the sources of fundamental knowledge to be presented subsequently and putting potential new advancements in proper perspective.

Finally, a newer requisite skill for expert-level performance of imaging consultants in head and neck cancer imaging is understanding the evolution of the radiology report. The need for consistency in the structure and content of the reports was discussed earlier. Expert-level sophistication beyond those basics requires the skill of not only constructing a succinct, complete, and accurate report but also a report that will not create and/or magnify unnecessary patient anxiety since patients now often read their reports. This skill is especially important in the reports of surveillance studies.

On the road to acquiring an expert level of performance, it is useful to study and understand the origins and documentation of knowledge that has become a substrate for our understanding the deep spread patterns of this disease. The modern anatomic basis for some of this understanding dates in the 1930s [3, 4] but goes back much further into the classics of anatomic exploration.

The tendencies of deep spread and deep volume of disease was well known before the modern imaging era. Those disease patterns are now visible to treatment planners on properly acquired and interpreted imaging studies. The initial description of the pathways of spread of primary head neck cancer was the work product of surgeons at the MD Anderson Cancer Center, Memorial Hospital, and Columbia Hospital in the 1940s–60s who chose to take on this challenging anatomic area. That effort was soon joined by early radiation oncologists. These individuals are clearly worthy of specific mention, independent of specific references to their publications. The "founding" group included Martin H (circa 1940 Memorial Sloan Kettering) [5], MacComb W, Jesse R, and Ballantyne AJ [6, 7] (all three of the MD Anderson Cancer Center circa 1960–70), J Conley (circa 1950 –Columbia) [8], and J Kirchner (circa 1970–Yale) [9]. All were extraordinary pioneers in modern head and neck surgery. G. Fletcher [7] and M. Lederman [10, 11], pioneering radiotherapists also contributed materially to our understanding of the natural history of this disease and its behavior as modified by radiotherapy and surgery in the same era. All chose to share this foundational knowledge through truly remarkable scientific publications and textbooks that will be more specifically referenced subsequently. It is sobering to realize that the surgeons developed much of their surgical skill by helping the wounded of World War II. The help provided for those injured soldiers turned into a gift for patients with head and neck cancer. Eventually the writings of these surgeons also became a gift to those wishing to understand how to develop modern imaging techniques to benefit our highly skilled surgeons and radiation oncology colleagues to offer their patients better outcomes.

These treating physicians of the "pre CT era" had to become students of this disease, which has the unavoidable specter of often tremendous functional and cosmetic consequences of both cancer growth and spread as well as the effects of a chosen treatment strategy. The inherent destructive growth of these cancers and the need for necessarily destructive, ablative therapy, in the pre-advanced imaging days, required great skill and understanding on the part of surgeons and early radiotherapists about whether highly morbid treatment plans would be worth the chance for cure. As students of the disease, they learned and documented the patterns of local/regional cancer spread by way of evaluating their successes and failures and honestly reporting these experiences (Martin [5], Fletcher, Ballantyne [7, 12], Conley

[8], Kirchner [9], Lederman [10, 11]). In doing so, those early investigators created the foundational material that allows us to recognize these predictable patterns of disease with CT and MRI. Given such proven fundamental knowledge, diagnostic radiologists have been challenged to fully exploit the capability of CT and MRI by providing imaging protocols that maximize information in the images. We must then make properly guided factual imaging observations, unique to each primary site, to fully inform the treatment decision-making process, which will in turn create the best cure to morbidity ratio.

1.3 The Fundamentals of Local and Regional Spread: The Basis of Eventual Expert Interpretive Skills and Appropriate Report Content

The foundational experience with regard to the local and regional spread of head and neck cancers were brought to us, as described earlier, by extraordinarily skilled general surgeons who ventured into this challenging problem without the benefit of modern imaging or the truly extraordinary options currently available for reconstruction with free vascularized bone and soft tissue flaps. Those surgeons presented this observational, fact-rich, experience to us through their writings, since the primary mode of therapy for treatment, especially before the coming of modern techniques in radiotherapy, was definitive and unfortunately, sometimes "exploratory" surgery. Their post–World War II surgical experience allowed them to record the spread patterns of head neck cancer as seen in the operative suite, in vividly descriptive terms, thereby creating the pathoanatomic foundation that diagnostic radiologist have exploited to explore the full potential of the modern imaging revolution mainly by way of CT and MRI. Simply put, their experience predicted observational opportunity beyond the limits of their physical examination that we now can provide noninvasively with our modern imaging tools. This descriptive surgical experience was sometimes supplemented by techniques such as whole organ sectioning of surgical specimens, especially in laryngeal and hypopharyngeal cancers [9], which allowed for an expanded understanding of disease spread patterns since these whole organ sections highly correlated with what was seen on even the earliest of the CT images at the beginning of the age of modern head and neck cancer imaging. These and other following observations are the foundational knowledge that inform a diagnostic radiologist, who wishes to become a true master student of these diseases and eventually expert enough to be a valued multidisciplinary team member.

The recorded experiences of these pioneers will be summarized in terms of the indispensable pathoanatomic local and regional spread of disease. Whether you explore these referenced materials in detail (which is highly recommended) or rely on more current interpretations of these experiences in textbooks on this topic [13], this knowledge is requisite for the acquisition of expert-level performance in the domain of head and neck cancer image interpretation. These observations are fundamental to treatment planning and, therefore, mandatory for image interpretation and proper reporting. The specific origins of this knowledge that must be mastered include:

Evaluation of the Primary Site

1. For anatomic patterns of local disease spread in cancers of the oral cavity and oropharynx, the writings of Martin [5], Conley [8], Lederman [11], and Ballantyne [7, 2] are essential reading.
2. For cancers of the hypopharynx and larynx, a study of the writings of Kirchner [9] supported by his extraordinary whole organ sectioning of excised specimens is an indispensable resource.
3. For anatomic patterns of local disease spread in parotid cancer and facial nerve vulnerability in surgical treatment, the writings of Conley [8] are an indispensable resource.
4. For anatomic patterns of local disease spread in cancers of the nasopharynx, the writings of Lederman [10] are an essential treatise.

Perineural Spread

1. Evaluation of perineural spread of cancer initially appreciated in the writings of Dodd [14]
2. Substantially augmented by experience in the modern imaging era with reported experience in the perineural spread of cutaneous malignancies [15] by J Batsakis in the pathology literature [16].

Regional Adenopathy

1. Anatomy: The foundational anatomical material for this, the work product in the writings of Rouvière [3] in the1930s augmented by Haagensen [17] in the 1970s.
2. Anatomy as altered by prior treatment: The truly extraordinary work in the MD thesis on cervical lymphangiography by Ugo Fisch [18] in 1966 fully documenting alterations in the spread of regional nodal disease due to surgery and/or RT. This work presents extraordinary concepts that must be taken into account both in initial and salvage treatment planning initially as well as in the context of surveillance imaging. This work is a must read and is the only work of its kind available. The observations of Fisch have been fully verified by our experience with CT and MRI over the last several decades [19].

3. Patterns of adenopathy that occur in squamous cell cancer of the oral cavity, oropharynx, larynx, and hypopharynx.
   (a) The risk of associated regional disease by primary site was established in the 1970s [20] and further substantiated in the 1980s [21] by our clinical colleagues working with pathology experts.
   (b) The work by Ballantyne [12] concerning the recognition and significance of retropharyngeal metastatic adenopathy in oral cavity and oropharyngeal cancer has subsequently saved untold amounts of unnecessary surgical morbidity when this pattern of adenopathy is confirmed on CT or MRI at these primary sites.
   (c) These studies of excised surgical specimens were done before the era of widespread combined surgery and preoperative RT, and eventual chemotherapy altered the natural history of the all- important regional component of head and neck cancer spread. In that way, they are the most significant resources that allow anticipation of metastatic nodal risk beyond those available from any current imaging study.
   (d) The recognition of the prognostic significance of extranodal extension especially when associated with carotid artery encasement or deep neck fixation by many authors.

1.4 Perspectives on Current Appropriate Use of Diagnostic Imaging in Head and Neck Cancers

This section represents the current practice of head and neck cancer imaging at the University of Florida College of Medicine in Gainesville, Florida. The imaging approaches suggested certainly may differ in other practices and the following suggestions may stimulate debate about preferred alternative approaches. There is no absolute right or wrong in such debate. The only truths are that expert professional behavior in planning and interpreting these studies must implement a knowledge of the potential spread patterns of this disease, generate and report the data necessary to make informed treatment decisions for our own referring clinician base, and in these pursuits, do the best we can for patients while respecting our responsibility for proper resource utilization.

1.4.1 Evaluation of the Primary Site and Perineural Spread

In general, contrast-enhanced CT of the maxillofacial region and neck performed in a balanced vascular phase is the preferred initial imaging examination for head and neck cancer. This study will show the soft-tissue extent of disease and related bone or cartilage invasion adequately for treatment planning in the vast majority of patients. Unavoidable degradation due to dental-related artifacts will sometimes limit the evaluation of soft-tissue extent in oral cavity and oropharyngeal cancer and also when necessary MRI can be used as a supplement.

The major exception to this is the superiority of MRI in showing the full extent of perineural spread of tumor. When perineural spread is in serious question and the presence or exclusion of imaging visible perineural cancer will alter treatment plans, MRI is used as a supplemental study.

Another exception may be nasopharyngeal cancer where MRI can certainly suffice entirely for primary and regional disease. In some cases, MRI is more informative than CT for evaluation of the primary site, especially with regard to perineural and intracranial spread. MRI may even be superior in evaluation of early skull base involvement in selected cases. Nasopharyngeal cancer disease differs biologically from squamous cell cancer of the oral cavity, oropharynx, larynx, and hypopharynx, and detailed evaluation of the regional disease is less critical in treatment planning.

The value of FDG-PET/CT as a routine pretreatment evaluation study with regard to the primary site varies with the particular clinical practice. In some practices, this expensive and somewhat complex study is considered an important tool for determining the possible radio responsiveness of tumor as well as providing added value in defining clinical and treatment planning target volumes. Other practices view the routine use of FDG-PET as an added and unnecessary expense for initial treatment planning. A full discussion of this variation in practice habits is beyond the scope of this chapter. It is my opinion that this test should only be used very selectively in pretreatment planning of head and neck cancers.

1.4.2 Regional Adenopathy

Contrast-enhanced CT in a balanced vascular phase combined with a maxillofacial CT represents the best overall approach to imaging of regional disease in the majority of head and neck cancers. Such a study provides all the information necessary for locoregional treatment decision-making in a high percentage of patients. Done with proper protocols, the morphologic rendering of early metastatic adenopathy is clearly superior with CT since CT is more likely to show focal metastatic defects in normal size nodes consistently better than any other anatomic imaging study.

The ongoing controversy with regard to the best approach to identify subclinical nodal metastatic disease will be discussed in a subsequent section of this chapter. At this point, it suffices to say that routine use of FDG-PET for nodal staging is not cost justified. While FDG-PET may reveal subclinical disease, such a discovery typically will not alter the treatment plan or outcome as established by clinical factors and the anatomic imaging studies employed for the initial evaluation of a known cancer. Moreover, no currently available imaging study can supplant the knowledge of the known risk of subclinical disease revealed in the studies of excised neck specimens in the 1970s and 1980s [20, 21]. Those risks must be accounted for, depending on the primary site in any rational treatment plan independent of imaging findings.

MRI anatomically can be used as a supplemental imaging study for confirmation of subtle retropharyngeal adenopathy and in situations where the risk of carotid artery encasement or deep neck fixation is the equivocal on a CT study and determination of that status will alter the treatment plan.

1.4.3 Distant Metastases

The need for evaluation of distant metastases is generally determined by the ordering clinical service. Occasionally, findings on initial head and neck imaging will suggest a higher risk that might be anticipated clinically. Such findings include, but are not limited to, occult low neck and supraclavicular adenopathy especially in the scalene nodes as well as unanticipated aggressive morphology of primary tumor and extranodal spread patterns of disease suggesting biological aggressiveness of the cancer.

The typical evaluation for distant metastases may be limited to a chest CT study but will often include whole body FDG-PET. There is also a rational basis for the use of either or both of these studies in patients who have multiple risk traditional factors for head and neck cancer including excessive alcohol use and smoking because of the association of second primary tumors especially of the lungs. This rationale does not include the HPV-related risk factor.

1.4.4 Surveillance

The initial choice for surveillance in majority of head and neck cancers is an anatomic study, typically contrast-enhanced maxillofacial and neck CT. The choice of CT is especially indicated when bone invasion or bone-related complications may be an issue in detection of disease or assessing for complications involving bone.

In nasopharyngeal and parotid cancer or when perineural spread is the primary concern, MRI is clearly the preferable anatomic imaging choice.

The use of FDG-PET for evaluating initial primary tumor responsiveness varies with clinical practice. In some practices, it is used to determine whether postradiation neck salvage will be instituted when a primary curative radiotherapy or chemoradiation plan is in place and the neck is considered at relatively high risk for persistent or recurrent disease. FDG-PET maybe used as a supplement in surveillance when anatomic imaging shows focal suspicious changes. Because of its relatively high negative predictive value, FDG-PET can encourage a reasonable wait-and-see approach with short interval anatomic imaging follow-up if salvage therapy for cure is a viable option. In the setting of suspicious anatomic findings and a positive FDG-PET study, decision-making is usually between short interval anatomic imaging follow-up or an imaging directed biopsy of the suspicious site, if the biopsy is at low risk for creating unwanted complications such as mandibular or laryngeal osteoradionecrosis. These already well-established practice trends have been embodied appropriately in the ACR NI-RADS guidelines.

1.5 Perspectives on Pitfalls, Distractions, and Ongoing Controversies in Head and Neck Cancer Imaging

The intent of this section is to put into perspective issues that have been constantly or newly raised in the literature over the last 40 years. These issues mainly focus on the potential value of imaging improving tissue specificity or other diagnostic tasks that might help in treatment planning and perhaps outcomes of patients with head and neck cancer. Some of the suggestions in the literature over the years have had a positive effect on these goals. Others represent a time investment on the part of the diagnostic radiologists that produces no marginal benefit toward altering medical decision-making or outcome. Use of these suggestions that do not alter the decision-making process may inappropriately commit human resource time as well as financial resources in a time in medicine when this is likely not an affordable option in the context of routine clinical care.

As with the suggestions for how to create structured reports or how to conduct a practice in head neck cancer imaging earlier in this chapter, some of this discussion would legitimately raise debate. The intent of presenting the offering of the following perspectives is to provide advice, based on 40 years of ongoing practice in this field to those who might wonder whether they can offer more to improve patients' outcome based on new inquires and reported data.

1.5.1 Pitfall: Forgetting the Fundamentals

An example of this was the urgently published experience of unexpected regional parotid node failure in patients irradiated with IMRT techniques for nasopharyngeal and oropharyngeal cancers with related nodal metastatic disease in 2007 [22, 23]. The IMRT planning in that report did not take into account the risk of re-routing of lymphatic drainage to the parotid nodes in the tonsillar cancer with ipsilateral cervical adenopathy based on knowledge available from Fisch's work [18]. The IMRT planning in the nasopharyngeal cancer patients either did not take into account possible re-routing of lymphatic flow due to related capillary obstruction from the presence of cervical adenopathy and/or by not considering knowledge from the writings of Rouvière [3] that here are variably present direct capillary lymphatics from the nasopharynx to the parotid lymph nodes. The IMRT technique thereby lowered the dose to the parotid nodes with the desire to reduce radiation sialoadenitis and gland atrophy and its unpleasant side effects but resulted in an "unusual" or "rare" pattern of failure for those primary sites.

Fundamental knowledge cannot be forgotten or ignored as we adopt newer and well-meaning alterations to previous therapies that had been proven over time not to encumber such a risk of and unusual failure pattern. The intent of sparing morbidity by adopting new approaches to therapy is admirable since morbidity is unfortunately not entirely unavoidable in the treatment of head neck cancer. Limiting treatment morbidity is a strong driving force for those who wish to advance the field. The fundamental natural history of the disease and its alterations due to therapy must be considered and studied to avoid circumstances similar to what occurred in these patients. If this ignorance of fundamental knowledge happened with the three patients in this report [22, 23], in a very sophisticated practice, it begs the question of what is happening on a more comprehensive scale in practices throughout the world. Even after this report, it appears that the "lessons learned" in this honestly reported unfortunate situation [22] still need to be learned unless a 4 or 5% failure rate in patients with otherwise curable disease is acceptable [24]. This is why it is so important for those who rely on imaging for planning to understand the original teachings of Rouvière [3] and Fisch [18] and others discussed earlier in this chapter and become students of the disease and not advocates for new techniques without considering this "old" knowledge.

Another example of neglecting the foundational early knowledge provided by surgeons in this field from the 1940s through the 1980s is evident in the relatively recent adoption of transoral resection (TORS) of oropharyngeal cancers, mainly those of the tonsil and tongue base. The advent of robotic surgery became a technique looking for indications. In head and neck surgery, robotic surgery found its home in this TORS domain. This led to a high level of adoption of this technique, perhaps prematurely, and without due consideration of the teachings of early pioneers in head and neck surgery with regard to the margins of tumor clearance. A significant number of patients following primary tumor resection using a robotic TORS approach required definitive radiotherapy after the TORS robotic procedure. Radiotherapy or a chemoradiation protocol would have been curative alone in the vast majority of these patients. Considering the spread patterns described by clinical colleagues and students of this disease such as Ballantyne, MacComb, Jesse, Martin, Conely, Lederman, and Fletcher [5–8, 10, 11] perhaps some study of imaging predictability of adequate margins, prior to widespread adoption of this technique, would have been in order. Would it have initially, based on those writings, better to consider that the penetration of the constrictor muscles of the pharynx to involve the parapharyngeal and retropharyngeal spaces to be a predictor of lack of adequate clearance of surgical margins? Could modern imaging especially with MRI reasonably predict penetration of the pharyngeal constrictor thus avoiding positive margins requiring definitive RT or chemoradiation salvage? Prospective evaluation considering the historical knowledge spread patterns combined with modern imaging capabilities may have, and still may, avoid situation of significant expense and morbidity of a larger surgical procedure than biopsy in many instances. Thoughtful attention to the teachings of our clinical colleagues who were pioneers in this field perhaps can avoid such pitfalls.

1.5.2 Potential Distraction: Tissue Specificity from Imaging Studies

The quest to derive tissue-specific information from diagnostic imaging studies is laudable. The intended variety of imaging approaches to this end suggested to be of potential value in several decision-making domains including: initial histologic diagnosis of masses that may represent primary cancers, regional lymph node metastasis diagnosis, and predictability of radio responsiveness of tumors and confident differentiation of post-treatment scarring and other reactive changes from recurrent cancer. The following list represents the physiologic data that can be derived from imaging studies as potential aids in improving tissue specificity:

1. CT and MRI perfusion including wash in and wash out characteristics
2. MR diffusion-weighted imaging
3. MR spectroscopy
4. Dual energy CT
5. PET/CT with FDG and perhaps more tumor-specific metabolic tracers

The only one of these which has proven reasonably useful in some situations is FDG-PET/CT. The rest remain techniques that require a substantial postprocessing and intense physician analysis of images, more scanning time on the unit, and more technologist input with regard to creation of datasets suitable for efficient analysis by the diagnostic radiologist.

Some of these suggested techniques are not useful, even aside from the human resource and perhaps direct financial costs, simply because they do not advance the treatment planning process that leads to a measurable improvement in outcome. In other settings an important reason for avoiding additive, but not meaningful data gathering, is that there is simply no reliable physiologic marker or surrogate that can replace tissue sampling or a strategy of watchful waiting with short interval anatomic imaging follow-up, depending on the clinical situation. Tissue sampling is safe and relatively easy using current imaging guided capabilities and has few pitfalls; the main one being situations where cases with low index of suspicion one avoids biopsies that may induce osteonecrosis of the mandible and/or osteonecrosis of an otherwise functional and disease-free larynx.

With regard to FDG-PET/CT (and perhaps PET/CT with more tumor-specific agents), there still is significant overuse of this technology. This is mainly because of this being one more nonspecific surrogate for tumor, based on metabolic activity. This technique became one of the initial indications for payment for PET as it replaced much of SPECT tumor imaging with FDG. That socioeconomic circumstance led to an ill-advised, ubiquitous, initial overuse of this technique in many patients presenting with head and neck cancer who did not need to study as part of their initial evaluation. This overuse persists to this day. While this technique can provide incremental data in some cases it is highly unusual that, as part of the initial evaluation, such incremental data will alter the treatment plan or even less so outcome.

There is a risk of other primary tumors (especially lung cancer) to arise in patients with risk factors for head and neck cancer; however, the question remains whether using FDG-PET for such a screening purpose is reasonable in all patients presenting with a known head and neck cancer.

With regard to the infrequent circumstance of identifying an occult primary pharyngeal cancer responsible for cervical adenopathy, FDG-PET offers only marginal improvement in diagnosis over the combination of well done and interpreted anatomic imaging and speculative or imaging directed biopsy of the tonsil and tongue base.

FDG-PET/CT is useful as a post-treatment surveillance tool; however, the technique is associated with a significant false positive rate related to metabolic activity which is often present as a result of reactive post-treatment changes. This is combined with the limitation of all imaging studies of not being able to detect low-volume macroscopic and microscopic disease in treatment beds. The balance between the use of this technique, clinical risk assessment, and imaging directed biopsy versus short interval follow-up was discussed earlier in this chapter with regard to surveillance issues. There is a reasonable approach to the surveillance role of FDG-PET/CT in the current ACR NI-RADS guidelines.

1.5.3 Ongoing Controversy: What Is the Best Imaging Study to Detect Regional Adenopathy?

Hayes Martin put the logical approach to surgical treatment of regional adenopathy in head neck cancer into clinical practice in the 1940s [5]. In 1970s and early 1980s, Lindberg and then Byers clearly defined the risk of subclinical neck disease and cancers of the oral cavity, oropharynx, larynx, and hypopharynx [20, 21]. The central argument in this longstanding controversy is whether there is an ideal imaging suite of tools that can definitively diagnose subclinical neck disease. A corollary argument being, can the results of such imaging be substituted for well-established, pathologically confirmed risk patterns of cervical metastatic disease in head and neck cancers in the clinical decision-making process [20, 21]. The simple answer to both questions is no. Imaging data is useful in planning and surveillance of regional nodal metastases but traditional knowledge about risk based on primary site should be the prime determinant of the basic approach to treatment of the neck combined with taking into account most appropriate choice of therapy for primary site management.

Since the earliest experience with the CT evaluation of cervical lymph node metastases, the question of whether imaging can improve on the clinical examination for treatment planning has been established [19]. CT imaging, even early in development, was at the outset proven to be an improvement over the physical examination. In addition, it was shown to be a major breakthrough with regard to the detection of nonpalpable lymph node groups such as the retropharyngeal lymph nodes, the importance of that group of nodes, and the retrostyloid group being first introduced by Ballantyne in the 1960s [12]. Subsequently, CT was confirmed in many following studies to be able to detect morphologically abnormal lymph nodes in groups one through six not clearly positive on physical examination as well as the presence and extent of extranodal extension. MRI has the same general capability of CT only with less overall accuracy, and MRI is typically not the initial study of choice in evaluating head neck cancer.

Other approaches to improving the accuracy of diagnosis of subclinical nodal disease proposed as possibly making a difference in treatment planning or treatment outcome include:

1. Physiologic parameters that may be derived from CT and MRI including perfusion data, dual energy CT data, and MRI diffusion-weighted imaging and spectroscopy. These were discussed earlier in this section and really are noncontributory to the routine practice of head neck cancer imaging for nodal staging.
2. Ultrasound with ultrasound directed biopsy of suspicious nodes: this technique is time-consuming, not patient

friendly and not shown to produce significant outcome or treatment planning benefit and is now relegated to niche use rather than as part of routine in initial staging as originally proposed.
3. Lymphoscintigraphy: this is mainly used in selected skin cancers.

This particular now 35 year-long controversy has likely reached a steady-state with contrast-enhanced CT of the neck combined with maxillofacial CT study as the basic approach to staging primary and regional disease. That approach can, in selected circumstances, be supplemented with MRI especially with regard to the detection of equivocal retropharyngeal lymph nodes and the extent of extranodal disease that might be showing equivocal carotid or deep neck fixation on CT.

Perhaps the future of tumor genetics or serum biomarkers will provide further insight into targeted therapies for both the primary site and regional disease and advance this discussion beyond the capability of modern imaging.

1.5.4 New Controversy: Is Routine Post-treatment Surveillance Justified?

The value of post-treatment surveillance should be measured against the likelihood of an effective "salvage" strategy. This risk-benefit analysis has become a more complex issue recently because targeted therapy options depending on both patient and tumor biology can be used to "manage" persistent disease as opposed to approaching salvage of a recurrence strictly with curative intent or supportive care only. It is important to remember three fundamental unanswered questions with regard to the value of surveillance imaging:

1. There is no uniform agreement about the preferred anatomic study of choice. Strategy with regard to this choice, as it exists in our practice, was discussed earlier in the section on surveillance and surveillance-related reporting.
2. There is no generalized agreement about the use of FDG-PET/CT. In our practice, it is used mainly for targeted problem-solving. It is part of the follow-up algorithm for a decision of whether to do a post RT or post chemoradiation neck dissection in patients who are categorized as high risk for neck failure during initial treatment decision-making for a primary amenable to RT or chemoRT control.
3. There is no agreed upon, much less proven, approach to appropriate surveillance intervals with a chosen imaging modality. The ACR NI-RADS guidelines do suggest appropriate intervals but these are not supported by prospective properly controlled studies. Some additional suggestions follow but reflect mainly how current practice is conducted rather than evidence-based practice.
4. There is no proof that surveillance has a significant overall survival benefit.

In spite of the four factors just presented, there is a clearly common and increasing trend to obtain a baseline anatomic study 3 months following the completion of all therapies. If the baseline study findings are consistent only with expected post-therapy changes, then typical follow-up intervals appear to be at 6 months, then 1 year. If findings remain stable over the first year, then follow-ups are extended to yearly intervals up to a total of 3 years.

When baseline studies are suspicious, a shorter interval follow-up with anatomic imaging interval of 3 months is typically adopted, and then depending on the stability of any worrisome findings, a tailored strategy emerges for most patients. These tailored strategies eventually tend to resemble those for more routine surveillance strategies just described once the findings are shown to be stable.

Of course, these practice trends are altered in the case of patients who become symptomatic. This is especially true of the occurrence of pain, progressive cranial nerve deficits, or signs and symptoms may be related anatomically to the primary site or nodal recurrence. Unfortunately, symptomatic recurrences tend to be less amenable to treatment by curative intent typically ending up in the category of recurrence management with the intent to control progression as much as possible.

Those who have a significant amount of surveillance in their practice of imaging of head and neck cancer will realize there is a substantial amount of heterogeneity in these imaging surveillance ordering practices. Some of the heterogeneity may be rationally based on clinical concerns and some may be on the basis of a patient's "need to know". There is simply no reliable data to sort out the rationale for the heterogeneity of current practice trends or surveillance provides any tangible benefit beyond patient reassurance in most cases.

If surveillance strategy regimens are adopted, 3 years of follow-up should prove adequate in the vast majority of head neck cancer, since 95% of recurrences will appear within 2 years. Some cancers have a different and more prolonged outside risk of recurrence and those plans can be individualized.

References

1. Mamlouk MD, Chang PC, Saket RR. Contextual radiology reporting: a new approach to neuroradiology structured templates. Am J Neuroradiol. 2018;39(8):1406–14. https://doi.org/10.3174/ajnr.A5697.
2. Muraki AS, Mancuso AA, Harnsberger HR, Johnson LP, Meads GB. CT of the oropharynx, tongue base, and floor of the mouth: normal anatomy and range of variations, and applications in staging carcinoma. Radiology. 1983;148(3):725–31.

3. Rouvière H. Anatomy of the human lymphatic system, Tobias MJ (trans), vol. 1–28. Ann Arbor, MI: Edwards Brothers; 1938. p. 77–8.
4. Grodinsky M, Holyoke EA. The fasciae and fascial spaces of the head, neck and adjacent regions. Am J Anat. 1935;63:367–408.
5. Martin H. Surgery of head and neck tumors. 1st ed. Hargestown, MD: Hoeber-Harper; 1957.
6. Jesse RH, Sugarbaker EV. Suquamous cell carcinoma of the oropharynx: why we fail. Am J Surg. 1976;132:435–8.
7. Ballantyne AJ. In: Fletcher GH, MacComb WS, editors. Routes of spread. Radiation therapy in the management of cancers of the oral cavity and oropharynx. Chap 3. Springfield: Charles C Thomas; 1962. p. 91–115.
8. Conley JJ. (1975) Salivary glands and the facial nerve. Grune & Stratton, New York: 12, 302, 349
9. Kirchner JA. What have whole organ sections contributed to the treatment of laryngeal cancer? Ann Otol Rhinol Laryngol. 1989;98(9):661–7.
10. Lederman M. Cancer of the nasopharynx: its natural history and treatment. Springfield: Charles C Thomas; 1961.
11. Lederman M. Cancer of the pharynx. J Laryngol. 1967;81:151.
12. Ballantyne AJ. Significance of retropharyngeal nodes in cancer of the head and neck. Am J Surg. 1964;108:500.
13. Mancuso AA, Hanafee WN. Head and neck radiology (2 volumes in print and another online). 1st ed. Philadelphia: Wolters Kluwer Health/Lippincott Williams & Wilkins; 2011.
14. Dodd GD, Dolan PA, Ballantyne AJ, et al. The dissemination of tumors of the head and neck via the cranial nerves. Radiol Clin North Am. 1970;8:445–62.
15. Williams LS, Mancuso AA, Mendenhall WM. Perineural spread of cutaneous squamous and basal cell carcinoma: CT and MR detection and its impact on patient management and prognosis. Int J Radiat Biol Phys. 2001;49:1061–9.
16. Batsakis J. Tumors of the head and neck: clinical and pathological considerations. 2nd ed. Baltimore: Williams and Wilkins; 1979.
17. Haagensen DC, Feind CR, Herter FP, Slanetz CA, Weinberg JA. The lymphatics in cancer. 1st ed. Philadelphia: WB Saunders; 1972. p. 60–208.
18. Fisch U. Lymphographische Untersuchungen uber das zervikale Lymphsystem (Fortschritte der Hals-Nasen-Ohrenheilkunde), vol. 14. Basel: Karger; 1968. p. 53–162. [English edition: Fisch U. Lymphography of the cervical lymphatic system. Philadelphia: WB Saunders; 1968. p. 47–146].
19. Mancuso AA, Maceri D, Rice D, Hanafee WN. CT of cervical lymph node cancer. Am J Roentgenol. 1981;136:381–5.
20. Lindberg RD. Distribution of cervical lymph node metastases from squamous cell carcinoma of the upper respiratory and digestive tracts. Cancer. 1972;29:1446–9.
21. Byers RM, Wolf PF, Ballantyne AJ. Rationale for elective modified neck dissection. Head Neck Surg. 1988;10:160–7.
22. Cannon DM, Lee NY. Recurrence in region of spared parotid gland after definitive intensity-modulated radiotherapy for head and neck cancer. Int J Radiat Oncol Biol Phys. 2008;70:660–5.
23. Mendenhall WM, Mancuso AA. Radiotherapy for head and neck cancer—is the "Next Level" down? Int J Radiat Oncol Biol Phys. 2009;73:645–6.
24. Xu Y, Zhang M, Yue Q, Zong J, Lin J, Sun R, Qiu S, Lin S, Pan J. Analysis of rare periparotid recurrence after parotid gland-sparing intensity-modulated radiotherapy for nasopharyngeal carcinoma. Cancer Radiother. 2016;20:377–83.

Diagnostic Imaging of Nasopharyngeal Carcinoma

2

Clement Yong, Justin Christopher Ng, Lih Khin Khor, Donovan Eu, Balamurugan A. Vellayappan, Timothy Cheo, and Vincent Fook-Hin Chong

Abstract

Our knowledge of nasopharyngeal carcinoma (NPC) is rapidly changing. This article is a snapshot of the present state of NPC imaging in relation to the latest staging system, current standards of care, and treatment complications. The article's emphasis on pathophysiology and important radiological anatomy will improve the interpretation of radiological findings and allow the radiologist to optimize the role of imaging in a multidisciplinary team.

Keywords

Nasopharyngeal carcinoma · Magnetic resonance imaging · Staging · Radiation · Complication · Pathophysiology · AJCC

2.1 Introduction

Nasopharyngeal carcinomas (NPC) are different from other head and neck malignancies in many ways: epidemiology, aetiology, histology and even treatment. For the radiologist, incidental detection of an NPC is not uncommon and the nasopharynx should always warrant close review (Figs. 2.1 and 2.2).

While rare in most parts of the world (0.6% of all cancer), NPC is found in high frequency in Southern China, Hong Kong, South-East Asia, and northern Africa, with these regions contributing over three quarters of newly diagnosed cases in 2012 [1]. Even within these endemic geographical clusters, there is a pronounced racial-ethnic bias. In South China for instance, exaggerated numbers are seen in the Cantonese population, where incidences of >20 per 100,000 person-years among males, double those in other dialect groups. Another example is the Bidayuh tribe in Sarawak, who are also unequally affected. Even mixed-race populations who report South Chinese ancestry show increased risk, while ethnicities with almost no intermingling with the Chinese (e.g., Indian Singaporeans) report low incidences [2, 3]. The results of these population studies point to an obvious genetic and epigenetic basis for the pathogenesis of NPC, and it was only through the early works of researchers including Epstein, Barr, Old, De Schryver, Zur Hausen, and Wolf that we can now link viral oncogenesis, and in particular the Epstein-Barr virus (EBV) with the development of NPC.

2.2 Anatomy

The nasopharynx is a post-nasal space that is limited anteriorly to the posterior edge of the nasal septum and inferiorly by the soft palate and an opposing pharyngeal muscular ridge known as Passavant's ridge (seen during swallowing). The lateral walls are formed by the upward continuation of the superior constrictor muscles (i.e., the pharyngobasilar fascia), while the sloping roof is formed in part by the sphenoid sinus, basisphenoid, and clivus. The nasopharynx is also in communication with the middle ear via the Eustachian tube. Some of the anatomical landmarks are shown in (Fig. 2.3), while other relevant anatomy will be discussed later in relation to staging.

C. Yong (✉) · J. C. Ng · V. F.-H. Chong
Department of Diagnostic Imaging, National University Cancer Institute Singapore (NCIS), National University Health System, Singapore, Singapore
e-mail: clement_yong@nuhs.edu.sg

L. K. Khor
Advanced Medicine Imaging Biopolis, Singapore, Singapore

D. Eu
Department of Otolaryngology Head and Neck Surgery, National University Cancer Institute Singapore (NCIS), National University Health System, Singapore, Singapore

B. A. Vellayappan · T. Cheo
Department of Radiation Oncology, National University Cancer Institute Singapore (NCIS), National University Health System, Singapore, Singapore

H. Ojiri (ed.), *Diagnostic Imaging in Head and Neck Cancer*, https://doi.org/10.1007/978-981-15-3188-0_2

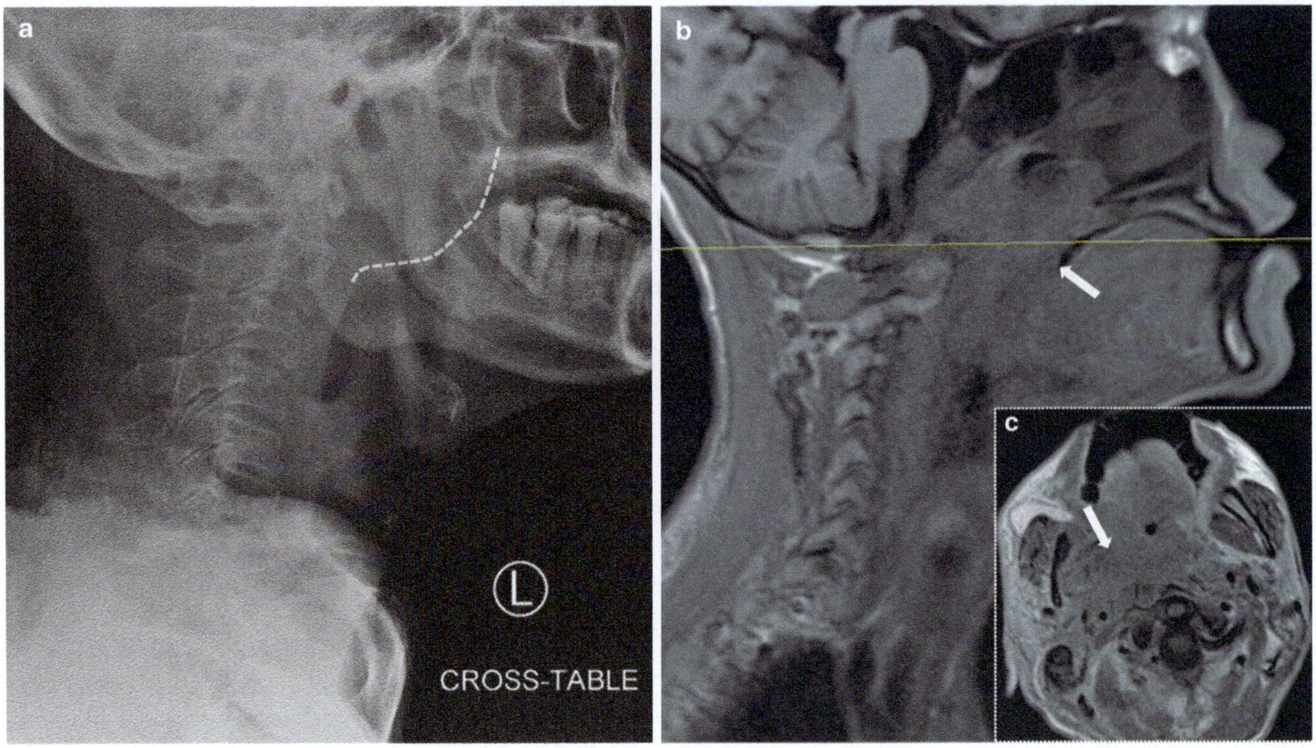

Fig. 2.1 Nasopharyngeal carcinoma. (**a**) Lateral neck radiograph with an incidental mass (dashed line) filling the posterior nasal space, (**b**) Sagittal T1 FLAIR, and (**c**) axial T1 post contrast images confirm a large nasopharyngeal carcinoma (solid arrow) invading the deep neck spaces

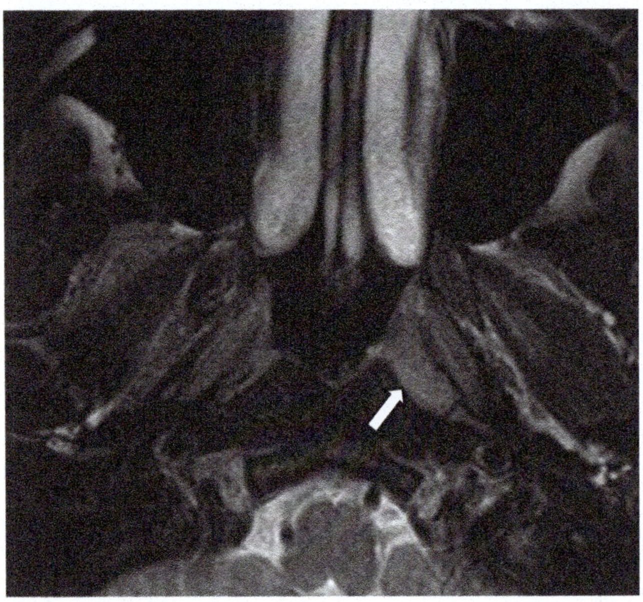

Fig. 2.2 Early nasopharyngeal carcinoma. Axial T2 image showing subtle increased signal at the left fossa of Rosenmuller (solid arrow). Subsequent endoscopic biopsy confirmed a nasopharyngeal carcinoma

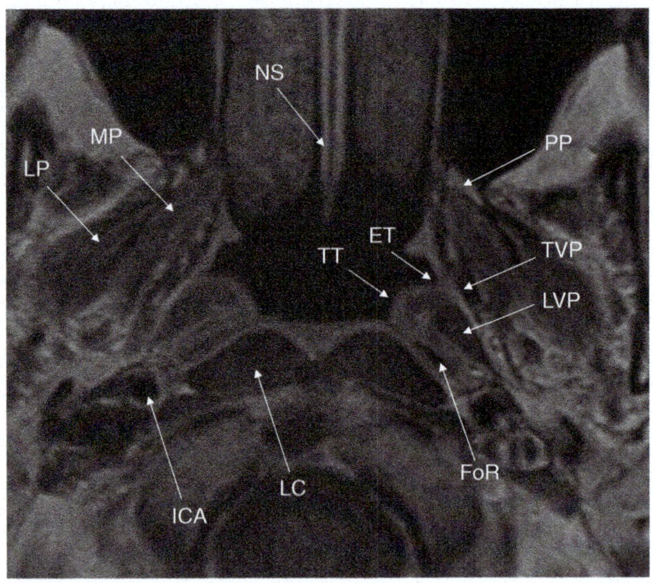

Fig. 2.3 Axial T1 image of the nasopharyngeal anatomy: lateral pterygoid muscle (LP); medial pterygoid muscle (MP); fossa of Rosenmuller (FoR); Eustachian tube opening (ET); Torus tubarius (TT); nasal septum (NS); longus capitis muscle (LC); levator veli palatini (LVP); tensor veli palatini (TVP); internal carotid artery (ICA); pterygoid process (PP)

2.3 Pathology

NPC is considered squamous in origin, but is often interspersed with lymphoid cells, giving rise to the term lymphoepithelioma. These NPC epithelial cells are unique, as they were the first discovered non-lymphatic cells to carry the EBV genome [4–6]. Since this discovery, population-based studies have found the virus consistently in nearly all NPC cells [7, 8], with the undifferentiated NPC subtype showing the highest viral association [9].

While latent EBV gene products are seen in all tumour cells, it is starkly absent from the surrounding lymphoid infiltrate [10]. Further analysis by Raab-Traub et al. [11] later showed that the EBV genome within the tumour was monoclonal, proving that the EBV infection precedes the growth of malignant cells and likely plays a direct role in the oncogenesis of nasopharyngeal carcinomas.

This oncogenic cascade is poorly understood and beyond the scope of this chapter, although it is worth noting that the interaction between both the EBV-infected epithelium and lymphoid stroma appears crucial for the clonal expansion of malignant cells [12].

Based on the World Health Organisation (WHO) 1991 classification, NPC is grouped into keratinising squamous cell carcinoma (KSCC) and non-keratinising carcinoma, which is further divided into non-keratinising differentiated carcinoma (NKDC) and non-keratinising undifferentiated carcinoma (NKUC) [13]. In endemic high risk areas, non-keratinising carcinoma make up 95% of cases [14], while the keratinising type is more common in low-risk areas [15].

2.4 AJCC/UICC TNM Classification

The American Joint Committee on Cancer (AJCC) and the Union for International Cancer Control (UICC) TNM classification is an anatomically driven staging system that uses epidemiological survival data to retrospectively identify prognostic anatomical features that impact survival. The staging of disease then allows a reproducible and objective way of determining treatment strategies. This cycle of staging, treatment, and survival are interdependent, and a change in one will affect the others.

The 7th edition of the AJCC TNM classification published in 2009 was based on survival data from two-dimensional radiotherapy (2D-RT), which has since been superseded by Intensity-modulated radiotherapy (IMRT) as the primary curative treatment for NPC. IMRT confers increased disease-specific survival (DSS) (85% with IMRT vs. 78% with 2D-RT) and overall survival (OS) (80% with IMRT vs. 71% with 2D-RT) that is consistent across various studies [16, 17]. A meta-analysis by Blanchard [18] further showed that the addition of concomitant chemotherapy to radiotherapy significantly improved DSS and OS in locoregionally advanced NPC.

The impact of these new treatment methods on survival outcomes questioned the utility of the 7th edition staging system. Not surprisingly, various studies later confirmed diminished survival benefits when applying the outmoded 7th edition to NPC treated with IMRT [19–21]. We are now onto the 8th edition, which was implemented in January 2018, and this will be used for the purpose of this text (Table 2.1).

Table 2.1 Changes in T classification of the American Joint Cancer Committee staging of nasopharyngeal carcinoma

AJCC 7th edition		AJCC 8th edition		Changes
TX	Primary tumour cannot be assessed	TX	Primary tumour cannot be assessed	
T0	No evidence of primary tumour	T0	No tumour identified, but EBV-positive cervical node(s) involvement	EBV+ nodes without a primary source presumed to be from the nasopharynx
T1	Tumour confined to the nasopharynx, or tumour extends to oropharynx and/or nasal cavity without parapharyngeal extension	T1	Tumour confined to nasopharynx, or extension to oropharynx and/or nasal cavity without parapharyngeal involvement	
T2	Tumour with parapharyngeal extension (posterolateral infiltration of tumour)	T2	Tumour with extension to parapharyngeal space, and/or adjacent soft tissue involvement (medial pterygoid, lateral pterygoid, pre-vertebral muscles)	Medial pterygoid, lateral pterygoid, pre-vertebral muscles down-staged to T2 from T4
T3	Tumour involves bony structures of skull base and/or paranasal sinuses	T3	Tumour with infiltration of bony structures at skull base, cervical vertebra, pterygoid structures, and/or paranasal sinuses	Clarification of bony structures to include cervical vertebrae, pterygoid plates, skull base, or paranasal sinuses
T4	Tumour with intracranial extension and/or involvement of cranial nerves, hypopharynx, or orbit, or with extension to the infratemporal fossa/masticator space	T4	Tumour with intracranial extension, involvement of cranial nerves, hypopharynx, orbit, parotid gland, and/or extensive soft tissue infiltration beyond the lateral surface of the lateral pterygoid muscle	

2.5 MRI Staging of the Primary Tumour (T-Classification)

2.5.1 T0 and T1

Tumour confined to nasopharynx, or extension to oropharynx, and/or nasal cavity without parapharyngeal involvement: The normal nasopharyngeal mucosa is thin and lined by lymphoid tissue. This can appear enlarged in young children and also in adults who smoke or suffer chronic rhinosinusitis [22]. As MRI is very sensitive in detecting small changes in the nasopharynx [23], a common radiological problem is differentiating nasopharyngeal lymphoid hyperplasia (NPLH) from early NPC (Fig. 2.4). Some features favouring NPLH may include: diffuse symmetrical thickening, vertical stripes on post-contrast T1-weighted (T1W) sequences, homogenous enhancement, mucosal bubbles, retention cysts, and serrated protrusions (Fig. 2.5) [24, 25]. However, endoscopic biopsy remains the best way of excluding NPC. MRI is often the first modality to detect small obscured tumours or those that are entirely submucosal [23], so any mucosal asymmetry should be assessed properly (Fig. 2.6).

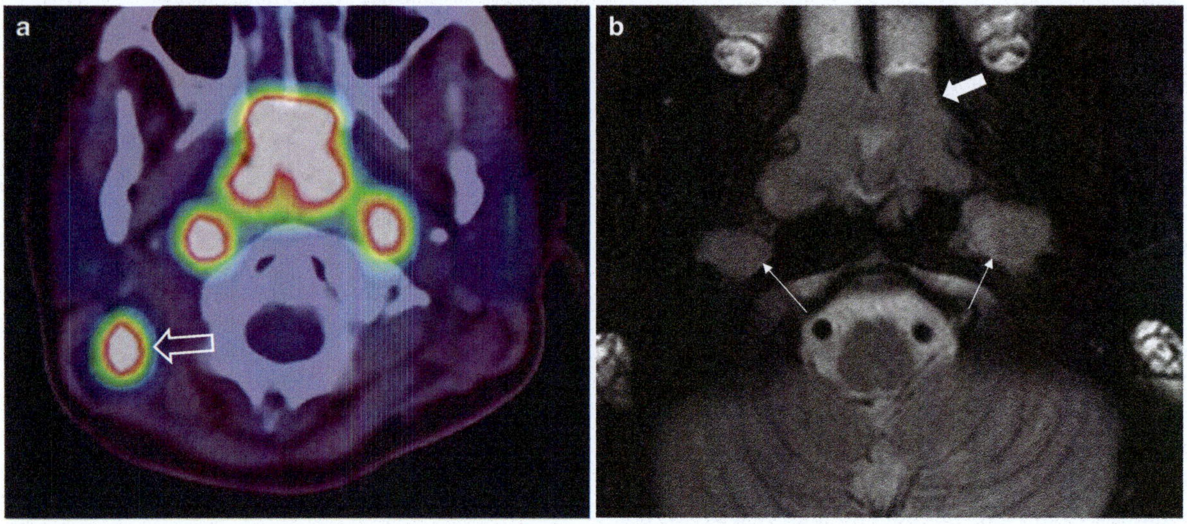

Fig. 2.4 Lymphoid hyperplasia mimicking an NPC. (**a**) Axial FDG PET/CT and (**b**) axial T2 fat saturated images showing a bulky nasopharynx (solid arrow) retropharyngeal nodes (thin arrows) and right posterior cervical lymph node (open arrow), with intense FDG avidity. Endoscopic biopsy showed this to be lymphoid hyperplasia

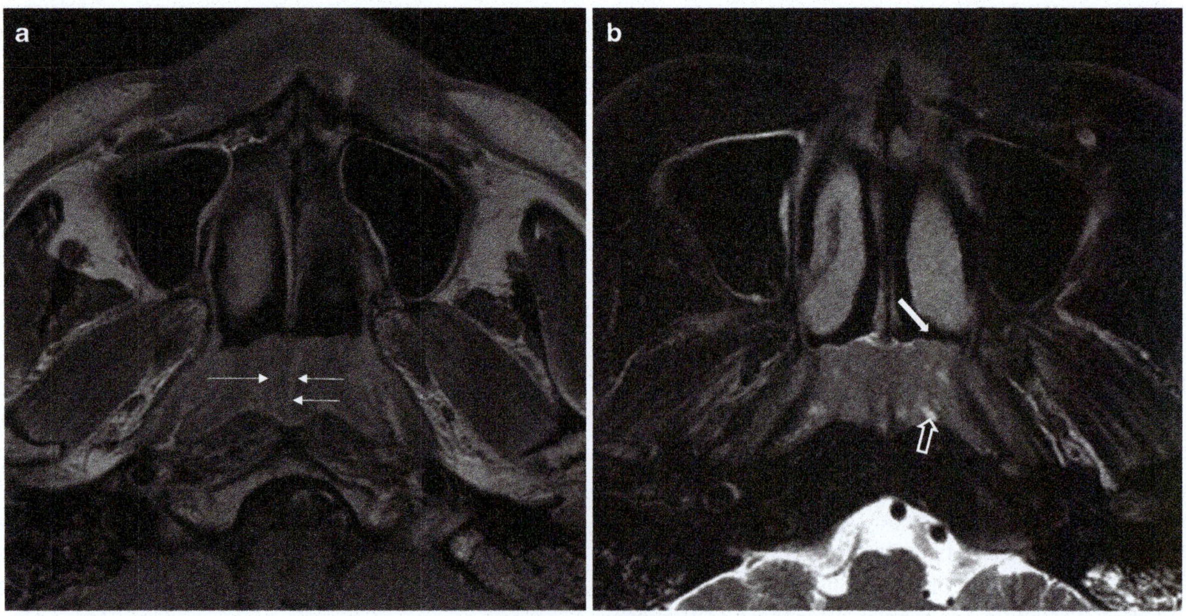

Fig. 2.5 Nasopharyngeal lymphoid hyperplasia. (**a**) Axial T1 post contrast and (**b**) axial T2 fat saturated images showing symmetrical mucosal thickening with vertical stripes (thin arrow), serrated margins (solid arrow), mucosal bubbles, and retained mucous (open arrow) that are characteristic of lymphoid hyperplasia

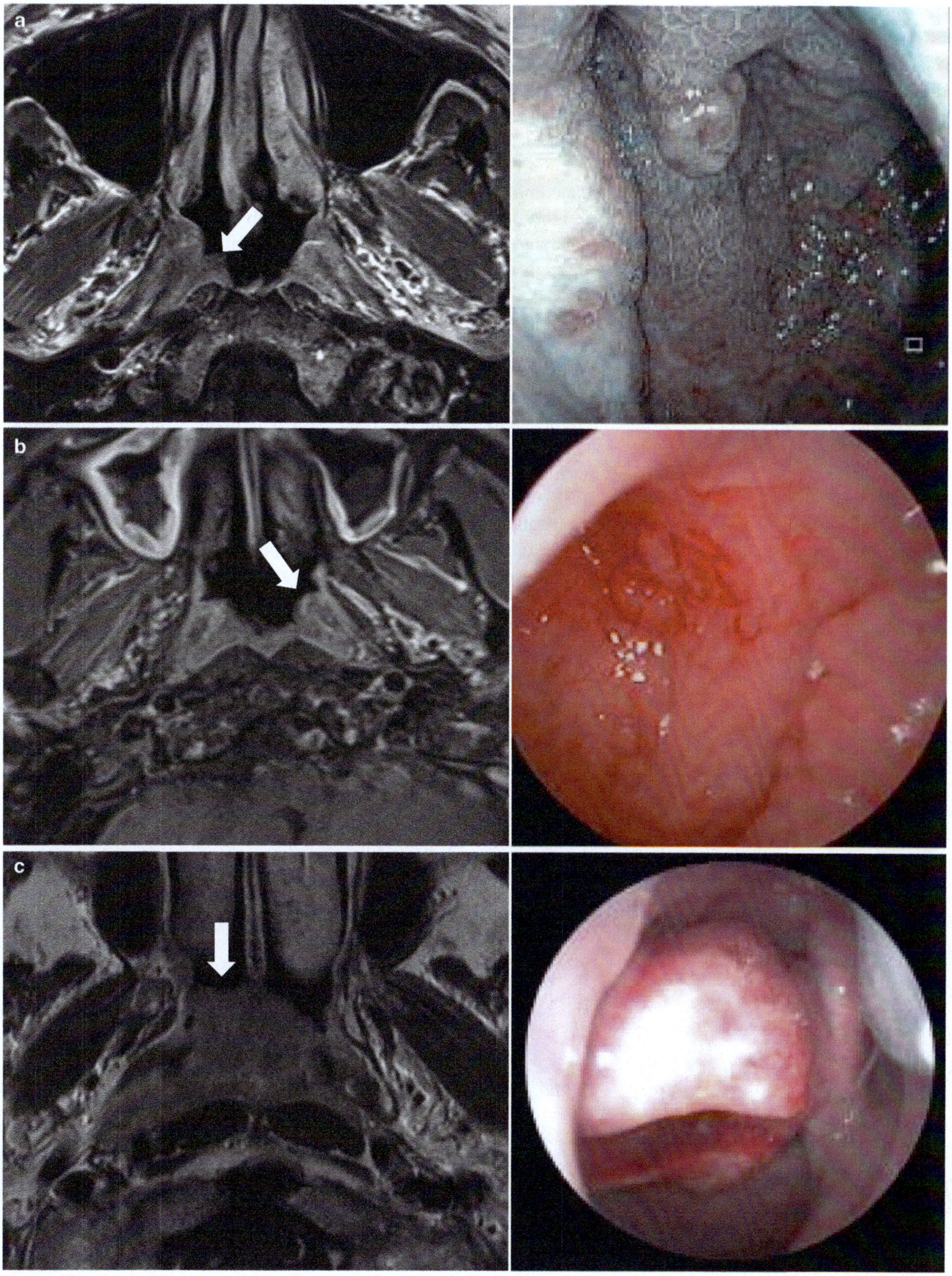

Fig. 2.6 Synergy of MRI and endoscopic assessment. MRI images (left column) and corresponding endoscopic pictures (right column) highlighting the importance of evaluating even subtle asymmetries. (Row **a**) Early right NPC (solid arrow) confined to the mucosa. (Row **b**) Early left infiltrative NPC (solid arrow) and (Row **c**) Large right exophytic NPC (solid arrow) filling the nasopharynx

The 8th edition now includes T0 when EBV-positive nodes are found in the absence of a primary lesion, presuming a nasopharyngeal origin. In T1 disease, the NPC is confined to the nasopharynx and arises most commonly within the fossa of Rosen Müller (FoR), a deep recess within the lateral nasopharynx that is posterior to the opening of the Eustachian tube (Fig. 2.3) [26]. This affinity for the FoR may be due to high concentrations of intermediate epithelium (a transitional zone between ciliated respiratory and squamous epithelium) that is particularly vulnerable to oncogenic stimuli [27]. Another area with dense intermediate epithelium is the nasopharyngeal roof.

An important anatomical structure to know is the pharyngobasilar fascia (PBF) [28]. It is a thick non-expansile aponeurosis between the mucous and muscular layer that attaches the pharynx to the skull base (hence its name) and acts as a barrier to the spread of NPC (Fig. 2.7). It maintains the shape of the nasopharynx and it thins caudally as the superior constrictor muscles come in. The Eustachian tube passes through the sinus of Morgagni within the PBF into the nasopharynx. The PBF also contains the levator veli palatini muscle (LVPM), which is inferior to and controls the opening of the Eustachian tube. The tensor veli palatini muscle (TVPM) however is outside the PBF in the parapharyngeal space (PPS), so identifying these muscles will help identify the limits of the PBF. NPC that is confined by the PBF is a classified T1 disease. Since the 8th edition designates tumour spread to the nasal cavity and oropharynx as T1 disease (Fig. 2.8), clear anatomical delineation of these spaces will not be discussed in this text.

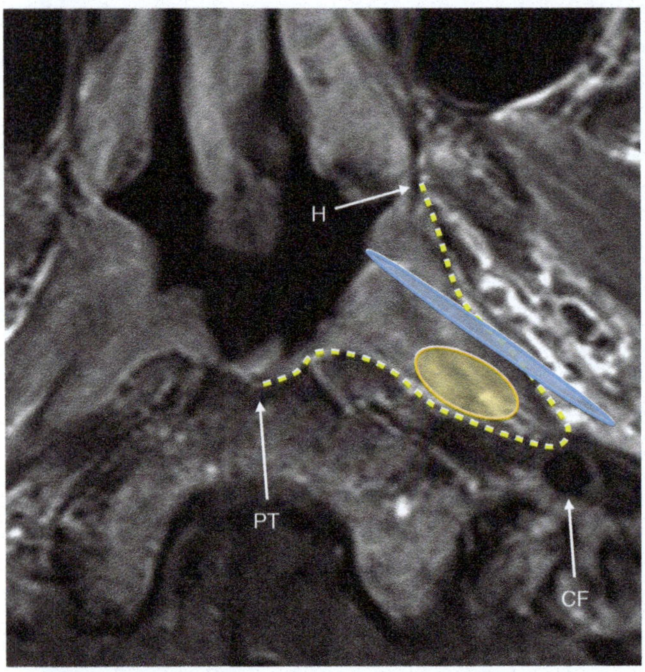

Fig. 2.7 Attachment of the pharyngobasilar fascia (dotted yellow line) to the pharyngeal tubercle (PT) on the occipital bone, behind the foramen lacerum (orange area), petrous bone just anterior to the carotid foramen (CF), cartilaginous Eustachian tube (blue area), and the free border of the pterygoid plate, known as the hamulus (H)

2.5.2 T2

Tumour with extension to parapharyngeal space and/or adjacent soft-tissue involvement (medial pterygoid, lateral pterygoid, pre-vertebral muscles): T2 disease comprise of tumour that has spread past the PBF into the parapharyngeal space and/or adjacent soft tissue (medial pterygoid, lateral pterygoid, pre-vertebral musculature). As mentioned before, involvement of the TVPM is T2 disease (Fig. 2.9).

The parapharyngeal space (PPS) is a fibrofatty space lateral to the nasopharynx that is best identified on the T1W sequence (Fig. 2.8). It is divided into the pre-styloid and post-styloid compartments by the tensor veli palatini fascia [29]. The post-styloid space is also called the carotid space and contains the internal carotid artery, internal jugular vein, sympathetic plexus and lower cranial nerves IX to XII.

The pre-vertebral space (PVS) contains the longus capitis, longus colli, and rectus capitis muscles and is separated from the pharyngeal mucosal space (PMS) by the thin fat-filled retropharyngeal space (RPS). The RPS is further

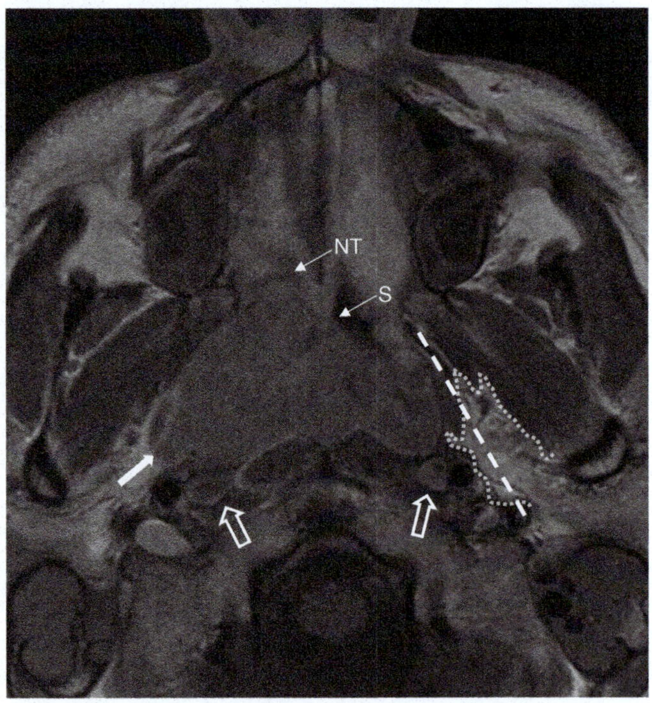

Fig. 2.8 Axial T1 post contrast image showing a T1 NPC invading the nasal turbinate (NT) and septum (S) but still confined by the pharyngobasilar fascia (solid arrow). Small bilateral retropharyngeal nodes (open arrow) should not be confused for pre-vertebral invasion. The parapharyngeal space fat (white dotted line) is divided by the tensor-vascular-styloid fascia (white dashed line)

divided by the thin alar fascia into the proper RPS anteriorly and the danger space posteriorly. While the proper RPS obliterates somewhere between T1 and T6, the danger space continues down to the diaphragm, providing a conduit from the pharynx to the posterior mediastinum [30].

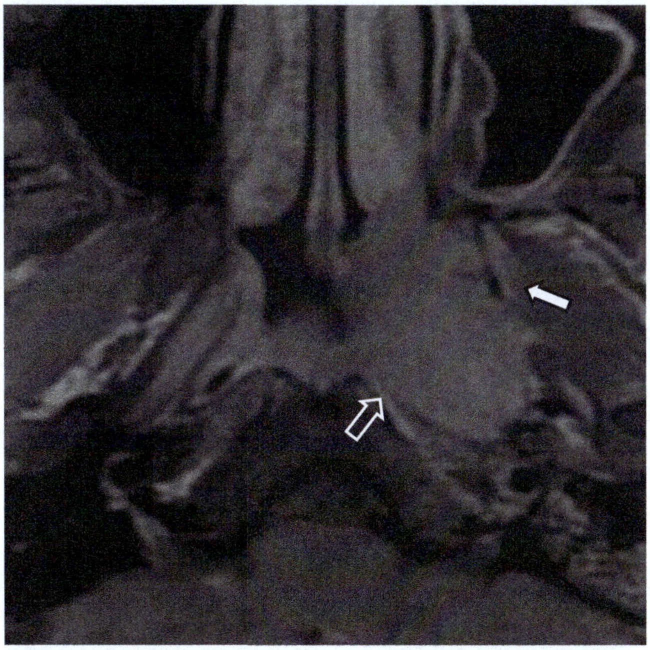

Fig. 2.9 T2 disease. Axial T1 post contrast fat saturated image showing a left nasopharyngeal carcinoma invading the left pre-vertebral space (open arrow) and medial pterygoid muscle (solid arrow)

PPS and PVS involvement are associated with increased risk of distant metastases and tumour recurrence due to the concentration of lymphatics and venous plexuses [31–33]. The inclusion of PVS involvement as T2 disease has received some debate, where a study of 506 patients [34] showed that NPC with PVS disease had similar OS and distant metastasis-free survival (DMFS) to T4 disease.

Infiltration of the medial and lateral pterygoid musculature were down-staged to T2 in the 8th edition due to studies showing good prognosis compared with tumour spread lateral to these muscles [35].

2.5.3 T3

Tumour with infiltration of bony structures at skull base, cervical vertebrae, and pterygoid structures: Tumour involvement of any bony structure or paranasal sinus is T3 disease. As NPC has a propensity for bony invasion, 60% of patients are already T3 at diagnosis [36]. The clivus, sphenoid body, pterygoid processes, and apices of the petrous temporal bones are most commonly involved and are seen on the T1W sequences as loss of the normal hyperintense fatty marrow (Fig. 2.10). Disease extension into the marrow is worrying as it is a route for haematogenous spread to the rest of the body [37]. Even early sclerosis of the pterygoid process may be enough to reflect tumour proximity or invasion [38].

The foramina and fissures within the central skull base also offer a direct pathway into the cranium and include the

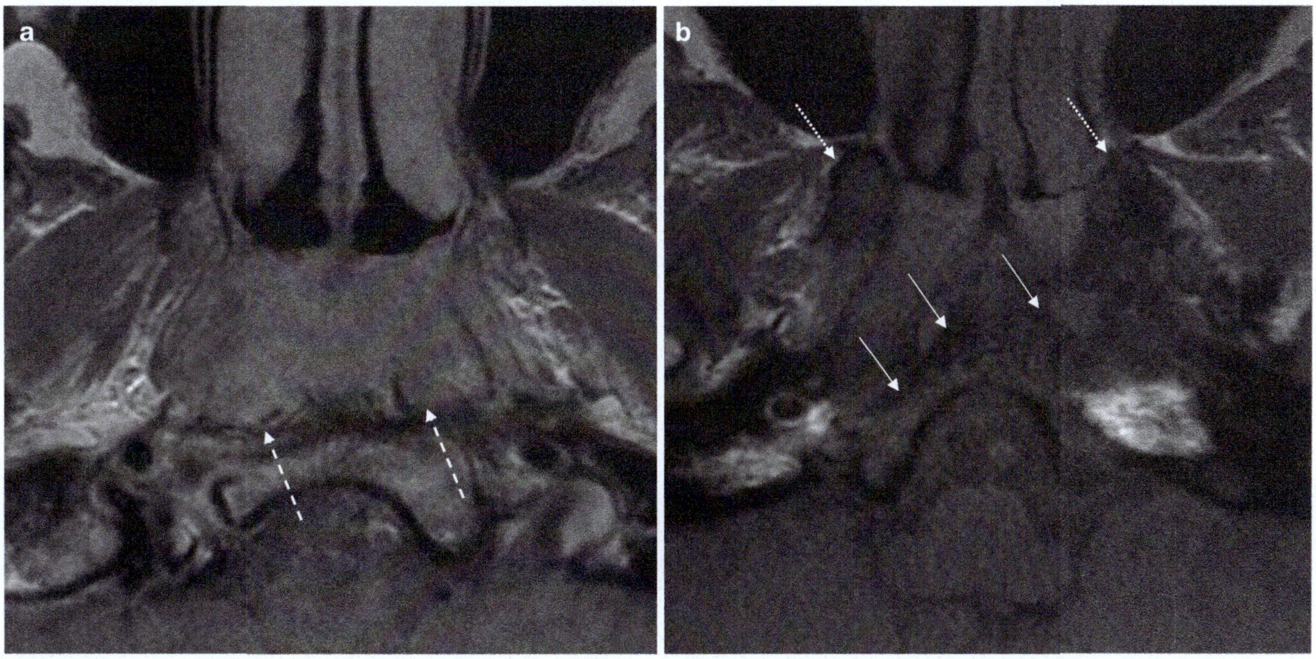

Fig. 2.10 T3 disease. (**a**) Axial T1 post contrast and (**b**) axial T1 images showing a nasopharyngeal carcinoma invading the pre-vertebral space (dashed arrows) with infiltration of bony structures at the clivus (thin arrows) and pterygoid plates (dotted arrows)

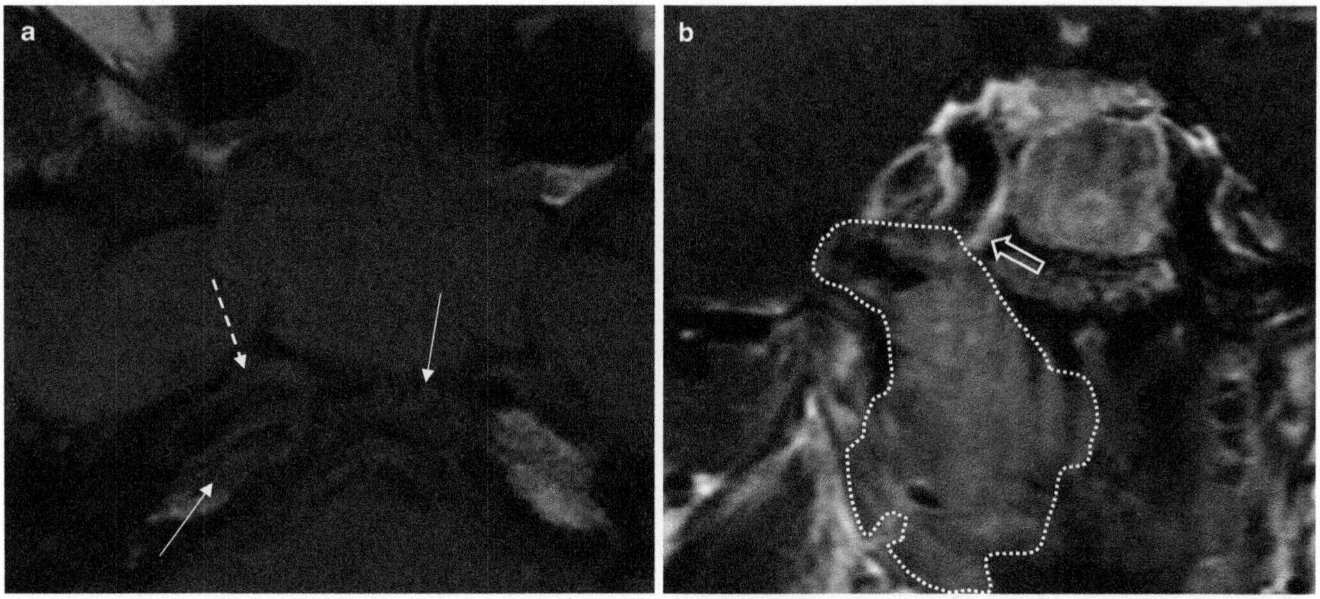

Fig. 2.11 Foramen lacerum involvement. (**a**) Axial T1 and (**b**) Coronal T1 post contrast images shows a right nasopharyngeal carcinoma (white dotted area) invading the foramen lacerum (dashed arrow) into the right cavernous sinus (open arrow). There is also loss of the normal marrow signal within the clivus and right petrous bone (thin arrows)

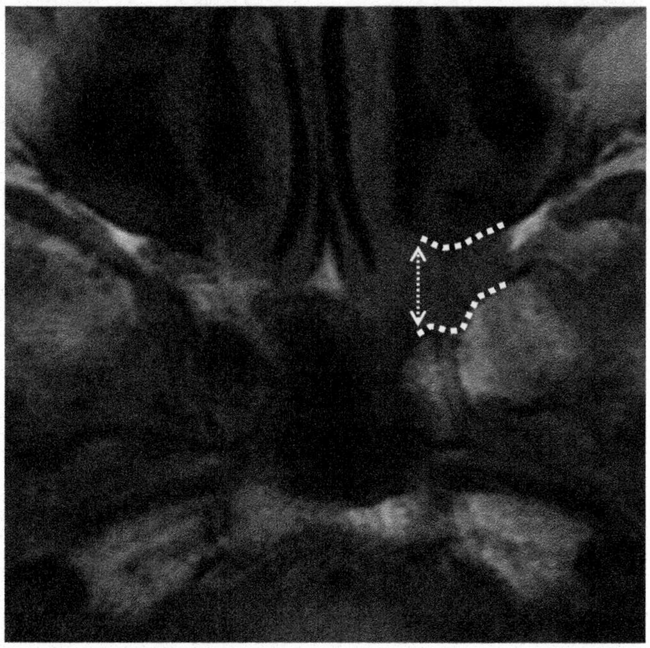

Fig. 2.12 Pterygopalatine fossa involvement. Axial T1 image shows soft tissue invading the sphenopalatine foramen (double arrow) with widening and loss of the normal fat within the pterygopalatine fossa (between dotted lines)

foramen ovale, foramen rotundum, Vidian canal, pterygopalatine fossa (PPF), petroclival fissure, jugular foramen, and hypoglossal canal. The foramen lacerum lies within the PBF and is directly below the internal carotid artery. Tumour seen here should be considered intracranial and classified as T4 disease (Fig. 2.11).

The pterygopalatine fossa is one of the most important neurovascular junction in the deep face, linking the nasal cavity (via sphenopalatine foramen), oral cavity (via pterygopalatine canal and greater palatine canal), orbit (via infraorbital fissure), masticator space (via pterygomaxillary fissure), and the middle cranial fossa (via foramen rotundum). The PPF is seen as a fat-filled inverted pyramid directly behind the maxillary sinus and is hyperintense on T1W imaging, with occasional flow voids (from the internal maxillary artery) and contrast enhancement (from emissary veins) [39]. NPC enters the PPF via the sphenopalatine foramen, and approximately 15% of patients have PPF invasion at time of diagnosis (Fig. 2.12) [40]. Chung et al. reported a 96.1% incidence of intracranial involvement once the pterygopalatine fossa and foramen ovale were involved [41], highlighting the importance of these channels.

Spread to the paranasal sinuses: Paranasal sinus invasion is more contentious. Although the 8th edition classifies this as T3 disease regardless of which sinus is involved [42], the Chinese 2008 staging system (TNMc2008) classifies this as T4, while authors like Zhang et al. contends that only ethmoid and maxillary sinus invasion should be considered T4 [43]. This is because the sphenoid sinus is relatively easily invaded as it sits above the nasopharynx with no intervening fascia or muscle. A small tumour load is enough to invade it, while the distant sinuses require a much larger tumour volume, with often simultaneous involvement of the sphenoid sinus. Zhang et al. showed that T3 disease with ethmoid or maxillary sinus invasion had similar local relapse-free survival as T4 disease [43].

If the ethmoid air-cells are invaded, there may also be a lower chance of shielding the optic nerves from the radiation field [44]. On MRI studies, tumours will often show enhancement and restricted diffusion, while mucous will not.

2.5.4 T4

Tumour with intracranial extension, involvement of cranial nerves: T4 involves the spread of tumour into the cranial vault. As the skull base foramina offer paths of least resistance, the cavernous sinuses and the dura at the floor of the middle cranial fossa are typically involved first (20% vs. 5% to the cranial fossa [41]). The cavernous sinus is of particular concern, containing the trigeminal ganglion (ophthalmic and maxillary branches), internal carotid artery and plexus, and multiple venous tributaries including the ophthalmic and some cerebral veins.

Unlike other staging features, cranial nerve involvement (CNI) is diagnosed clinically, with the majority of cases presenting with upper CN palsies, particularly of the trigeminal and abducens nerves [45]. CNI can be detected on MRI. Some of the imaging features include: abnormal thickening and enhancement of the nerve, widening and obliteration of the neural foraminal fat, atrophy or hyperintensities within the affected musculature and asymmetrical effacement of Meckel's cave or gasserian ganglion (Fig. 2.13) [46]. These features, however, are also often seen in asymptomatic patients, and the decision

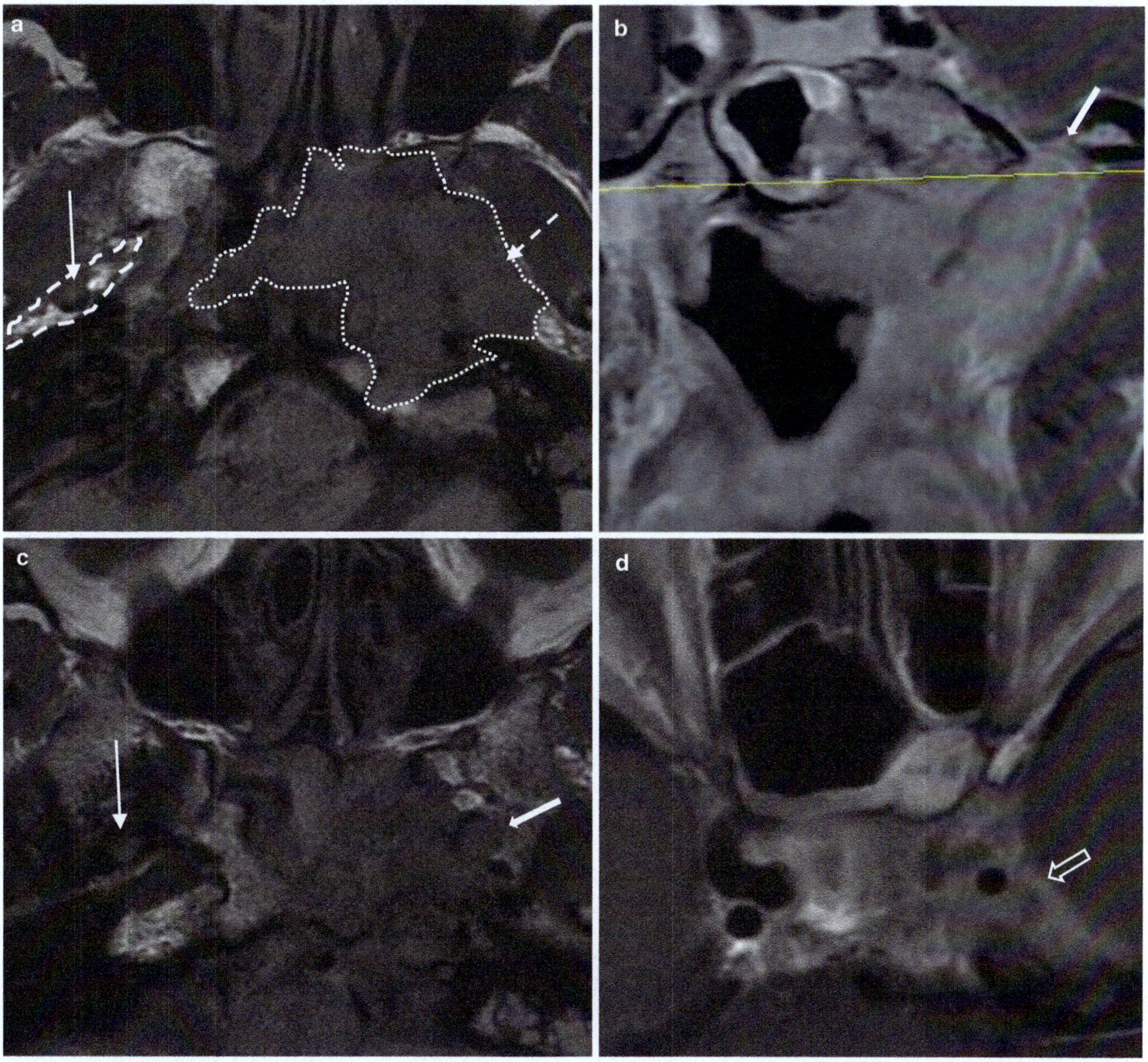

Fig. 2.13 Perineural disease. (**a**) Axial T1, (**b**) Coronal T1 post contrast, (**c**) Axial T1 at the level of the yellow line in (**b**), and (**d**) Axial T1 post contrast images. This patient with a large left NPC (white dotted area) has invaded the left mandibular branch of the trigeminal nerve CNV3. This is seen as loss of fat around the nerve (dashed arrow) compared with the normal parapharyngeal fat on the right (white dashed area). There is also enlargement of the nerve (thick solid arrows) through the foramen ovale and bulkiness of the left cavernous sinus (thick open arrow). The normal right CNV3 is shown in (**a + c**) as (thin arrows)

to classify this as T4 disease requires further evaluation. Zong et al. recently showed MRI-detected CNI had no effect on prognosis [46], while older studies suggested the opposite [47].

Spread to the hypopharynx, orbit, parotid gland, and/or extensive soft-tissue infiltration beyond the lateral surface of the lateral pterygoid muscle: An important change in the AJCC 8th edition is the subdivision of masticator space involvement. In the 7th edition, this space was designated as T4 disease. However, after Pan et al. [35] reported good prognosis of lateral pterygoid involvement compared to disease beyond these muscles, only disease lateral to the lateral surface of the lateral pterygoid muscle is now classified as T4 (Figs. 2.14 and 2.15).

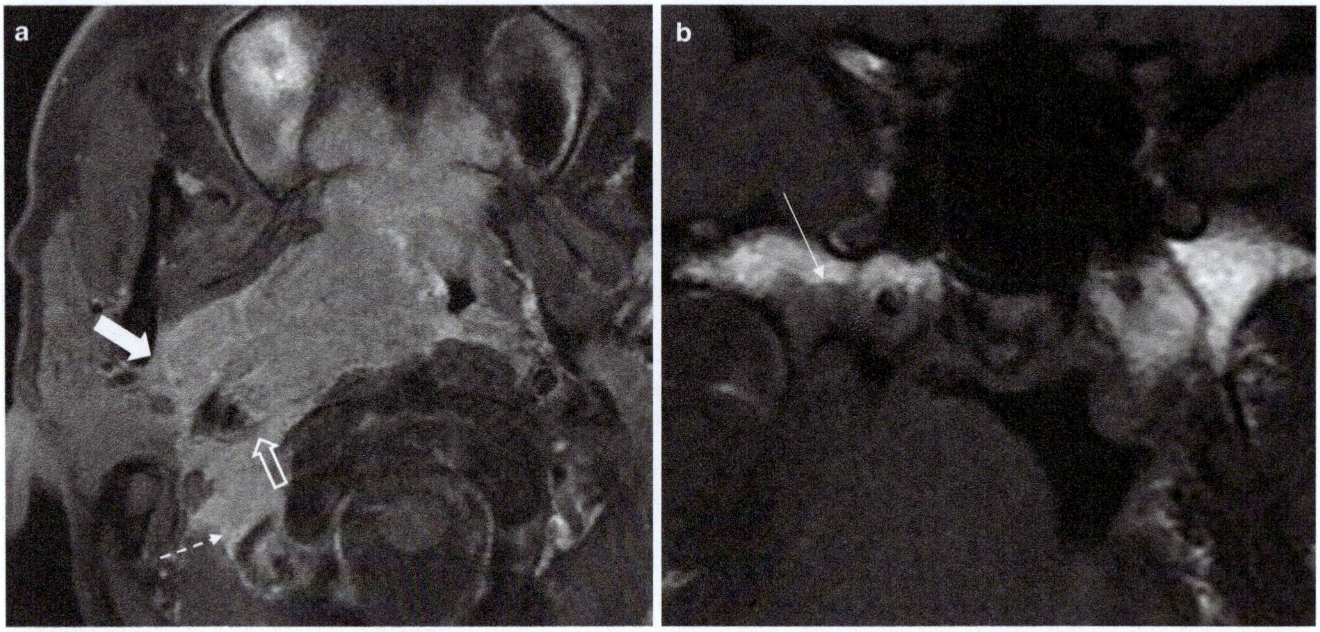

Fig. 2.14 T4 disease. (**a**) Axial T1 post contrast fat saturated and (**b**) coronal T1 images showing a large right nasopharyngeal carcinoma involving the right skull base (thin arrow), right carotid space (open arrow), right parotid gland and posterior cervical space (dashed arrow)

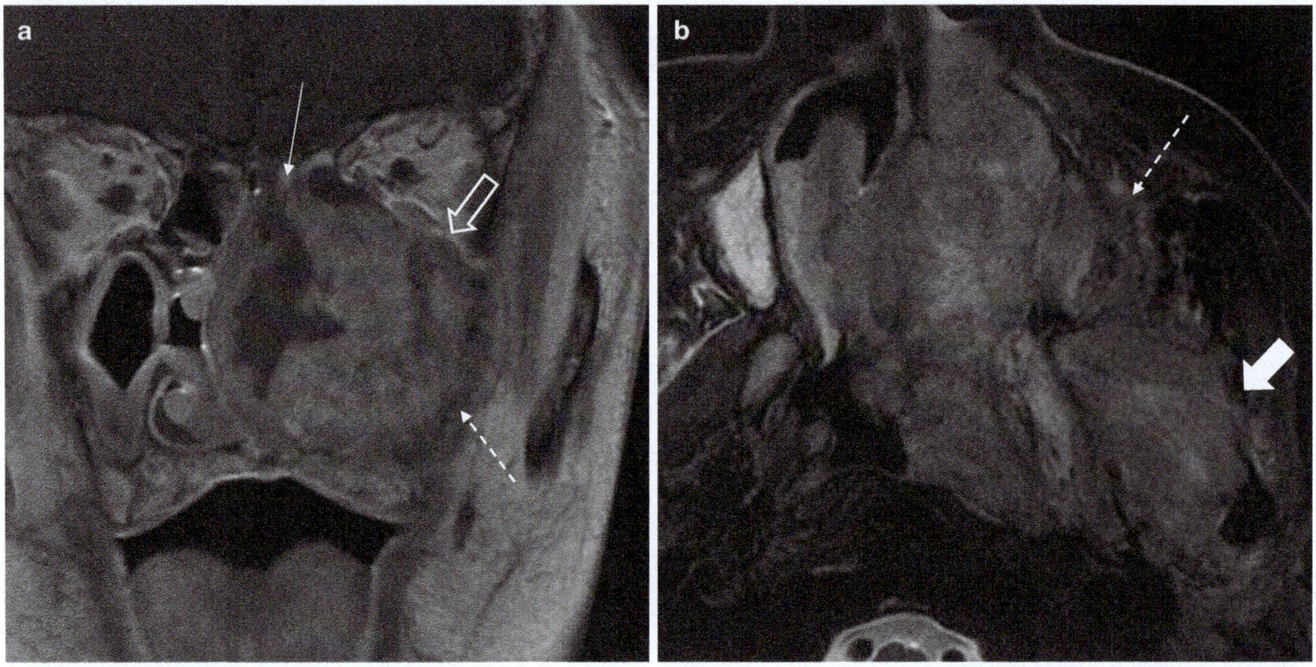

Fig. 2.15 T4 disease. (**a**) Coronal T1 post contrast and (**b**) axial T2 fat saturated images show a left nasopharyngeal carcinoma invading past the left lateral pterygoid musculature (solid arrows), ethmoid (thin arrow), left maxillary sinus (dashed arrow), and left orbital floor (open arrow)

2.6 MRI Staging of Nodal Disease (N Classification) (Table 2.2)

The majority of patients present with nodal metastases, with some series quoting incidences as high as 96%. This commonly involves the lateral retropharyngeal nodes (RLN) aka nodes of Rouvière, which lie medial to the carotid arteries from the skull base down to C3 in up to 80% of patients [44, 48]. Other studies note equal or higher sentinel spread to the level II nodes [49, 50], suggesting direct lymphatic pathways to both RLN and internal jugular chains [44, 49]. The lymphatic drainage of the nasopharynx can be divided into [51]:

Table 2.2 Changes in N classification of the American Joint Cancer Committee staging of nasopnaryngeai carcinoma

AJCC 7th edition		AJCC 8th edition		Changes
NX	Regional nodes cannot be assessed	NX	Regional lymph nodes cannot be assessed	
N0	No regional lymph node metastasis	N0	No regional lymph node metastasis	
N1	Unilateral metastasis m cervical lymph node(s), 6 cm in greatest dimension, above the supraclavicular fossa, and/or unilateral or bilateral retropharyngeai lymph nodes, 6 cm in greatest dimension (midline nodes are considered ipsilateral nodes)	N1	Unilateral metastasis m cervical lymph node(s) and/or unilateral or bilateral metastasis in retropharyngeai lymph node(s), 6 cm or smaller in greatest dimension, above the caudal border of cricoid cartilage	Supraclavicular nodes redefined as nodes extending below the caudal border of the cricoid cartilage
N2	Bilateral metastasis in cervical lymph node(s), 6 cm in greatest dimension, above the supraclavicular fossa (midline nodes are considered ipsilateral nodes)	N2	Bilateral metastasis in cervical lymph node(s), 6 cm or smaller in greatest dimension, above the caudal border of cricoid cartilage	
N3	Metastasis in a lymph node or nodes >6 cm and/or to the supraclavicular fossa	N3	Unilateral or bilateral metastasis in cervical lymph node(s), larger than 6 cm in greatest dimension, and/or extension below the caudal border of cricoid cartilage	N3a and N3b combined under N3
N3a	> 6cm in dimension			
N3b	Extension to the supraclavicular fossa			

- Primary lateral pathway into the RLN and upper internal jugular chain (level II nodes). Prominent RLN are normal in children before puberty, after which they involute.
- Secondary medial pathway from the roof and posterior wall into the median retropharyngeal node, located anterior to the medial parts of the longus colli muscles [30]. These do not form a discrete nodal chain and are not consistently present.
- Rare pathway into the intraparotid nodes if the Eustachian tube is involved.

MRI eases detection of these nodal metastases [52] and are considered positive if the minimum axial diameter is ≥6 mm (92% positive predictive value) for RLN, ≥10 mm for cervical nodes, and ≥11 mm for the jugulodigastric nodes or if it shows central necrosis (100% specificity) [53] or extracapsular spread regardless of size. Grouping of RLN is rare and should always be considered malignant, while a borderline (1–2 mm below threshold) group of ≥3 cervical nodes can be used as a diagnostic criterion for nodal metastasis [53]. FDG PET/CT also shows good accuracy in nodal staging for newly diagnosed NPC and is part of the routine staging investigation in many centres (Fig. 2.16) [54].

2.6.1 N1, N2

Unilateral (N1)/Bilateral (N2) cervical and/or unilateral or bilateral retropharyngeal node(s), ≤6 cm in greatest dimension, above caudal border of cricoid cartilage: For staging of the cervical nodes, N1 refers to unilateral nodes, while N2 refers to bilateral nodes which have not reached the criteria for N3 staging. The greatest dimension (i.e. long axis) is used when measuring metastatic nodes.

2.6.2 N3

Unilateral or bilateral metastasis in cervical lymph node(s) >6 cm in greatest dimension and/or extension below the caudal border of cricoid cartilage: A welcome change in the AJCC 8th edition is the combination of N3a and N3b into a single designation of N3. The 8th edition also recategorised the supraclavicular nodes, which was previously determined by identifying the clavicle on the same axial slice. This was confusing, as it depended on the varying positions of the clavicle. N3 disease is now neatly defined as extension below the caudal edge of the cricoid cartilage.

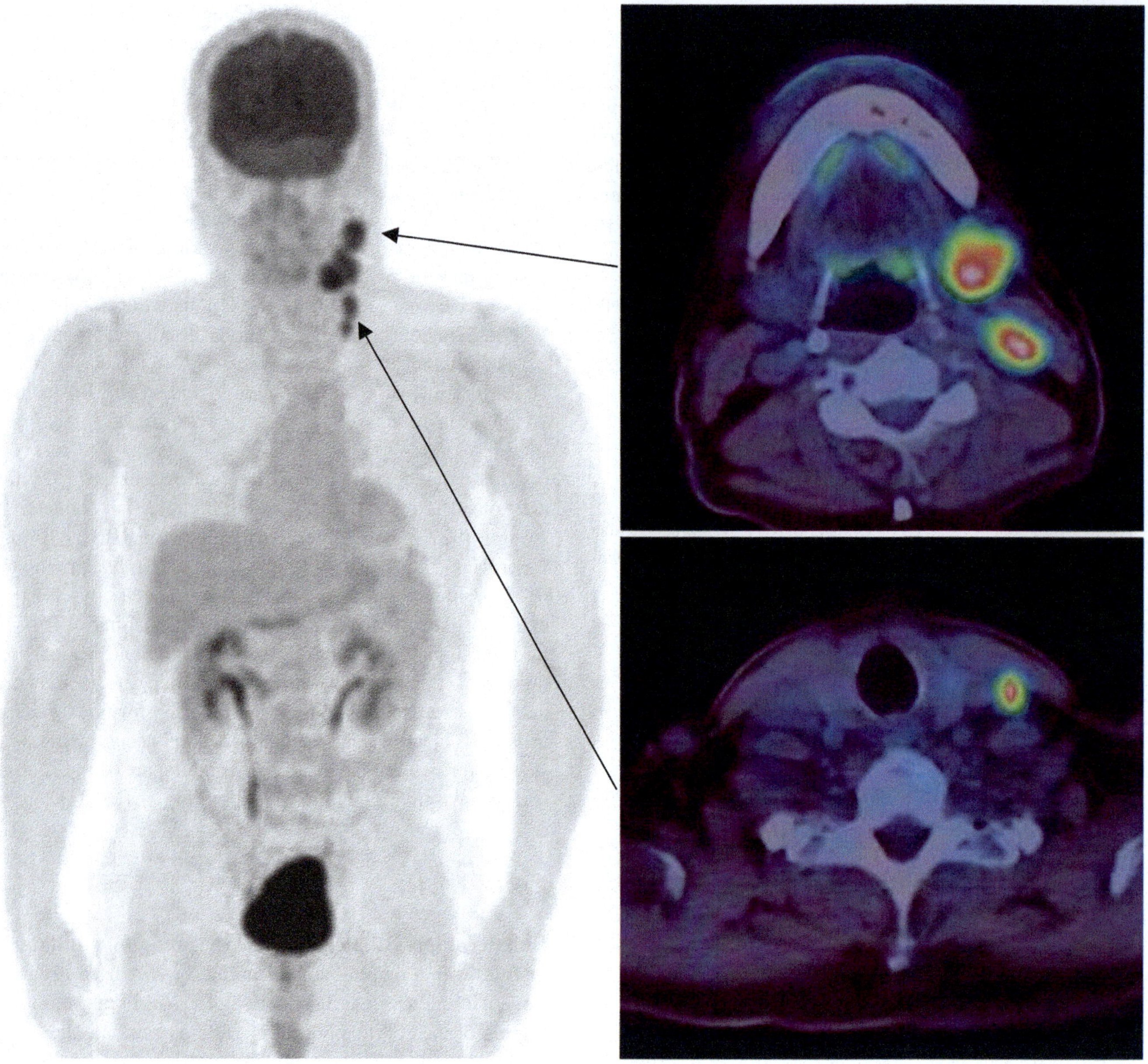

Fig. 2.16 FDG PET/CT used for nodal staging. Intensely FDG avid left level 1b, level II, and left infracricoid lymph nodes are noted, in keeping with nodal metastases. No suspicious FDG-avid lesion is seen elsewhere

The nodal spread of NPC tends to follow a stepwise fashion down the internal jugular (level II – IV) and spinal accessory chains (level V) which converge at the high internal jugular node (level II). However, unusual spread patterns to the anterior neck (level VI and VII), submandibular (level I), and parotid nodes have also been reported. This is likely due to disruption in the normal lymphatic drainage and subsequent retrograde flow into the aforementioned nodes [49]. A careful search for these metastatic nodes is important in radiotherapy planning (Fig. 2.17).

2.7 MRI Staging of Distant Metastates (M Classification)

Distant metastasis (DM) carries a poor prognosis and is also a major cause of IMRT failure. Large cohort studies found DM in up to 20% of patients, mostly within the skeleton, which far outweighs the thorax and liver (in decreasing frequency). Bony metastases are lytic in 66%, sclerotic in 21%, and mixed in 13% of cases [55], with a rare diffusely sclerotic pattern that can be confused with myelofibrosis or other osteoblastic metastases (e.g. prostatic carcinoma) [56].

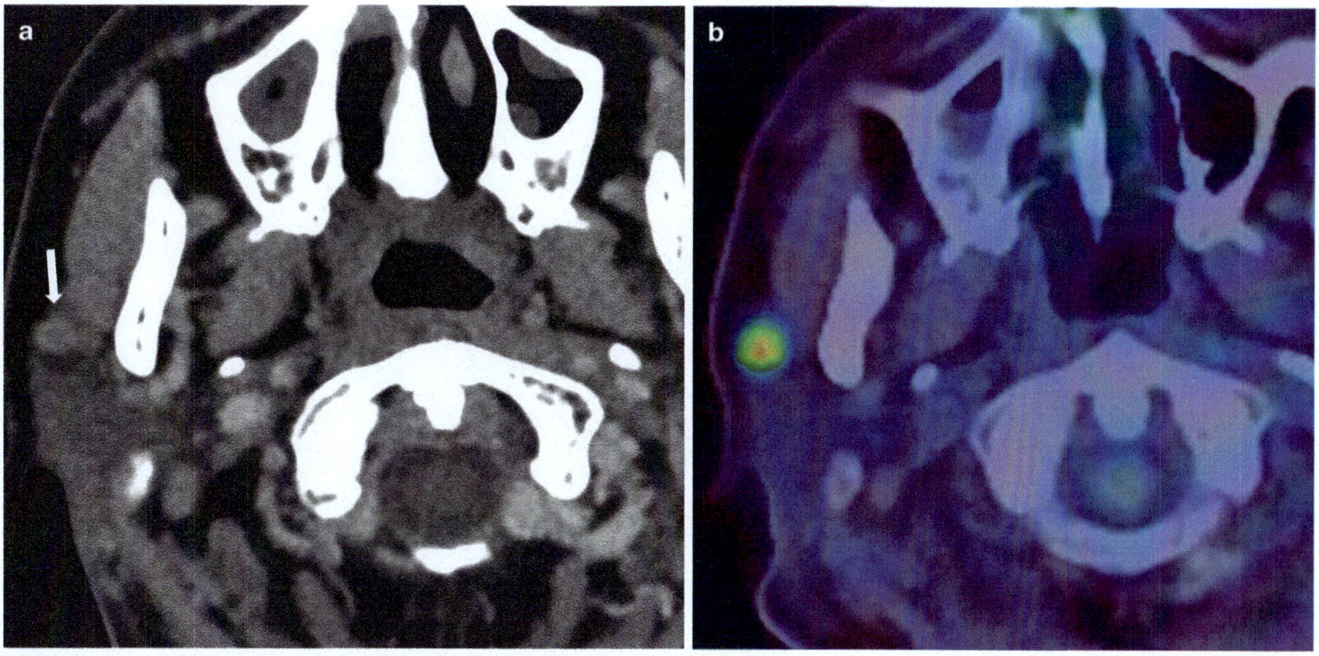

Fig. 2.17 Parotid nodal metastasis. (**a**) Axial contrast enhanced CT shows an inconspicuous right intraparotid node (solid arrow). (**b**) Subsequent FDG PET/CT shows high FDG avidity in keeping with nodal metastasis. This highlights the importance of FDG PET/CT in detection of nodal disease

Not surprisingly, the incidence of DM increases with nodal spread, from 14% in N2 to 48% in N3 [57]. Even with excellent locoregional control using IMRT, 1 in 6 patients continue to develop DM, often within a year of treatment [58]. This can perhaps be explained by subclinical micrometastases at initial staging.

In addition to MRI, a conventional metastatic workup (CMW) may also include an abdominal ultrasound, a chest radiograph, and a skeletal scintigraphy (Fig. 2.18), which require multiple examinations. This is increasingly being replaced by FDG PET/CT; a single albeit costlier alternative. A systemic review by Xu et al. [59] showed that PET/CT had better pooled sensitivity (85.7% vs. 38.0%) and specificity (98.1% vs. 97.6%) than CMW. This is primarily due to its better performance in detecting bone metastasis. However, the same study also concluded suboptimal PET/CT sensitivity (72.7%) in detecting liver metastasis.

In addition to detection, the intensity of FDG uptake can also serve as a prognostic biomarker. Tumours demonstrating a high FDG uptake usually denotes a more aggressive tumour biology and a higher incidence of distant metastasis [60]. It is well documented from experience with other head and neck cancers that areas of high FDG uptake are frequently associated with a higher rate of local failure post radiotherapy. In this context, FDG PET/CT can also be utilised for the purpose of dose painting in radiotherapy [61].

2.8 Radiotherapy for the Radiologist

Unlike many other tumours, the first line of treatment for NPC is radiotherapy (RT). RT is integral in curative-intent treatment, with radiobiological experiments showing that 66–70 Gy of fractionated radiation (in 2 Gy fractions) is required to control grossly visible disease in the nasopharynx and lymph nodes [62]. Microscopic disease in the tumour peripheries or at high-risk nodes requires a lower dose of 50–60 Gy, owing to lower tumour cell density.

Historically, RT was delivered using unsophisticated techniques (2D or 3D) based on bony landmarks from radiographs. This allowed for only simple beam arrangements that lead to significant toxicity [63] as large portions of uninvolved structures were included in the radiation portal. Signs of toxicity can be seen acutely in rapidly proliferating tissues (e.g. mucositis) or as a late complication months to years later (e.g. pituitary dysfunction).

IMRT was developed in the early 2000s and utilises computer-controlled algorithms for dose-painting and highly conformal dose distributions to allow for improved tumour coverage, while keeping dose in adjacent tissue at a safe level [64] (Fig. 2.19). Tumours directly abutting structures like the brainstem and optic chiasm may force a reduction in dose due to unacceptable morbidity. In such cases, induction chemotherapy can be offered in the hope of tumour shrinkage prior to RT.

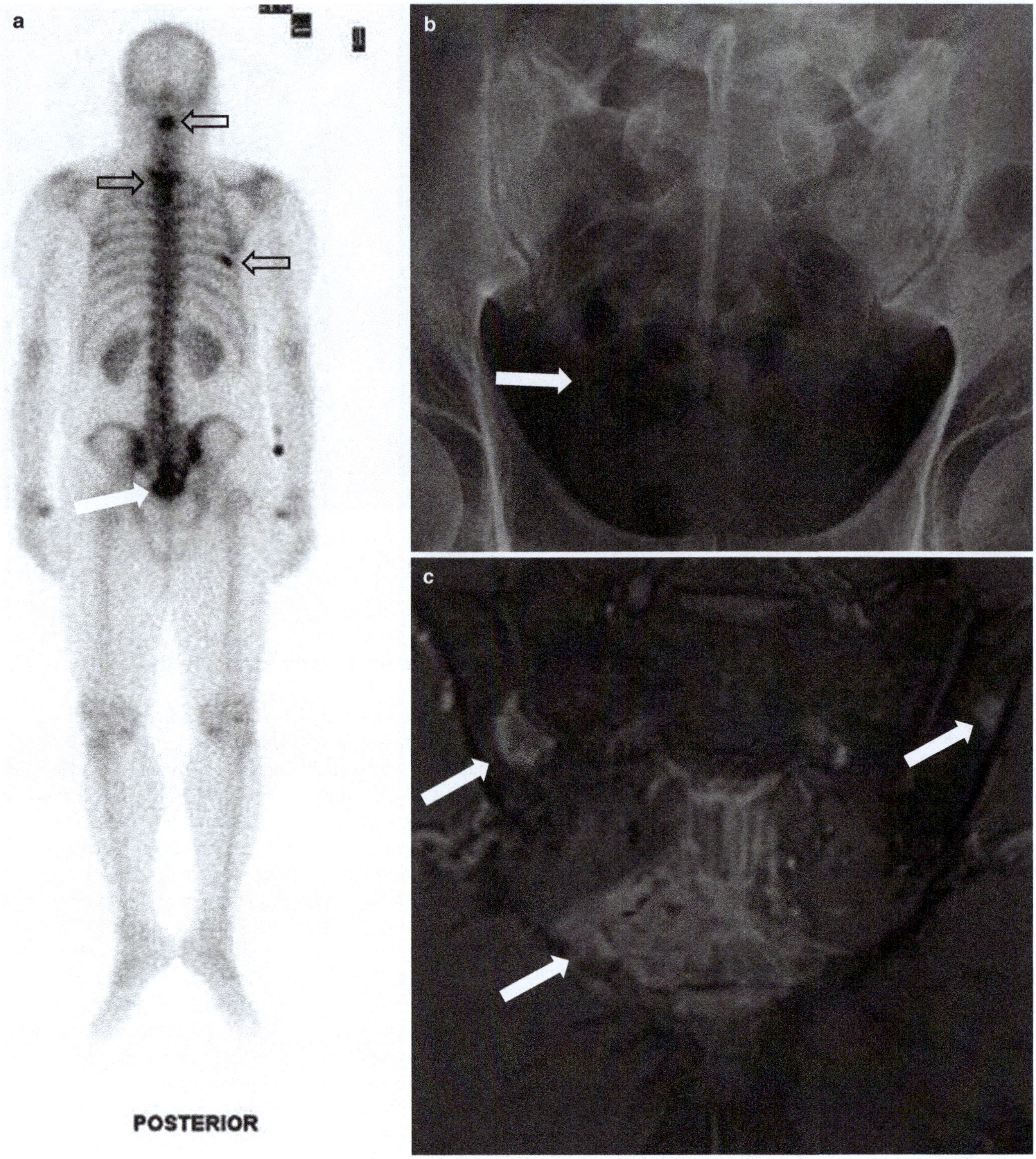

Fig. 2.18 Bony metastases: (**a**) Bone scintigraphy, (**b**) pelvic radiograph, and (**c**) coronal T1 post contrast fat saturated images show large destructive osseous lesions seen within the sacrum and iliac bones (white solid arrows), while the bone scan also shows other sites within the axial skeleton and rib (black open arrows)

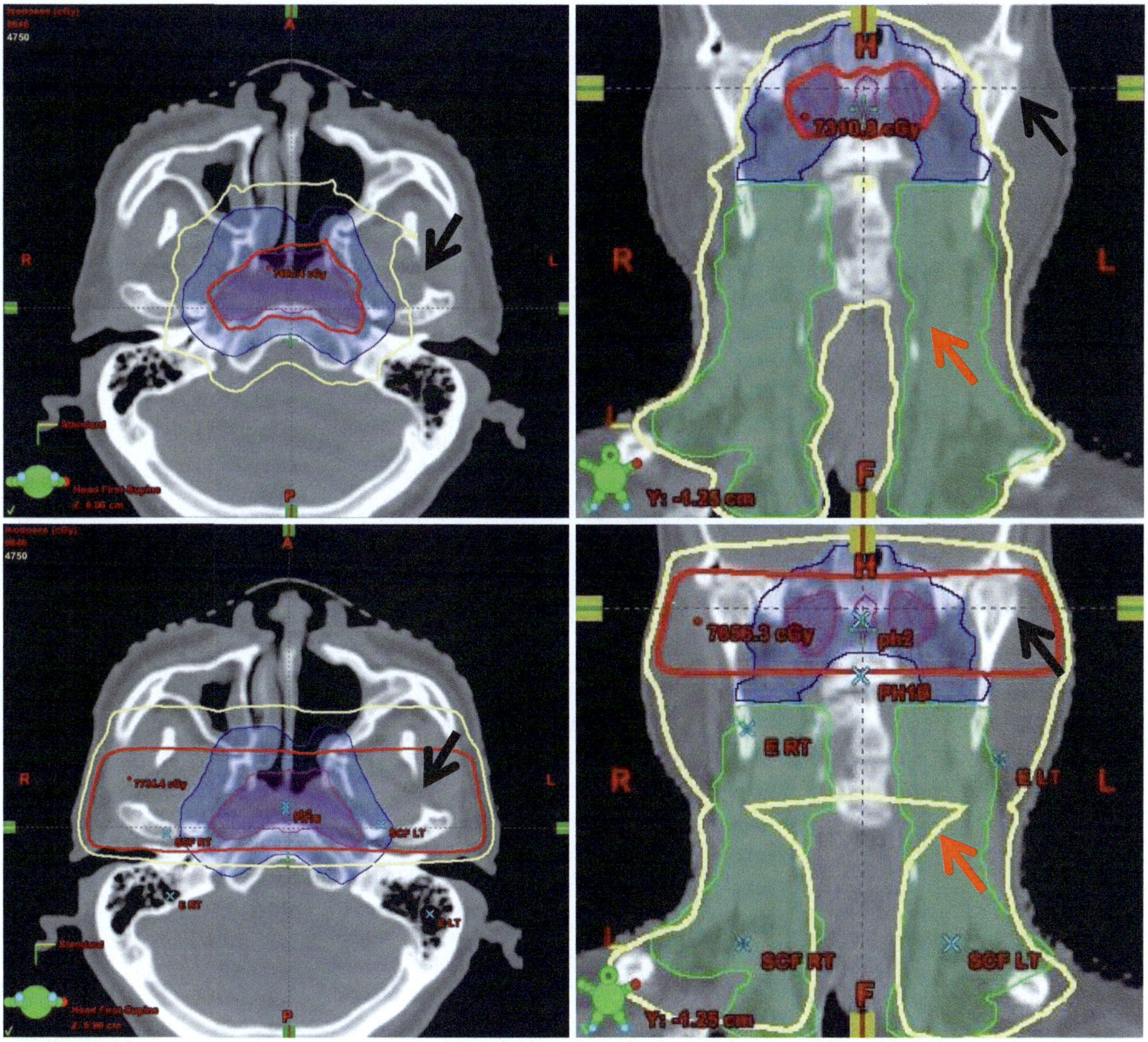

Fig. 2.19 Comparison of IMRT (top row) vs. 3DCRT (bottom row). Note the black arrows indicating areas of unintended high dose (including mandible, skull base) with 3DCRT that is spared with IMRT. Red arrows indicate areas of inadequate low dose coverage with 3DCRT that receives good coverage with IMRT. *Key: Pink Cloud: High dose target volume. Blue and green Clouds: Low dose target volume. Red Line: Area receiving high dose (>66 Gy). Yellow Line: Area receiving low dose (>47 Gy)*

Radiotherapy Planning: Radiotherapy planning is done primarily on a contrast- enhanced CT dataset with the patient in treatment position: lying supine (with a neck rest) and immobilized with a rigid custom-made thermoplastic mask that is mounted and referenced to the scanning couch (Fig. 2.20). This allows for reproducible positioning throughout the treatment duration (7 weeks). As the target delineation is only performed on CT (which has poor soft tissue contrast), incorporation of clinical information, endoscopic findings, MRI and PET/CT is crucial for margin accuracy.

MRI sequences can even be overlaid with the CT-simulation dataset in a process known as co-registration or simply 'fusion'. In cases where the MRI and CT-simulation dataset are not aligned, software permitting deformable registration or preferential alignment at the nasopharynx may be favoured. Some centres may choose to have the CT simulation done prior to an MRI with the patient in the thermoplastic mask to ensure satisfactory MRI–CT fusion.

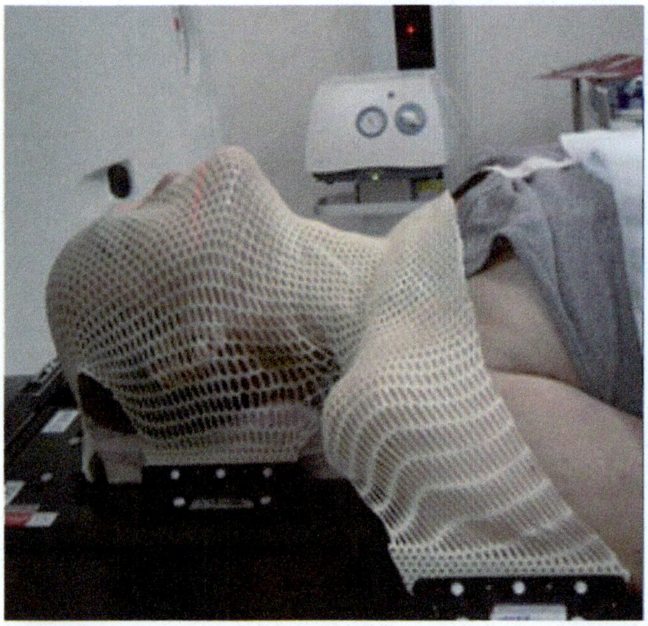

Fig. 2.20 CT scan simulation. Five-point head and neck thermoplastic shell used for immobilisation during head and neck radiotherapy treatments

2.9 Tumour Recurrence

Despite the success of RT, residual or recurrent disease remains a problem. Salvage treatment is largely dependent on the sites of recurrence which can broadly be divided into local, regional, or distant disease.

2.9.1 Local Failure

Local failure following RT occurs in 10–36% of patients [65], and subsequent treatment is largely divided into surgery, radiotherapy, or chemotherapy.

For most patients, especially those with small recurrent tumours, surgical extirpation is preferred as recurrent tumours tend to be resistant to radiotherapy. Surgery further avoids compounding radiation toxicities that can occur in up to 70% of re-irradiated patients [66, 67]. Key features for surgical consideration include:

- Encasement and proximity to the carotid artery. While there has been no large prospective studies to determine this, most surgeons would consider a carotid encasement of 180° to be unresectable. Despite this, some specialized centers have demonstrated feasibility of resection using novel techniques such as a extracranial–intracranial bypass [68].
- Lateral extension to the infratemporal fossa and invasion of the cavernous sinus/intracranial space may be considered unresectable in view of the difficulty in achieving oncologically clear margins [69]. In general, these features are indicators of advanced disease and pose significant perioperative morbidity and mortality.
- Tumour involvement in unusual areas such as the paranasal sinus (Fig. 2.21) should also be evaluated to allow for comprehensive treatment plans. In certain cases, orbital involvement may require exenteration to achieve adequate tumour clearance (Fig. 2.22).

Surgery may be performed using conventional open approaches such as the maxillary swing, lateral rhinotomy, facial translocation, and craniofacial approaches or via minimally invasive approaches, such as endoscopic or robotic nasopharyngectomies. These surgical approaches are determined by institutional practice and available surgical expertise. While there is no evidence-based guideline as to the selection of approaches, most surgeons would tend to favour an endoscopic approach for small volume disease largely confined to the nasopharynx. Lateral extension to the parapharyngeal space with close proximity to the carotid vasculature (within 1cm) would favour an open approach [70]. In some centers, the use of facial translocation and craniofacial approach has been favoured for resection of tumours with skull base involvement, thereby allowing for a combined approach with the neurosurgeons [69].

SUVmax on FDG PET combined with plasma EBV values have proved to be useful in determining the prognosis of cases treated by surgery. Chan et al. [71] looked at recurrent tumours treated with nasopharyngectomy and discovered that those with a curative outcome had significantly lower preoperative log plasma EBV DNA values (2.2 vs. 3.4) and mean SUVmax (4.3 vs. 6.9) than patients with further recurrence.

Surgically unresectable tumours may be considered for re-irradiation, with various techniques like brachytherapy, IMRT, stereotactic radiosurgery, and proton beam therapy being employed. Patients who are unsuitable for either surgery or re-irradiation are subsequently treated with palliative chemotherapy.

2.9.2 Regional Failure

Regional failure mostly presents with nodal metastasis in the upper cervical nodal basins, such as level II and Va stations, and accounts for approximately 5–13% of patients [14, 72]. Surgery is again the treatment of choice, especially when the

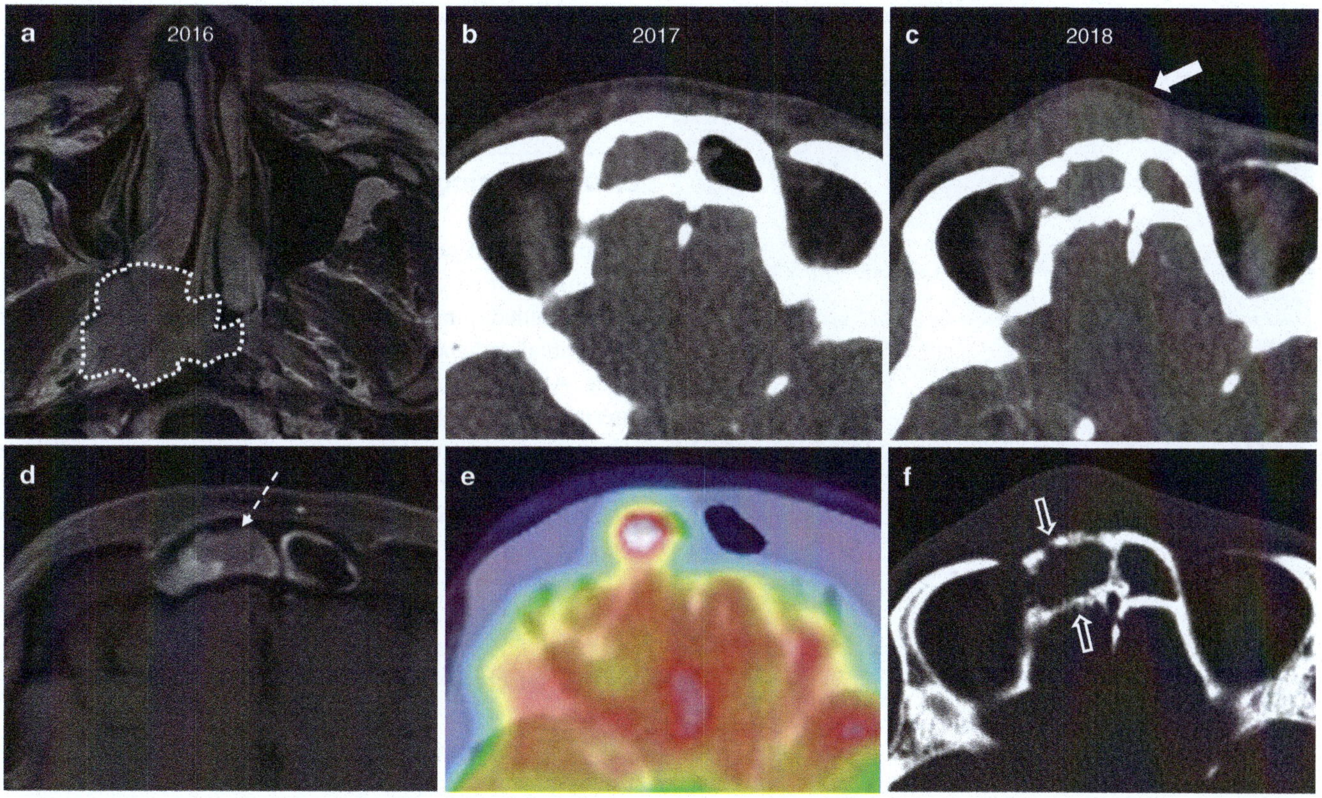

Fig. 2.21 Frontal sinus metastasis. (**a**, **d**) A patient with a right T2N2M0 NPC (white area) had right frontal sinusitis (dashed arrow). (**b**, **e**) 1 year post treatment, the sinusitis showed FDG avidity suggesting active inflammation. (**c**, **f**) 2 years post treatment, an enlarging forehead swelling (solid arrow) was thought to represent a Pott's puffy tumour with erosion of the inner and outer tables (open arrow). This was later biopsy proven to be metastatic NPC

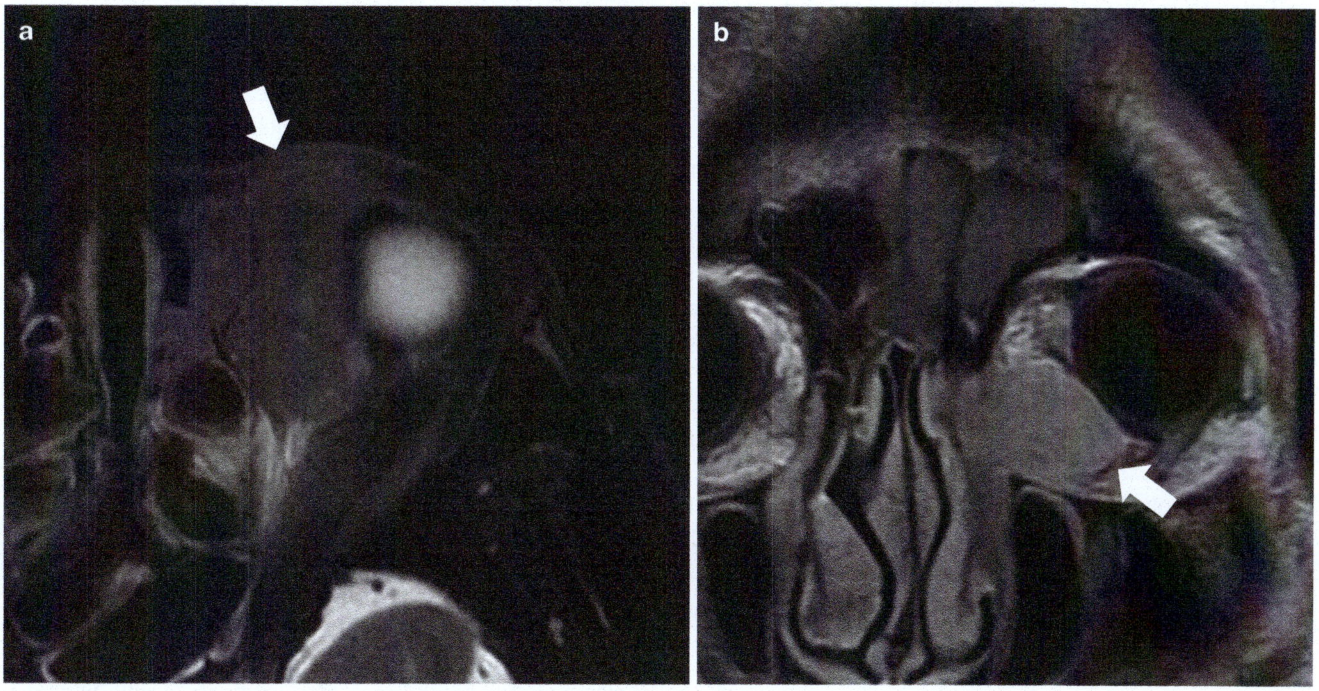

Fig. 2.22 Orbital metastasis. (**a**) Axial T2 fat saturated and (**b**) coronal T1 post contrast images show metastasis (solid arrow) into the left orbit

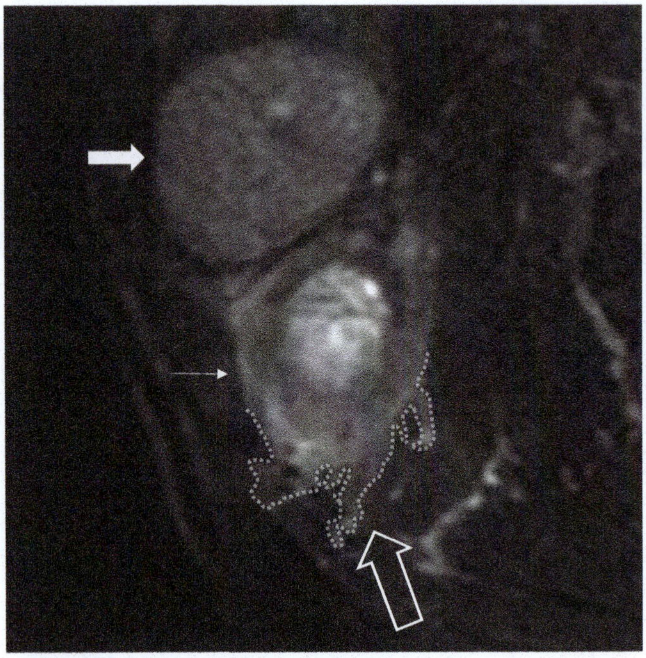

Fig. 2.23 Extracapsular spread. Axial T2 fat saturated image of a necrotic lymph node with extracapsular spread (thin arrow). It shows an indistinct capsular outline (white dotted line), loss of the surrounding fat plane, and infiltration of adjacent structures (thick open arrow). A second enlarged lymph node is seen anteriorly (solid arrow) without extracapsular spread

nodes are situated in the lateral neck. Key imaging features include:

- Relation to the carotid arteries, invasion of the internal jugular vein, and the metastasis to the parotid, which impact the nature of neck dissection.
- Extra-nodal extension which is not uncommon following chemoradiation (Fig. 2.23).
- The presence of a retropharyngeal node should also be evaluated during pre-treatment planning. The treatment of residual/recurrent retropharyngeal lymph node still remains inconclusive due to the difficulties of surgical access to this location. As such, radiation is typically employed for treatment of these nodes. Surgical extirpation of these nodes have also been demonstrated in some centers [73].

Conventional treatment of lateral nodal disease in recurrent/residual nasopharyngeal carcinoma includes a radical neck dissection. This is often due to the presence of significant extra-nodal extension and the extensive nature of nodal disease in these patients [74].

2.9.3 Distant Metastases

Distant metastasis following primary treatment is largely targeted using systemic treatment regimes such as chemotherapy. Other novel approaches include treatment with immunotherapy agents, which is unfortunately beyond the scope of this chapter.

2.10 Imaging Tumour Recurrence

There is lack of consensus around the timing of follow-up imaging, with an early baseline study at 3–6 months often recommended. Any enlarging or new soft tissue lesion or intracranial enhancement is suspicious for tumour recurrence. After radiotherapy, however, the tumour site is often intermixed with inflammation, fibroplasia, and scarring that more often result in persistent soft tissue distortion than a normalised anatomy. This makes it difficult in separating NPC recurrence from the surrounding mash. Even endoscopic assessment and deep biopsies can prove difficult due to sampling errors.

2.10.1 Nuclear Medicine

FDG PET/CT excels in this setting as metabolic changes usually precede morphological changes. Liu et al. [75] conducted a meta-analysis comparing FDG PET, CT, and MRI in detecting residual/recurrent NPC in 1813 patients. The pooled sensitivity and specificity was FDG PET (95% and 90%), CT (76% and 59%), and MRI (78% and 76%). The superior diagnostic accuracy of FDG PET/CT is contrasted against its high cost and poor soft-tissue contrast.

Due to the high cost of FDG PET in most countries, there is a need for a cost-effective method in selecting patients who will benefit from surveillance scans. A risk adaptive approach where high risk patients are scanned more frequently is often employed. However, a more attractive option is to use tumour biomarkers to detect evidence of disease and then utilise FDG PET for localisation of disease sites. This approach was described by Wang et al. [76], who analysed plasma EBV DNA levels every 3–6 months post treatment, then performed FDG PET when EBV DNA levels were positive. Using this method, plasma EBV DNA levels detected NPC recurrence with 100% accuracy, while FDG PET had an accuracy of 79%.

Another major pitfall of FDG PET is the false-positive uptake in infective and inflammatory conditions during the early post-radiotherapy period which take up glucose and mimic active disease. In light of this, the time to scanning is an important factor in reducing the number of false-positive findings; the current practice is to wait 3–4 months after treatment before the first follow-up FDG PET study. False-negative results may also occur if: (1) the patient is scanned too early, (2) the recurrent tumour is too small or has a low metabolic rate, (3) the recurrence is at a site with physiologically high metabolism, or (4) the FDG uptake is obscured by artefacts from adjacent metal ware (e.g. dental crowns and fillings).

2.10.2 MRI

MRI has superior soft tissue contrast to FDG PET/CT, and its use helps improve diagnostic confidence. Mature scar tissue will show low T2 signal, delayed enhancement, and contraction over time, while recurrent tumour will show intermediate T1 and T2 signals, intermediate enhancement, and expand over time. In contrast, inflammatory tissue has higher T2 signal and avid enhancement compared to tumour. Unfortunately in practice, these features tend to overlap, particularly within the early post-treatment period where inflammation, infection, and immature scar tissue can all appear expansile [77].

DWI is also useful in increasing the conspicuity of remnant tumour (Fig. 2.24). Xu et al. [78] described lower ADC values (~1.097×10^{-3} mm^2/s) in tumours compared to the lateral pterygoid muscle (~1.501×10^{-3} mm^2/s), while non-tumoural tissue show higher ADC values (~1.843×10^{-3} mm^2/s). The use of conventional echo-planar DWI at the skull base is limited by magnetic field inhomogeneity, complex anatomy, and image drift. While these limitations can be overcome by using non-echo-planar DWI (e.g. HASTE and PROPELLAR), the disadvantages include longer scan time and lower signal-to-noise ratio [79].

In the assessment of nodal recurrence, the reader should also be aware of anatomical mimics such as the cervical sympathetic ganglia. These comprise of three interconnected ganglia: the stellate, middle cervical, and superior cervical ganglia (SCG) that lie within the pre-vertebral fascia medial to the carotid sheath. In particular, the SCG (the largest of the three) can enlarge post RT and mimic a RLN. The SCG can be recognized by a few characteristic features (Fig. 2.25) [80]: (1) Homogeneous enhancement due to large surrounding capillaries and lack of a blood-nerve barrier. (2) T2 hyperintense with an internal hypointense spot (venule) or fat (an interneural space not to be confused with lymph node hilar fat). (3) Elongated with cranio-caudal tapering.

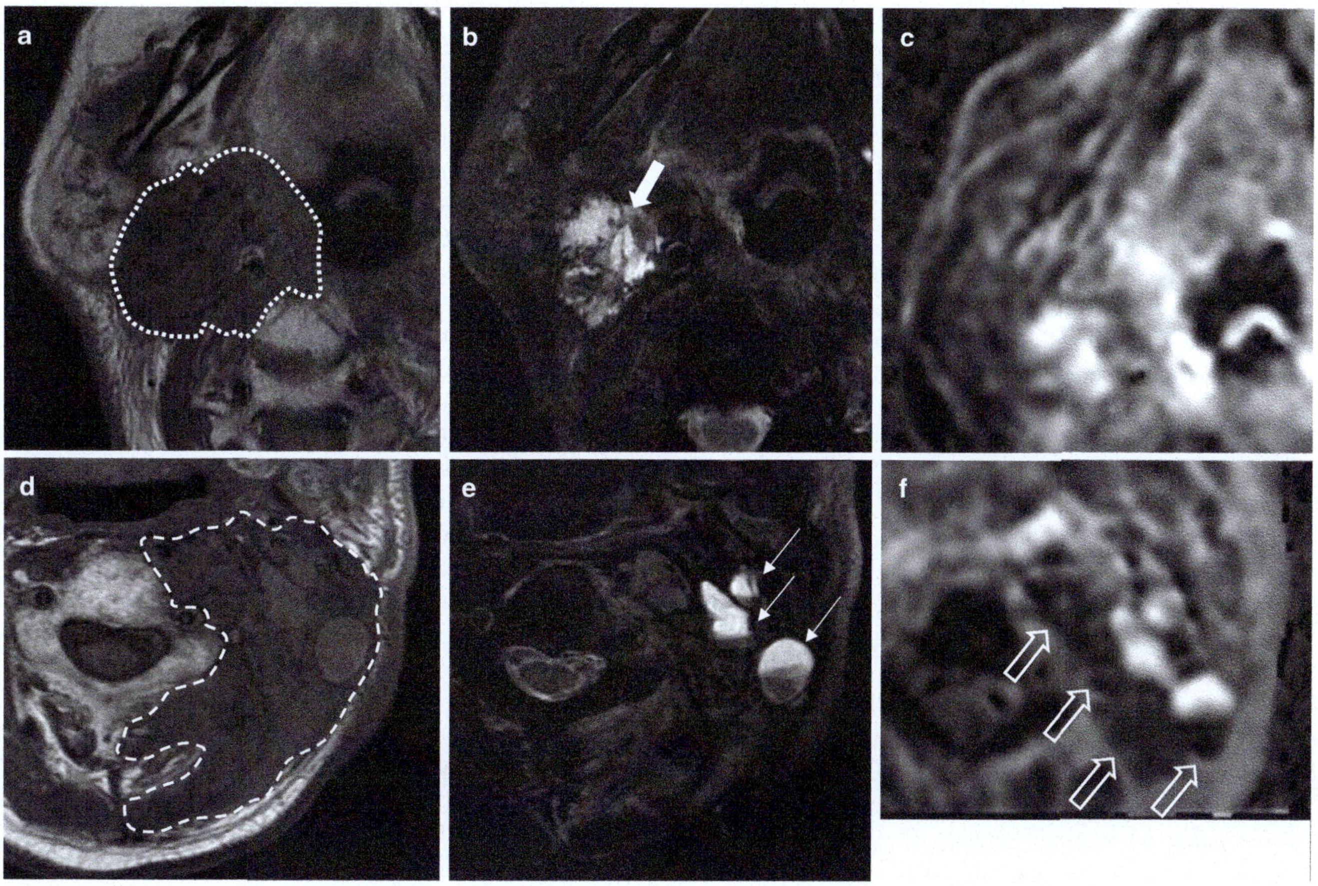

Fig. 2.24 Post-operative infection vs. recurrence. (**a**, **d**) Axial T1 images (**b**, **e**) Axial T2 fat saturated images and (**c**, **f**) ADC maps. The upper row (**a** + **b** + **c**) shows inflammatory tissue (white dotted area) with cysts (solid arrow) and no restricted diffusion, while the lower row (**d** + **e** + **f**) shows a tumour recurrence (white dashed area) with cysts (thin solid arrow) and restricted diffusion (open arrows)

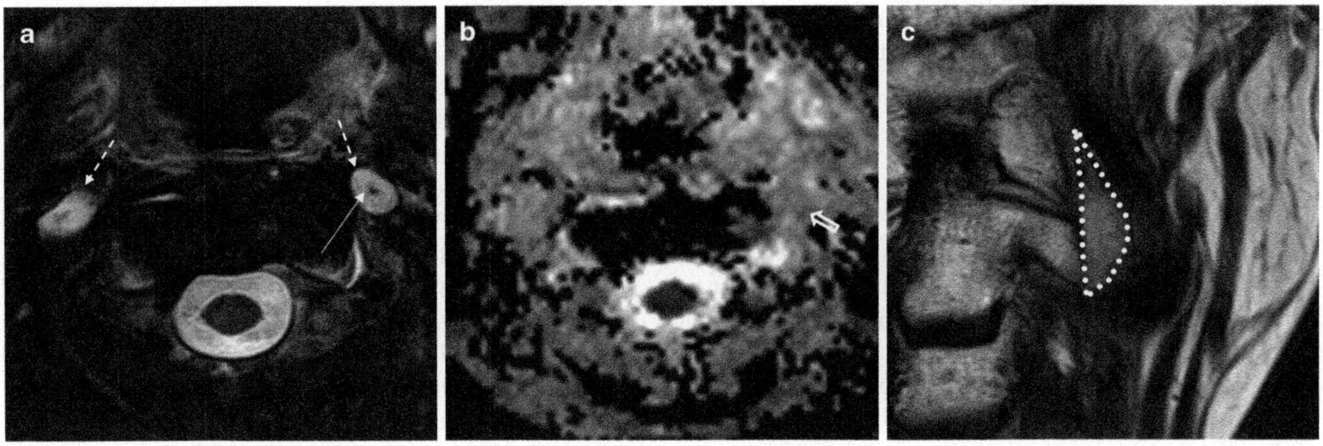

Fig. 2.25 Superior cervical ganglions. (**a**) Axial T2 fat saturated, (**b**) ADC map, and (**c**) coronal T1 images. There are bilateral enlarged superior cervical ganglions showing high T2W signal (dashed arrows), a central dot (thin arrow), no restricted diffusion (open arrow), and cranio-caudal tapering (white area) that is in keeping with a superior cervical ganglion

2.11 Complications of Radiotherapy

Despite IMRT's ability to better conform to the tumour target, unintended radiation exposure to adjacent anatomical structures remains inevitable. Understanding the biological effects of radiation can help the radiologist anticipate and recognise complications when they occur.

2.11.1 Radiation-Induced Central Nervous System (CNS) Injury

Our CNS was once thought to be extremely radio-resistant due to the low rate of neuronal cell division. However, both structural and functional injuries are now well documented, occurring at a median of 5 years post exposure and in up to 20% of cases [81, 82]. This is the single most debilitating complication of RT.

2.11.1.1 Injury to the Brain

While earlier simplified theories suggested either vascular ischemia or direct parenchymal damage [83], the model proposed by Tofilon and Fike [84] is perhaps the most plausible. Here, radiation causes acute cell death, inciting a cytokine-led 'protective-reparatory' response that triggers a cycle of persistent oxidative stress and chronic inflammation leading to tissue death. The CNS is particularly susceptible to oxidative stress due to its high rate of oxidative metabolism (forming superoxides) and poor antioxidant levels (especially in oligodendrocytes, neurons, and endothelial cells). Radiation-induced CNS injury can generally be divided into two stages:

1. Reversible acute/early-delayed phase (1–6 months) with oedema and demyelination. This is seen as T2 hyperintensities that gradually become confluent, often sparing the subcortical U-fibers (Fig. 2.26). The myelin membrane is thought to be particularly susceptible to oxidative injury. This in combination with the loss of oligodendrocytes (interrupts myelin synthesis) [85] can explain the early preference of radiation injury for white matter.
2. Irreversible late-delayed phase (>6 months) characterised by endothelial cell loss, and ultimately white matter necrosis [86]. This typically occur in areas with the highest radiation exposure – usually the medial temporal lobes and seen as liquefied T2W hyperintense areas with a 'spreading wavefront' pattern enhancement and haemorrhage (Fig. 2.26) [87]. In some cases, this can also lead to tumefactive cyst formation (Fig. 2.27) [88].

The clinical and imaging features of radiation injury should help differentiate it from residual tumour. In equivocal cases, a multidisciplinary approach with review of the radiotherapy plan (Fig. 2.28), adjunct use of EBV DNA, and serial imaging are helpful. Advanced imaging techniques like MR spectroscopy (MRS) and perfusion can also be utilised. MRS features of radiation necrosis include markedly elevated lactate and lipid, reduced choline and corresponding reduced choline: creatine ratio. This can be further supported by MR perfusion showing reduced cerebral blood volume (Fig. 2.29) [89] or FDG PET/CT showing decreased radiotracer uptake [90].

2.11.1.2 Injury to the Cranial Nerves

Radiation-induced cranial nerve palsy (CNP) is a delayed complication, with a latency period measured in years. Cranial nerves are relatively radio-resistant owing to their large vasa nervorum and dural arterial network that prevent ischaemia [91]. However, up to 30% of patients still experience CNP, particularly of the lower cranial nerves [92]. This was presumably due to their smaller rootlet form but may also

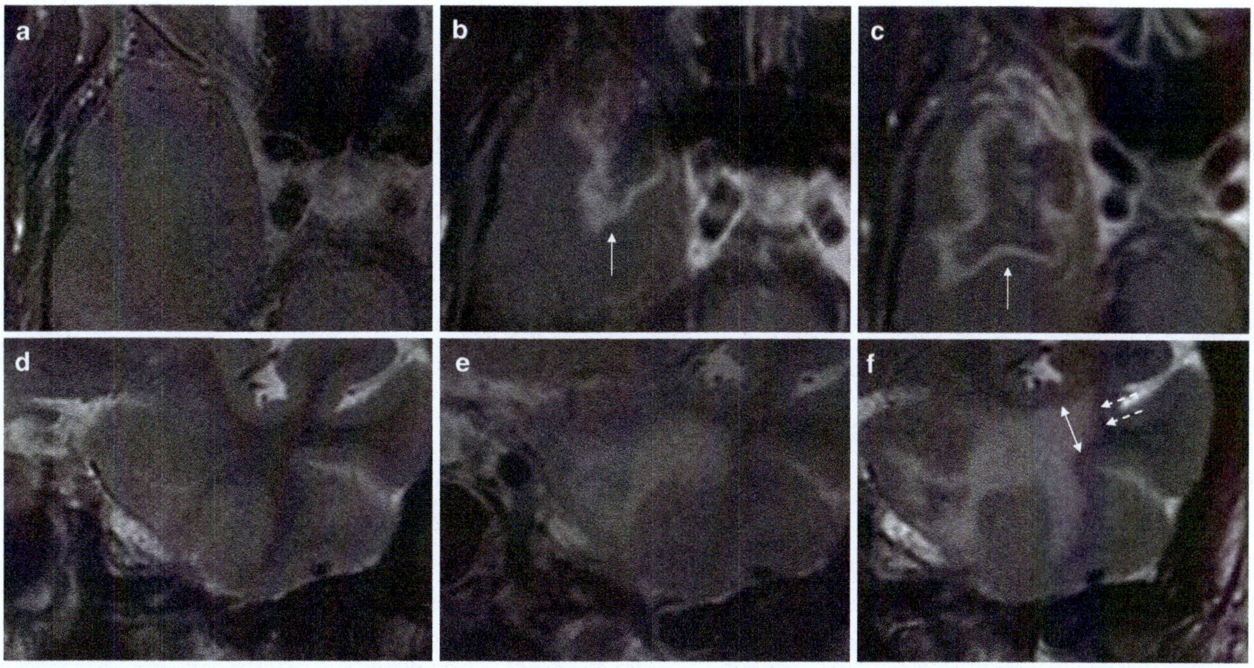

Fig. 2.26 Radiation necrosis. (**a–c**) Axial T1 post contrast images show a 'spreading wavefront' pattern of enhancement. (**d–f**) Coronal T2 images of a different patient show a growing T2W hyperintense area of early demyelination and oedema exerting mass effect and widening the gyrus (double arrow head). Note the sparing of the subcortical U-fibers (dashed arrows)

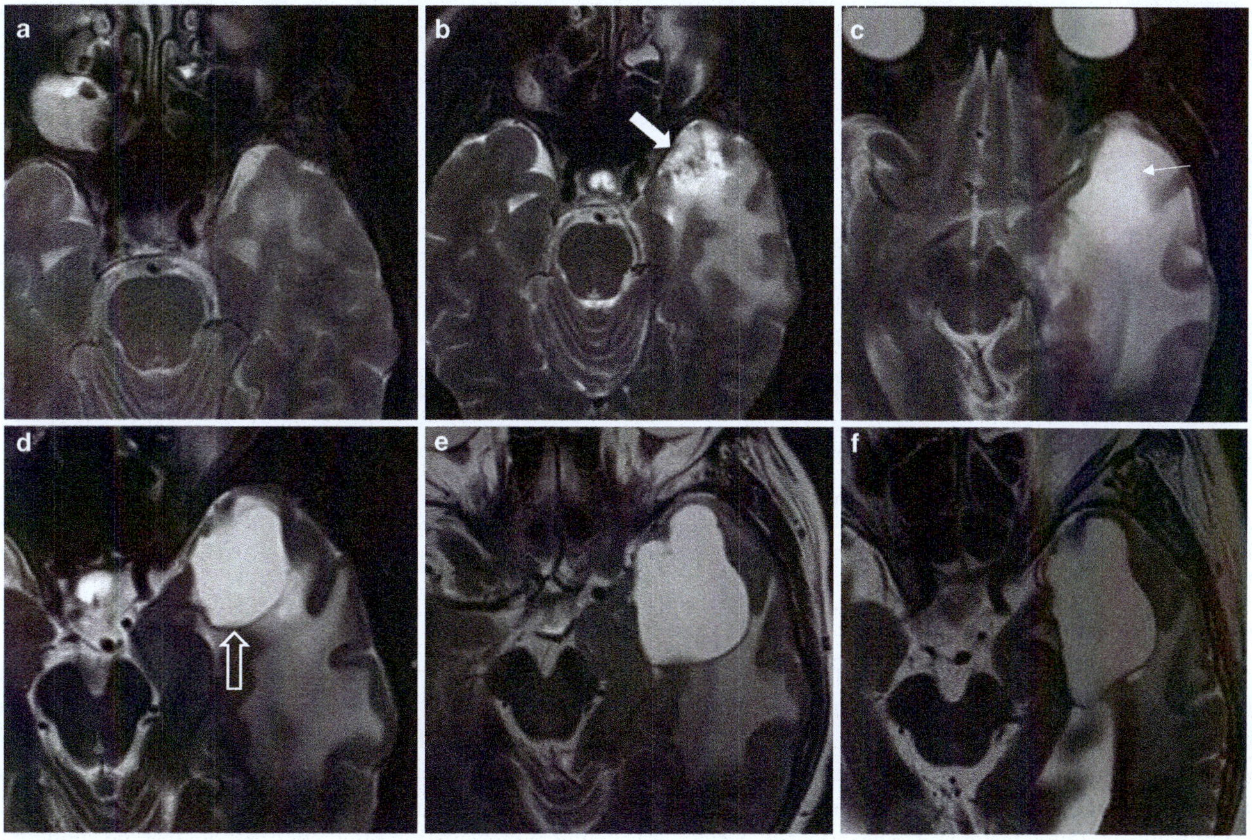

Fig. 2.27 Radiation-induced delayed cyst formation. (**a–d**) Axial T2 fat saturated and (**e, f**) Axial T2 images showing development of a tumefactive cyst over the course of 4 years post RT. (**a**) Early demyelination and oedema with (**b**) a focus of radiation necrosis (solid arrow) and (**c**) subsequent enlargement of a liquefied T2 hyperintense area (thin arrow) and oedema. (**d–f**) Follow-up MRI showed formation of a tumefactive cyst (open arrow) which continued to grow over 2 years

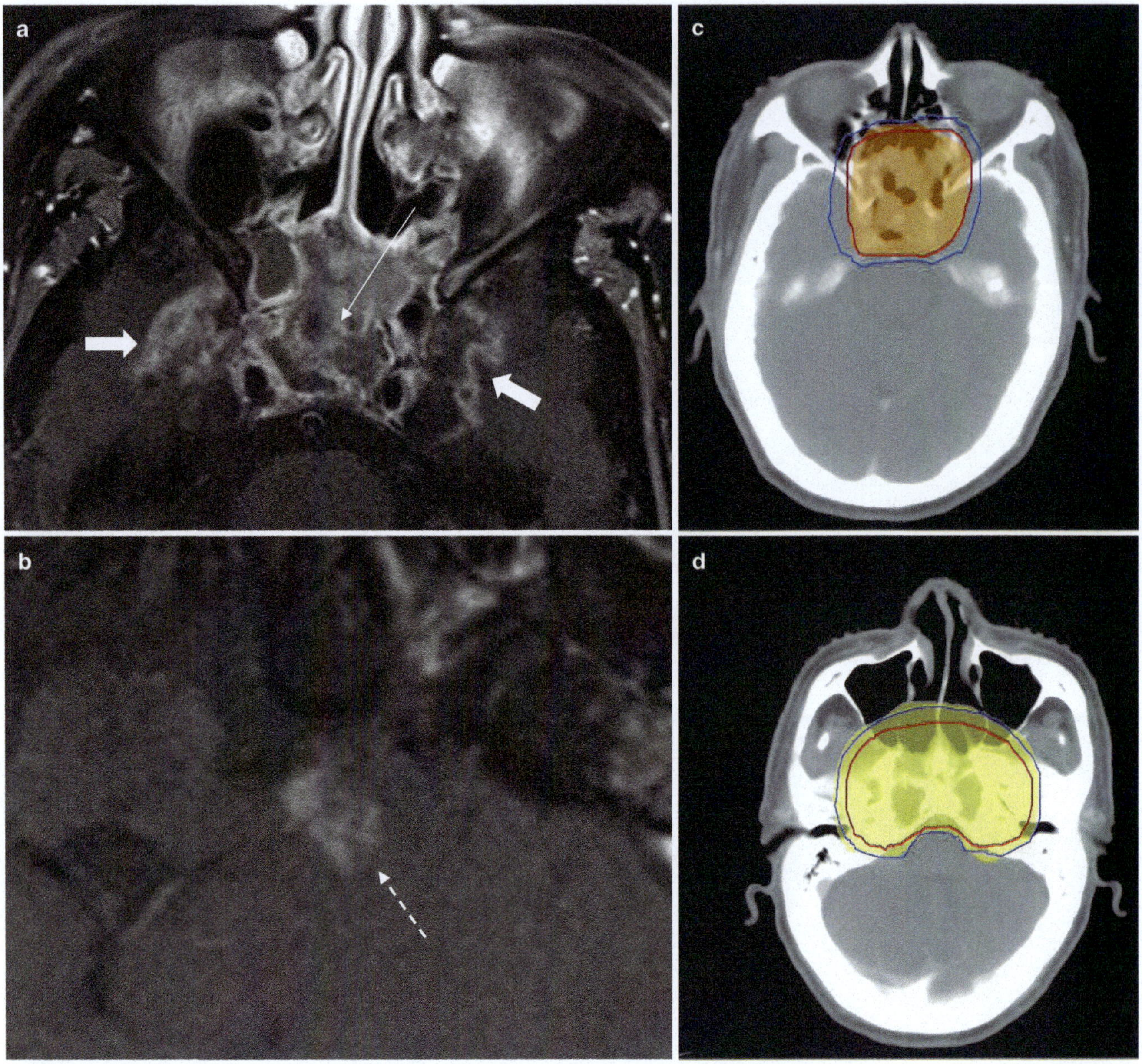

Fig. 2.28 Reviewing treatment plans. (**a**) Axial T1 post contrast fat saturated, (**b**) axial T1 post contrast image at the cerebellum, (**c**) radiation treatment plan showing 66 Gy isodose line (orange colour wash), and (**d**) radiation treatment plan showing ~60 Gy isodose line (yellow colour wash). Osteoradionecrosis of the basisphenoid (thin arrow) is noted. Reviewing the treatment plans increases confidence in diagnosing radiation necrosis of the temporal lobes (solid arrows) and cerebellum (dashed arrow) which is rare but occurred in this case as the hypoglossal canal was treated to a full dose corresponding with the ~60 Gy iso dose line (yellow colour wash). Adhering to large cooperative group protocols, we allow a maximum dose of up to 65 Gy to the temporal lobes

be partly caused by extrinsic factors, as their longer course through the neck exposes them to infiltration and compression by surrounding muscle fibrosis. This causal link is supported by autopsy cases showing perineural fibrosis and fibrous infiltration of the nerve fibres themselves [93].

While the imaging features of the affected nerves are often subtle (mild enlargement, enhancement, and increased T2 hyperintensity), more apparent findings can be seen in target organs. For example, radiation injury to the hypoglossal nerve typically results in oedema, fatty infiltration, and atrophy of the affected hemi-tongue (Fig. 2.30). Radiation-induced optic neuropathy, on the other hand, can present with acute and irreversible loss of vision [94]. The stark clinical presentation often contrasts against the subtle imaging findings, highlighting the importance of obtaining good clinical history.

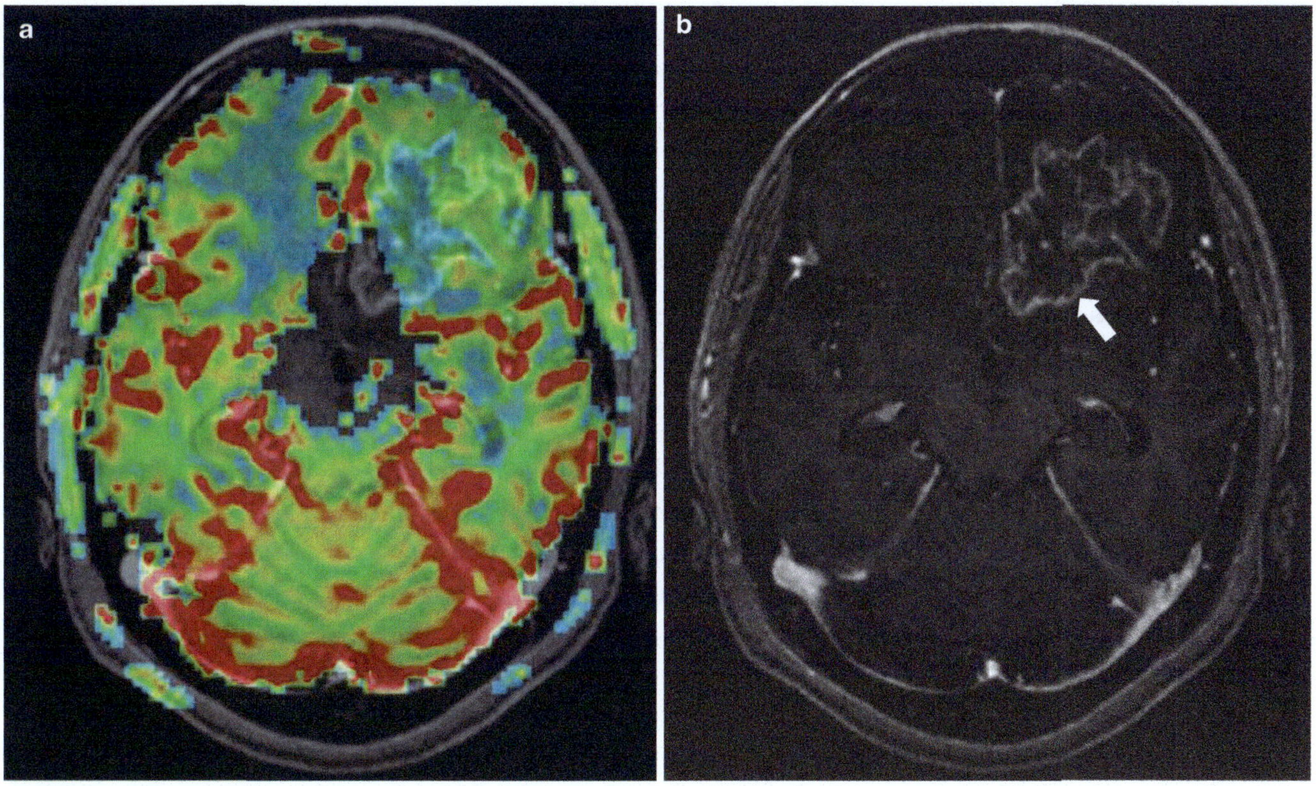

Fig. 2.29 DSC MR perfusion of radiation necrosis. (**a**) Cerebral blood volume and (**b**) axial T1 post contrast images showing 'spreading wavefront' enhancement (solid arrow) with no increased CBV (coloured red) that is in keeping with radiation necrosis

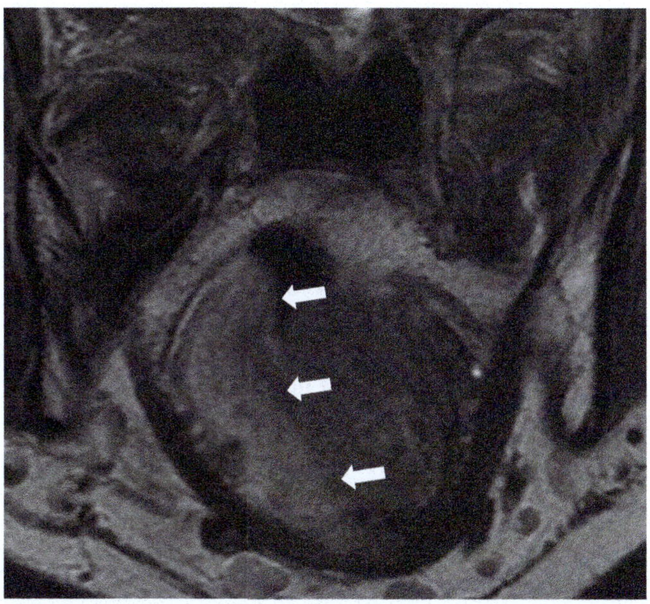

Fig. 2.30 Hypoglossal nerve palsy. Coronal T1 image shows hemiatrophy of the right hemi-tongue (solid arrow), with fatty replacement seen as T1 hyperintensities

2.11.2 Radiation-Induced Bone and Cartilage Injury

Changes in irradiated bone is dose dependent and can be seen as low as 8 Gy [83]. These changes range from early oedema and haemorrhage, to severe forms that include osteoradionecrosis (ORN).

Days after irradiation, the marrow shows oedema and haemorrhage (decreasing T1 signal). After 3 weeks, the depleted red marrow is replaced by fat (increasing T1 signal) in two distinct patterns; homogeneous (Fig. 2.31) or bandlike surrounding the basivertebral veins. Bone marrow receiving 50 Gy is irreversibly damaged due to the ablation of vascular sinusoids, while those receiving <50 Gy may regenerate normal red marrow in a year or two (decreasing T1 signal) [95].

ORN is seen in approximately 7% of treated NPC [96] and is rare in those receiving <60 Gy [97]. Once thought to be due to osteomyelitis within irradiated bone, ORN is now theorised to be due to an imbalance of bone metabolism (resorption and deposition) caused by bony atrophy and infiltrative fibrosis [98].

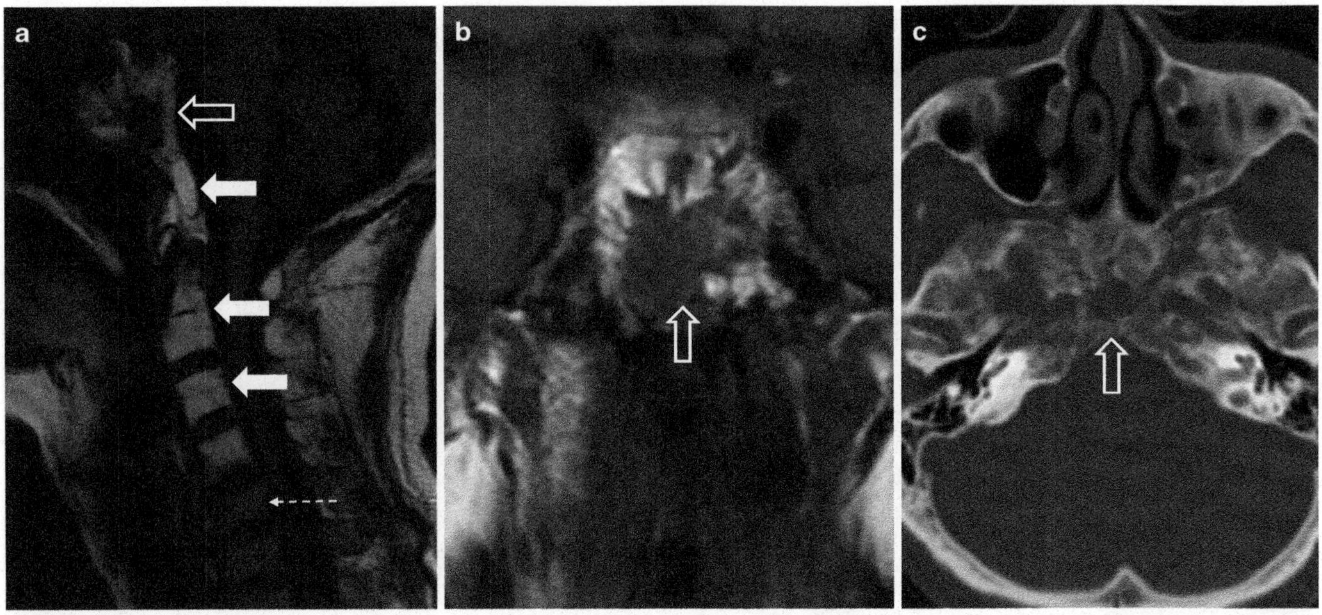

Fig. 2.31 Radiation-induced bone changes. (**a**) Sagittal T1 image shows fatty marrow replacement in the skull base and upper cervical spine (solid arrows). Note the normal red marrow in the lower cervical spine (dashed arrow) showing higher T1 signal than the adjacent disc. (**b**) Coronal T1 and (**c**) axial CT images show osteoradionecrosis of the basisphenoid (open arrows) with mottling of the bone and cortical defects

CT may show focal osteopenia, cortical interruptions, and decreased trabeculation with patchy sclerosis that reflect reactive new bone formation. MRI typically shows a heterogeneously high T2 signal and patchy enhancement that later turn into bony destruction with varying degree of bone dehiscence that increases the risk of infection, pneumocephaly, and CSF leakage [82].

ORN is extremely difficult to distinguish from osteomyelitis and tumour recurrence, and the diagnosis is often made histologically, with ORN showing an absence of osteoblastic activity and inflammatory cells as opposed to osteomyelitis [99].

Radiation to cartilaginous structures may similarly result in early perichondritis or delayed chondronecrosis with fragmentation and structural collapse [100]. In the context of NPC, this typically involves the torus tubarius and the temporomandibular joints, leading to trismus and speech impairment [101]. Rarely, ORN can also affect the external auditory canal (Fig. 2.32) [102].

2.11.3 Radiation-Induced Vascular Injury

Radiation-induced vasculopathies are more likely to involve the small vessels than the large vessels.

Radiation-induced small vessel disease in the brain manifests as telangiectasia and cavernous malformations. Previous theories suggested a release of vascular endothelial growth factor (VEGF) in response to radiation injury, thereby inducing angiogenesis [103]. Subsequent hyalinisation and fibrinoid necrosis of the vascular walls lead to thrombosis and occlusion, resulting in further recruitment of collateral blood supply. This vicious cycle ultimately drives the gradual enlargement of these vascular malformations, which are seen on MRI as scattered blooming artefacts on the gradient-weighted sequences [87]. They are usually asymptomatic.

Large vessel vasculopathy is often multifactorial [104–106], where damage to the endothelium and vasa vasorum drives an ischaemic and fibrotic response. As the internal elastic lamina and endothelium become scarred, they culminate in luminal narrowing of the vessel (Fig. 2.33). It is also believed that arterial stenosis contributes to accelerated atherosclerosis, which is often more diffuse with less calcification and seen in arterial segments that are not usually involved in atherosclerotic patients (i.e. common carotid and internal carotid arteries, rather than carotid bifurcation).

Pseudoaneurysms and carotid blowouts are rare but well-established complications of RT (Fig. 2.34). They confer significant mortality and require emergency endovascular or surgical treatment. The exact mechanism of pseudoaneurysm formation is unclear, but is believed to be an extension of the aforementioned arterial wall injury [107].

2.11.4 Radiation-Induced Mucosal Injury

After RT, the irradiated mucosa and soft tissue invariably show signs of inflammation [82]. Patients can present with mucositis and pharyngitis with oedema within the deep neck spaces and non-enhancing retropharyngeal fluid showing

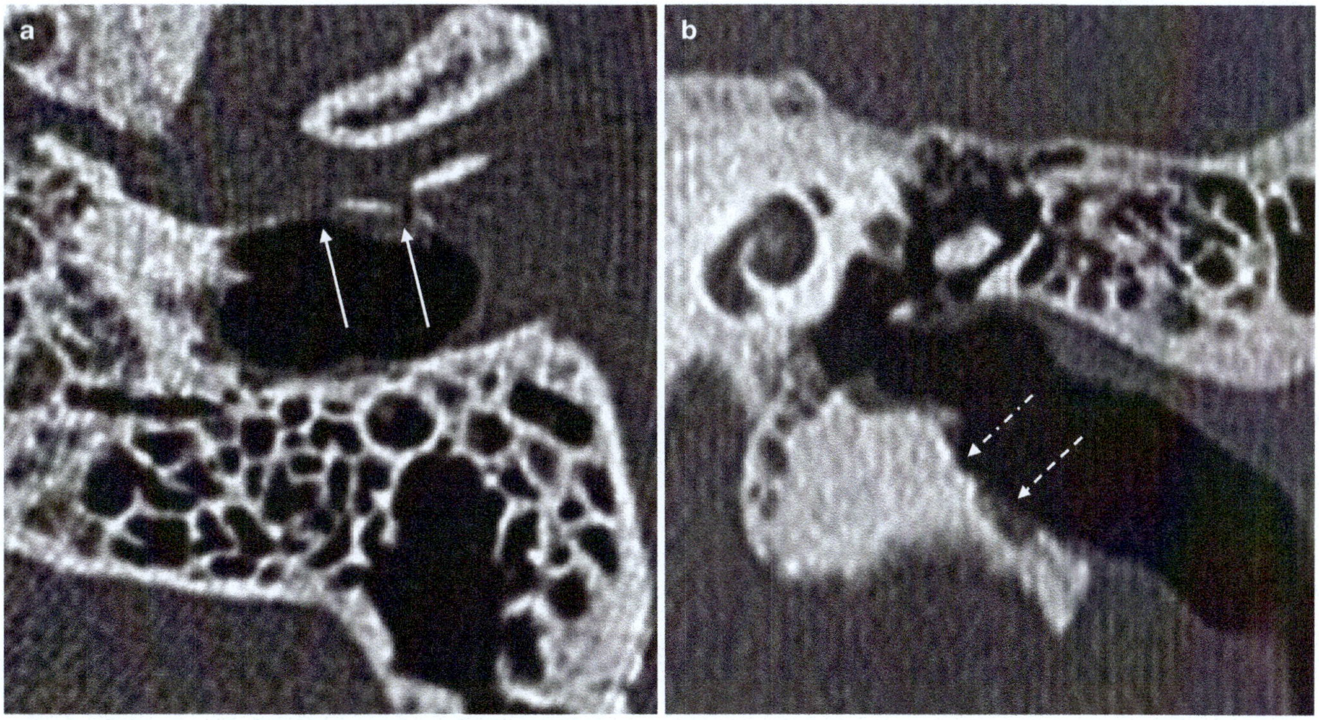

Fig. 2.32 Osteoradionecrosis of the temporal bone. (**a**) Axial CT and (**b**) Coronal CT images showing erosion (dashed arrows) and dehiscence (thin arrows) of the antero-inferior external auditory canal. Seeing exposed necrotic bone (dot dash arrow) is a hallmark feature of osteoradionecrosis of the external auditory canal

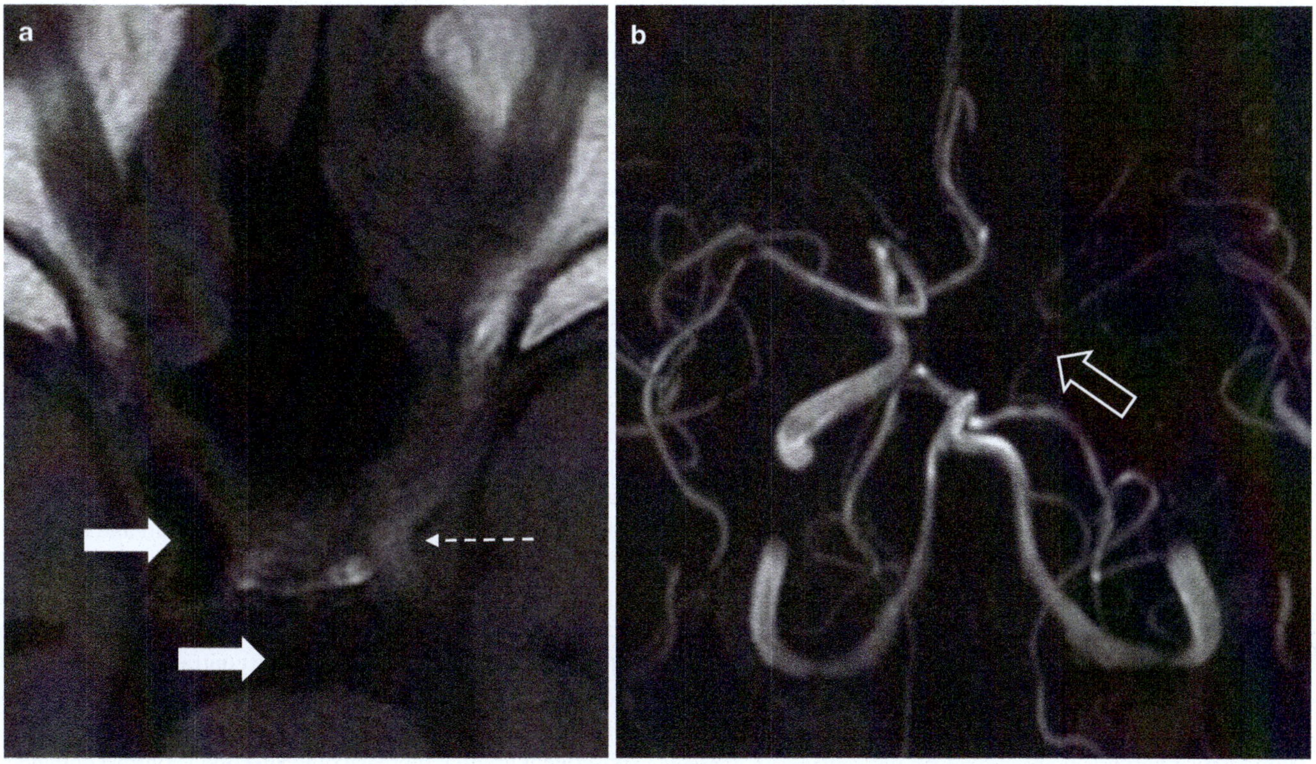

Fig. 2.33 Radiation-induced vascular disease. (**a**) Axial T1 and (**b**) 3D Time of Flight MR angiography images showing loss of flow void in the left ICA (dashed arrow) compared to the other cerebral vessels (solid arrows). This suspicion of radiation-induced vascular thrombosis was supported by the MRA showing no flow within the left intracranial ICA

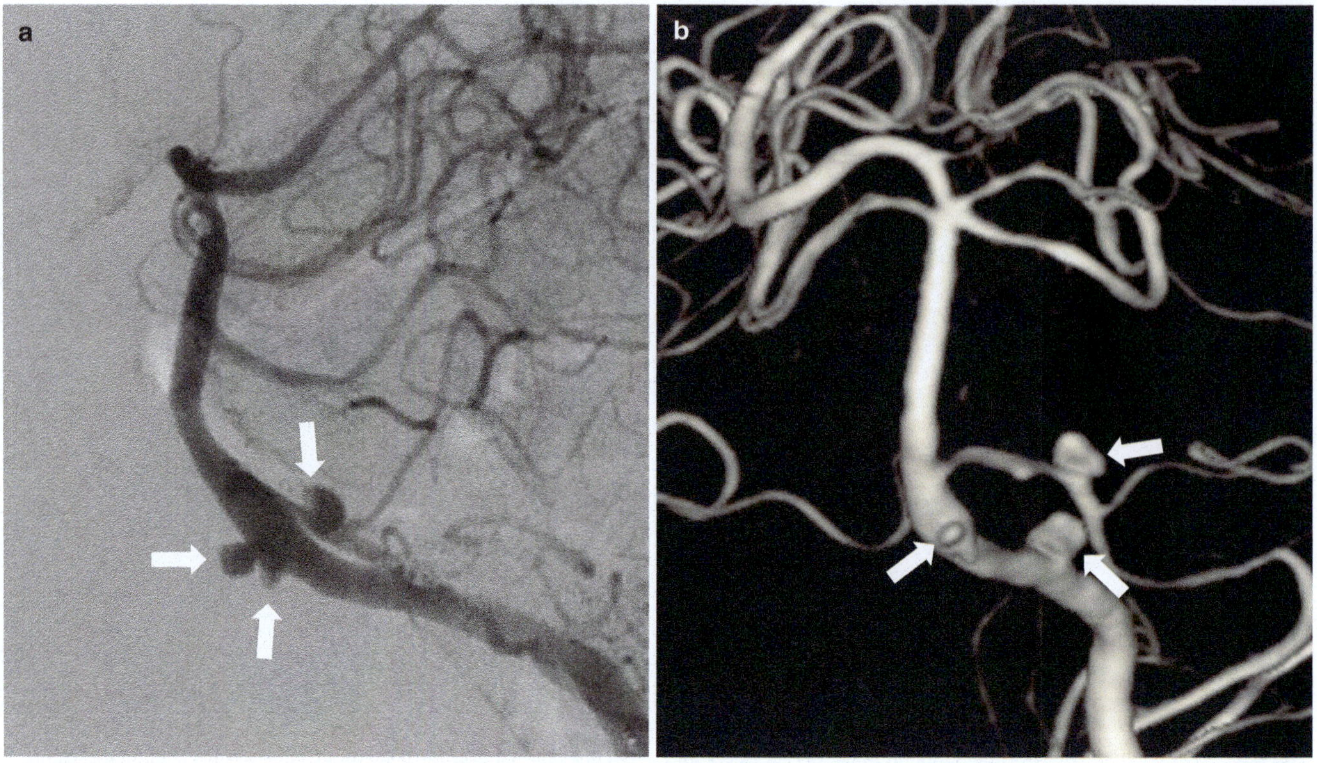

Fig. 2.34 Radiation-induced pseudoaneurysms. (**a**) Selective catheter angiogram of the left vertebral artery and its (**b**) 3D reconstruction shows three pseudoaneurysms (solid arrows) in the basilar artery, AICA, and PICA vessels. This patient was treated with conventional 2D radiotherapy with radiation portals designed based on bony landmarks, over 30 years ago. Although she has been cured of her disease, the location of the pseudoaneurysm is consistent with arterial structures within the high dose area (~60 to 70 Gy)

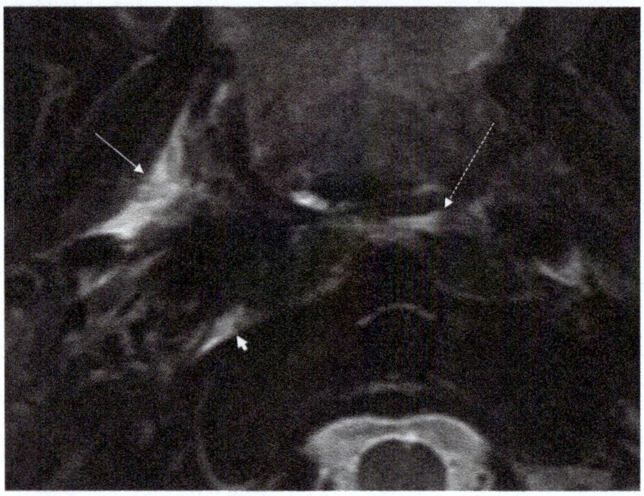

Fig. 2.35 Interstitial oedema post radiation. Axial T2 fat saturated image showing T2 hyperintense oedema within the right parapharyngeal space (thin arrow), retropharyngeal space (dashed arrow), and prevertebral space (arrowhead)

concave margins like a 'bow-tie' (Fig. 2.35). This is different from a retropharyngeal abscess which has enhancing convex margins [108].

While MRI is useful for assessing deep-seated infection, it is important to remember that 'normal' mucosa can also show hyperenhancement and hyperemia that persist for months to years after RT [82, 83]. In some cases, chronic mucositis with developing fibrosis can result in pharyngeal stenosis, while prominent granulation tissues may form polyps that mimic tumour recurrence.

2.11.5 Radiation-Induced Glandular (Exocrine and Endocrine) Injury

Historically, almost all patients undergoing RT experience glandular changes, with the incidence of xerostomia approaching 98% in some studies [81]. This however is much reduced with IMRT, which now spares the parotid glands (Fig. 2.19) [109]. The irradiated parotid and submandibular glands typically show early hyperenhancement and hyperemia (Fig. 2.36), with subsequent gradual atrophy and fatty infiltration. Recently, this glandular dysfunction can also be imaged [110, 111]; Dynamic contrast-enhanced MRI and DWI show loss of the normal biphasic response to glandular stimulation (i.e. Initial drop in ADC value with subsequent gradual increase) and sustained contrast enhancement with delayed washout possibly due to fibrosis.

With regard to the pituitary gland, damage to the hypothalamic-pituitary axis (HPA) is due to several mecha-

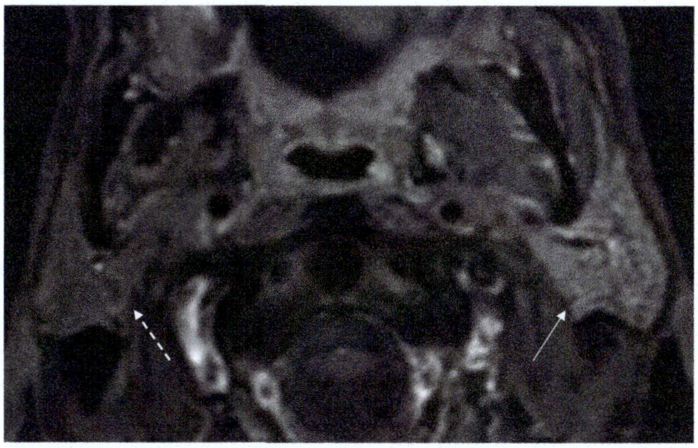

Fig. 2.36 Radiation-induced glandular injury. Axial T1 contrast enhanced image showing asymmetrical hyperenhancement of the left parotid gland (thin arrow) compared to the normal right side (dashed arrow)

nisms and most commonly involves the anterior pituitary lobe [112, 113]. This includes microstructure alteration with demyelination and axonal loss in the hypothalamus, as well as injury to the small vessels supplying the HPA. Progressive microangiopathy and ischaemia is the underlying cause for hormonal imbalance, with growth hormone deficiency being the most prevalent [114]. While these changes are clinically apparent, they are often radiologically occult.

2.11.6 Radiation-Induced Neoplasms

Radiation-induced neoplasms are rare, but are now seen in part due to increased overall survival. For a confident diagnosis to be made, the neoplasm must be within the radiation port, must occur with higher prevalence in irradiated patients, must have a different histology to the treated primary, and must only occur after a latency period of at least 3 years [115]. While meningiomas are the most common intracranial radiation-induced neoplasms, sarcomas and squamous cell carcinomas (SCC) are the two most aggressive [83].

Radiation-induced sarcomas tend to occur 10–15 years after RT and are often very aggressive. These include osteosarcomas, chondrosarcomas, malignant fibrous histiocytomas, and malignant nerve sheath tumours. SCC, however, tends to occur more than 10 year after RT and typically involves the external auditory canals and temporal bones. Both sarcomas and SCC confer poor prognosis and requires early detection and prompt surgical resection for definitive cure.

Other less common radiation-induced neoplasms include osteochondromas and thyroid malignancies, although very few studies have established causality of these thyroid cancers.

2.12 Future Imaging Techniques

68Ga-Dotapeptides are Octreotide analogues used for imaging somatostatin receptor (SSTR) expressing tumours (e.g. pheochromocytomas, paragangliomas, and small cell lung carcinomas). Undifferentiated NPC have now been reported to also express SSTR, highlighting the potential of a new imaging biomarker [116–119]. The absence of tracer uptake within the brain parenchyma on Dotapeptide PET/CT (usually intensely avid on FDG PET/CT) results in more accurate detection of intracranial disease. SSTR expression in NKUC also opens the possibility of new treatment alternatives such as peptide receptor radionuclide therapy (PRRT) that is used to treat neuroendocrine tumours.

18F-Fluoromisonidazole (FMISO) for imaging hypoxia is another example of PET tracers with emerging applications in NPC imaging. Hypoxia is an adverse prognostic factor usually associated with radio resistance, treatment failure, and decreased overall survival. FMISO PET/CT can identify areas of tumour hypoxia, enabling radiotherapy dose boosting to these regions potentially resulting in better local control [120].

Looking forward, in this era of rapid development in genomics, epigenomics, and proteomics, there is an evolving need to image tumour-specific biomarkers that can predict resistance to treatment, detect tumour heterogeneity, and guide targeted therapy. Radiomics as well as the development of biomarker-specific radionuclides are paving the way towards this future. These can affect treatment choice and outcome, and the specialist must continue to keep abreast with these changes, so as to be able to understand and interpret the imaging findings and support clinical advancement in the field.

References

1. Ferlay J, et al. Cancer incidence and mortality worldwide: sources, methods and major patterns in GLOBOCAN 2012. Int J Cancer. 2015;136(5):E359–86.
2. Armstrong RW, Kutty M, Dharmalingam SK. Incidence of nasopharyngeal carcinoma in Malaysia, with special reference to the State of Selangor. Br J Cancer. 1974;30(1):86–94.
3. Chang ET, Adami H-O. The enigmatic epidemiology of nasopharyngeal carcinoma. Cancer Epidemiol Biomarkers Prev. 2006;15(10):1765–77.
4. Zur Hauzen H. EBV DNA in biopsies of Burkitt tumours and anaplastic carcinomas of the nasopharynx. Nature. 1970;228:1956–8.
5. Old L, et al. Precipitating antibody in human serum to an antigen present in cultured Burkitt's lymphoma cells. Proc Natl Acad Sci. 1966;56(6):1699–704.
6. De Schryver A, et al. Epstein–Barr virus-associated antibody patterns in carcinoma of the post-nasal space. Clin Exp Immunol. 1969;5(5):443.
7. De Martel C, et al. Global burden of cancers attributable to infections in 2008: a review and synthetic analysis. Lancet Oncol. 2012;13(6):607–15.

8. Zeng Y, et al. Prospective studies on nasopharyngeal carcinoma in epstein-barr virus IgA/VCA antibody-positne persons in Wuzhou City, China. Int J Cancer. 1985;36(5):545–7.
9. Neel HB III, Pearson GR, Taylor WF. Antibodies to Epstein-Barr virus in patients with nasopharyngeal carcinoma and in comparison groups. Ann Otol Rhinol Laryngol. 1984;93(5):477–82.
10. Wolf H, Zur Hausen H, Becker V. EB viral genomes in epithelial nasopharyngeal carcinoma cells. Nat New Biol. 1973;244(138):245–7.
11. Raab-Traub N, Flynn K. The structure of the termini of the Epstein-Barr virus as a marker of clonal cellular proliferation. Cell. 1986;47(6):883–9.
12. Young LS, Dawson CW. Epstein-Barr virus and nasopharyngeal carcinoma. Chin J Cancer. 2014;33(12):581.
13. Shanmugaratnam K, Sobin LH. International histological classification of tumours. In: Shanmugaratnam K, Sobin LH, editors. Histological typing of tumours of the upper respiratory tract and ear. Geneva: World Health Organisation; 1991. p. 32–3.
14. Wei WI, Sham JS. Nasopharyngeal carcinoma. Lancet. 2005;365(9476):2041–54.
15. Tse LA, et al. Incidence rate trends of histological subtypes of nasopharyngeal carcinoma in Hong Kong. Br J Cancer. 2006;95(9):1269–73.
16. Peng G, et al. A prospective, randomized study comparing outcomes and toxicities of intensity-modulated radiotherapy vs. conventional two-dimensional radiotherapy for the treatment of nasopharyngeal carcinoma. Radiother Oncol. 2012;104(3):286–93.
17. Lee AW, et al. Evolution of treatment for nasopharyngeal cancer–success and setback in the intensity-modulated radiotherapy era. Radiother Oncol. 2014;110(3):377–84.
18. Blanchard P, et al. Chemotherapy and radiotherapy in nasopharyngeal carcinoma: an update of the MAC-NPC meta-analysis. Lancet Oncol. 2015;16(6):645–55.
19. Zong J, et al. Impact of intensity-modulated radiotherapy on nasopharyngeal carcinoma: validation of the 7th edition AJCC staging system. Oral Oncol. 2015;51(3):254–9.
20. Lee N, et al. Intensity-modulated radiotherapy in the treatment of nasopharyngeal carcinoma: an update of the UCSF experience. Int J Radiat Oncol Biol Phys. 2002;53(1):12–22.
21. Mao Y-P, et al. Re-evaluation of 6th edition of AJCC staging system for nasopharyngeal carcinoma and proposed improvement based on magnetic resonance imaging. Int J Radiat Oncol Biol Phys. 2009;73(5):1326–34.
22. Kamel RH, Ishak EA. Enlarged adenoid and adenoidectomy in adults: endoscopic approach and histopathological study. J Laryngol Otol. 1990;104(12):965–7.
23. King A, et al. Magnetic resonance imaging for the detection of nasopharyngeal carcinoma. Am J Neuroradiol. 2006;27(6):1288–91.
24. Bhatia KS, et al. Nasopharyngeal mucosa and adenoids: appearance at MR imaging. Radiology. 2012;263(2):437–43.
25. Wang M-L, et al. Value of contrast-enhanced MRI in the differentiation between nasopharyngeal lymphoid hyperplasia and T1 stage nasopharyngeal carcinoma. Radiol Med. 2017;122(10):743–51.
26. Chong VF, Khoo JB, Fan YF. Imaging of the nasopharynx and skull base. Neuroimaging Clin N Am. 2004;14(4):695–719.
27. Poh SS, Chua MLK, Wee JT. Carcinogenesis of nasopharyngeal carcinoma: an alternate hypothetical mechanism. Chin J Cancer. 2016;35(1):9.
28. Maheshwar AA, et al. Roof of the parapharyngeal space: defining its boundaries and clinical implications. Ann Otol Rhinol Laryngol. 2004;113(4):283–8.
29. Curtin HD. Separation of the masticator space from the parapharyngeal space. Radiology. 1987;163(1):195–204.
30. Debnam JM, Guha-Thakurta N. Retropharyngeal and prevertebral spaces: anatomic imaging and diagnosis. Otolaryngol Clin North Am. 2012;45(6):1293–310.
31. Teo P, Lee W, Yu P. The prognostic significance of parapharyngeal tumour involvement in nasopharyngeal carcinoma. Radiother Oncol. 1996;39(3):209–21.
32. Ho H-C, et al. Prognostic influence of parapharyngeal extension in nasopharyngeal carcinoma. Acta Otolaryngol. 2008;128(7):790–8.
33. Lee CC, et al. The prognostic influence of prevertebral space involvement in nasopharyngeal carcinoma. Clin Otolaryngol. 2008;33(5):442–9.
34. Zhou G-q, et al. Prognostic value of prevertebral space involvement in nasopharyngeal carcinoma based on intensity-modulated radiotherapy. Int J Radiat Oncol Biol Phys. 2012;82(3):1090–7.
35. Pan JJ, et al. Prognostic nomogram for refining the prognostication of the proposed 8th edition of the AJCC/UICC staging system for nasopharyngeal cancer in the era of intensity-modulated radiotherapy. Cancer. 2016;122(21):3307–15.
36. King A, et al. MRI of local disease in nasopharyngeal carcinoma: tumour extent vs tumour stage. Br J Radiol. 1999;72(860):734–41.
37. Tang L-L, et al. Prognostic value and staging categories of anatomic masticator space involvement in nasopharyngeal carcinoma: a study of 924 cases with MR imaging. Radiology. 2010;257(1):151–7.
38. Shatzkes DR, et al. Sclerosis of the pterygoid process in untreated patients with nasopharyngeal carcinoma. Radiology. 2006;239(1):181–6.
39. Tashi S, et al. The pterygopalatine fossa: imaging anatomy, communications, and pathology revisited. Insights Imaging. 2016;7(4):589–99.
40. Chong VF, Fan YF. Pterygopalatine fossa and maxillary nerve infiltration in nasopharyngeal carcinoma. Head Neck. 1997;19(2):121–5.
41. Chung NN, et al. Impact of magnetic resonance imaging versus CT on nasopharyngeal carcinoma: primary tumour target delineation for radiotherapy. Head Neck. 2004;26(3):241–6.
42. Tian L, et al. Nasopharyngeal carcinoma with paranasal sinus invasion: the prognostic significance and the evidence-based study basis of its T-staging category according to the AJCC staging system. BMC Cancer. 2014;14(1):832.
43. Zhang Y, et al. Should all nasopharyngeal carcinoma with paranasal sinus invasion be staged as T3 in the intensity-modulated radiotherapy era? a study of 1811 cases. J Cancer. 2016;7(10):1353.
44. King AD, Bhatia KSS. Magnetic resonance imaging staging of nasopharyngeal carcinoma in the head and neck. World J Radiol. 2010;2(5):159.
45. Huang C-C, et al. Therapeutic outcome of nasopharyngeal carcinoma with cranial nerve palsy: a single institution experience of 104 patients. OncoTargets Ther. 2017;10:2069.
46. Zong J, et al. Does MRI-detected cranial nerve involvement affect the prognosis of locally advanced nasopharyngeal carcinoma treated with intensity modulated radiotherapy? PLoS One. 2014;9(6):e100571.
47. Liu L, et al. Prognostic impact of magnetic resonance imaging-detected cranial nerve involvement in nasopharyngeal carcinoma. Cancer. 2009;115(9):1995–2003.
48. Ng WT, et al. N-staging by magnetic resonance imaging for patients with nasopharyngeal carcinoma: pattern of nodal involvement by radiological levels. Radiother Oncol. 2007;82(1):70–5.
49. Ng S-H, et al. Nodal metastases of nasopharyngeal carcinoma: patterns of disease on MRI and FDG PET. Eur J Nucl Med Mol Imaging. 2004;31(8):1073–80.
50. Lu L, et al. Sentinel node necrosis is a negative prognostic factor in patients with nasopharyngeal carcinoma: a magnetic resonance imaging study of 252 patients. Curr Oncol. 2017;24(3):e220.
51. Mukherji SK, Armao D, Joshi VM. Cervical nodal metastases in squamous cell carcinoma of the head and neck: what to expect. Head Neck. 2001;23(11):995–1005.

52. Kato H, et al. Metastatic retropharyngeal lymph nodes: comparison of CT and MR imaging for diagnostic accuracy. Eur J Radiol. 2014;83(7):1157–62.
53. Zhang G-Y, et al. Radiologic criteria of retropharyngeal lymph node metastasis in nasopharyngeal carcinoma treated with radiation therapy. Radiology. 2010;255(2):605–12.
54. Vellayappan BA, et al. Accuracy of 18F-flurodeoxyglucosepositron emission tomography/computed tomography in the staging of newly diagnosed nasopharyngeal carcinoma: a systematic review and meta-analysis. Radiol Oncol. 2014;48(4):331–8.
55. Sham JS, et al. Nasopharyngeal carcinoma: pattern of skeletal metastases. Br J Radiol. 1990;63(747):202–5.
56. Tan KC, et al. Unusual endocrine presentations of nasopharyngeal carcinoma. Cancer. 1996;77(10):1967–72.
57. Liu F-Y, et al. 18F-FDG PET can replace conventional work-up in primary M staging of nonkeratinising nasopharyngeal carcinoma. J Nucl Med. 2007;48(10):1614–9.
58. Li A-C, et al. Distant metastasis risk and patterns of nasopharyngeal carcinoma in the era of IMRT: long-term results and benefits of chemotherapy. Oncotarget. 2015;6(27):24511.
59. Xu C, et al. Optimal modality for detecting distant metastasis in primary nasopharyngeal carcinoma during initial staging: a systemic review and meta-analysis of 1774 patients. J Cancer. 2017;8(7):1238.
60. Aktan M, et al. Prognostic value of pre-treatment 18 F-FDG PET uptake for nasopharyngeal carcinoma. Radiol Med. 2017:1–9.
61. Liu F, et al. PET/CT-guided dose-painting versus CT-based intensity modulated radiation therapy in locoregional advanced nasopharyngeal carcinoma. Radiat Oncol. 2017;12(1):15.
62. Vikram B, et al. Patterns of failure in carcinoma of the nasopharynx: I. Failure at the primary site. Int J Radiat Oncol Biol Phys. 1985;11(8):1455–9.
63. Leung TW, et al. Treatment results of 1070 patients with nasopharyngeal carcinoma: an analysis of survival and failure patterns. Head Neck. 2005;27(7):555–65.
64. Taylor A, Powell M. Intensity-modulated radiotherapy—what is it? Cancer Imaging. 2004;4(2):68.
65. Na'ara S, et al. Outcome of patients undergoing salvage surgery for recurrent nasopharyngeal carcinoma: a meta-analysis. Ann Surg Oncol. 2014;21(9):3056–62.
66. Teo PML, et al. How successful is high-dose (≥ 60 Gy) reirradiation using mainly external beams in salvaging local failures of nasopharyngeal carcinoma? Int J Radiat Oncol Biol Phys. 1998;40(4):897–913.
67. Chua DT, et al. Reirradiation of nasopharyngeal carcinoma with intensity-modulated radiotherapy. Radiother Oncol. 2005;77(3):290–4.
68. Chan JYW, et al. Extracranial/intracranial vascular bypass and craniofacial resection: New hope for patients with locally advanced recurrent nasopharyngeal carcinoma. Head Neck. 2016;38(S1):E1404–12.
69. Hao S-P, et al. Nasopharyngectomy for recurrent nasopharyngeal carcinoma: a review of 53 patients and prognostic factors. Acta Otolaryngol. 2008;128(4):473–81.
70. Chen MY, et al. Endoscopic nasopharyngectomy for locally recurrent nasopharyngeal carcinoma. Laryngoscope. 2009;119(3):516–22.
71. Chan JYW, et al. Prediction of surgical outcome using plasma epstein–barr virus dna and 18F-FDG PET-CT scan in recurrent nasopharyngeal carcinoma. Head Neck. 2012;34(4):541–5.
72. Lee AW, et al. Retrospective analysis of 5037 patients with nasopharyngeal carcinoma treated during 1976–1985: overall survival and patterns of failure. Int J Radiat Oncol Biol Phys. 1992;23(2):261–70.
73. Chan JYW, et al. Surgical salvage for recurrent retropharyngeal lymph node metastasis in nasopharyngeal carcinoma. Head Neck. 2013;35(12):1726–31.
74. Wei WI, Mok VW. The management of neck metastases in nasopharyngeal cancer. Curr Opin Otolaryngol Head Neck Surg. 2007;15(2):99–102.
75. Liu T, et al. FDG-PET, CT, MRI for diagnosis of local residual or recurrent nasopharyngeal carcinoma, which one is the best? A systematic review. Radiother Oncol. 2007;85(3):327–35.
76. Wang WY, et al. Plasma Epstein-Barr virus DNA screening followed by 18F-fluoro-2-deoxy-D-glucose positron emission tomography in detecting post-treatment failures of nasopharyngeal carcinoma. Cancer. 2011;117(19):4452–9.
77. Razek AAKA, King A. MRI and CT of nasopharyngeal carcinoma. Am J Roentgenol. 2012;198(1):11–8.
78. Xu J-F, et al. Value of diffusion-weighted magnetic resonance imaging on the follow-up of nasopharyngeal carcinoma after radiotherapy. J Xray Sci Technol. 2014;22(5):605–12.
79. Yamauchi H, Srinivasan A. Diffusion imaging of the head and neck. Curr Radiol Rep. 2014;2(5):49.
80. Yokota H, et al. MR imaging of the superior cervical ganglion and inferior ganglion of the vagus nerve: structures that can mimic pathologic retropharyngeal lymph nodes. Am J Neuroradiol. 2018;39(1):170–6.
81. Siala W, et al. Late toxicities after conventional radiotherapy for nasopharyngeal carcinoma: incidence and risk factors. J Radiother. 2014;2014:268340.
82. King A, et al. Delayed complications of radiotherapy treatment for nasopharyngeal carcinoma: imaging findings. Clin Radiol. 2007;62(3):195–203.
83. Small W, Woloschak GE. Radiation toxicity: a practical medical guide, vol. 128. Berlin: Springer Science & Business Media; 2006.
84. Tofilon PJ, Fike JR. The radioresponse of the central nervous system: a dynamic process. Radiat Res. 2000;153(4):357–70.
85. Shaw EG, Robbins ME. The management of radiation-induced brain injury. In: Radiation toxicity: a practical guide. Berlin: Springer; 2008. p. 7–22.
86. Stephens L. Invited review: permanent radiation myelopathy. Br J Radiol. 1992;65:737–53.
87. Heckl S, Aschoff A, Kunze S. Radiation-induced cavernous hemangiomas of the brain: a late effect predominantly in children. Cancer. 2002;94(12):3285–91.
88. Fang W, et al. Late-onset cystic brain necrosis after radiotherapy for nasopharyngeal carcinoma. Jpn J Clin Oncol. 2017;47(6):499–504.
89. Nael K, et al. Multiparametric MRI for differentiation of radiation necrosis from recurrent tumour in patients with treated glioblastoma. Am J Roentgenol. 2018;210(1):18–23.
90. Langleben DD, Segall GM. PET in differentiation of recurrent brain tumour from radiation injury. J Nucl Med. 2000;41(11):1861–7.
91. Chong V. Imaging the cranial nerves in cancer. Cancer Imaging. 2004;4 Spec No A:S1–5.
92. Kong L, et al. Radiation-induced cranial nerve palsy: a cross-sectional study of nasopharyngeal cancer patients after definitive radiotherapy. Int J Radiat Oncol Biol Phys. 2011;79(5):1421–7.
93. Stoll BA, Andrews JT. Radiation-induced peripheral neuropathy. Br Med J. 1966;1(5491):834.
94. Archer EL, Liao EA, Trobe JD. Radiation-induced optic neuropathy: clinical and imaging profile of twelve patients. J Neuroophthalmol. 2019;39(2):170–80.
95. Ollivier L, et al. Improving the interpretation of bone marrow imaging in cancer patients. Cancer Imaging. 2006;6(1):194.
96. Tang CL, et al. Late temporal lobe extensive osteoradionecrosis post radiation for nasopharyngeal carcinoma: case series. Indian J Otolaryngol Head Neck Surg. 2017;69(3):409–14.
97. Hanley ME, Cooper JS. Osteoradionecrosis. In: StatPearls [Internet]. Treasure Island, FL: StatPearls Publishing; 2017.
98. Rivero JA, Shamji O, Kolokythas A. Osteoradionecrosis: a review of pathophysiology, prevention and pharmacologic management

using pentoxifylline, α-tocopherol, and clodronate. Oral Surg Oral Med Oral Pathol Oral Radiol. 2017;124(5):464–71.

99. Reuther T, et al. Osteoradionecrosis of the jaws as a side effect of radiotherapy of head and neck tumour patients—a report of a thirty year retrospective review. Int J Oral Maxillofac Surg. 2003;32(3):289–95.
100. Debnam JM. Imaging of the head and neck following radiation treatment. Patholog Res Int. 2011;2011:607820.
101. Wu VW, Ying MT, Kwong DL. A study on the post-radiotherapy changes of temporomandibular joint in nasopharyngeal carcinoma patients. Br J Radiol. 2017;90(1080):20170375.
102. Hao S, et al. Osteoradionecrosis of external auditory canal in nasopharyngeal carcinoma. Chang Gung Med J. 2007;30(2):116.
103. Cutsforth-Gregory JK, et al. Characterization of radiation-induced cavernous malformations and comparison with a nonradiation cavernous malformation cohort. J Neurosurg. 2015;122(5):1214–22.
104. Xu J, Cao Y. Radiation-induced carotid artery stenosis: a comprehensive review of the literature. Interv Neurol. 2013;2(4):183–92.
105. Okamura H-o, et al. Histopathological examination of ruptured carotid artery after irradiation. J Otorhinolaryngol Relat Spec. 2002;64(3):226–8.
106. Ye J, et al. A study of radiation-induced cerebral vascular injury in nasopharyngeal carcinoma patients with radiation-induced temporal lobe necrosis. PLoS One. 2012;7(8):e42890.
107. Kong F, et al. Long-term survival and late complications of intensity-modulated radiotherapy for recurrent nasopharyngeal carcinoma. BMC Cancer. 2018;18(1):1139.
108. Hoang JK, et al. Multiplanar CT and MRI of collections in the retropharyngeal space: is it an abscess? Am J Roentgenol. 2011;196(4):W426–32.
109. Nutting CM, et al. Parotid-sparing intensity modulated versus conventional radiotherapy in head and neck cancer (PARSPORT): a phase 3 multicentre randomised controlled trial. Lancet Oncol. 2011;12(2):127–36.
110. Zhang Y, et al. Evaluation of salivary gland function using diffusion-weighted magnetic resonance imaging for follow-up of radiation-induced xerostomia. Korean J Radiol. 2018;19(4):758–66.
111. Dirix P, et al. Diffusion-weighted magnetic resonance imaging to evaluate major salivary gland function before and after radiotherapy. Int J Radiat Oncol Biol Phys. 2008;71(5):1365–71.
112. Pekic S, Miljic D, Popovic V. Hypopituitarism following cranial radiotherapy. In: Endotext [Internet]. South Dartmouth, MA: MDText.com; 2018.
113. Ratnasingam J, et al. Hypothalamic pituitary dysfunction amongst nasopharyngeal cancer survivors. Pituitary. 2015;18(4):448–55.
114. Appelman-Dijkstra NM, et al. Pituitary dysfunction in adult patients after cranial radiotherapy: systematic review and meta-analysis. J Clin Endocrinol Metabol. 2011;96(8):2330–40.
115. Cahan W. Sarcoma arising in irradiated bone. Report of eleven cases. Cancer. 1948;1:3–29.
116. Loh K, et al. Somatostatin receptors in nasopharyngeal carcinoma. Virchows Arch. 2002;441(5):444–8.
117. Schartinger VH, et al. 68 Ga-DOTA 0-Tyr 3-octreotide positron emission tomography in nasopharyngeal carcinoma. Eur J Nucl Med Mol Imaging. 2015;42(1):20–4.
118. Khor LK, et al. Correlation between^ sup 68^ Ga-DOTA-NOC PET/CT and^ sup 18^ F-FDG PET/CT in EBV-positive undifferentiated nasopharyngeal carcinoma. Eur J Nucl Med Mol Imaging. 2015;42(7):1162.
119. Khor LK, et al. 68Ga-DOTA-peptide: A novel molecular biomarker for nasopharyngeal carcinoma. Head Neck. 2016;38(4):E76–80.
120. Qiu J, et al. 18F-Fluoromisonidazole positron emission tomography/CT-guided volumetric-modulated arc therapy-based dose escalation for hypoxic subvolume in nasopharyngeal carcinomas: a feasibility study. Head Neck. 2017;39(12):2519–27.

Diagnostic Imaging of Oropharyngeal Cancer

3

Akifumi Fujita

Abstract

Despite a steady decline in the incidence of head and neck cancers in the last few decades, the incidence of oropharyngeal cancer has shown an overall increase that is largely attributable to the rise in infections with the human papilloma virus (HPV). Oropharyngeal cancer has become the leading site for HPV-associated cancers in humans. Typically, HPV-associated oropharyngeal cancer presents in a younger, healthier population with a different set of risk factors and a good prognosis for survival. It is important for physicians and radiologists to become familiar with the features of epidemic HPV-associated oropharyngeal cancer, as well as the characteristic imaging finding differences between HPV-associated and non-HPV-associated oropharyngeal cancers, which are critical for patient management.

Keywords

Oropharynx · HPV-associated · Non-HPV-associated

3.1 Introduction

The most common histologic type of oropharyngeal carcinoma is squamous cell carcinoma (SCCa), which represents more than 95% of oropharyngeal malignancies [1, 2]. Traditionally, oropharyngeal carcinoma was closely related to tobacco and alcohol exposure. The incidence of carcinoma in the oropharynx was similar to that of the other sites of the upper aerodigestive tract those that all shared common exposure to the carcinogens in tobacco. Whereas the overall incidence of head and neck SCCa has been decreasing, mostly attributable to the decline in smoking, oropharyngeal SCCa incidence has been relatively stable, which is explained by the increasing incidence of human papillomavirus (HPV)-associated oropharyngeal SCCa [3–5]. In this chapter, we mainly describe the anatomy, demographics and epidemiology, histopathology, imaging findings, and management of HPV-associated and non-HPV-associated oropharyngeal cancers.

3.2 Oropharyngeal Squamous Cell Carcinoma

3.2.1 Demographics and Epidemiologic Features (Table 3.1)

There are well-established risk factors for head and neck cancers such as smoking and alcohol abuse, both separately and synergistically. Poor oral hygiene and radiation exposure

Table 3.1 Clinical characteristics of human papillomavirus-associated (HPV-positive) and non-human papillomavirus-associated (HPV-negative) oropharyngeal cancer

	HPV positive	HPV negative
Tumor location	Mostly Palatine tonsils (lateral wall) and Lingual tonsil (anterior wall)	Frequently Palatine tonsils (lateral wall) and Lingual tonsil (anterior wall)
Age	Young to middle	Middle to elder
Gender	Male	Male
Risk factor	Sexual habits	Smoking Alcohol
Histopathology	Poorly differentiated	Well-differentiated Keratinized
Immunochemistry	p16 positive	p53 positive
Primary lesion	Small Well-circumscribed	Various Ill-defined
Lymph node metastasis	Frequent multiple Cystic Extranodal spread	Various
Double cancer	Rare	Frequent
Incidence	Increasing	Decreasing
Prognosis	Good	Poor

A. Fujita (✉)
Department of Radiology, Jichi Medical University School of Medicine, Shimotsuke, Tochigi, Japan
e-mail: akifuji@jichi.ac.jp

H. Ojiri (ed.), *Diagnostic Imaging in Head and Neck Cancer*, https://doi.org/10.1007/978-981-15-3188-0_3

are also known risk factors. The landscape of head and neck cancer has experienced dramatic changes over the past decades in many Western countries [2, 3, 6]. Although head and neck cancer has been decreasing, mostly attributable to the decline in smoking, the incidence of oropharyngeal SCCa has been increasing in many countries, likely attributable to the influence of HPV-associated oropharyngeal SCCa [7–9]. The incidence of HPV-associated oropharyngeal SCCa in the United States has increased by a startling 225% from 1988 to 2004 [5]. During the past two decades, oropharyngeal SCCa also increased among men and/or women in different European nations [2]. HPV-16 and, less often, HPV-18 are the most frequent oncologic viral agents [10].

HPV-associated oropharyngeal SCCa patients tend to be younger, nonsmoking, nondrinking, white males of higher than average socioeconomic backgrounds, often with a history of multiple sexual partners. Because HPV-associated SCCa commonly arises in nonsmokers, a lack of significant tobacco or alcohol exposure does not provide evidence against malignancy. Initial symptoms of oropharyngeal SCCa are a neck mass and sore throat. The non-HPV-associated cohort had a significantly higher proportion of patients without nodal spread compared to the HPV-positive cohort [11]. Importantly, in contrast to non-HPV-associated disease, HPV-associated SCCa with lymph node spread has excellent survival rates, ranging from approximately 80% to 90% for early-stage disease. Patients with HPV-associated SCCa have improved outcomes [12], and this prognostic difference has prompted changes in the latest 8th edition AJCC guideline [13], as well as attempts to reduce the long-term toxicity resulting from standard therapy with reduction of radiation doses, elimination of chemotherapy, or minimally invasive robotic surgery. Currently, these de-escalated treatment options are being evaluated in multiple clinical trials [14]. Although HPV-associated SCCa has a reliably better prognosis than non-HPV-associated SCCa, deleterious somatic alterations resulting from tobacco exposure worsen the prognosis of HPV-positive smokers relative to HPV-positive nonsmokers [15].

3.2.2 Anatomical Considerations

The oropharynx is posterior to the oral cavity, between the nasopharynx and hypopharynx, the latter being separated from the oropharynx by the superior aspect of the hyoid bone. The anterior limit is defined by a plane formed by the circumvallate papillae, the anterior tonsillar pillars, and the soft palate. The posterior pharyngeal wall is its posterior limit. Laterally it is bounded by the palatine tonsils and the anterior and posterior tonsillar pillars. The oropharynx is composed of the anterior wall (base of the tongue/lingual tonsils), lateral walls (palatine tonsils), posterior wall, and superior wall (soft palate). The soft palate extends from the posterior aspect of the hard palate to the uvula. The base of the tongue consists of the tonsillar tissue in the posterior third of the tongue. The palatine tonsils are lymphoid tissues nestled between the anterior and posterior tonsillar pillars, which are mucosal folds created by the palatoglossus and palatopharyngeal muscles, respectively. The posterior wall is between the soft palate superiorly and the hyoid bone inferiorly [13]. Within these subsites of the oropharynx, the tonsil and tongue base are the most common sites to be affected by carcinoma. These sites differ from the other subsites because they have a high density of lymphoid cells and show a strong association with HPV-associated squamous carcinoma [16]. The strong predilection of HPV for the oropharynx is due to the microanatomy of the reticulated epithelium of the base of the tongue and tonsils. HPV infects the reticulated epithelium lining of the deep tonsillar crypts. The deep crypts of the tonsils are immune-privileged sites, which means they can tolerate the introduction of antigens without eliciting an inflammatory immune response. This results in inhibition of the effector function of the HPV-specific T cells and thereby facilitates immune evasion at the time of initial HPV infection [17].

3.2.3 Staging of Oropharyngeal Cancer

Since HPV-related oropharyngeal SCCa is now well established as a distinct entity compared to non-HPV-related oropharyngeal SCCa, the American Joint Committee on Cancer (AJCC) 8th edition staging system has changed significantly, intending to reflect the improved prognosis associated with HPV-related oropharyngeal SCCa [13]. In addition, the new system provides clinicians with prognostication based on more refined clinical and pathologic features unique to HPV-related oropharyngeal SCCa.

The HPV-related oropharyngeal SCCa clinical T classification no longer includes a T4b category, because 5-year overall survival was similar for patients classed as T4a and T4b according to the 7th edition of TNM staging system. One of the most significant changes was the inclusion of extranodal extension for non-HPV-related oropharyngeal SCCa. In addition, the new system clearly states the pathologic definition of extranodal extension [13].

3.2.4 Imaging Features

The most important roles of imaging in head and neck malignancies including oropharyngeal carcinoma are to clarify the extension of the primary lesion and to investigate for metastases. Oropharyngeal SCCa may spread in several ways, such as by direct extension over mucosal surfaces and by dissemination via lymphatic drainage pathways [18]. Since superficial mucosal lesions are not often radiographically evident, the extent of mucosal spread is best estimated with a physical examination. However, the overall extent of a tumor is often underestimated at physical examination because of the inability to detect submucosal spread and direct invasion of adjacent structures (Figs. 3.1 and 3.2). Evaluation of SCCa of the base of tongue should also include a determination of the involvement of the intrinsic muscle of the tongue (Fig. 3.3), crossing of the midline of the tongue, and invasion of the pre-epiglottic fat. Evaluation of a tonsillar SCCa should include a determination of the involvement of the pterygoid muscles and extension along the pterygomandibular raphe to the skull base [18].

Presuming the histopathological diagnosis by imaging is not usually required, but there are several reports describing the imaging features for differentiating between HPV-associated and non-HPV-associated oropharyngeal SCCa [19–24]. Chan et al. reported the radiologic features of primary tumors comparing 397 cases of HPV-associated and 148 cases of non-HPV-associated oropharyngeal SCCa [24].

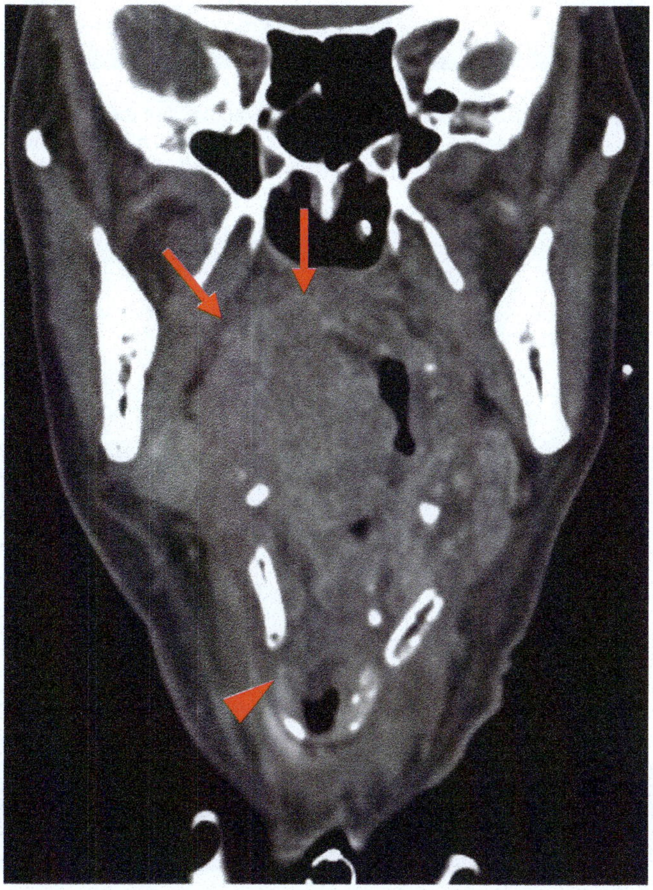

Fig. 3.1 Non-HPV-associated oropharyngeal SCCa of the right tonsil. Contrast-enhanced CT coronal image shows an ill-defined margin of the invasive mass at the right lateral wall of the oropharynx extending to the soft palate (arrows) and larynx (arrowhead)

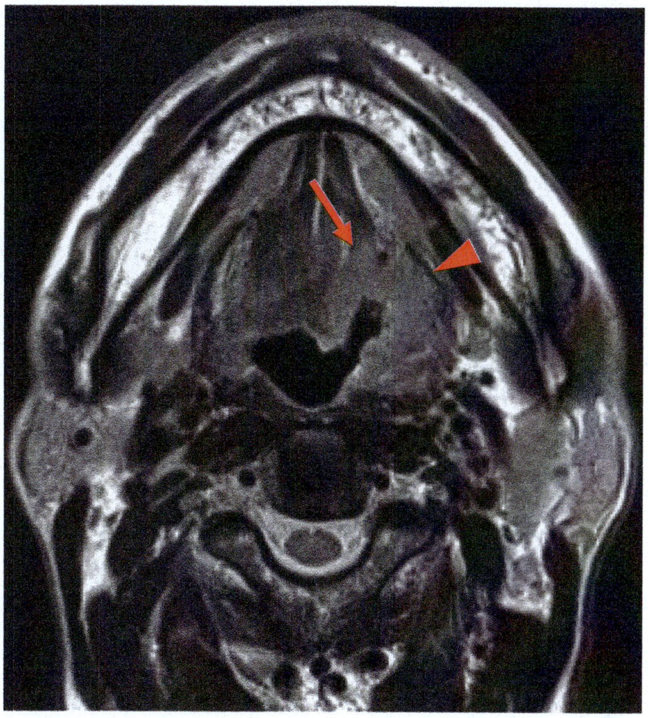

Fig. 3.2 Non-HPV-associated oropharyngeal SCCa of the left base of the tongue. T2W image shows an ill-defined mass with ulceration at the left anterior wall of the oropharynx invading genioglossus muscle (arrow) and hyoglossus muscle (arrowhead)

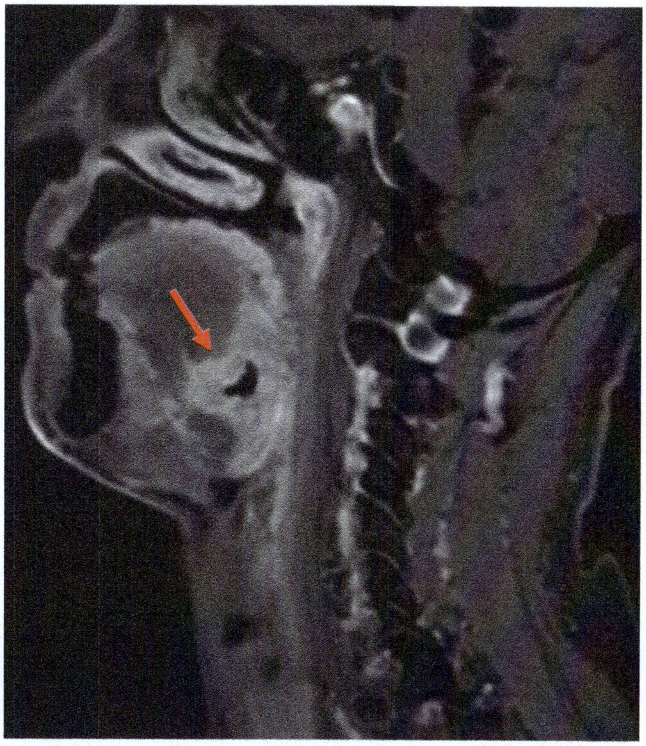

Fig. 3.3 Non-HPV-associated oropharyngeal SCCa of the left base of the tongue. Contrast-enhanced, fat-saturated T1W sagittal image shows an ill-defined mass with ulceration (arrow) at the left anterior wall of the oropharynx invading the intrinsic muscle of the tongue

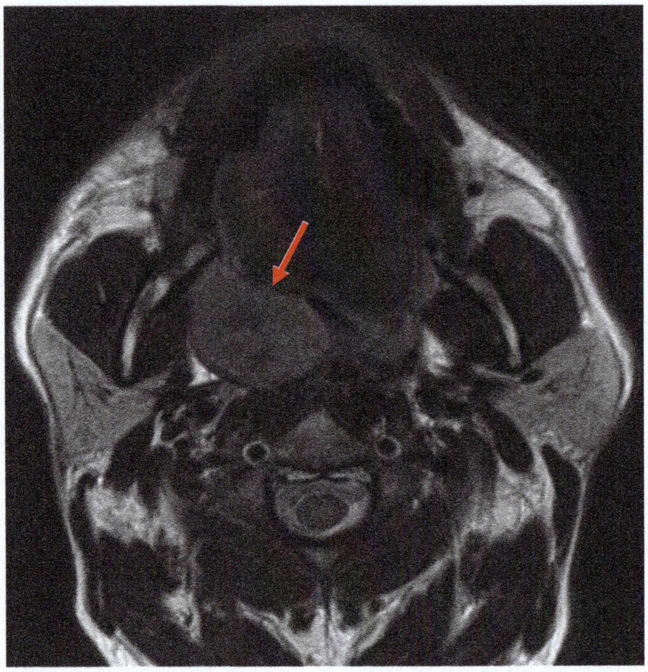

Fig. 3.4 HPV-associated oropharyngeal SCCa of the right lateral palatine tonsil. T2W MR image shows a well-defined exophytic appearance of the mass at the right lateral wall of the oropharynx (arrow)

HPV-associated oropharyngeal primary tumors had significantly smaller size at presentation in the axial dimensions, including the anterior–posterior dimension, although no difference was demonstrated in the superior–inferior dimension. In addition, HPV-associated primary tumors were more likely to have an exophytic appearance (Fig. 3.4). Although ulceration and necrosis were uncommon in both groups, a significantly lower proportion of HPV-associated SCCa cases demonstrated these features (Figs. 3.2 and 3.5). Notably, of HPV-associated never-smokers, only 5% had ulcerations, whereas 13% of HPV-associated smokers had ulcerations. Cantrell et al. reported the CT imaging differences between HPV-associated and non-HPV-associated oropharyngeal SCCa cases, and a greater percentage of HPV-associated SCCa demonstrated primary tumors with well-defined borders (Figs. 3.4 and 3.6), whereas non-HPV-associated tumors demonstrated ill-defined borders and increased invasion of adjacent muscle (Figs. 3.1, 3.3, and 3.7) [21].

Despite the overall improved prognosis of HPV-associated SCCa relative to non-HPV-associated SCCa, there is no significant difference in the incidence of extracapsular spread or matted appearance of nodal metastases [21, 23, 24], a well-established predictor of poor prognosis in SCCa of the head and neck (Fig. 3.7). HPV-associated oropharyngeal SCCa demonstrates an increased incidence of cystic and clustered nodal metastases (Fig. 3.8) [21, 24]. A common imaging finding in HPV-associated SCCa, cystic metastases caused by a small or poorly visualized primary, highlights a common

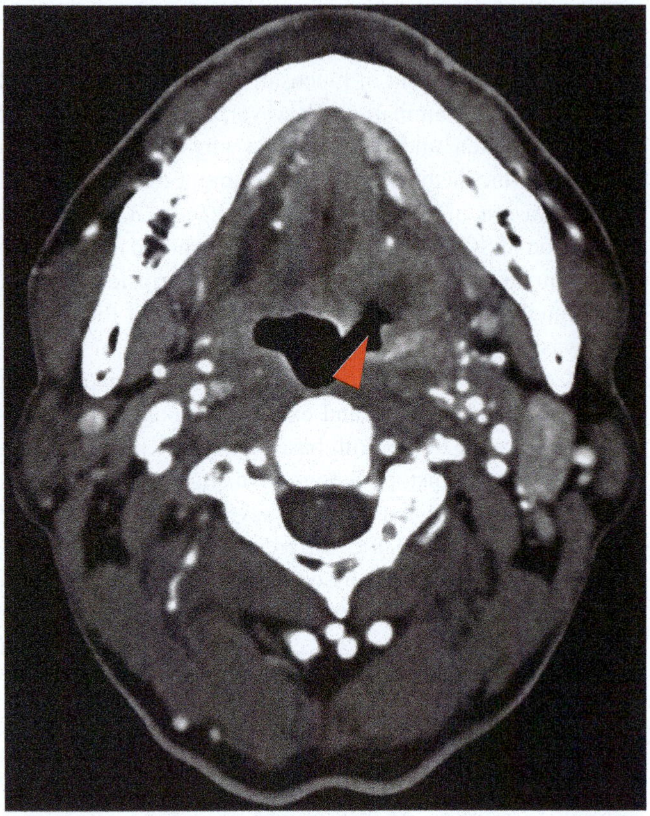

Fig. 3.5 Non-HPV-associated oropharyngeal SCCa of the left base of the tongue. Contrast-enhanced CT image shows an ill-defined mass with ulceration (arrowhead) at the left anterior wall of the oropharynx

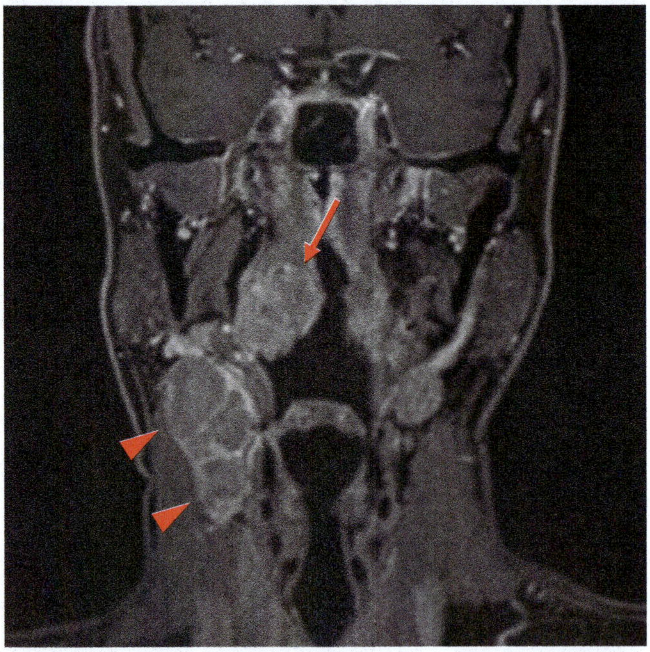

Fig. 3.6 HPV-associated oropharyngeal SCCa of the right base of the tongue. Contrast-enhanced CT image shows an ill-defined margin of the invasive mass at the right anterior wall of the oropharynx extending to the floor of the mouth (arrows). Associated lymph node metastasis is invading the carotid artery and the jugular vein (arrowhead)

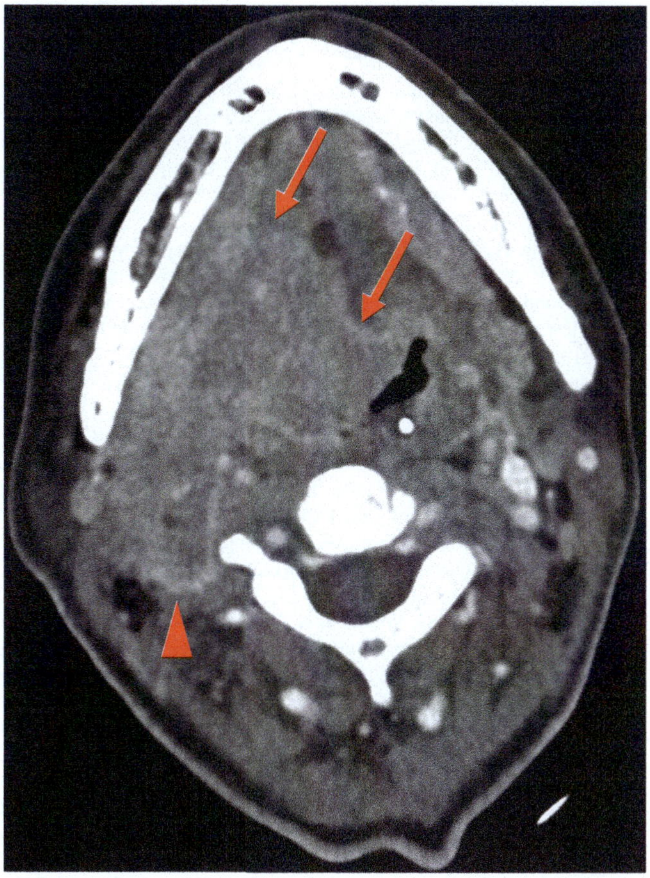

Fig. 3.7 Non-HPV-associated oropharyngeal SCCa of the right palatine tonsil with multiple lymph node metastases. Contrast-enhanced, fat-saturated T1W coronal image shows an enhanced mass at the right lateral wall of the oropharynx (arrow), and multiple lymph node swelling with extracapsular spread (matted nodes; arrowheads) at the right level II region

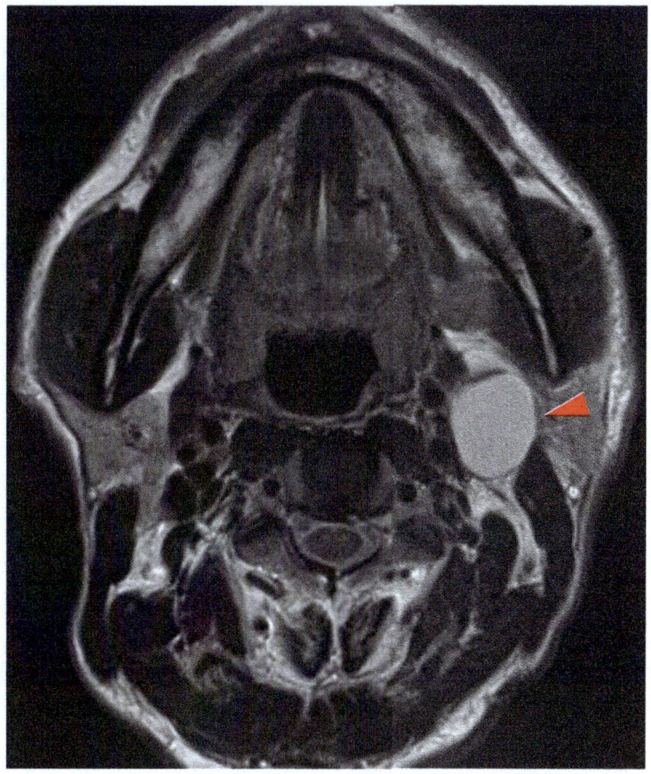

Fig. 3.8 HPV-associated oropharyngeal SCCa of the left palatine tonsil with cystic lymph node metastasis. T2W image shows a well-defined cystic-appearing lymph node at the left level II region (arrowhead)

clinical/radiologic pitfall that is of particular concern, given the rapidly rising incidence of oropharyngeal SCCa attributable to HPV. Because HPV-associated SCCa is commonly, clinically, and radiologically occult at the primary site, radiologists must recognize that cystic neck masses in adult patients should be considered cystic metastases until proven otherwise; a branchial cleft cyst should be considered the exception rather than the rule for an adult with a cystic neck mass.

These imaging differences between HPV-associated SCCa and non-HPV-associated SCCa are congruent with the understanding that HPV-associated SCCa represents a separate clinical entity, driven by different somatic molecular events and with a different clinical phenotype.

3.3 Differential Diagnosis

As mentioned earlier, SCCa is the most common histologic type of malignancy arising in the oropharynx, but there are some other malignancies we should consider in the differential diagnosis. There are also benign tumors or inflammatory diseases that mimic malignant tumors.

3.3.1 Malignant Lymphoma

Malignant lymphoma is also common and the second most common neoplasm of the head and neck. Although pretreatment imaging evaluation is critical for tumor staging and treatment planning, both SCCa and lymphoma of the oropharynx usually arise from the same anatomic sites, such as the palatine tonsils and the tongue base, and they show similar imaging characteristics. Generally, malignant lymphoma demonstrates a well-defined mass and homogeneous internal density/intensity on CT/MR imaging (Fig. 3.9) [25], but these characteristics are also common findings in HPV-associated SCCa. Diffusion-weighted imaging and dynamic contrast-enhanced MR imaging have the potential to differentiate the two malignancies, but there is overlap in ADC values and dynamic enhancing patterns [26, 27]. Associated lymph node swellings in the cervical region or other sites with homogeneous density/intensity may help make the diagnosis, but lymphoma also shows necrosis or cystic changes of the lymph node lesions, which may mimic metastatic lymph nodes of SCCa. Histopathological examination is necessary for diagnosis,

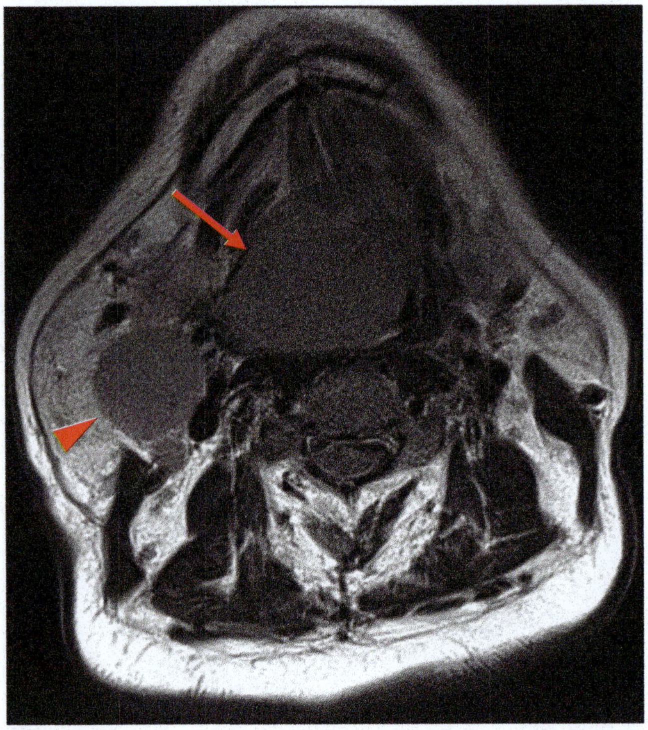

Fig. 3.9 Malignant lymphoma, diffuse large B-cell of the right palatine tonsil with cervical lymph node involvement. T2W image shows a well-defined exophytic appearance of the mass at the right lateral wall of the oropharynx (arrow). Right cervical lymph node at level II region is also noted with well-defined homogeneous intensity (arrowhead)

but it is important to inform the clinicians or pathologists of the possibility of lymphoma.

3.4 Summary

Since other oropharyngeal tumors, such as minor salivary gland tumors, sarcomas, and papillomas, are extremely rare compared to SCCa and lymphoma, it is important to be familiar with oropharyngeal SCCa and lymphoma both clinically and radiographically. We should be especially aware of the recently established HPV-related cancers. However, since imaging findings are mostly nonspecific, it is difficult to differentiate them from each other. Biopsy is always necessary to manage oropharyngeal tumors.

References

1. Landry D, Glastonbury CM. Squamous cell carcinoma of the upper aerodigestive tract: a review. Radiol Clin North Am. 2015;53(1):81–97.
2. Chaturvedi AK, Anderson WF, Lortet-Tieulent J, Curado MP, Ferlay J, Franceschi S, et al. Worldwide trends in incidence rates for oral cavity and oropharyngeal cancers. J Clin Oncol. 2013;31(36):4550–9.
3. Gillison ML, Chaturvedi AK, Anderson WF, Fakhry C. Epidemiology of human papillomavirus-positive head and neck squamous cell carcinoma. J Clin Oncol. 2015;33(29):3235–42.
4. Chaturvedi AK. Global burden of human papillomavirus-positive head and neck cancers. Lancet Oncol. 2014;15(12):1282–3.
5. Chaturvedi AK, Engels EA, Pfeiffer RM, Hernandez BY, Xiao W, Kim E, et al. Human papillomavirus and rising oropharyngeal cancer incidence in the United States. J Clin Oncol. 2011;29(32):4294–301.
6. Mehanna H, Beech T, Nicholson T, El-Hariry I, McConkey C, Paleri V, et al. Prevalence of human papillomavirus in oropharyngeal and nonoropharyngeal head and neck cancer—systematic review and meta-analysis of trends by time and region. Head Neck. 2013;35(5):747–55.
7. Hama T, Tokumaru Y, Fujii M, Yane K, Okami K, Kato K, et al. Prevalence of human papillomavirus in oropharyngeal cancer: a multicenter study in Japan. Oncology. 2014;87(3):173–82.
8. De Felice F, Tombolini V, Valentini V, de Vincentiis M, Mezi S, Brugnoletti O, et al. Advances in the management of HPV-related oropharyngeal cancer. J Oncol. 2019;2019:9173729.
9. You EL, Henry M, Zeitouni AG. Human papillomavirus-associated oropharyngeal cancer: review of current evidence and management. Curr Oncol. 2019;26(2):119–23.
10. Marur S, D'Souza G, Westra WH, Forastiere AA. HPV-associated head and neck cancer: a virus-related cancer epidemic. Lancet Oncol. 2010;11(8):781–9.
11. Khalid MB, Ting P, Pai A, Russo JL, Bakst R, Chai RL, et al. Initial presentation of human papillomavirus-related head and neck cancer: a retrospective review. Laryngoscope. 2019;129(4):877–82.
12. Ang KK, Harris J, Wheeler R, Weber R, Rosenthal DI, Nguyen-Tan PF, et al. Human papillomavirus and survival of patients with oropharyngeal cancer. N Engl J Med. 2010;363(1):24–35.
13. Amin MB, American Joint Committee on Cancer, American Cancer Society. AJCC cancer staging manual. Eight edition/editor-in-chief, Mahul B. Amin, editors, Stephen B. Edge, and 16 others; Donna M. Gress, RHIT, CTR—Technical editor; Laura R. Meyer, CAPM—Managing editor. ed. Chicago IL: American Joint Committee on Cancer, Springer; 2017. xvii, 1024 p.
14. Wu CC, Horowitz DP, Deutsch I, Rahmati R, Schecter JM, Saqi A, et al. De-escalation of radiation dose for human papillomavirus-positive oropharyngeal head and neck squamous cell carcinoma: a case report and preclinical and clinical literature review. Oncol Lett. 2016;11(1):141–9.
15. Gillison ML, Zhang Q, Jordan R, Xiao W, Westra WH, Trotti A, et al. Tobacco smoking and increased risk of death and progression for patients with p16-positive and p16-negative oropharyngeal cancer. J Clin Oncol. 2012;30(17):2102–11.
16. Tham T, Wotman M, Roche A, Kraus D, Costantino P. The prognostic effect of anatomic subsite in HPV-positive oropharyngeal squamous cell carcinoma. Am J Otolaryngol. 2019;40(4):567–72.
17. Duensing S, Munger K. Mechanisms of genomic instability in human cancer: insights from studies with human papillomavirus oncoproteins. Int J Cancer. 2004;109(2):157–62.
18. Trotta BM, Pease CS, Rasamny JJ, Raghavan P, Mukherjee S. Oral cavity and oropharyngeal squamous cell cancer: key imaging findings for staging and treatment planning. Radiographics. 2011;31(2):339–54.
19. Goldenberg D, Begum S, Westra WH, Khan Z, Sciubba J, Pai SI, et al. Cystic lymph node metastasis in patients with head and neck cancer: an HPV-associated phenomenon. Head Neck. 2008;30(7):898–903.
20. Corey AS, Hudgins PA. Radiographic imaging of human papillomavirus related carcinomas of the oropharynx. Head Neck Pathol. 2012;6(Suppl 1):S25–40.

21. Cantrell SC, Peck BW, Li G, Wei Q, Sturgis EM, Ginsberg LE. Differences in imaging characteristics of HPV-positive and HPV-negative oropharyngeal cancers: a blinded matched-pair analysis. Am J Neuroradiol. 2013;34(10):2005–9.
22. Morani AC, Eisbruch A, Carey TE, Hauff SJ, Walline HM, Mukherji SK. Intranodal cystic changes: a potential radiologic signature/biomarker to assess the human papillomavirus status of cases with oropharyngeal malignancies. J Comput Assist Tomogr. 2013;37(3):343–5.
23. Fujita A, Buch K, Truong MT, Qureshi MM, Mercier G, Jalisi S, et al. Imaging characteristics of metastatic nodes and outcomes by HPV status in head and neck cancers. Laryngoscope. 2016;126(2):392–8.
24. Chan MW, Yu E, Bartlett E, O'Sullivan B, Su J, Waldron J, et al. Morphologic and topographic radiologic features of human papillomavirus-related and -unrelated oropharyngeal carcinoma. Head Neck. 2017;39(8):1524–34.
25. Aiken AH, Glastonbury C. Imaging Hodgkin and non-Hodgkin lymphoma in the head and neck. Radiol Clin North Am. 2008;46(2):363–78, ix-x.
26. Park M, Kim J, Choi YS, Lee SK, Koh YW, Kim SH, et al. Application of dynamic contrast-enhanced MRI parameters for differentiating squamous cell carcinoma and malignant lymphoma of the oropharynx. Am J Roentgenol. 2016;206(2):401–7.
27. Ichikawa Y, Sumi M, Sasaki M, Sumi T, Nakamura T. Efficacy of diffusion-weighted imaging for the differentiation between lymphomas and carcinomas of the nasopharynx and oropharynx: correlations of apparent diffusion coefficients and histologic features. Am J Neuroradiol. 2012;33(4):761–6.

Diagnostic Imaging of Oral Cavity Cancer

4

Takashi Hiyama

Abstract

Oral cancer is one of the universally prevalent cancer type, and squamous cell carcinomas account for more than 90%. Fundamental knowledge such as the epidemiology and etiology of the oral cancer, imaging anatomy of oral cavity, and AJCC/UICC (American Joint Committee of Cancer/International Union Against Cancer) TNM classification is needed for image interpretation. The new concept of depth of invasion in T classification and extranodal extension in N classification is added from AJCC/UICC 8th edition. These items will be described earlier in this chapter.

The oral cavity is divided into eight subsites (mucosal lips, oral tongue, upper alveolar ridge, lower alveolar ridge, retromolar trigone, floor of mouth, buccal mucosa, and hard palate). The invasion pattern of oral cavity cancer differs depending on the primary site of involvement. The invasion pattern of oral cancer according to the primary involvement of each subsite is discussed later in this chapter. We also discuss lymph node metastasis, post-treatment imaging results, treatment complications, and recurrence in oral cancer.

Keywords

Oral cancer · Tongue · Hard plate · Alveolar ridge · Lip · Buccal mucosa · Oral floor · Retromolar trigone · MRI · CT

T. Hiyama (✉)
Department of Diagnostic Radiology, National Cancer Center Hospital East, Kashiwa, Chiba, Japan
e-mail: thiyama@east.ncc.go.jp

4.1 Epidemiology and Etiology

There is an estimated incidence of 355,000 cases of oral cavity cancer worldwide each year, which contributes to an estimated mortality of 177,000 cases per year [1]. Overall oral cancer including oropharyngeal involvement is the sixth most common cancer in the world [2]. A high incidence of oral cancer is found in Southern Asia (India, Pakistan, Sri Lanka, Taiwan, and China). More than 90% of cancers in the oral cavity are squamous cell carcinoma [2]. The other common types of oral cancer are salivary gland malignancies and sarcomas. Tobacco smoking, betel quid chewing, alcohol use, poor oral hygiene, and mechanical irritation are the known risk factors for developing squamous cell carcinoma of the oral cavity [3]. Symptoms include discomfort, pain, reduced mobility of the tongue, and irritation from wearing dentures, although early squamous cell cancers may be asymptomatic.

4.2 Anatomy of Oral Cavity: An Overview

The oral cavity extends from the junction of the skin and the vermilion border of the lips to the junction of the hard palate and the soft palate above, to the line of circumvallate papillae below, and to the anterior tonsillar pillars laterally. The oral cavity is divided into the following subsites: mucosal lips, oral tongue (anterior two-thirds), upper alveolar ridge, lower alveolar ridge, retromolar trigone, floor of mouth, buccal mucosa, and hard palate (Fig. 4.1) [4].

The mucosal lip begins at the junction of the vermilion border with the skin and includes only the vermilion surface or the portion of the lip that comes in contact with the opposing lip. The anterior two-thirds of the tongue is the freely mobile portion of the tongue that extends anteriorly from the line of circumvallate papillae to the undersurface of the tongue at the junction with the floor of the mouth. The lower alveolar ridge is the mucosa overlying the alveolar process of the mandible, which extends from the line of attachment of

H. Ojiri (ed.), *Diagnostic Imaging in Head and Neck Cancer*, https://doi.org/10.1007/978-981-15-3188-0_4

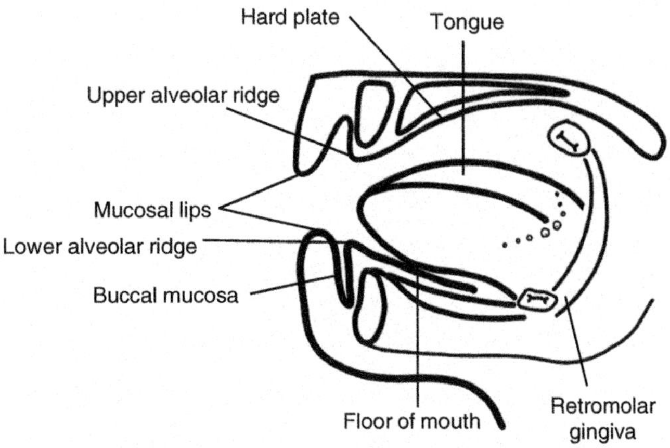

Fig. 4.1 Subsite of the oral cavity according to the AJCC 8th edition. Oral cavity divided into the mucosal lip, tongue, lower and upper alveolar ridge, retromolar gingiva, floor of mouth, buccal mucosa, and hard plate

mucosa in the lower gingivobuccal sulcus to the line of attachment of the floor of mouth. The upper alveolar ridge is the mucosa overlying the alveolar process of the maxilla, which extend from the line of attachment of mucosa in the upper gingivobuccal sulcus to the junction of the hard palate. The floor of the mouth is the mucosa overlying the mylohyoid and hyoglossus muscles, extending from the inner surface of the lower alveolus to the undersurface of the tongue. The retromolar trigone is the mucosa overlying the ascending ramus of the mandible. The buccal mucosa includes the mucosa of the inner surface of the cheeks and the lips from the line of contact of the opposing lips to the line of attachment of mucosa of the upper and lower alveolar ridge. The hard plate extends from the inner surface of the superior alveolar ridge to the posterior edge of the palatine bone. Further detailed anatomy is explained under imaging sections of each subhead.

Table 4.1 TNM classification of the American Joint Committee of Cancer (AJCC), International Union Against Cancer (UICC) 8th edition (2017)

T classification	
T1	Tumor ≤2 cm with depth of invasion (DOI) ≤5 mm
T2	Tumor ≤2 cm with DOI >5 mm or tumor >2 cm and ≤4 cm with DOI ≤10 mm
T3	Tumor >2 cm and ≤4 cm with DOI >10 mm or tumor >4 cm with DOI ≤10 mm
T4a	Moderately advanced local disease, tumor >4 cm with DOI >10 mm or tumor invades adjacent structures only (e.g., through cortical bone of the mandible or maxilla or involves the maxillary sinus or skin of the face) Note: Superficial erosion of bone/tooth socket (alone) by a gingival primary is not sufficient to classify a tumor as T4
T4b	Very advanced local disease, tumor invades masticator space, pterygoid plates, or skull base, and/or encases the internal carotid artery

N Classification	
NX	Regional lymph nodes cannot be assessed
N0	No regional lymph node metastasis
N1	Metastasis in a single ipsilateral lymph node, 3 cm or smaller in greatest dimension, ENE (−)
N2	Metastasis in a single ipsilateral node larger than 3 cm but not larger than 6 cm in greatest dimension and ENE (−); or metastases in multiple ipsilateral lymph nodes, none larger than 6 cm in greatest dimension and ENE(−); or in bilateral or contralateral lymph nodes, none larger than 6 cm in greatest dimension and ENE (−)
N2a	Metastasis in a single ipsilateral node larger than 3 cm but not larger than 6 cm in greatest dimension and ENE (−)
N2b	Metastases in multiple ipsilateral nodes, none larger than 6 cm in greatest dimension and ENE (−)
N2c	Metastases in bilateral or contralateral lymph nodes, none larger than 6 cm in greatest dimension and ENE (−)
N3	Metastasis in a lymph node larger than 6 cm in greatest dimension and ENE (−); or Metastasis in any node(s) and clinically overt ENE (+)
N3a	Metastasis in a lymph node larger than 6 cm in greatest dimension and ENE (−)
N3b	Metastasis in any node(s) and clinically overt ENE (+)

4.3 TNM Classification

TNM classification for oral cancer on AJCC/UICC (American Joint Committee of Cancer/International Union Against Cancer) 8th edition (2017) is shown in Table 4.1.

4.3.1 T Classification

Although there were several minor changes in the 8th edition of AJCC and UICC, T1–3 classification is determined by the depth of invasion (DOI) and tumor size. Pathologically, DOI is measured by identification of the "horizon" of the basement membrane of the adjacent squamous mucosa. A perpendicular "plumb line" is dropped from this horizon to the deepest point of tumor invasion, which represents the DOI [4]. Multiple studies have shown a strong relationship of DOI to disease-free survival, overall survival, and development of neck metastases [5, 6].

T4a includes tumor size more than 4 cm with DOI more than 10 mm, invasion through the cortical bone of the mandible or maxilla, and involvement of the maxillary sinus or the skin. T4b includes invasion of the masticator space, pterygoid plates, or skull base and/or encasement of the internal carotid artery. A superficial erosion of the mandible or maxilla by a primary gingival lesion is notably not sufficient to classify as T4. Radiologists need to assess these structures, especially the deep structures, which are inaccessible by a physical examination.

4.3.2 N classification

N classification is determined mainly by the size, number, and distribution of lymph node involvement. In addition, extra-nodal extension (ENE) is classified as N3b by the AJCC 8th edition [4]. Clinical ENE in AJCC 8th edition is defined as unquestionable ENE by physical examination that is supported by radiological evidence. Therefore, radiologists need to evaluate ENE for clinical N staging. If ENE with invasion of adjacent structures is strongly suspected on imaging but is physically undetectable, a second-look physical examination is recommended.

4.4 Imaging Techniques

4.4.1 CT

Computed tomography can take a wide range of body images in a short time, and CT is the standard method for radiologic evaluation of primary tumors and lymph node and distant metastases in head and neck cancer. CT is also excellent for the evaluation of erosion or destruction of cortical bone. However, dental artifacts sometimes create difficulty in assessment of oral cancer. Iterative metal artifact reduction algorithm and dual-energy CT with monochromatic image reconstruction have been investigated to reduce metal artifacts [7–9].

Slice thickness should be 3 mm or less for evaluation of the primary tumor and lymph node metastases. Coronal reconstruction is useful for evaluation of oral cancer. For evaluation of the bone, slice thickness should be 1 mm or less. Bone invasion can be evaluated more accurately by cross-sectional images using multiplanar reconstruction (MPR) for the anterior part of the mandible and long and short axis reconstruction for the posterior part. In addition, CT-generated panoramic view clearly shows the range of bone destruction [10]. An example of a CT protocol is shown in Table 4.2.

Table 4.2 Example of CT protocol

Range of reconstruction	Plane	Window	Slice thickness	FOV
From the skull base to thoracic inlet	Axial	Soft	3 mm	24 cm
Oral cavity(primary)	Axial	Soft/bone	1 mm	16 mm
	Coronal[a]	Soft/bone	1 mm	16 mm
	Sagittal[a]	Soft/bone	1 mm	16 mm

[a]Oblique coronal and sagittal images are also reconstructed if bone invasion is suspected. Panoramic view is generated if necessary

Table 4.3 Example of MRI protocol

Sequence	Plane	Slice thickness	FOV	Matrix
T1WI	Axial	3 mm	25 mm	512 × 512
T2WI	Axial Coronal	3 mm	25 mm	512 × 512
DWI	Axial	3 mm	25 mm	128 × 128
STIR	Coronal	3 mm	25 mm	512 × 512
3D-T1WI	Axial[a]	1 mm	23 mm	320 × 320
Gd-FS-T1WI	Axial Coronal	3 mm	25 mm	512 × 512
3D-Gd FS-T1WI	Axial[a]	1 mm	23 mm	320 × 320

[a]Coronal and axial images are also reconstructed from 3D sequence

4.4.2 MRI

Magnetic resonance imaging has excellent soft-tissue contrast and is useful for the evaluation of primary tumor extension. Furthermore, MRI is less susceptible to metal artifacts compared with CT in general. However, MRI may have motion artifacts due to swallowing motion or movement of jaw.

The slice thickness in MRI is 3 mm or less. Routinely, T1-weighted, T2-weighted, STIR, and DWI images are obtained on axial and/or coronal plane. Thin slice 3D T1-weighted images and reconstruction images are useful for precise evaluation [11]. Usually, fat-suppression is used for contrast-enhanced T1-weighted images. Example of an MRI protocol is shown in Table 4.3.

4.5 Imaging of Oral Cancer

4.5.1 Mucosal Lip

Cancer involving only the mucosal part of lips is classified as oral cancer, while cancer involving the rest of lip is classified as skin cancer. The mucosal lip is subdivided into the upper lip, the lower lip, and the commissures of the mouth. Lower lip cancer is more common as compared to upper lip cancer. Squamous cell carcinomas that arise in the upper lip and the oral commissures have a worse prognosis than those originating in the lower lip [12].

The extension pattern of cancer of the lips and its related anatomy on MRI is shown in Fig. 4.2. Lower lip cancer may invade the skin anteriorly, the submucosal fat and orbicularis oris muscle inferiorly, and the mandible and buccal mucosa posteriorly (Fig. 4.3). Upper lip cancers have the potential for invasion into the premaxillary region and the nasal cavity. Lower and upper lip cancers are well evaluated in sagittal images, and the commissures are easily depicted in coronal images in CT scan. Carcinoma of the oral commissures easily invades the upper and lower lips and the buccal mucosa (Fig. 4.4).

Fig. 4.2 Extension pattern of the lip cancer and related anatomy in MRI. (**a**) Sagittal T2-weighted image and (**b**) Axial T2-weighted image. Extension pattern is indicated by arrows and a lower letter corresponding with the bullet. (1) Skin, (2) orbicularis oris muscle, (3) mandible, (4) maxilla, (5) buccinator muscle, (6) levator anguli oris muscle

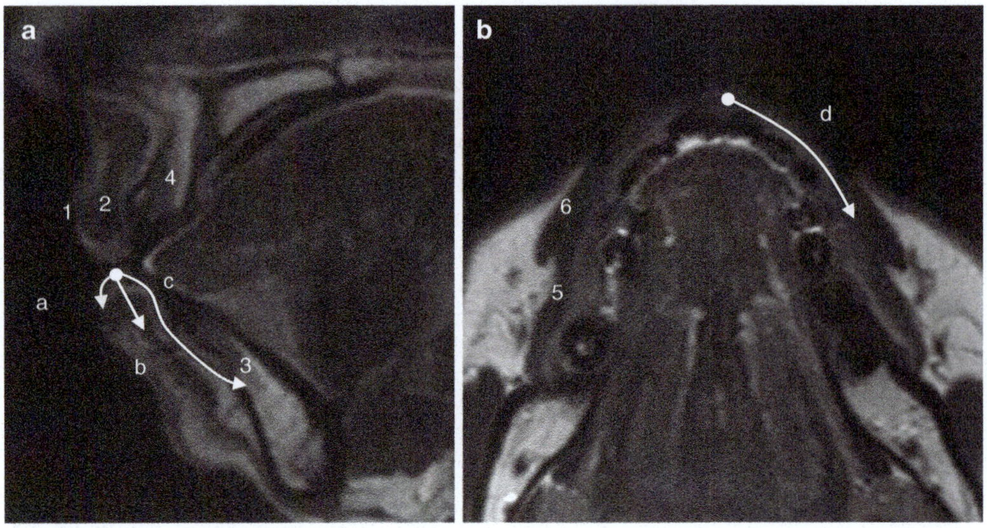

a. Anterior
   Direct invasion to the skin
b. Inferior
   Direct invasion to the submucosal fat or orbicularis oris muscle
c. Posterior
   Direct invasion to the buccal mucosa, mandible or maxilla
d. Lateral
   Direct invasion to the buccal mucosa, buccinator muscle or levator anguli oris muscle

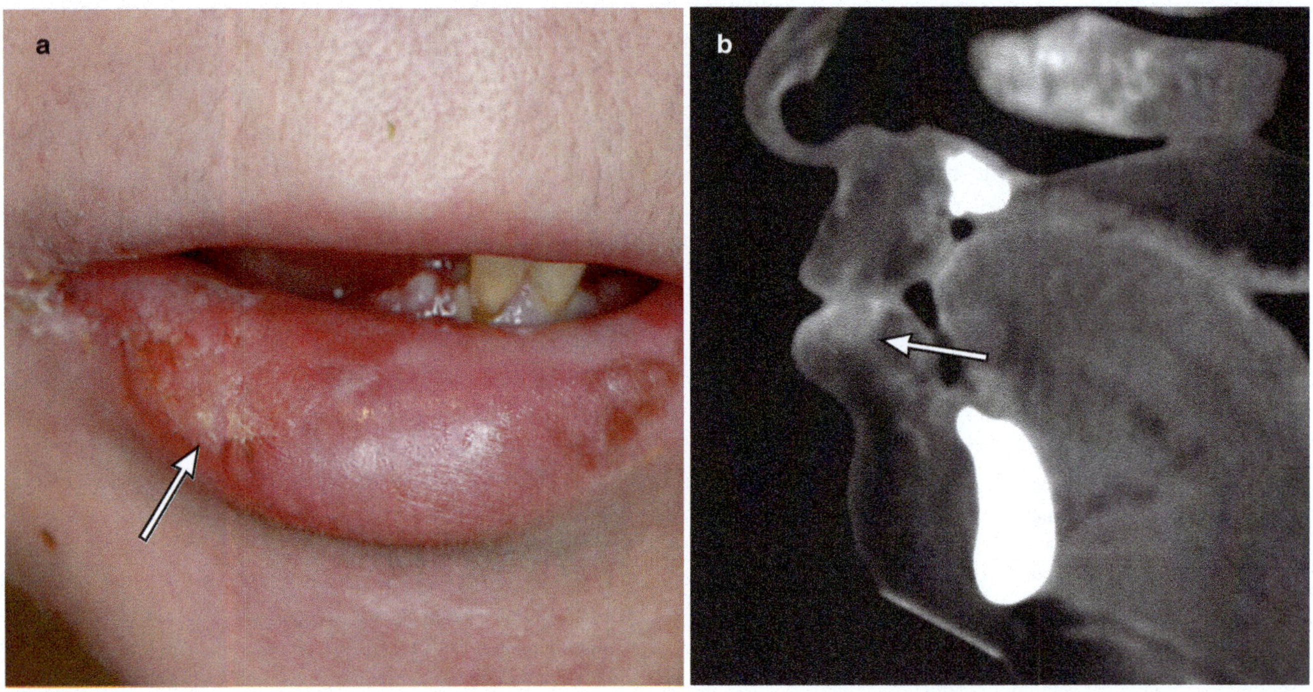

Fig. 4.3 A 59-year-old woman with squamous cell carcinoma of the lower lip. (**a**) The tumor is seen at the vermilion of the lip (arrow). (**b**) Sagittal contrast-enhanced CT shows tumor invasion into the submucosal fat and contact with the orbicularis oris muscle (arrow)

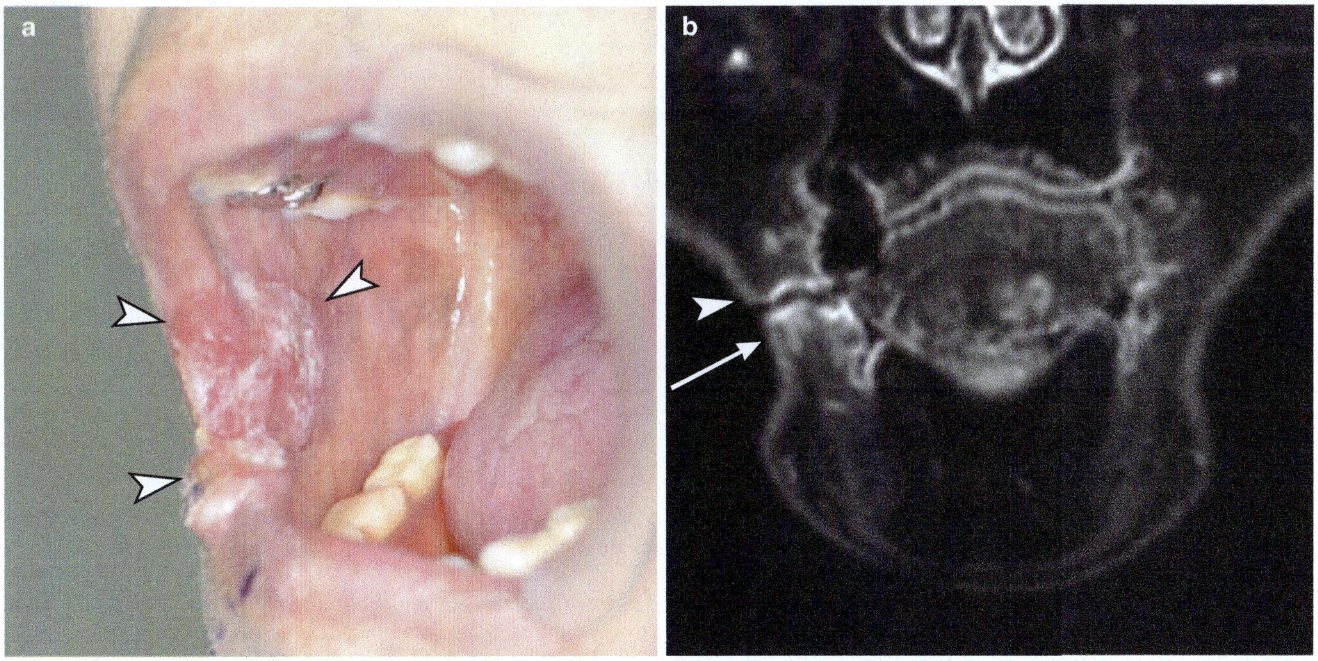

Fig. 4.4 A 73-year-old woman with squamous cell carcinoma of the right commissure of the mouth. (**a**) The tumor extends from commissure of the mouth to the lower and upper vermilion of the lip and buccal mucosa (arrowheads). (**b**) Post-contrast T1-weighted image with fat suppression shows tumor extension to the lower lip (arrow) and upper lip (arrowhead)

Surgical excision is generally preferred for the treatment of lip carcinoma. Defects that involve less than two-thirds of the lip may be closed primarily, while defects involving up to three-quarters of the lip need to be reconstructed with full thickness pedicled flaps from the uninvolved lip (Abbe-Estlander flaps) [13].

4.5.2 Tongue

The tongue consists of intrinsic and extrinsic muscles. The intrinsic muscles are the transverse, vertical, superior longitudinal, and inferior longitudinal muscles. These muscles originate and insert within the tongue. The extrinsic muscles include the genioglossus, hyoglossus, styloglossus, and palatoglossus muscles. These muscles have external bony origins and terminate in the tongue. Hence, tongue carcinoma has the potential to spread along the extrinsic muscles to external regions. Neurovascular bundles run medial and lateral to the hyoglossus muscle. The lingual nerve and the hypoglossal nerve run lateral to the hyoglossus muscle. Tongue cancer most frequently originates in the lateral borders but also occurs on the dorsum, apex, and the undersurface of tongue. Extension pattern of carcinoma of the tongue and its related anatomy on MRI are shown in Fig. 4.5.

In tongue cancer, T classification is mainly determined by the tumor size and DOI. Pathologically, DOI is measured using a perpendicular "plumb line" from the basement membrane of adjacent normal mucosa to the deepest point of tumor invasion. Although measurement method of DOI is not radiologically defined, the measurement is performed considering the pathological DOI. The reference line is determined as that which connects the junction of both side point of tumor and the normal mucosa on imaging (Fig. 4.6). The length of the perpendicular line from the reference line to the deepest invasion point represents the radiologic DOI. In MRI, the normal mucosa is easily defined on contrast-enhanced T1-weighted images. Another method of DOI measurement is to subtract the distance between the deepest points of tumor invasion and the lingual septum from the distance between the lingual septum and the border of tongue of the intact side (Fig. 4.6c). DOI measurements recorded in MRI are 1–3 mm larger than those recorded in the pathologic examination [14, 15]. In ulcerative lesions and elevated lesions, the thickness of the tumor and the DOI are different (Fig. 4.6d).

In addition to tumor size and DOI, accurate assessment of extent of tumor is important for treatment planning. Tongue cancers easily infiltrate the hyoglossus muscle under the mucosa (Fig. 4.7). When it infiltrates further, it invades the neurovascular bundles, genioglossus muscle, and lingual septum and may also invade to the opposite side of the tongue. Invasion of the neurovascular bundles affects treatment and prognosis [16]. Tumors may extend deep along the transverse

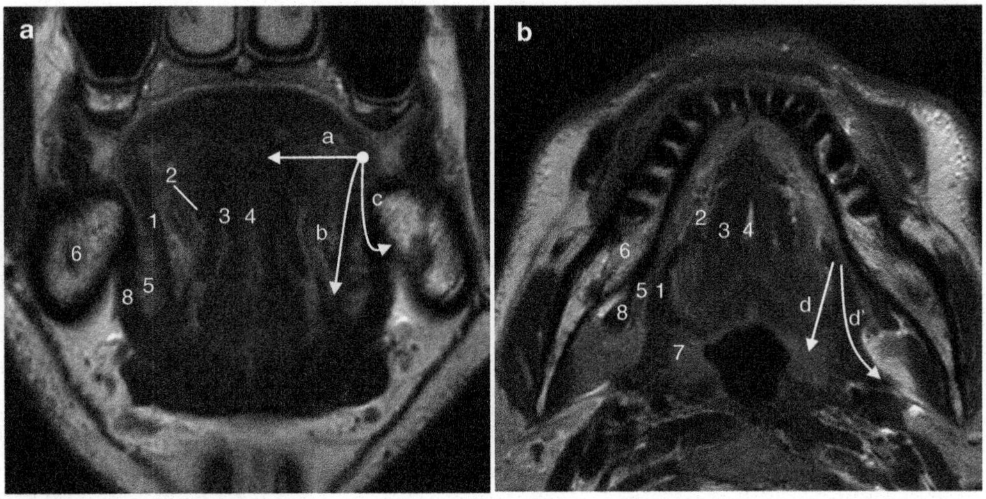

Fig. 4.5 Extension pattern of tongue cancer and related anatomy in MRI. (**a**) Coronal T2-weighted image and (**b**) Axial T2-weighted image. Extension pattern is indicated by arrows and a lower letter corresponding with the bullet. (1) hyoglossus muscle, (2) neurovascular bundle, (3) genioglossus muscle, (4) tongue septum, (5) glosso-mylohyoid gap, (6) mandible, (7) tonsil, (8) mylohyoid muscle

a. Medial
   Direct invasion to the hyoglossus muscle, neurovascular bundle, genioglossus muscle, lingual septum
   Extension along the intrinsic (transverse) muscles of the tongue
b. Inferior
   Direct invasion to the sublingual space, neurovascular bundles, glosso-mylohyoid gap or mylohyoid muscle
   Extension along the hyoglossus muscle to the sublingual space and hyoid bone
   Perineural spread along the hypoglossal or lingual nerves
c. Lateral
   Direct invasion to the oral floor, lower gingiva or mandible
   Mandibular invasion from tumor extension along the mylohyoid muscle
d. Posterior
   Direct invasion to the base of tongue, palatoglossus muscle or tonsils
   Extension to the anterior palatine arch and soft palate along the palatoglossal muscle
   Extension to the parapharyngeal space along the styloglossus muscle (d')

muscles. Tumors may spread downward along the hyoglossus muscle and reach the sublingual space and the hyoid bone. Perineural extension along the lingual or hypoglossal nerve may also be seen. Additionally, tumors may also extend to glosso-mylohyoid gap, a space between the hyoglossus and the mylohyoid muscles, and may invade the submandibular gland or ducts. Obstruction of the submandibular duct due to tumor invasion causes secondary submandibular adenitis. Lingual tumors may further extend to the floor of the mouth, the gingiva, and the mandible. Mandibular invasion along the mylohyoid muscle may be seen. Posteriorly, tumors may extend along the styloglossus muscle to the parapharyngeal space (Fig. 4.8). Less frequently, extension to the palatoglossus muscle (anterior palatine arch) may occur. The tumor also extends to the oropharynx (lingual base and tonsils) and the supraglottic region.

4.5.3 Lower Alveolar Ridge (Lower Gingival Cancer)

The lower gingiva covers the alveolar process of the mandible. The retromolar trigone is located posteriorly, the buccal mucosa laterally, and the oral floor medially. Gingival cancer may occur in any part of the lower gingiva, but it occurs frequently in the molar area and is often present at the alveolar crest. Gingival cancer sometimes reveals as an area of incomplete healing after tooth extraction [17]. Extension pattern of carcinoma of the lower gingiva and its related anatomy on MRI are shown Fig. 4.9.

Gingival cancer invades the cortex of the mandible located under the gum and extends into the bone marrow (Fig. 4.10). Superficial erosion of bone or tooth socket by a gingival cancer is not enough to classify the tumor as T4 according to the AJCC 8th edition. All tumors of the oral cavity have the ability to invade the mandible. The prevalence of mandibular bone invasion in head and neck cancer ranges from 12 to 56% [18, 19]. The sensitivity and specificity of detection of mandibular bone infiltration are 72% and 90% on CT and 78% and 83% on MRI, respectively [20].CT can easily detect bone erosion or destruction, but the evaluation of bone marrow infiltration often presents a challenge. Gingival cancer tends to invade bone marrow in areas without bone cortex, such as the alveolar crest, extraction socket, and nutrition canal.

MRI is superior to CT for assessment of bone marrow invasion, and accurate evaluation of tumor extension to the

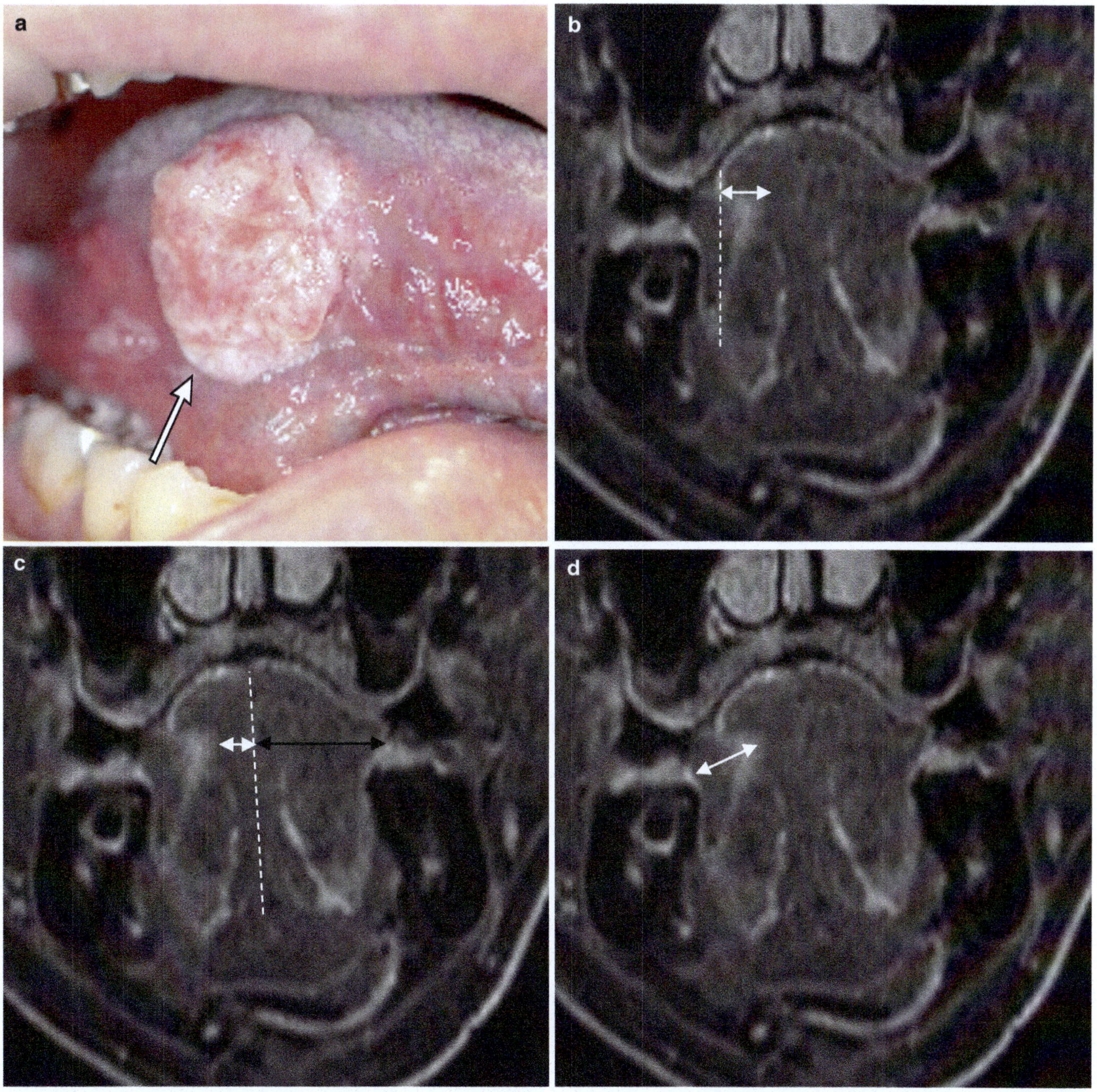

Fig. 4.6 Example of the measurement of DOI and tumor thickness. A 63-year-old man with squamous cell carcinoma of the tongue (right boarder). (**a**) The tumor protrudes from the tongue surface (arrow). (**b**) Presumable reference line (dashed line) and perpendicular line from the reference line to the deepest invasion point (double-headed arrow) represents DOI (9 mm). (**c**) Another method of measurement of DOI is subtracting the distance between the deepest point of tumor invasion and tongue septum (white double-headed arrow) from the distance between the tongue septum and the opposite tongue border (black double-headed arrow, DOI = 12 mm). Dashed line: tongue septum. (**d**) The tumor thickness (white double-headed arrow, 16 mm) is different from DOI. Pathological DOI was 11 mm

bone marrow is essential for optimal treatment. Vertical and horizontal extension of mandibular bone marrow infiltration needs to be assessed. Similar intensities in the bone marrow as the tumors on T2WI and T1WI are considered as tumor invasion. In case the signal intensity is reduced on T1WI, and weak enhancements as compared to tumors are shown on MRI, it is difficult to identify the signal change if it caused by tumor infiltration or inflammation due to periodontitis or post-extraction alveolitis. Assessment of vertical extension is needed to determine whether marginal resection can be performed. Usually, marginal resection is possible if the tumor limits itself within the upper two-thirds of the mandible. When the tumor reaches the mandibular canal, perineural spread along the mandibular nerve may occur (Fig. 4.10e, f).

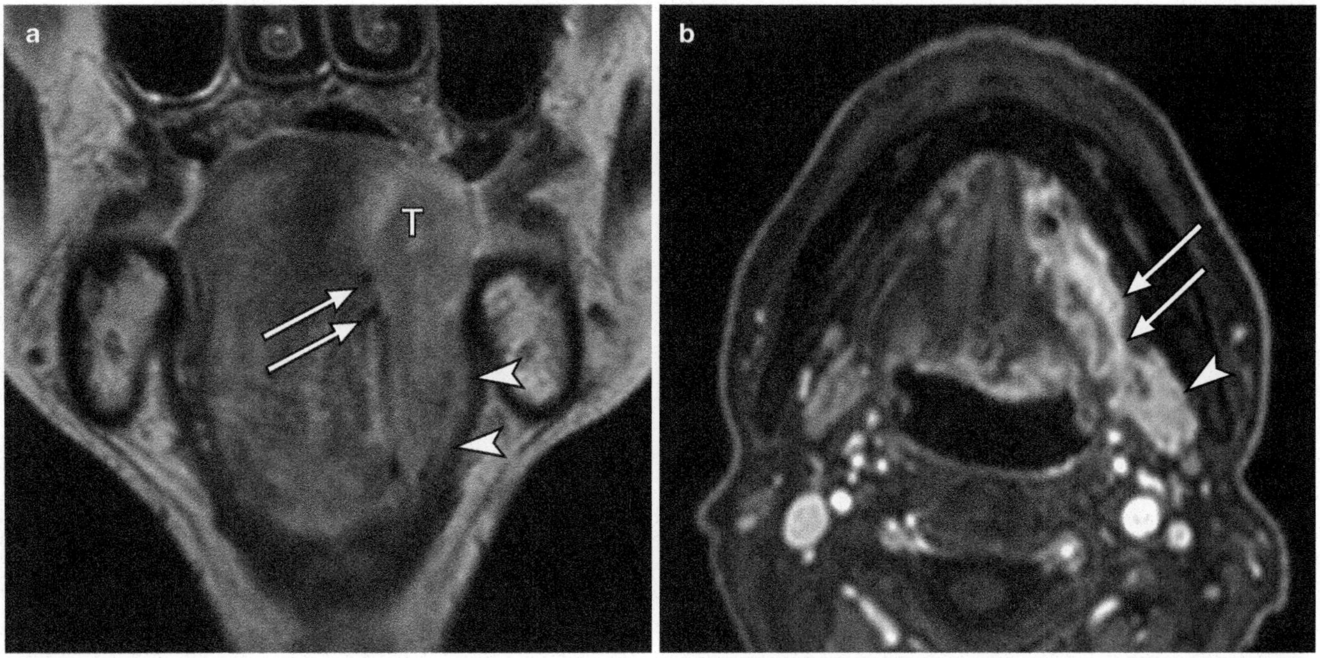

Fig. 4.7 A 70-year-old man with squamous cell carcinoma of the tongue. (**a**) The tumor (T) invades the hyoglossus muscle and is in contact with the neurovascular bundle, shown as flow void on T2-weighted image (arrow). The tumor extends along the hyoglossus muscle to the glosso-mylohyoid gap (arrowhead). (**b**) Post-contrast T1-weighted image with fat suppression shows tumor invasion into the sublingual space and glosso-mylohyoid gap (arrow). Secondary submandibular adenitis is also seen (arrowhead)

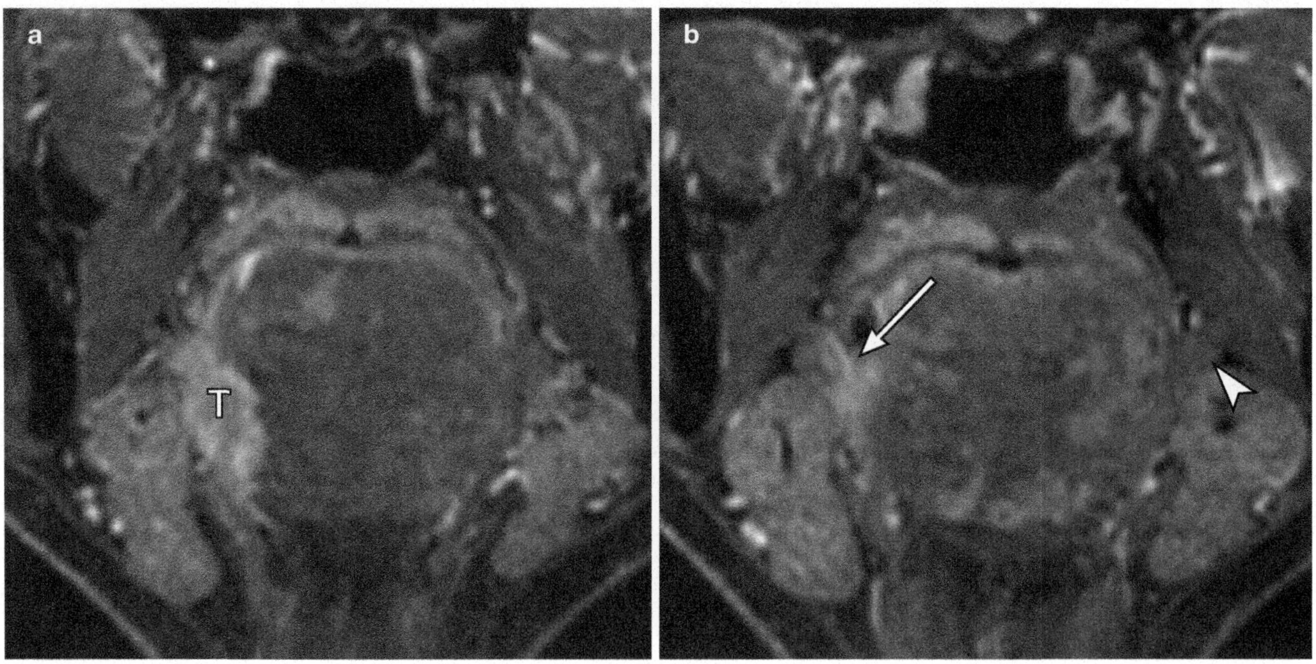

Fig. 4.8 A 65-year-old man with squamous cell carcinoma of the tongue. (**a**, **b**) Post-contrast T1-weighted image with fat suppression shows the tongue cancer (T) invading the hyoglossus muscle and spread along the styloglossus muscle (arrow) posteriorly. Normal styloglossus muscle on the unaffected side (arrowhead)

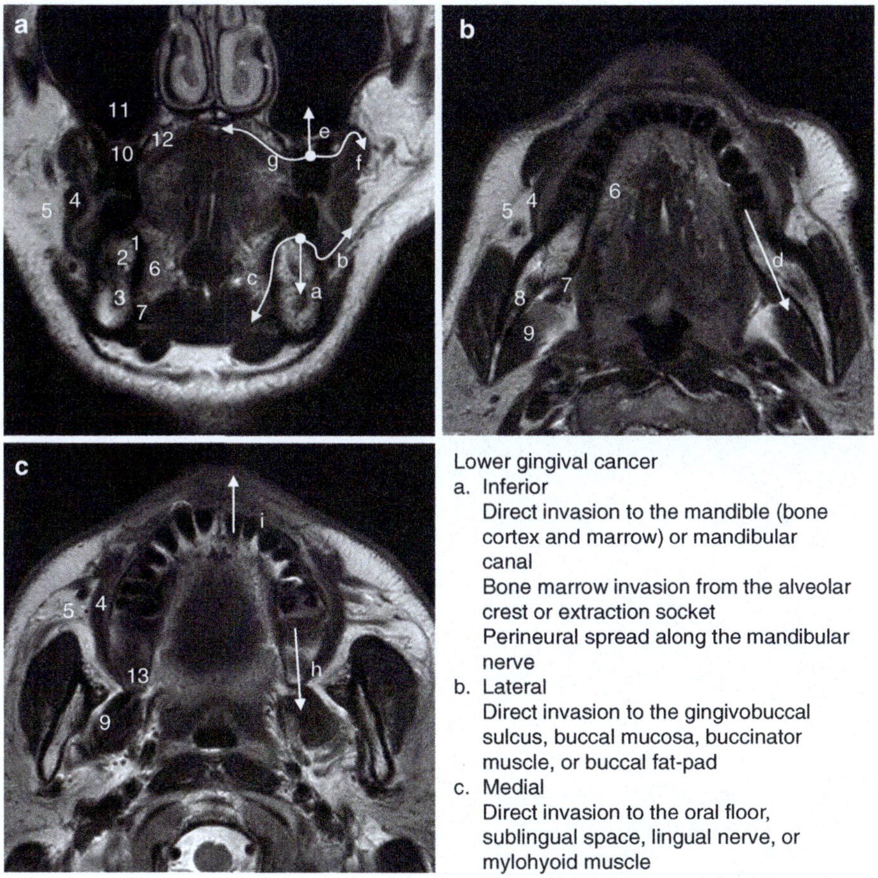

Lower gingival cancer

a. Inferior
   Direct invasion to the mandible (bone cortex and marrow) or mandibular canal
   Bone marrow invasion from the alveolar crest or extraction socket
   Perineural spread along the mandibular nerve
b. Lateral
   Direct invasion to the gingivobuccal sulcus, buccal mucosa, buccinator muscle, or buccal fat-pad
c. Medial
   Direct invasion to the oral floor, sublingual space, lingual nerve, or mylohyoid muscle
   Extension along the mylohyoid muscle towards the hyoid bone
d. Posterior
   Direct invasion to the retromolar area, mandibular ramus, or masticator space

Upper gingival caner

e. Superior
   Direct invasion to the alveolar process (bone cortex and marrow or maxillary sinus)
f. Lateral
   Direct invasion to the gingivobuccal sulcus, buccal mucosa, buccinator muscle, or buccal fat-pad
g. Medial
   Direct invasion to the hard palate
   Perineural spread along the palatine nerves
h. Posterior
   Direct invasion to the maxillary tuberosity, retromolar trigone, masticator space, pterygoid process, or pterygopalatine fossa
   Perineural spread along the posterior superior alveolar nerve
i. Anterior
   Direct invasion of the upper lip or floor of the nasal cavity

Fig. 4.9 Extension pattern of the lower and upper gingival cancer and related anatomy. (**a**) Coronal T2-weighted image, (**b**, **c**) Axial T2-weighted image. Extension pattern is indicated by arrows and a lower letter corresponding with the bullet. (1) mandible (bone cortex), (2) mandible (bone marrow), (3) mandibular canal, (4) buccinator muscle, (5) buccal fat-pad, (6) sublingual space, (7) mylohyoid muscle, (8) mandibular ramus, (9) masticator space, (10) alveolar process, (11) maxillary sinus, (12) hard plate, (13) maxillary tuberosity

Perineural spread (PNS) is seen in MRI as an enlargement of the mandibular canal, enlargement of the mandibular foramen, and thickening and enhancement of the nerve.

Gingival cancer may invade the oral floor or the sublingual space along the mylohyoid muscle medially and the buccal mucosa and the buccinator muscle laterally. Posteriorly, the tumor extends to the retromolar trigone, the mandibular ramus, and the masticator space.

4.5.4 Upper Alveolar Ridge (Upper Gingival Cancer)

The upper gingiva covers the alveolar ridge of the maxilla. The maxillary tuberosity is located posteriorly, the buccal mucosa laterally, and the hard palate medially. Upper gingival cancer may occur in any part of the upper gingiva, but it most often occurs in the molar area and is often present at the alveolar crest [21]. Upper gingival cancer is sometimes difficult to distinguish from cancer of the hard palate or the maxillary sinus. Extension pattern of carcinoma of the upper gingiva and its related anatomy on MRI are shown in Fig. 4.9.

Upper gingival cancer invades alveolar process superiorly. When maxillary sinus is well pneumatized, the bone of alveolar process becomes thin and tumors easily invade into maxillary sinus. As stated earlier, superficial erosion of bone or tooth socket by a gingival cancer is not enough to classify a tumor as T4. Posteriorly, upper gingival cancer extends to the maxillary tuberosity, which may be infiltrated through the alveolar foramen. Cancer also may extend to the retromolar

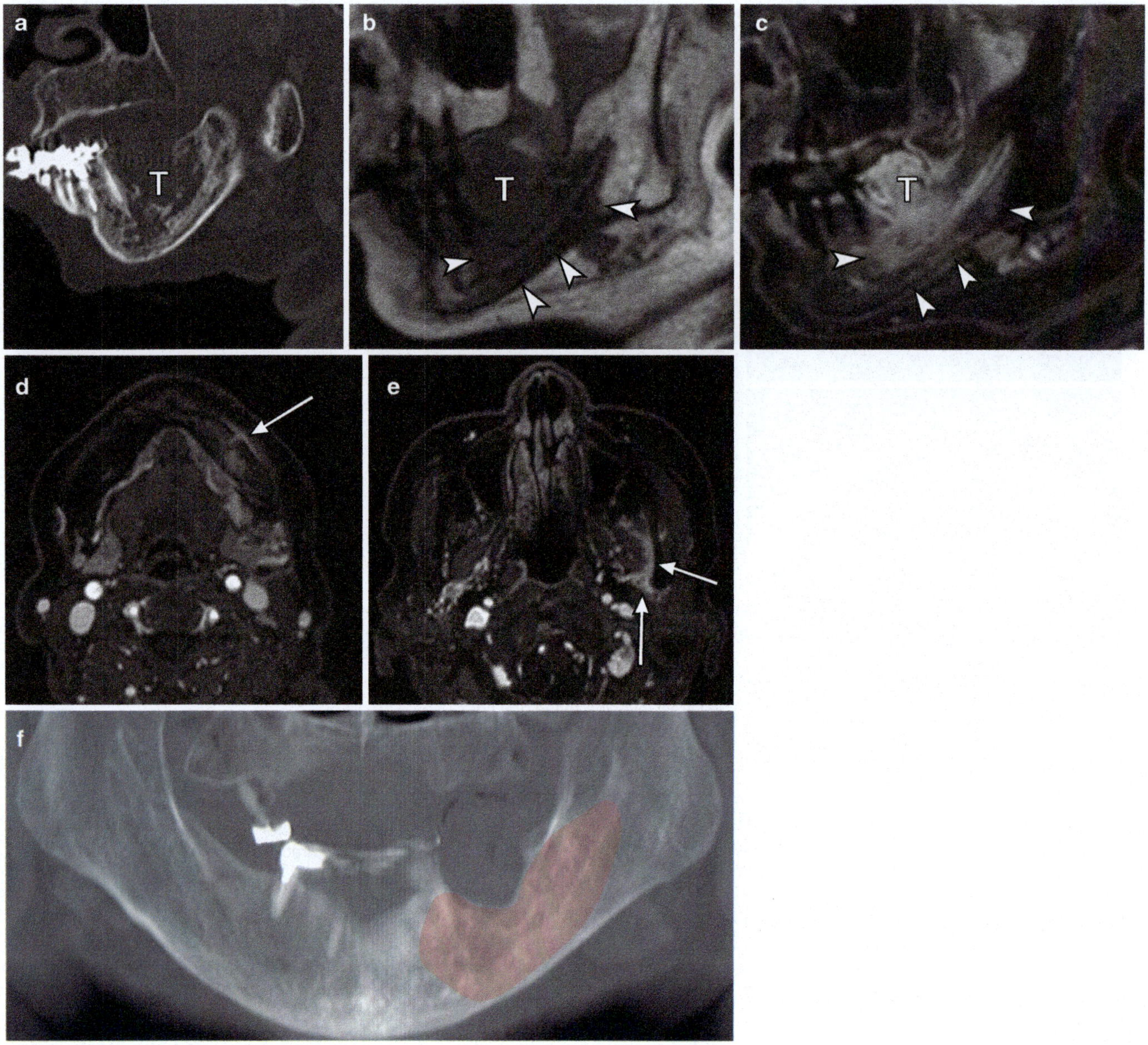

Fig. 4.10 A 74-year-old woman with squamous cell carcinoma of the lower gingiva. (**a**) CT shows bone destruction by the tumor (T), but the extension of tumor could not be assessed. (**b, c**) Lower gingival cancer located at molar lesion invades into the bone marrow, which shows low signal intensity on the T1-weighted image (**b**) and post-contrast T1-weighted image with fat suppression (**c**). Range of tumor extension could be evaluated on the MRI (arrowheads in **b**, **c**), and the mandibular canal is also involved. (**d**, **e**) Axial post-contrast T1-weighted image shows perineural spread along the mandibular nerve to the mental foramen anteriorly (arrow in **d**) and masticator space posteriorly (arrow in **e**). (**f**) Extension of bone marrow infiltration overlaid on panoramic view is useful for surgical planning

area, pterygoid plate, pterygoid muscles, retroantral fat, and pterygopalatine fossa (Fig. 4.11). Carcinoma of the anterior part of the upper gingiva may invade the inner mucosa of the upper lip or the nasal cavity (Fig. 4.12). Medially, the tumor extends to the hard palate and may extend beyond the midline. Laterally, the tumor extends from the gingival buccal groove to the buccal mucosa, buccinator muscle, and buccal fat-pad. PNS along the posterior superior alveolar nerve and the greater and lesser palatine nerves (V2) may be seen.

4.5.5 Retromolar Trigone

Retromolar trigone is a triangular mucosa overlying the vertical ramus of the mandible extending up to the maxillary tuberosity (Fig. 4.1). The lower part of the retromolar trigone corresponds to retromolar fossa which is bounded by the internal oblique ridge medially and the buccinator crest laterally. The pterygomandibular raphe is a tendinous band between the hamulus of the medial pterygoid plate and the posterior end of the mylohyoid line of the mandible [22].

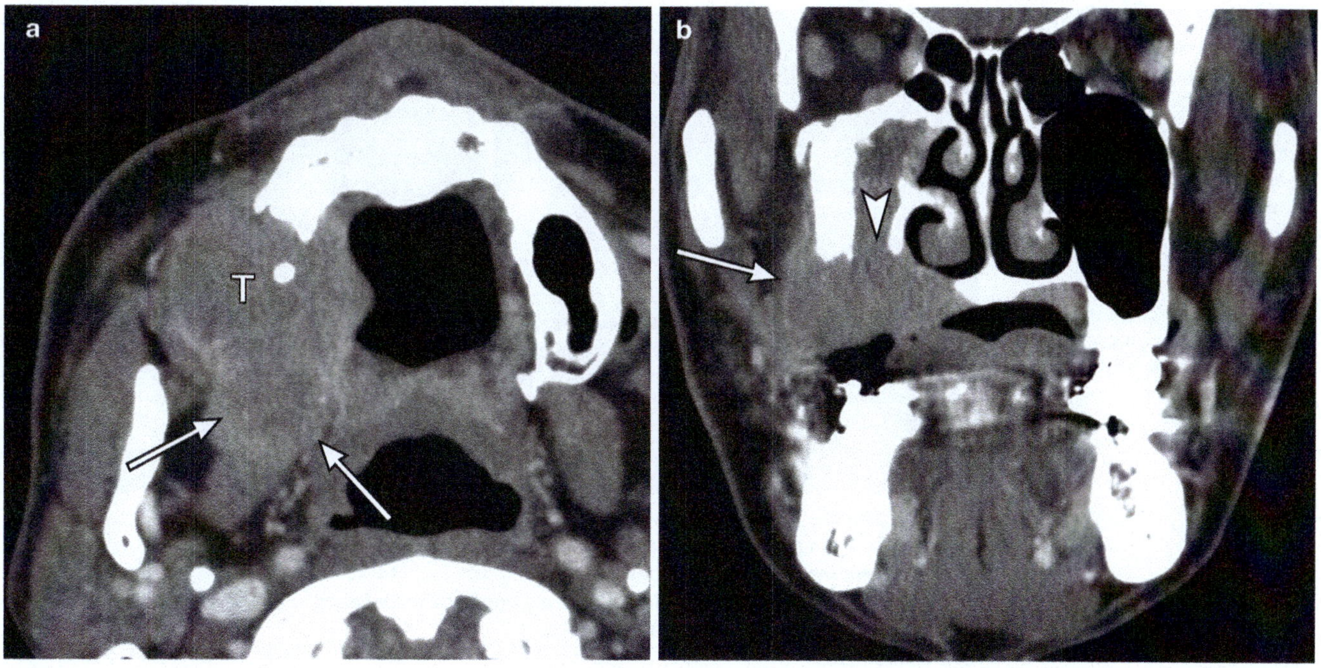

Fig. 4.11 A 67-year-old man with squamous cell carcinoma of the upper gingiva. (**a**) Axial contrast-enhanced CT shows that the tumor (T) replaces the right posterior part of the alveolar process including the maxillary tuberosity and invades the pterygoid plate and pterygoid muscle (arrow). (**b**) Coronal contrast-enhanced CT image shows tumor invasion into the gingivobuccal sulcus and superior part of the buccinator muscle laterally (arrow) and the maxillary sinus superiorly (arrowhead). Involvement of the right hard plate is also seen

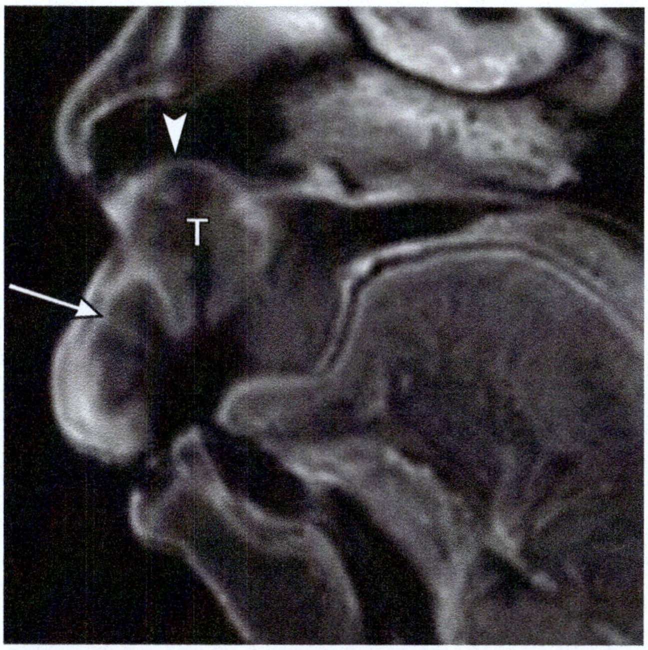

Fig. 4.12 A 71-year-old woman with squamous cell carcinoma of the upper gingiva. Sagittal post-contrast T1-weighted image with fat suppression shows tumor (T) invasion into the inner mucosa of the upper lip and orbicularis oris muscle anteriorly (arrow), and floor of the nasal cavity superiorly (arrowhead)

It gives attachment to buccinator and superior constrictor muscles. It is recognized as a pterygomandibular fold in the mouth. The palatoglossus muscle runs more medially and forms the anterior palatine arch. Extension pattern of carcinoma of the retromolar area and its related anatomy on MRI are shown in Fig. 4.13.

Since the mandible is located directly beneath the submucosa of the retromolar area, a retromolar gingival cancer easily invades the mandible (Fig. 4.14). The incidence of bone invasion in retromolar gingival cancer ranges from 14 to 75% of cases [23]. The oblique CT image with bone reconstruction algorithm is useful for detection of bone invasion of retromolar area. A study reported the sensitivity, specificity, and accuracy of CT for mandibular cortical and for bone marrow invasion to be 94, 90, and 91.8% and 83, 92, and 89%, respectively [23]. Posteriorly, tumors extend to the medial pterygoid muscle from the pterygomandibular space between the medial pterygoid muscle and the medial surface of ramus of the mandible (Fig. 4.15). Invasion to the pterygoid muscles cause trismus. Tumors may extend to the anterior palatine arch and tonsillar fossa. During upward extension along the pterygomandibular raphe, tumors extend to the pterygoid process and the maxillary tuberosity. Laterally, tumors extend to the buccal mucosa, buccinator muscle, and buccal fat-pad. Medially, tumors may invade the oral floor and the mylohyoid muscle.

4.5.6 Floor of the Mouth

The floor of the mouth is a horizontally aligned U-shaped space situated in the oral cavity [24]. Carcinoma of the floor

Fig. 4.13 Extension pattern of the cancer of the retromolar area and related anatomy. (**a**) Axial T2-weighted image, (**b**) Coronal T2-weighted image. Extension pattern is indicated by arrows and a lower letter corresponding with the bullet. (1) mandible ramus, (2) masticator space, (3) anterior palatine arch, (4) tonsil, (5) buccinator muscle, (6) buccal fat-pad, (7) lower gingiva, (8) mylohyoid muscle, (9) maxillary tuberosity

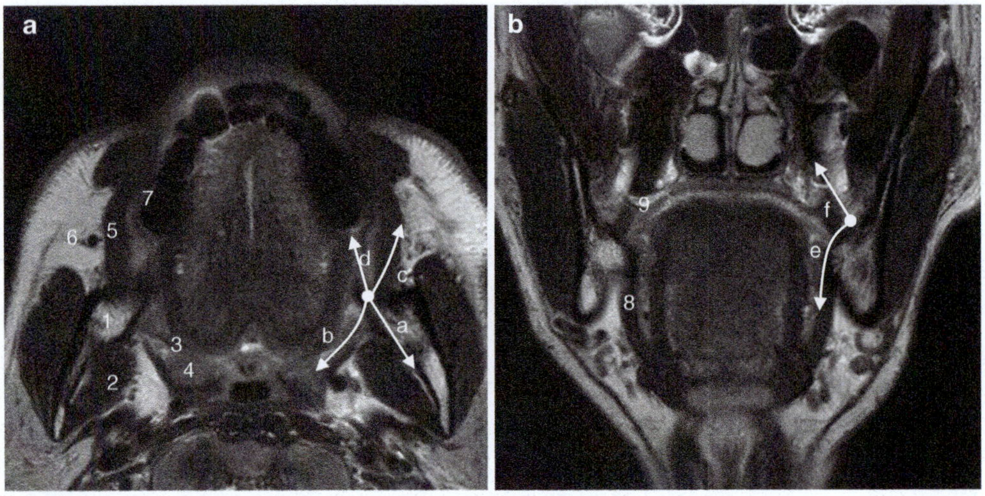

a. Posterolateral
   Direct invasion to the mandibular ramus, fat tissue in front of the mandibular ramus, or masticator space
   Invasion of the pterygoid muscle from the pterygomandibular space
   Perineural spread along the mandibular nerve
b. Posteromedial
   Direct invasion to the pterygomandibular raphe, anterior palatine arch, or pharyngeal constrictor muscle
c. Anterolateral
   Direct invasion to the buccal mucosa, buccinator muscle, or buccal fat-pad
d. Anterior
   Direct invasion to the lower gingiva
e. Medial
   Direct invasion to the oral floor or mylohyoid muscle
f. Superior
   Direct invasion to the maxillary tuberosity or upper gingiva
   Extension to the pterygoid process along the pterygomandibular raphe
   Perineural spread along the posterior superior alveolar nerve to the retro-antral fat

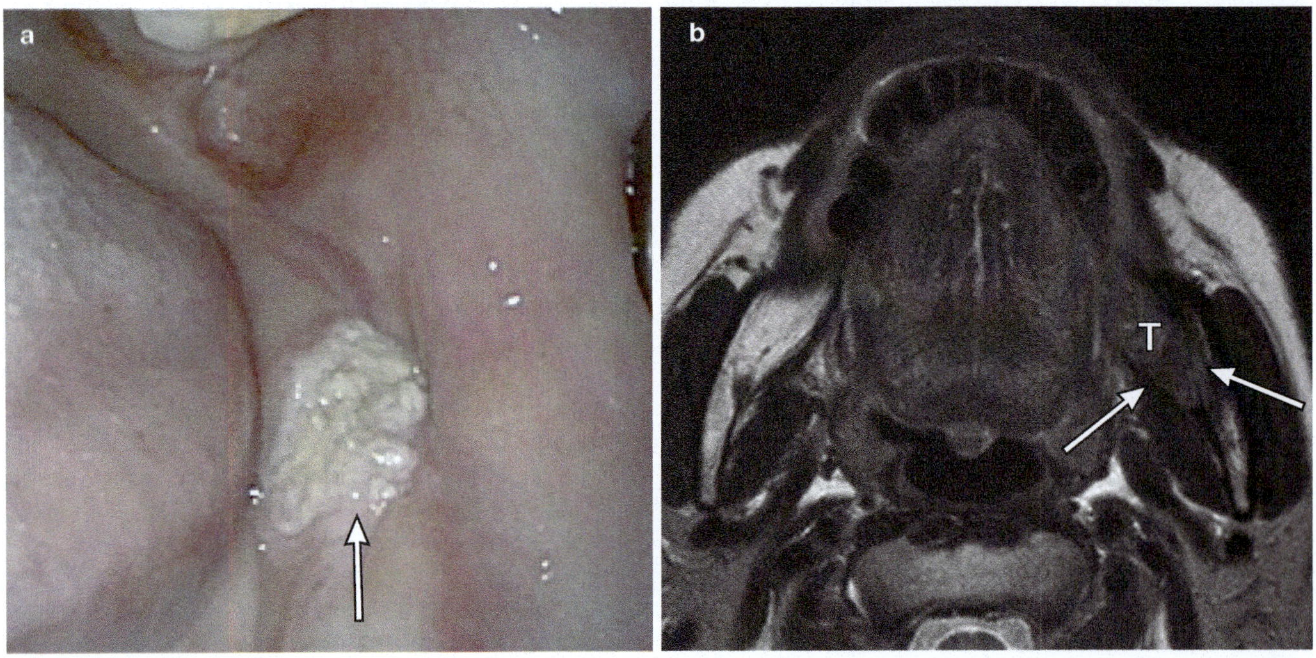

Fig. 4.14 A 71-year-old woman with squamous cell carcinoma of the retromolar area. (**a**) The tumor (T) is located at left retromolar area. (**b**) T2-weighted image shows tumor invading the mandibular ramus (arrow), which is not detected in the intraoral findings

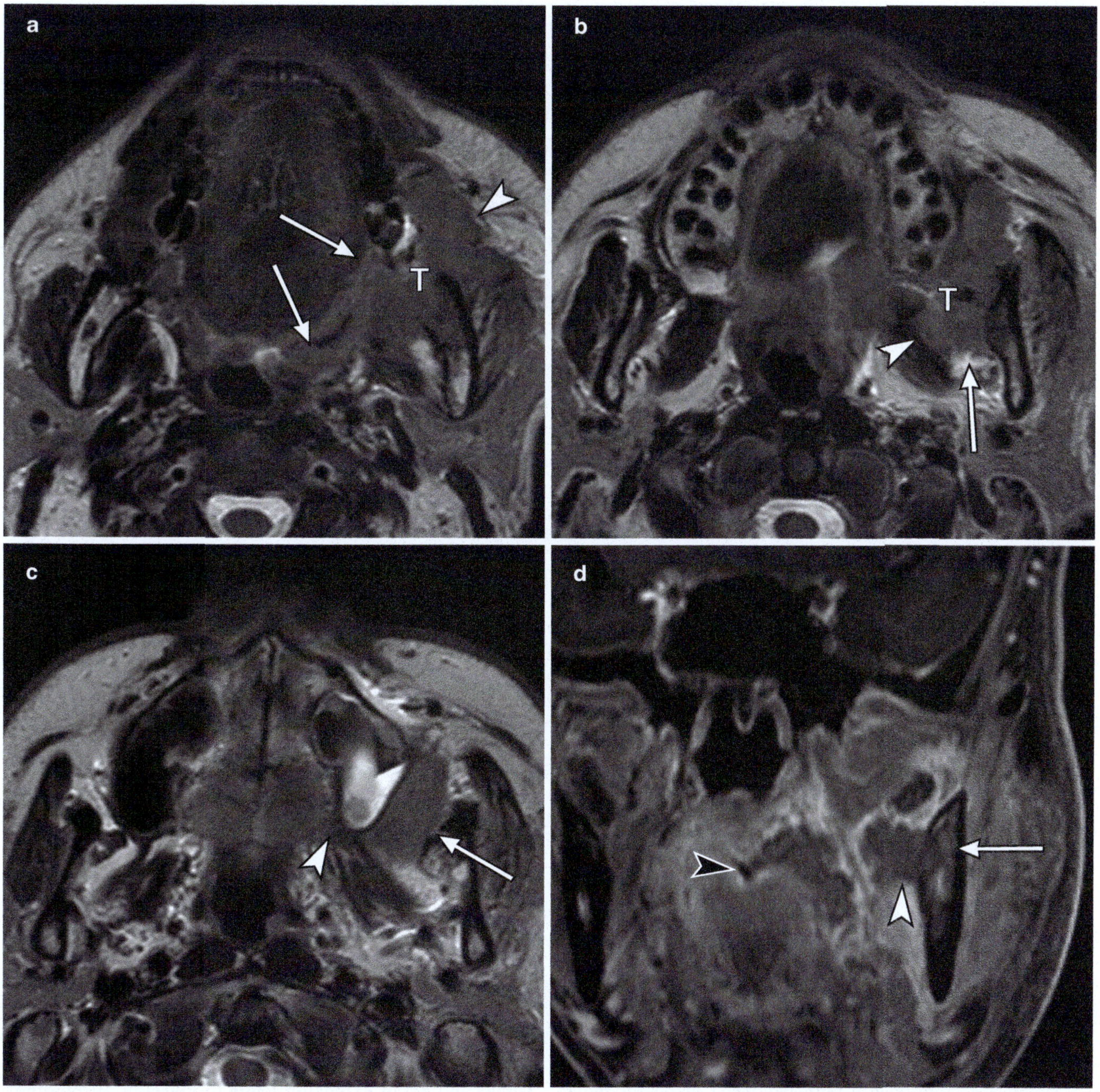

Fig. 4.15 A 55-year-old woman with squamous cell carcinoma of the retromolar area. (**a**) T2-weighted image show tumor of the retromolar trigone (T) extending to the buccinator muscle anteriorly (arrowhead), pterygomandibular raphe, constrictor muscle, and anterior palatine arch posteriorly (arrows). (**b**) The tumor (T) also invades the pterygomandibular space of the masticator space (arrow) and the medial pterygoid muscle (arrowhead) on T2-weighted image. (**c**) Tumor extends around the pterygoid plates and retroantral fat superiorly (arrowhead) on T2-weighted image. (**d**) Coronal post-enhanced T1-weighted image with fat suppression shows the tumor extends to the bone marrow of the mandible (arrow), pterygomandibular space (white arrowhead), and soft palate of the oropharynx (black arrowhead)

of mouth is classified as anterior and lateral types. Anterior type carcinoma is more common than the lateral type. It is often difficult to distinguish oral floor cancer from sublingual gland tumors on imaging analysis; however, sublingual tumor is identifiable as a submucosal lesion on clinical examination. Extension pattern of carcinoma of the oral floor and its related anatomy on MRI are shown in Fig. 4.16.

The sublingual space is located under the mucosa of the oral floor, which contains the sublingual gland and the hyoglossus muscle. Therefore, cancers of the floor of the mouth invade early into the sublingual space. Tumors may invade the genioglossus muscle, geniohyoid muscle, and hyoglossus muscle and may extend along these muscles to the mandible or the hyoid bone (Fig. 4.17). Laterally, tumors may

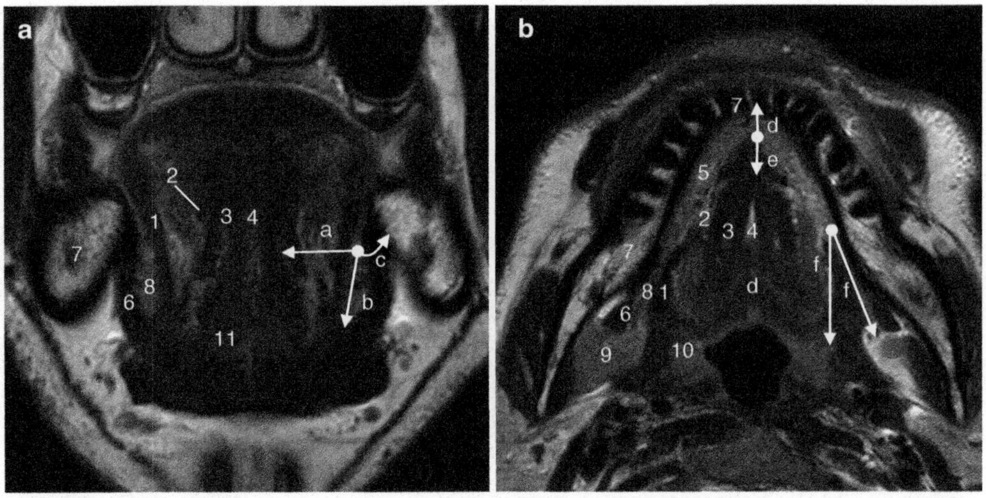

Fig. 4.16 Extension pattern of the cancer of the oral floor and related anatomy. (**a**) Coronal T2-weighted image, (**b**) Axial T2-weighted image. Extension pattern is indicated by arrows and a lower letter corresponding with the bullet. (1) hyoglossus muscle, (2) neurovascular bundle, (3) genioglossus muscle, (4) tongue septum, (5) sublingual gland, (6) mylohyoid muscle, (7) mandible, (8) glosso-mylohyoid gap, (9) submandibular gland, (10) tonsil, (11) geniohyoid muscle

a. Medial
   Direct invasion to the hyoglossus muscle, neurovascular bundle, genioglossus muscle, or lingual septum
b. Inferior
   Direct invasion to the sublingual gland, mylohyoid muscle, or neurovascular bundle
   Perineural spread along the lingual or hypoglossal nerve
c. Lateral
   Direct invasion to the mandible
   Extension along the mylohyoid muscle to the mandible
d. Anterior (anterior type)
   Direct invasion to the mandible
   Extension along the genioglossus muscle to the mandible
e. Posterior (anterior type)
   Direct invasion to the genioglossus muscle, geniohyoid muscle
f. Posterior (lateral type)
   Direct invasion to the glosso-mylohyoid gap, submandibular gland, base of tongue, and tonsils

invade the mandible from the gingival mucosa or along the mylohyoid muscle (Fig. 4.18). Posterolaterally, tumors invade the submandibular space from the glosso–mylohyoid gap and the lateral wall of oropharynx from the base of tongue or the tonsillolingual sulcus. Tumor invasion of the Wharton ducts results in obstructive submandibular sialoadenitis (Fig. 4.18b).

There is a significantly high incidence of occult metastatic disease (21%) for T1 floor of mouth tumors [25]. Anterior type cancer may metastasize to bilateral lymph nodes.

4.5.7 Buccal Mucosa

Buccal cancer may develop in any part of the buccal mucosa, but it often occurs near the buccal mucosal ridge where the upper and lower teeth meet [21, 26]. Buccal cancer includes cancer of the inner surface of the lip [4]. Extension pattern of buccal carcinoma and its related anatomy on MRI are shown in Fig. 4.19.

Buccal mucosal cancers invade the submucosal fat, buccal muscle, and/or orbicularis oris muscle and extend into the buccal fat-pad (Fig. 4.20). As it progresses, it invades the skin and the masticator space. Patients with a tumor thickness less than 6 mm may have a better survival rate [27]. Invasion of the parotid duct or its opening may result in secondary obstructive parotitis (Fig. 4.20c). Upper and lower extension leads to invasion of the gingival buccal groove and the mandible and maxilla, respectively. The confirmation of extension to the gingiva is necessary for evaluation of invasion of mandible or maxilla; however, such confirmation is difficult on imaging analysis. Puffed check technique is useful for distinction of cancers of buccal mucosa from that of gingival mucosa and makes determination of extension of cancer easier (Fig. 4.20b). Tumors also extend to the mandible or maxilla along the buccinator muscles. Skin invasion is seen in 11% of cases and bone involvement in 39.9% [28]. Cancer of the buccal mucosa may extend to the retromolar area, showing the same invasion pattern as a cancer of the retromolar trigone.

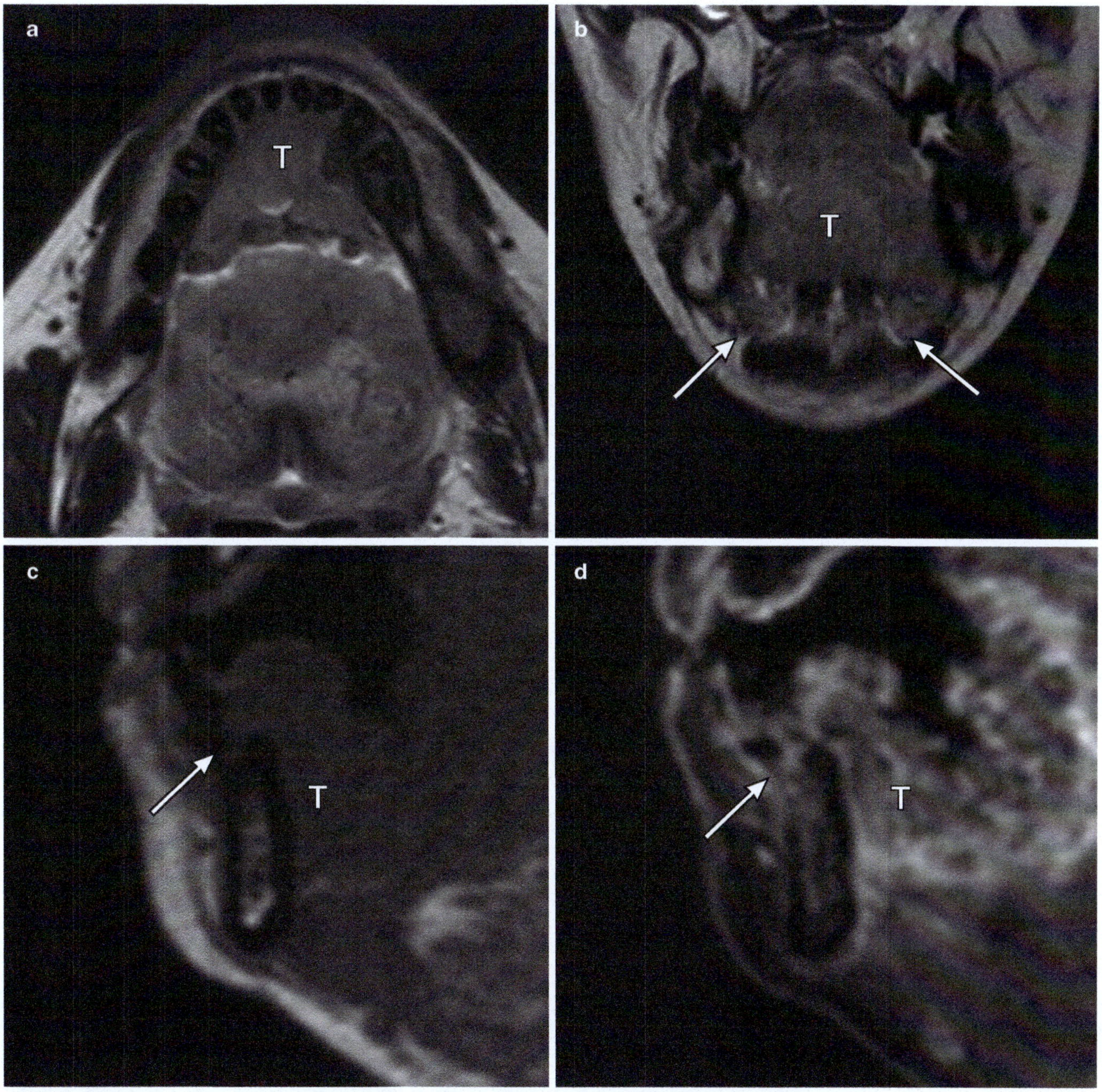

Fig. 4.17 A 55-year-old woman with squamous cell carcinoma of the oral floor (anterior type). (**a**) Axial T2-weighted image shows the tumor (T) is located anterior part of the floor of the oral cavity. (**b**) Coronal T2-weighted image shows bilateral genioglossus muscle is replaced by the tumor (T). Bilateral sublingual glands are preserved (arrow). (**d**, **e**) On the sagittal T1-weighted image and post-contrast T1-weighted image with fat suppression, the tumor (T) invades into the bone marrow of the mandible from the tooth socket (arrow)

4.5.8 Hard Palate

The hard palate forms the upper wall of the oral cavity. Its bony wall consists of the maxilla anteriorly and the palatine bone posteriorly. Hard palate has a greater and a lesser palatine foramen through which the greater and lesser palatine nerves pass. Nasopalatine foramen is located at the anterior part which transmits the nasopalatine nerve, originating from the maxillary nerve. The hard palate contains minor salivary glands which show slightly higher signal intensity on T2-weighted images. Alveolar processes are present bilaterally and are continuous with the gingival mucosa. Among the various types of hard palate cancer, the proportions of minor salivary grand malignancies such as adenoid cystic carcinoma or mucoepidermoid carcinoma are higher than that of squamous cell carcinoma [29]. Moreover, benign salivary

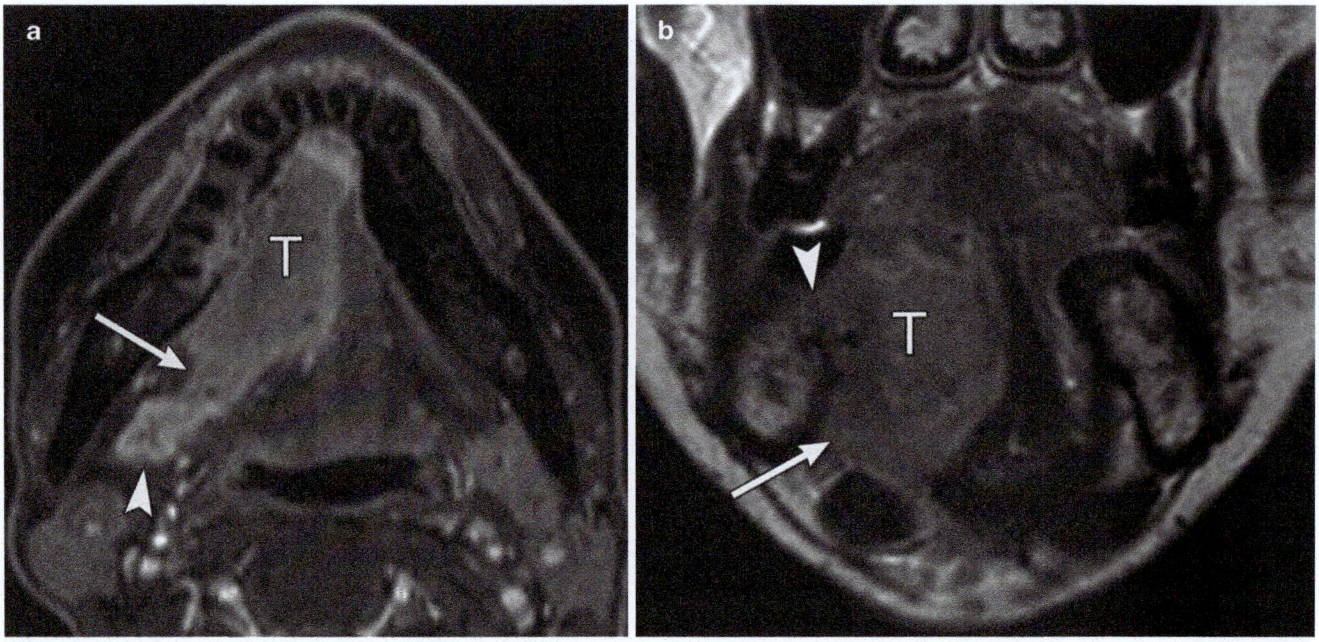

Fig. 4.18 A 61-year-old woman with squamous cell carcinoma of the oral floor (lateral type). (**a**) The tumor (T) is located at the lateral part of the floor of the oral cavity on the post-contrast T1-weighted image with fat suppression. The tumor extends to the glosso-mylohyoid gap posteriorly (arrow). The stronger enhancement of the right submandibular gland compared with the left one reveals the obstructive sialadenitis (arrowhead). (**b**) On coronal T2-weighted image, the tumor (T) invades the mylohyoid muscle (arrow) and extends to the mandible along the mylohyoid muscle (arrowhead)

Fig. 4.19 Extension pattern of the cancer of the buccal mucosa and related anatomy. (**a**) Axial T2-weighted image, (**b**) Coronal T2-weighted image. Extension pattern is indicated by arrows and a lower letter corresponding with the bullet. (1) mandibular ramus, (2) masticator space, (3) submucosal fat, (4) buccinator muscle, (5) buccal fat-pad, (6) lower gingivobuccal sulcus, (7) mandible, (8) upper gingivobuccal sulcus, (9) alveolar process, and (10) maxillary sinus

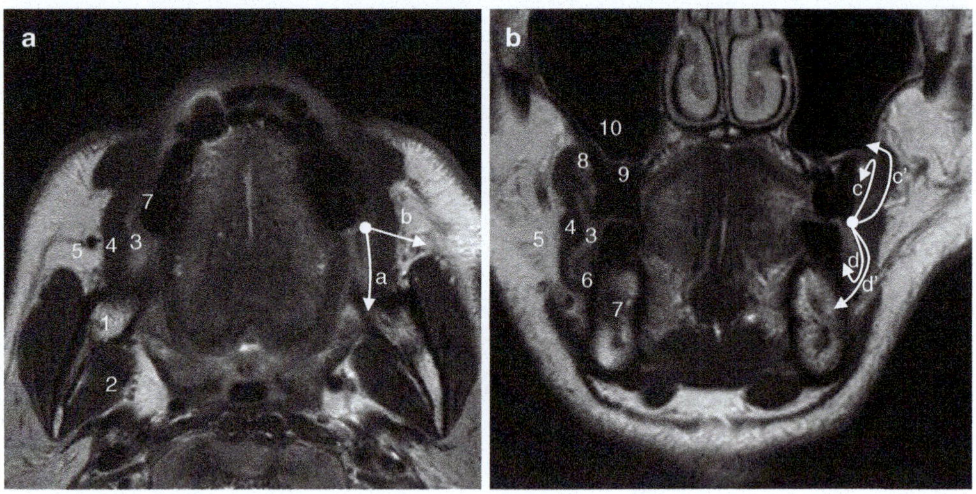

a. Posterior
   Direct extension to the retromolar area and invasion of the mandibular ramus, pterygomandibular raphe, or masticator space
   Extension to the infratemporal fossa from buccal space
b. Lateral
   Direct invasion to the submucosal fat, buccinator muscle, buccal fat-pad, parotid duct, or skin
c. Superior
   Direct invasion to the upper gingivobuccal sulcus, upper gingiva, or maxilla
   Extension along the buccinator muscle to the maxilla (c')
d. Inferior
   Direct invasion to the upper gingivobuccal sulcus, lower gingiva, or mandible
   Extension along the buccinator muscle to the mandible (d')

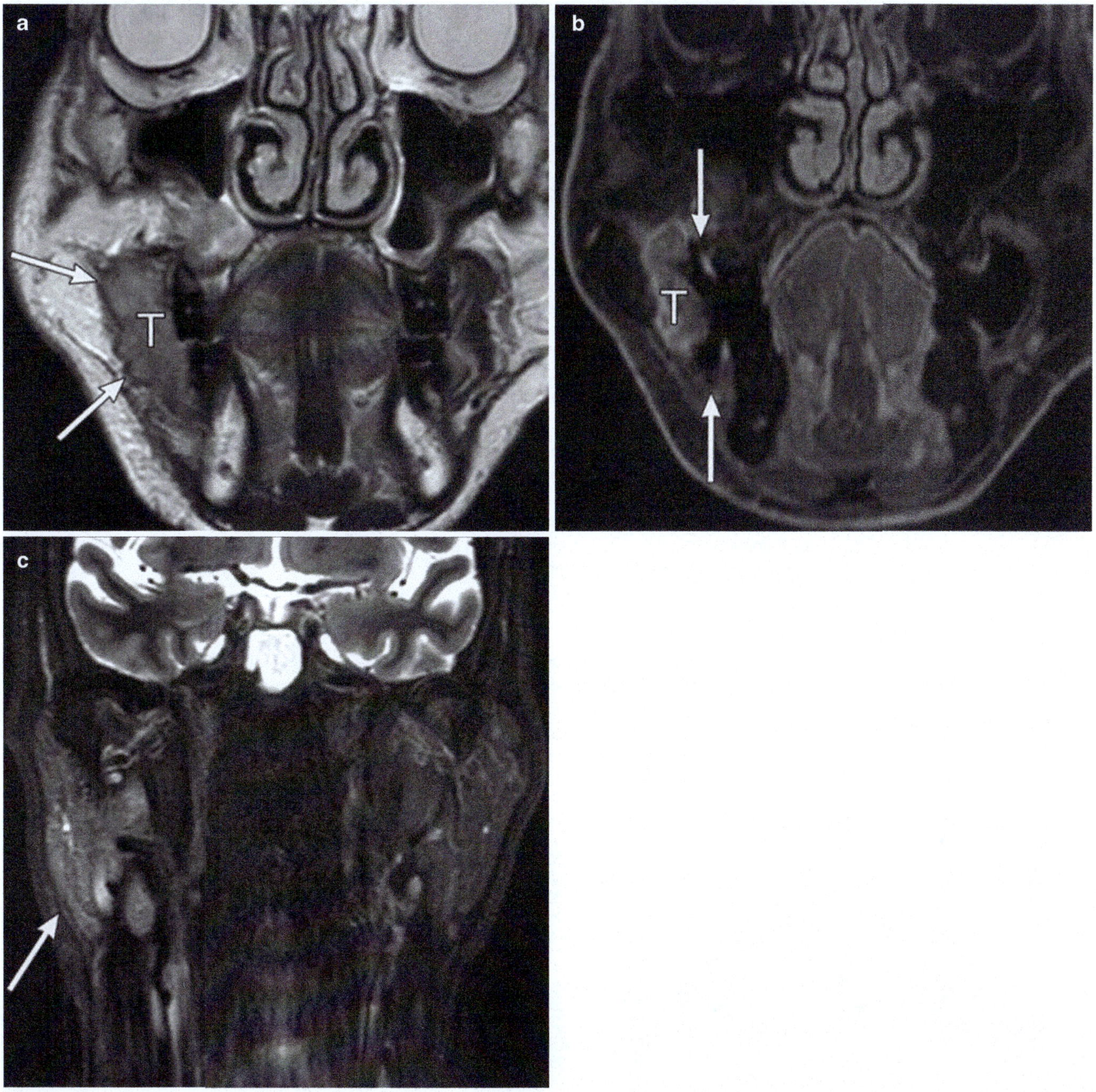

Fig. 4.20 A 60-year-old woman with squamous cell carcinoma of the buccal mucosa. (**a**) Coronal T2-weighted image shows the tumor (T) invading submucosal fat and buccinator muscle but does not extend to the buccal fat (arrow). (**b**) Post-enhanced T1-weighted image with puffed cheek technique shows the tumor does not extends to the upper and lower gingivobuccal sulcus (arrow). (**c**) STIR image shows secondary parotitis (arrow) due to invasion of the parotid duct

gland tumors, such as pleomorphic adenoma, may also occur. Extension pattern of carcinoma of the hard palate and its related anatomy on MRI are shown in Fig. 4.21.

Carcinoma of hard plate invades the bone of hard palate superiorly and may extend to the nasal cavity and the maxillary sinus (Fig. 4.22). Laterally, it invades the gingival and alveolar processes; in this scenario, evaluation of extent of bone marrow invasion becomes necessary. Cancers may extend along the greater and lesser palatine nerves from the palatine foramen to the pterygopalatine fossa (Fig. 4.23). Perineural spread is visualized as an enlarged foramen and fat obliteration of the pterygopalatine fossa. Posterolaterally, tumors extend to the maxillary tuberosity, the pterygoid process, and pterygoid muscles. The posterior part of the hard palate is continuous with the soft palate, which belongs to the oropharynx.

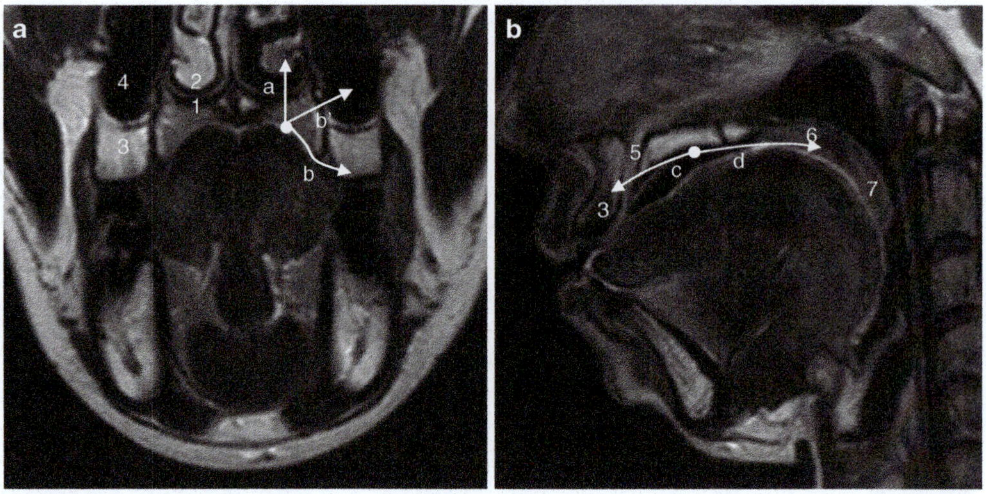

Fig. 4.21 Extension pattern of the cancer of the hard plate and related anatomy. (**a**) Coronal T2-weighted image, (**b**) Sagittal T2-weighted image. Extension pattern is indicated by arrows and a lower letter corresponding with the bullet. (1) hard plate, (2) nasal cavity, (3) alveolar process, (4) maxillary sinus, (5) nasopalatine canal, (6) soft palatine, (7) uvula

a. Superior
   Direct invasion of the hard palate, floor of the nasal cavity, or greater and lesser palatine nerves
   Perineural spread along the maxillary nerve
b. Lateral
   Direct invasion of the upper gingiva, alveolar process, maxillary tuberosity, or maxillary sinus (b')
c. Anterior
   Direct invasion of the nasopalatine canal, upper gingiva, or alveolar process
d. Posterior
   Direct invasion of the soft palate, uvula, pterygoid process, pterygopalatine fossa, or masticator space

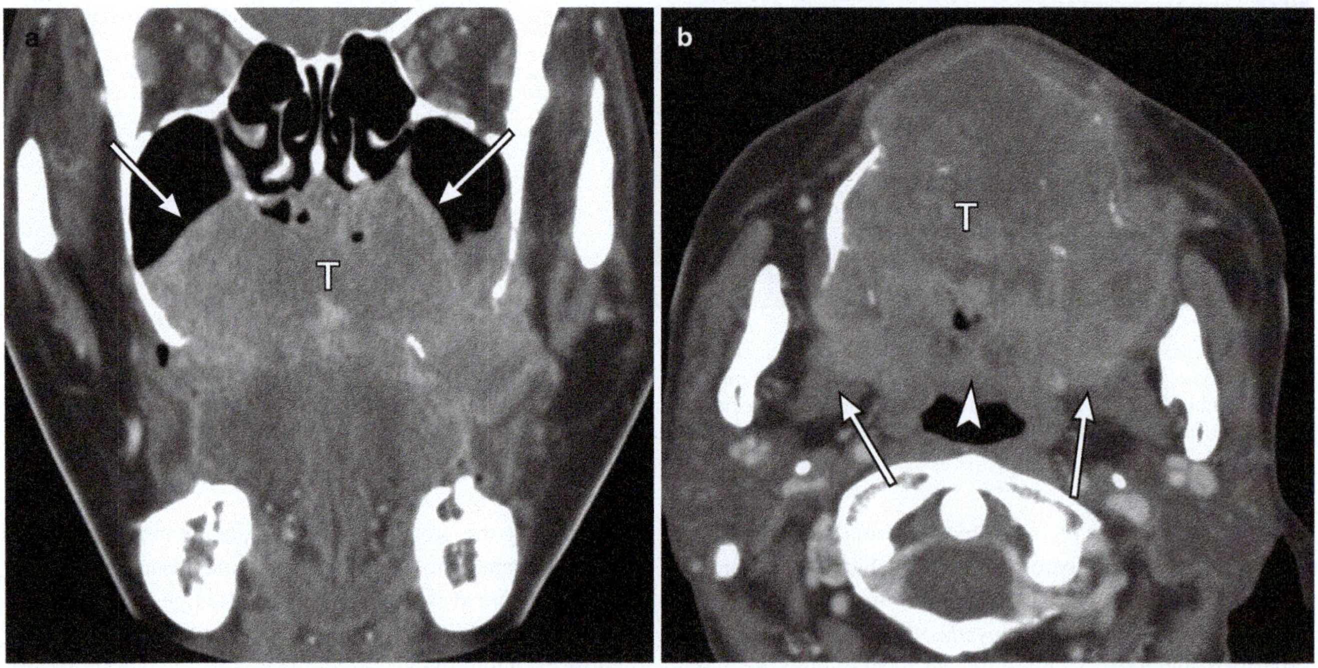

Fig. 4.22 A 57-year-old woman with squamous cell carcinoma of the hard plate. (**a**) Coronal contrast-enhanced CT shows the tumor (T) invading the bilateral nasal cavity and maxillary sinus superiorly (arrow). (**b**) Axial contrast-enhanced CT shows that the tumor (T) replaces the maxillary process and invades the bilateral pterygoid process and medial pterygoid muscles posteriorly (arrow). The tumor extends to the soft palate (arrowhead)

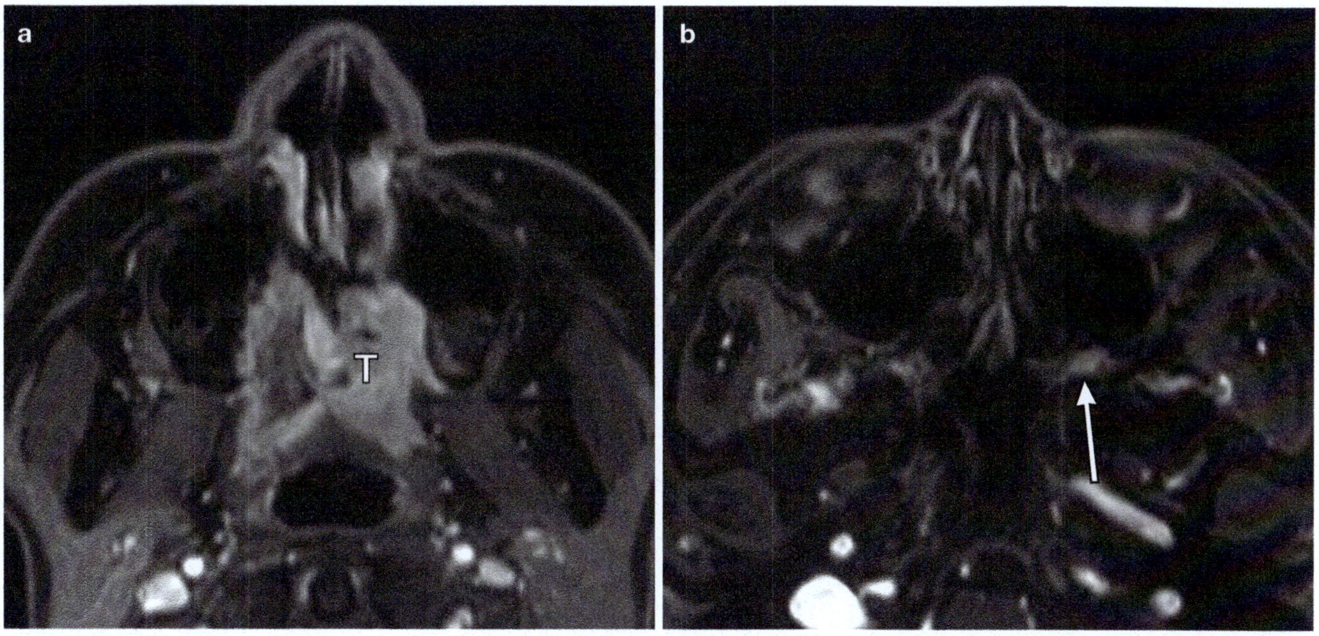

Fig. 4.23 A 57-year-old woman with adenoid cystic carcinoma of the hard plate. (**a**, **b**) On post-enhanced T1-weighted image with fat suppression, the tumor (T) in the left hard plate spread to the left pterygopalatine fossa along the second division of the trigeminal nerve (arrow)

4.5.9 Lymph Node Metastasis

Lymph node metastases occur in about 40% of patients with oral cancer [30]. Clinical manifestation is hidden in 15–34% of cases. Oral cancer has a tendency to spread to levels I and II. However, the lower nodal stations may be involved (levels III or IV) without involvement of Level II (skip metastasis), especially in tongue cancer [31]. Lymph nodes which are less frequently involved but are nevertheless significant includes the lateral and medial lingual nodes, mandibular nodes, buccinator lymph node, and the retropharyngeal lymph nodes [21] (Fig. 4.24).

According to the AJCC 8th edition, clinical ENE is classified as N3b. Definition of clinical ENE is unquestionable ENE by physical examination which is supported by radiological evidence. In oral cancer, Level I lymph node metastasis may invade the mandible, submandibular gland, mylohyoid muscle, and platysma (Fig. 4.24d). Level IIA lymph nodes may invade the carotid artery, deep layer of deep cervical fascia, submandibular gland, and hypoglossal nerve.

4.6 Imaging of Post-treatment Change, Complication, and Recurrence

4.6.1 Post-treatment Change

When surgery is performed without reconstruction, the surgical defect is seen on imaging. Edema which is visualized as hyperintensity on T2WI is observed during the early postoperative phase. Fibrosis progresses in about 6 months, and reduced signal intensity on T2-weighted images and weakened contrast enhancement is observed with progressing time. After surgery with reconstruction, myocutaneous flap is visible at site of surgical defect (Fig. 4.25a). Enhancement at the site of anastomosis of surgical flaps can be seen over a long period [32]. Atrophy of the muscle in the transplanted flap with fatty infiltration may be seen.

After radiotherapy, thickening of the skin and the platysma muscle, reticulation of the fat tissue, and increased enhancement of the major salivary glands may be seen on imaging [33]. These post-treatment changes become stable at approximately 6–8 weeks.

4.6.2 Complications

Early surgical complications are abscess and fistula formation (Fig. 4.25). Mandibular osteoradionecrosis is a late complication. The imaging findings of mandibular osteoradionecrosis include cortical interruptions, bone absorption, bone sequestration, pathological fractures, soft tissue swellings, and fistula formation [33]. Radiologically, the diagnosis of tumor recurrence may sometimes be difficult.

4.6.3 Recurrence

Recurrence of superficial lesions can be confirmed clinically, but recurrence at deep locations may be identified only radiologically. Recurrence is likely to occur at limits of

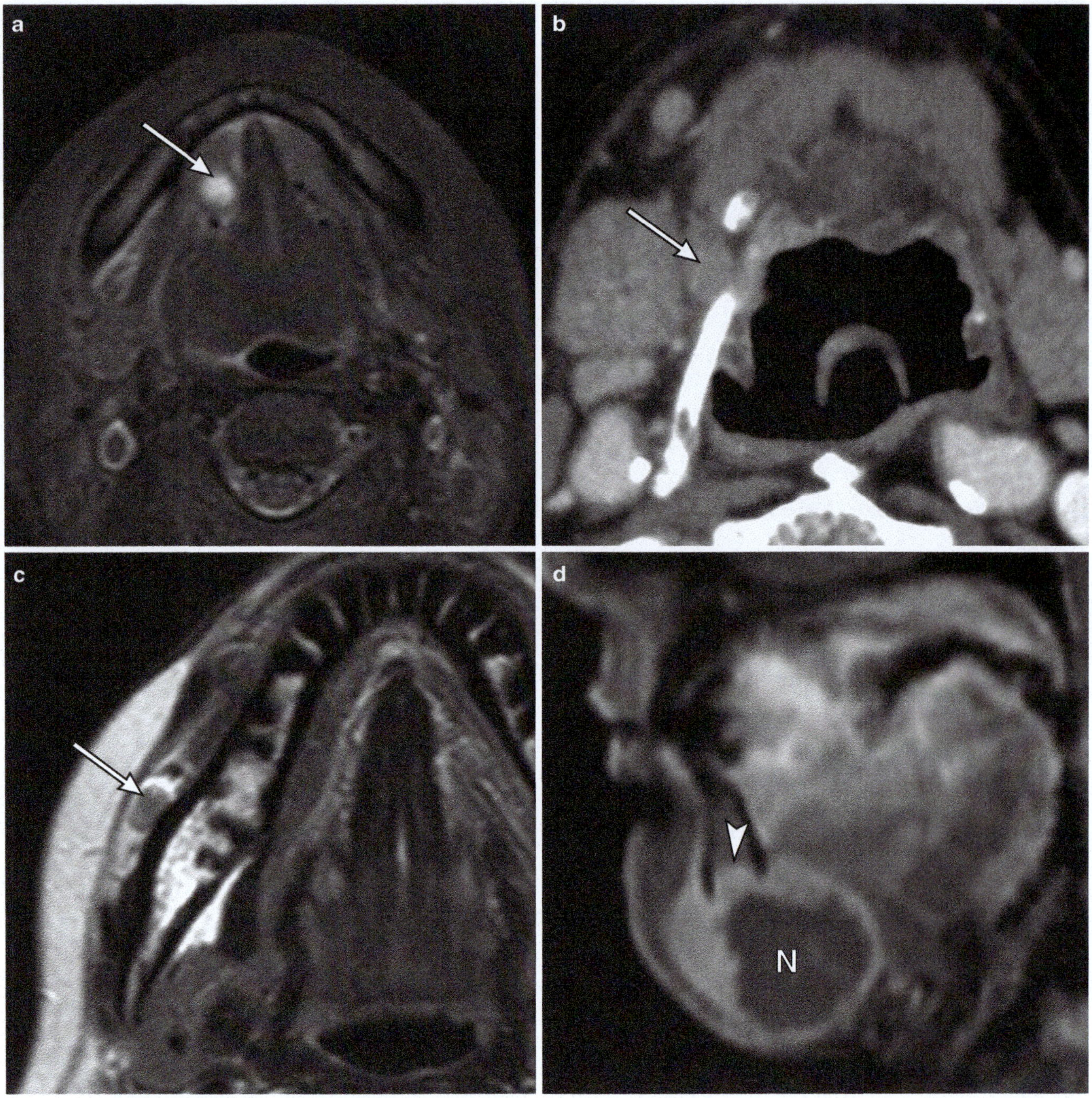

Fig. 4.24 Example cases of lymph node metastasis. (**a**) Right lateral lingual lymph node metastasis (arrow) from tongue cancer is seen on the STIR image. (**b**) Contrast-enhanced CT shows right para-hypoid lymph node metastasis (arrow). (**c**) T2-weighted image shows mandibular node metastasis (arrow) from buccal cancer. Nodal metastasis was pathologically proven. (**d**) Nodal metastasis (N) invading into the mandibular bone (arrow) is classified as clinical N3b with physical findings

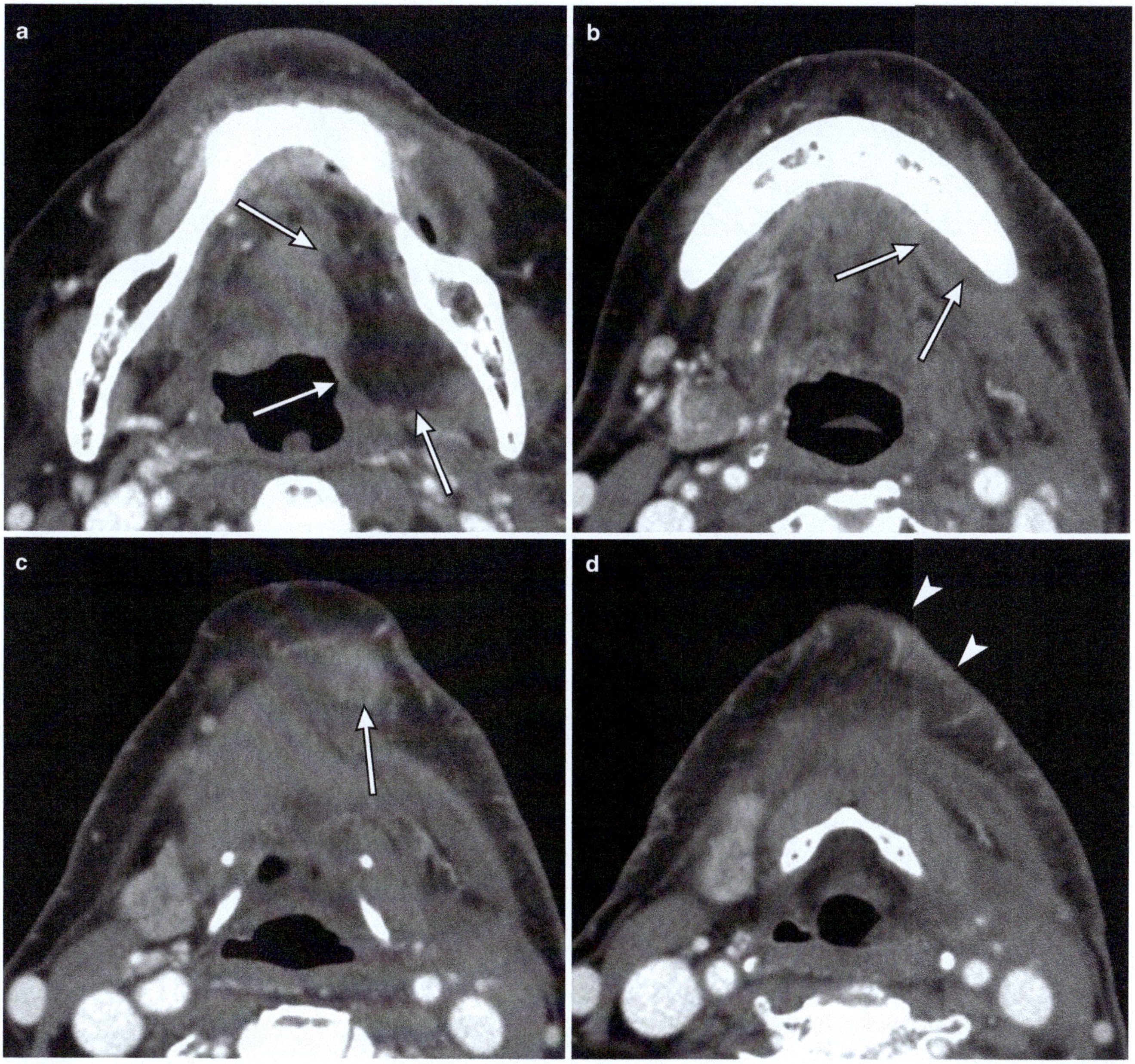

Fig. 4.25 Post-operative image of a 73-year-old woman with tongue cancer, complaining of discharge of pus at the submental region. (**a**) Contrast-enhanced CT image shows fat tissue on the left side of the oral cavity due to reconstruction (arrow). (**b**) A small amount of fluid collection is seen along the inner surface of the mandible (arrow) on the contrast-enhanced CT image. (**c**, **d**) Fistula formation (arrow) and skin swelling (arrow head) are seen on contrast-enhanced CT images

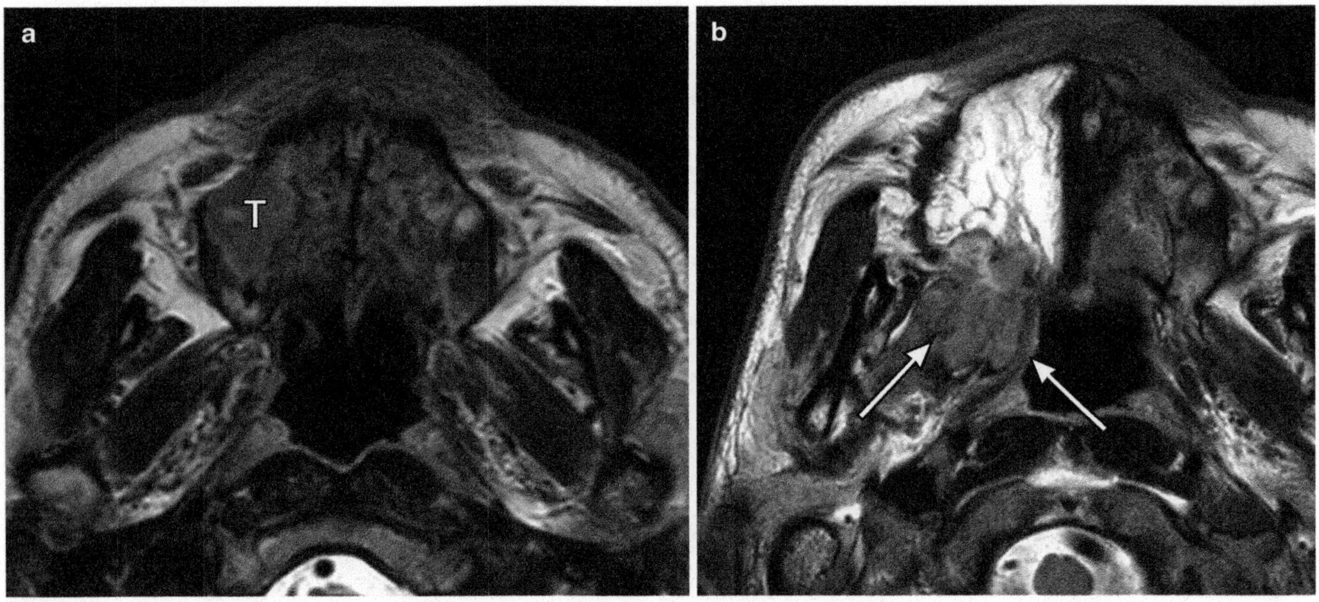

Fig. 4.26 A 78-year-old man with a recurrence of upper gingival squamous cell carcinoma. (**a**) Upper gingival cancer (T) is seen on the preoperative T2-weighted image. (**b**) Routine follow-up MRI after surgery shows mass formation with hyperintensity on the T2-weighted image at the deep margin of the reconstructed fat tissue (arrow)

the surgical margins (oral base, extrinsic lingual muscles, mandible, perineural region, or lingual base) and at the edges of the surgical flaps (Fig. 4.26) [34]. In addition, when new symptoms, such as ear aches, occur, they may be caused by referred otalgia due to local recurrence, and in these cases, careful radiological evaluation is necessary [35]. The primary finding of recurrence on CT is a soft tissue mass with contrast enhancement. The main findings of recurrence on MRI is soft tissue mass with high signal intensity on T2-weighted images, intermediate intensity on T1-weighted images, and contrast enhancement [32]. The apparent diffusion coefficient values may be useful for differentiation of recurrent tumors from post-treatment changes [36].

References

1. Ferlay J, Soerjomataram I, Ervik M, Dikshit R, Eser S, Mathers C. GLOBOCAN 2012 v1.0, Cancer Incidence and monality worldwide: IARC Cancer Base No. 11. Lyon: IARC, World Health Organ; 2012.
2. Sloan P, Gale N, Hunter K, Lingen M, Nylander K, Reibel J, et al. Tumour of the oral cavity and mobile tongue. In: Swerdlow SH, editor. WHO classification of tumours of haematopoietic and lymphoid tissues (World Health Organ Classification of Tumours). 4th ed. Lyon: International Agency for Research on Cancer; 2017. p. 105–31.
3. Kumar M, Nanavati R, Modi T, Dobariya C. Oral cancer: etiology and risk factors: a review. J Cancer Res Ther. 2016;12(2):458.
4. Amin MB, Edge SB. In: Amin MB, editor. AJCC Cancer Staging Manual. 8th ed. New York: Springer; 2017.
5. Ebrahimi A, Gil Z, Amit M, Yen T-C, Liao C-T, Chaturvedi P, et al. Primary tumor staging for oral cancer and a proposed modification incorporating depth of invasion: an international multicenter retrospective study. JAMA Otolaryngol Head Neck Surg. 2014;140(12):1138–48.
6. Huang SH, Hwang D, Lockwood G, Goldstein DP, O'Sullivan B. Predictive value of tumor thickness for cervical lymph-node involvement in squamous cell carcinoma of the oral cavity: a meta-analysis of reported studies. Cancer. 2009;115(7):1489–97.
7. De Crop A, Casselman J, Van Hoof T, Dierens M, Vereecke E, Bossu N, et al. Analysis of metal artifact reduction tools for dental hardware in CT scans of the oral cavity: kVp, iterative reconstruction, dual-energy CT, metal artifact reduction software: does it make a difference? Neuroradiology. 2015;57(8):841–9.
8. Hakim A, Slotboom J, Lieger O, Schlittler F, Giger R, Michel C, et al. Clinical evaluation of the iterative metal artefact reduction algorithm for post-operative CT examination after maxillofacial surgery. Dentomaxillofac Radiol. 2017;46(4):20160355.
9. Hirata K, Utsunomiya D, Oda S, Kidoh M, Funama Y, Yuki H, et al. Added value of a single-energy projection-based metal-artifact reduction algorithm for the computed tomography evaluation of oral cavity cancers. Jpn J Radiol. 2015;33(10):650–6.
10. Fagelman D, Huang AB. Prospective evaluation of lesions of the mandible and maxilla: findings on multiplanar and three-dimensional CT. Am J Roentgenol. 1994;163(3):693–8.
11. Suzuki N, Kuribayashi A, Sakamoto K, Sakamoto J, Nakamura S, Watanabe H, et al. Diagnostic abilities of 3T MRI for assessing mandibular invasion of squamous cell carcinoma in the oral cavity: comparison with 64-row multidetector CT. Dentomaxillofac Radiol. 2019;48(4):20180311.
12. Zitsch RP, Park CW, Renner GJ, Rea JL. Outcome analysis for lip carcinoma. Otolaryngol Head Neck Surg. 1995;113(5):589–96.
13. Coppit GL, Lin DT, Burkey BB. Current concepts in lip reconstruction. Curr Opin Otolaryngol Head Neck Surg. 2004;12(4):281–7.
14. Murakami R, Shiraishi S, Yoshida R, Sakata J, Yamana K, Hirosue A, et al. Reliability of MRI-derived depth of invasion of oral tongue cancer. Acad Radiol. 2019;26(7):e180–6.
15. Park J-O, Jung S-L, Joo Y-H, Jung C-K, Cho K-J, Kim M-S. Diagnostic accuracy of magnetic resonance imaging (MRI)

in the assessment of tumor invasion depth in oral/oropharyngeal cancer. Oral Oncol. 2011;47(5):381–6.

16. Mukherji SK, Weeks SM, Castillo M, Yankaskas BC, Krishnan LA, Schiro S. Squamous cell carcinomas that arise in the oral cavity and tongue base: can CT help predict perineural or vascular invasion? Radiology. 1996;198(1):157–62.
17. Suzuki K, Shingaki S, Nomura T, Nakajima T. Oral carcinomas detected after extraction of teeth: a clinical and radiographic analysis of 32 cases with special reference to metastasis and survival. Int J Oral Maxillofac Surg. 1998;27(4):290–4.
18. Tsue TT, McCulloch TM, Girod DA, Couper DJ, Weymuller EAJ, Glenn MG. Predictors of carcinomatous invasion of the mandible. Head Neck. 1994;16(2):116–26.
19. Ebrahimi A, Murali R, Gao K, Elliott MS, Clark JR. The prognostic and staging implications of bone invasion in oral squamous cell carcinoma. Cancer. 2011;117(19):4460–7.
20. Li C, Yang W, Men Y, Wu F, Pan J, Li L. Magnetic resonance imaging for diagnosis of mandibular involvement from head and neck cancers: a systematic review and meta-analysis. PLoS One. 2014;9(11):e112267.
21. Kimura Y. Oral cavity. In: Sakai O, Ojiri H, editors. CT MRI head neck. 3rd ed. Tokyo: Medical Science International; 2019. p. 465–510.
22. Monteiro M. Face and scalp. In: Standring S, editor. Gray's anatomy. 40th ed. Amsterdam: Elsevier; 2008. p. 467–98.
23. Arya S, Rane P, Sable N, Juvekar S, Bal M, Chaukar D. Retromolar trigone squamous cell cancers: a reappraisal of 16 section MDCT for assessing mandibular invasion. Clin Radiol. 2013;68(12):e680–8.
24. La'porte SJ, Juttla JK, Lingam RK. Imaging the floor of the mouth and the sublingual space. Radiographics. 2011;31(5):1215–30.
25. Hicks WLJ, Loree TR, Garcia RI, Maamoun S, Marshall D, Orner JB, et al. Squamous cell carcinoma of the floor of mouth: a 20-year review. Head Neck. 1997;19(5):400–5.
26. Ojiri H. Oral cavity. In: Ojiri H, editor. Head neck imaging. 3rd ed. Tokyo: Nankodo; 2016. p. 189–242.
27. Urist MM, O'Brien CJ, Soong SJ, Visscher DW, Maddox WA. Squamous cell carcinoma of the buccal mucosa: analysis of prognostic factors. Am J Surg. 1987;154(4):411–4.
28. Bobdey S, Sathwara J, Jain A, Saoba S, Balasubramaniam G. Squamous cell carcinoma of buccal mucosa: an analysis of prognostic factors. South Asian J Cancer. 2018;7(1):49–54.
29. Aydil U, Kızıl Y, Bakkal FK, Köybaşıoğlu A, Uslu S. Neoplasms of the hard palate. J Oral Maxillofac Surg. 2014;72(3):619–26.
30. Noguti J, De Moura CFG, De Jesus GPP, Da Silva VHP, Hossaka TA, Oshima CTF, et al. Metastasis from oral cancer: an overview. Cancer Genomics Proteomics. 2012;9(5):329–35.
31. Patel S, Sakthivel P, Singh I, Gulati A, Gupta D. Frequency of skip metastases in oral cancer: an overview. Int J Head Neck Surg. 2016;6:80–5.
32. Lell M, Baum U, Greess H, Nomayr A, Nkenke E, Koester M, et al. Head and neck tumors: imaging recurrent tumor and post-therapeutic changes with CT and MRI. Eur J Radiol. 2000;33(3):239–47.
33. Hermans R. Posttreatment imaging in head and neck cancer. Eur J Radiol. 2008;66(3):501–11.
34. Som PM, Urken ML, Biller H, Lidov M. Imaging the postoperative neck. Radiology. 1993;187(3):593–603.
35. Hiyama T, Sekiya K, Kuno H, Oda S, Kusumoto M, Minami M, et al. Imaging of extracranial head and neck lesions in cancer patients: a symptom-based approach. Jpn J Radiol. 2019;37(5):354–70.
36. Hwang I, Choi SH, Kim Y-J, Kim KG, Lee AL, Yun TJ, et al. Differentiation of recurrent tumor and posttreatment changes in head and neck squamous cell carcinoma: application of high b-value diffusion-weighted imaging. Am J Neuroradiol. 2013;34(12):2343–8.

Diagnostic Imaging of Laryngeal and Hypopharyngeal Cancers

5

Hirofumi Kuno

Abstract

Laryngeal and hypopharyngeal cancers need to be precisely evaluated as treatment can have a substantial impact on patients' quality of life. Treatment strategies are determined based on each primary site, subsite, and degree of local tumor spreading, taking into consideration the curability and predicted functional prognosis. Imaging plays a crucial role in the staging of laryngeal and hypopharyngeal cancers, particularly when distinguishing the absence or presence of laryngeal cartilage invasion by the tumor and extralaryngeal spread. To define the optimal treatment strategies, a thorough understanding of the tumor spreading patterns with related anatomies, imaging technique including the potential applications, limitations, and advantages of existing and evolving imaging technologies is necessary. In this chapter, we present a concise overview of imaging procedures for staging and common tumor spreading patterns of laryngeal and hypopharyngeal cancers in each subsite. We also discuss imaging findings of posttreatment changes, treatment complications, and recurrence.

Keywords

Larynx · Hypopharynx · Squamous cell carcinoma · TNM · MRI · CT · PET

5.1 Introduction

Laryngeal and hypopharyngeal cancers are common malignant tumors in the head and neck. Most of these cases are squamous cell carcinomas (SCCs). The hypopharynx and larynx are organs essential for the functions necessary to maintain life, such as breathing and eating, and also for vocalizations which are important for sociality. Therefore, laryngeal and hypopharyngeal cancers need to be precisely evaluated as treatment can have a substantial impact on patients' quality of life.

Accurate staging of laryngeal and hypopharyngeal cancer requires imaging modalities such as computed tomography (CT) and magnetic resonance imaging (MRI). As with other early laryngeal and hypopharyngeal lesions, T1 and T2 lesions are often best staged with endoscopy. The role of imaging is to determine cranial, caudal, and deep extension and staging. In view of the functional and social importance of the larynx, any decision on the optimal management strategy for laryngeal or hypopharyngeal cancer must involve consideration of both potential survival and functional consequences of any given treatment approach. Since treatment is selected based on the precise recognition of extent and invasion pattern of a tumor, imaging plays a crucial role in any multidisciplinary approach for management of laryngeal and hypopharyngeal cancers. Clinical information including endoscopic findings given by clinicians supports imaging diagnosis. As such, collaboration among radiologists, surgeons, and radiation oncologists is important.

5.2 Epidemiology

More than 95% of the malignancies that arise in laryngeal and hypopharyngeal carcinomas are SCCs and are closely associated with tobacco and alcohol. Men are affected 5–10 times more frequently than women, and incidence increases with advancing age, with median age at diagnosis of 65 years [1, 2]. The patient population is similar to that affected by lung cancer and increased incidence in patients of low socioeconomic status. Other risk factors for laryngeal carcinoma include passive tobacco smoke exposure, occupational exposure to chemical irritants, chronic irritation caused by reflux, and viral exposure.

H. Kuno (✉)
Department of Diagnostic Radiology, National Cancer Center Hospital East, Kashiwa, Chiba, Japan

H. Ojiri (ed.), *Diagnostic Imaging in Head and Neck Cancer*, https://doi.org/10.1007/978-981-15-3188-0_5

5.3 Anatomy

The larynx and hypopharynx have closely interrelated anatomy. The structure of the "laryngeal box" consists of the epiglottis, thyroid cartilage, cricoid cartilage, and arytenoid cartilage (Fig. 5.1). The hyoid bone is part of the laryngeal skeleton. The "laryngeal box" is immediately anterior to the hypopharynx, forming the anterior wall of the hypopharynx. The larynx bulges into the anterior aspect of the hypopharynx, and boundaries of the hypopharynx are described as laryngeal subsites. Posteriorly, the larynx is separated from the hypopharynx by the aryepiglottic folds (Fig. 5.2). Figure 5.3 shows an image dissection of laryngoscopy and endoscopy. Laryngoscopy and endoscopy are usually inverted vertically and horizontally. Radiologists should understand both fiber imaging and cross-sectional imaging.

The hypopharynx is the portion of the aerodigestive tract between the oropharynx (superior) and proximal cervical esophagus (inferior). The superior boundary lies in a plane at the hyoid bone level, and the inferior boundary is the lower border of the cricoid cartilage. Immediately posterior and deep to the hypopharynx is the retropharyngeal space.

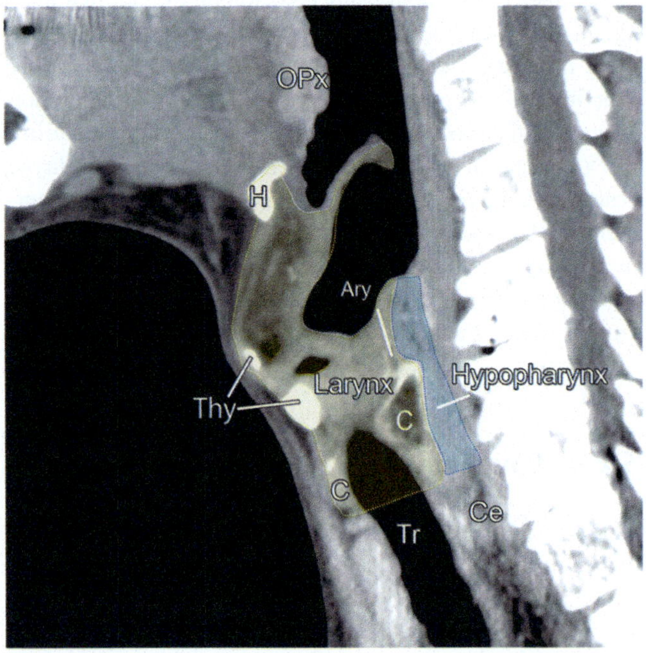

Fig. 5.1 Overview of the anatomy of the larynx and hypopharynx. Laryngeal box (yellow) and hypopharynx (blue). The "laryngeal box" is immediately anterior to the hypopharynx, forming the anterior wall of the hypopharynx. *Thy* thyroid cartilage, *C* cricoid cartilage, *Ary* arytenoid cartilage, *H* hyoid bone, *Ce* cervical esophagus, *Tr* trachea

5.3.1 Anatomy of the Larynx

The superior border of the larynx is the free edge of the epiglottis, dividing it from the oropharynx. The inferior extent is the lower border of the cricoid cartilage (Fig. 5.1). The larynx is divided into supraglottic, glottic, and subglottic subsites (Figs. 5.2 and 5.3).

1. The supraglottic larynx can be subdivided into suprahyoid and infrahyoid regions, divided by the hyoid bone. The supraglottic larynx includes the epiglottis (suprahyoid and infrahyoid components), aryepiglottic folds, arytenoids, and false vocal cords. The lateral aspect of the aryepiglottic folds forms the medial wall of the pyriform sinus.
2. The glottic larynx is composed of the true vocal folds, extending from the apex of the lateral ventricle (the inferior boundary of the supraglottic larynx and superior margin of the true vocal fold) to the inferior margin of the true vocal folds. The glottis comprises an area 1 cm in height, extending caudal to the plane of the mid-ventricle. The subsites of the glottic larynx include the anterior and posterior commissures and the right and left true vocal cords. The thyroarytenoid muscle also forms the vocalis muscle medially. The anterior commissure is the site of attachment of the vocal ligaments to the thyroid cartilage via the anterior commissure tendon (Broyles ligament). The posterior commissure is the posterior space between the vocal cords, at the vocal process of each arytenoid cartilage.
3. The subglottic larynx extends from the inferior margin of the true vocal cord (approximately 1 cm below the laryngeal ventricle anteriorly), through the inferior border of the cricoid cartilage. On axial cross-sectional imaging, the immediate subglottic mucosa is usually smooth, thin, and symmetric, without any significant soft tissue between the cricoid cartilage and air column. Any abnormal soft tissue in the subglottic lumen should raise the possibility of tumor extension. Subglottic tumors are difficult to assess endoscopically. Detection by radiologists is important, as it will impact treatment planning and prognosis.

5.3.2 Anatomy of Hypopharynx

The hypopharynx is the portion of the pharynx extending from the plane of the superior border of the hyoid bone (or vallecula) to the plane corresponding to the lower border of the cricoid cartilage. The hypopharynx is divided into the pyriform sinuses (right and left), posterior hypopharyngeal walls, and postcricoid region (Figs. 5.2 and 5.3).

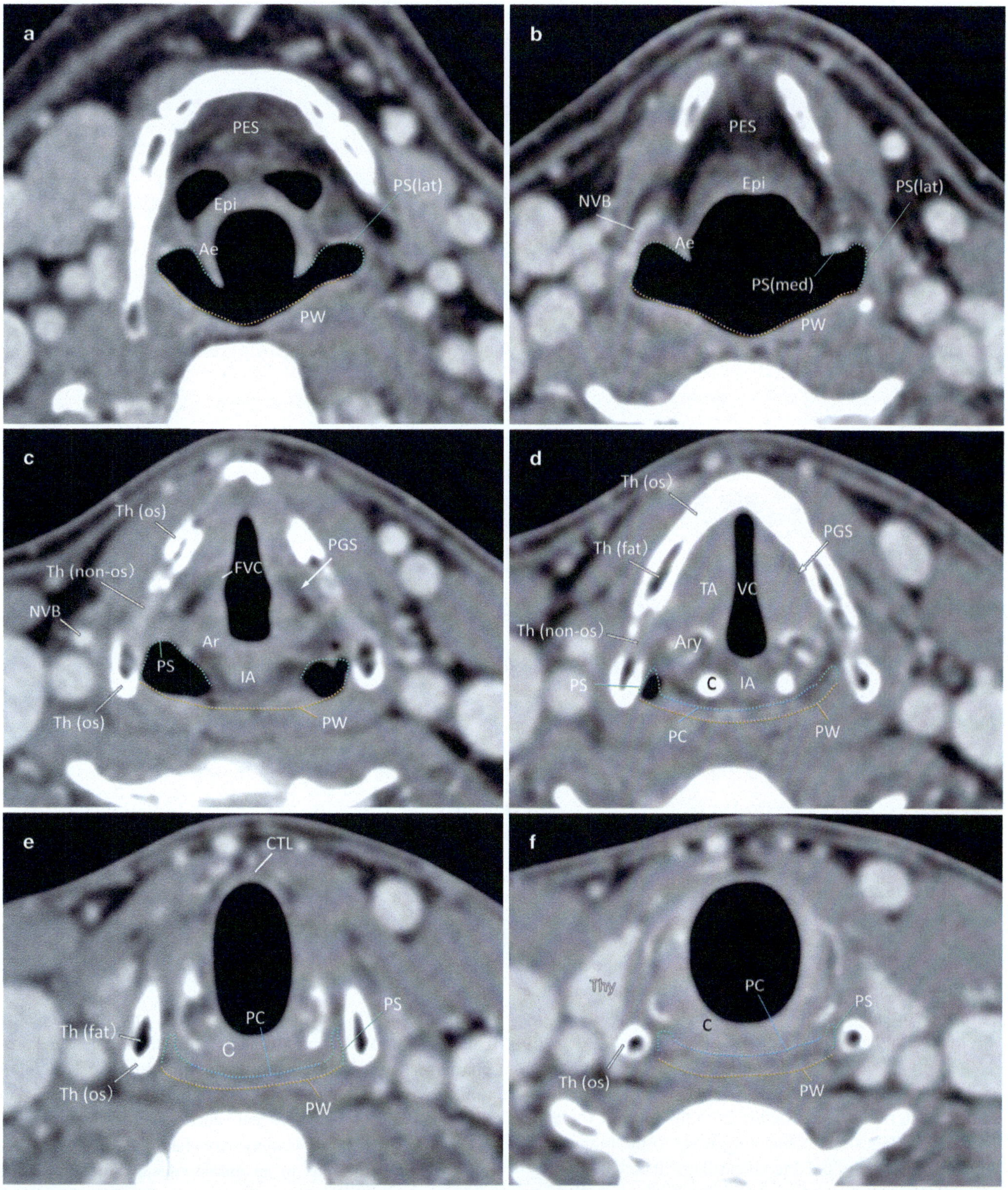

Fig. 5.2 CT anatomy of larynx and hypopharynx (**a-f**). The hypopharynx is divided into the pyriform sinuses (green), posterior hypopharyngeal walls (orange), and postcricoid region (blue). *Th (os)* ossified thyroid cartilage, Th *(non-os)* non-ossified thyroid cartilage, Th *(fat)* fat marrow orf the thyroid cartilage; PES, preepiglottic space; Epi, epiglottis; Ar, arytenoid cartilage; TA, true vocal cord; FVC, false vocal cord; PGS, paraglottic space; IA, inter-arytenoid; Thy, thyroid gland; CTL, cricothyroid ligament; C, cricoid cartilage

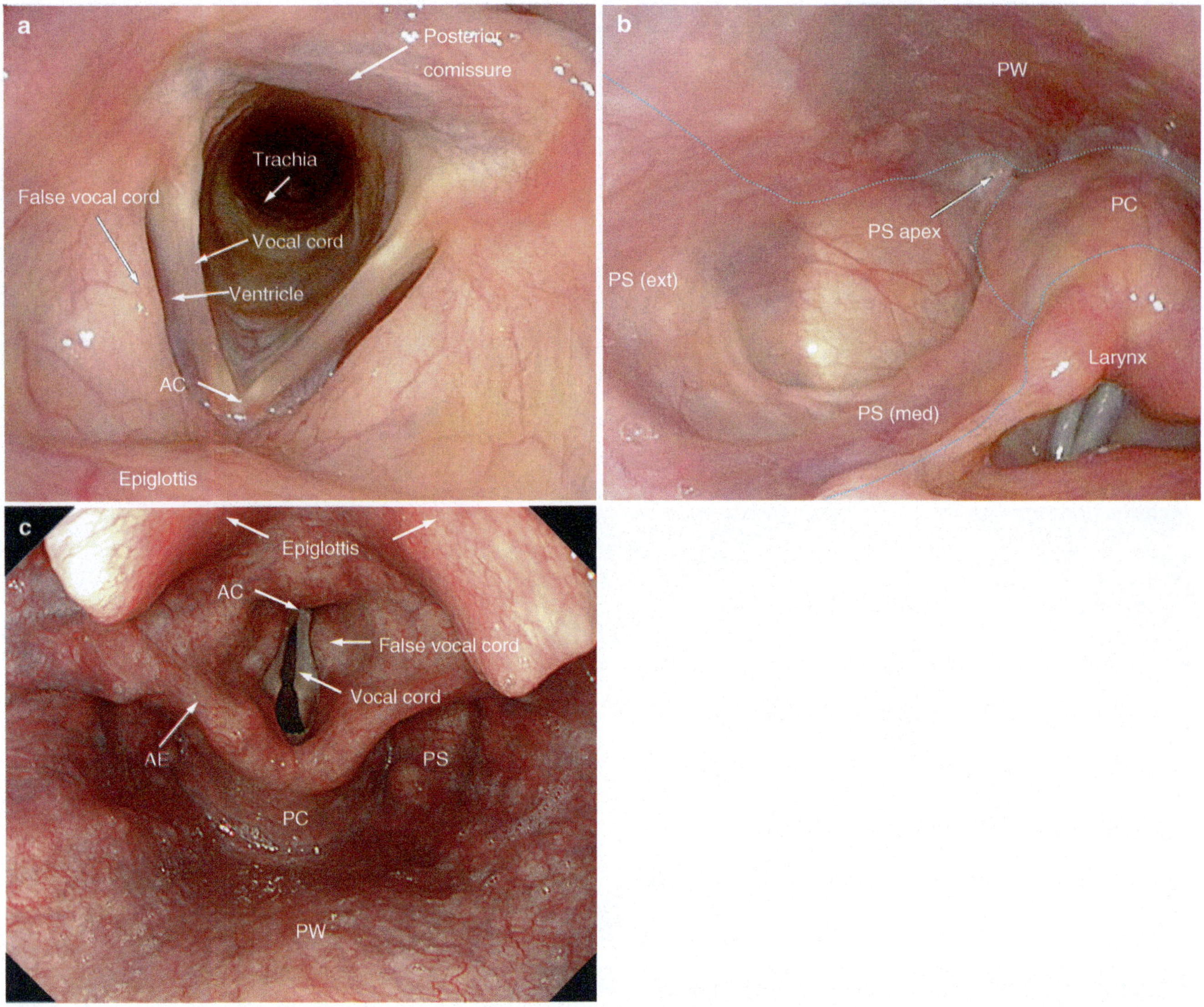

Fig. 5.3 Laryngoscopic (**a**, **b**) and endoscopic (**c**) anatomy of larynx and hypopharynx. Note the laryngoscopy (**a**, **b**) and endoscopy (**c**) are usually inverted vertically and horizontally. *AC* anterior commissure, *PS* pyriform sinus, *PW* posterior wall

1. The pyriform sinus extends from the pharyngoepiglottic fold to the upper end of the esophagus at the lower border of the cricoid cartilage. It is bounded laterally by the lateral pharyngeal wall and medially by the lateral surface of the aryepiglottic fold and arytenoid and cricoid cartilages.
2. The postcricoid area extends from the level of the arytenoid cartilages and connecting folds to the plane of the inferior border of the cricoid cartilage. It connects the two pyriform sinuses, which form the anterior wall of the hypopharynx.
3. The posterior pharyngeal wall extends from the level of the superior surface of the hyoid bone (or vallecula) to the inferior border of the cricoid cartilage and from the apex of one pyriform sinus to the other.

5.3.3 Deep Space of Larynx

Deep spaces (Fig. 5.4) of the larynx are important potential paths of submucosal tumor spread from both laryngeal and oropharyngeal tumors and cannot be identified on clinical examination. The preepiglottic space and paraglottic space are related to the T classification of laryngeal cancer. The paraglottic space also serves as a pathway leading hypopharyngeal cancer involving the pyriform sinus in an intralaryngeal direction. These spaces are one of the routes for metastasis of laryngeal and hypopharyngeal carcinoma, as many blood vessels are present.

5.3.3.1 Preepiglottic Space (PES)

The preepiglottic space is a fat-containing potential space anterior to the epiglottis, extending superiorly to the hyoid

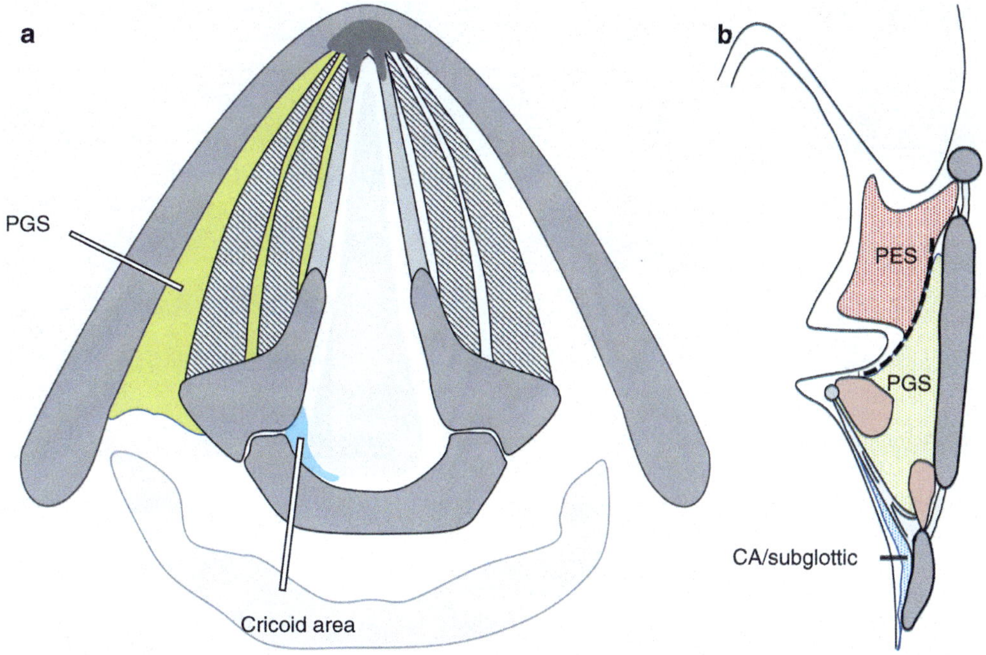

Fig. 5.4 Schema of the deep space of larynx. Axial at the glottic level (**a**) and coronal of the larynx (**b**). *PGS* paraglottic space, *PES* preepiglottic space, *CA* cricoid area

bone (Fig. 5.4b). It is bordered superiorly by the hyoepiglottic ligament; anteriorly by the hyoid bone, thyrohyoid membrane, and thyroid cartilage; and posteroinferiorly by the thyroepiglottic ligament and epiglottic cartilage. The preepiglottic space is adjacent to the paraglottic space (PGS) posteroinferiorly and is separated from it by fibrous tissue termed the thyroglottic ligament. Posterosuperiorly, the two spaces are not clearly delineated from each other [3]. Although this space can be seen in the axial plane, the preepiglottic space is best evaluated in the sagittal plane on both CT and MR imaging.

5.3.3.2 Paraglottic Space (PGS)

The paraglottic space is a paired, fat-filled potential space between the mucosa and laryngeal cartilage framework (Fig. 5.4) and is contiguous superiorly with the preepiglottic space [4]. Laterally, the paraglottic space is surrounded by the thyroid lamina. Posteriorly, the paraglottic space is surrounded by the mucosa of the hypopharynx (pyriform sinus). Medially, the PGS is surrounded by the thyroglottic ligament, thyroarytenoid muscle, and aryepiglottic muscle at the supraglottic level; thyroarytenoid muscle at the glottic level; and thyroarytenoid muscle, lateral cricoarytenoid muscle, and conus elasticus at the subglottic level. Inferiorly, the paraglottic space is surrounded by the cricothyroid muscle. The paraglottic space is mostly fat containing at the level of the supraglottis, surrounding the laryngeal ventricle and containing the thyroarytenoid (or vocalis) muscle at the level of the glottis, with a thin sliver of fat laterally deep to the thyroid cartilage. The paraglottic space can be seen in the axial plane but is more visible in the coronal plane in both CT reformations and MR imaging.

5.3.3.3 Cricoid Area/Subglottic Space

The cricoid area/subglottic space of the human larynx is a loose connective tissue (areolar tissue) area in the subglottis composed of adipose tissue, loose elastic, and collagen fibers (Fig. 5.4) [5, 6]. The cricoid area is the region of areolar tissue medial to the internal perichondrium of the cricoid. The cricoid area is bounded by the subglottic area and is fused with the conus elasticus above and first tracheal ligament below. The cricoid area is one of the routes for subglottic spread and prelaryngeal spread and/or paratracheal metastasis of laryngeal cancer [7]. Since many blood vessels, including the superficial branch of the cricothyroid artery, are present in the cricoid area, tumor invasion into the cricoid area and intravascular tumor invasion facilitate metastasis to the prelaryngeal, pretracheal, and/or paratracheal regions.

5.3.4 Laryngeal Cartilage

The laryngeal cartilages are frameworks and compartments of the larynx. The major laryngeal cartilages are the thyroid, cricoid, arytenoid, and epiglottic cartilages. The thyroid, cricoid, and arytenoid cartilages are composed of varying amounts of ossified and non-ossified hyaline cartilage. Ossified cartilage appears similar to the bone on CT, with a peripheral hyperdense cortex and central hypodense medullary cavity, whereas non-ossified bone has an appearance of soft tissue (Figs. 5.2 and 5.5a). On MR imaging, ossified cartilage is hypointense peripherally on all sequences (similar to cortical bone), with the medullary cavity similar to fat on all sequences. Conversely, non-ossified hyaline cartilage appears as an intermediate-to-low signal on both T1- and

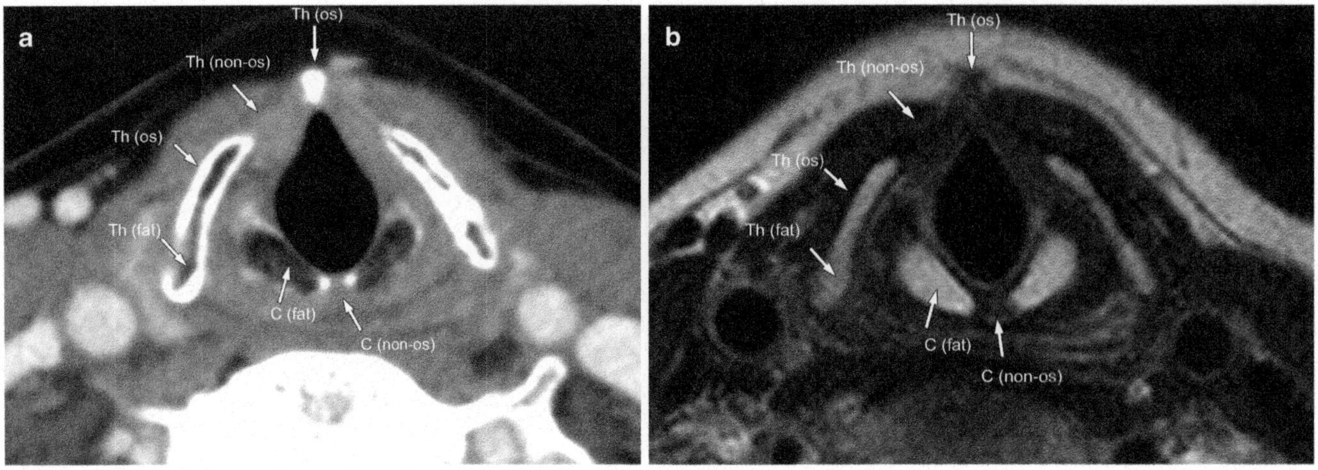

Fig. 5.5 Anatomy of the laryngeal cartilage. Contrast-enhanced CT (**a**) and T2-weighted image (**b**). *Th* thyroid cartilage, *C* cricoid cartilage, *os* ossified, *non-os fat* fat marrow

T2-weighted sequences (Fig. 5.5b). There should be no post-contrast enhancement within the medullary cavity of either ossified or non-ossified cartilage. The trend is toward increased cartilage ossification with advancing age; however, these findings are extremely variable and irregular, often making determination of laryngeal cartilage erosion or penetration by adjacent tumors difficult, particularly on CT [8]. The epiglottis and vocal process of the arytenoid are composed of yellow fibrocartilage and do not ossify (Fig. 5.2).

5.4 Imaging Techniques

5.4.1 CT

CT is the preferred initial imaging method for staging of laryngeal and hypopharyngeal cancer. The images are obtained with the patient supine and during quiet respiration (not while holding the breath). The neck should be in slight extension, and the head is aligned along the cephalocaudal axis to allow comparison of symmetrical structures. Malpositioning may create an appearance that simulates disease. Every effort should be made to make the patient feel comfortable. Typically, a 100-mL injection of 300 mgI/mL iodinated contrast medium is injected at a rate of 2.5–3.0 mL/s, and the scan is initiated 60–70 s after the start of the injection, proceeding in a craniocaudal direction. The scan range is set from the base of the skull to the bottom of the neck. Reconstructed images are generated as frontal and coronal sections parallel and vertical to the vocal cords from 1 cm above the hyoid bone to the inferior margin of the cricoid cartilage. The vocal cords are identified in sagittal sections on a separate workstation, and an axial image is created according to the inclination. The identification of the glottic level is a good indicator of "arytenoid cartilage (especially the vocal process)." The slice thickness should be 1–2 mm according to the performance of the device with small (typically 16-cm) field of view.

When dual-energy CT is available, an iodine overlay (IO) image (blending iodine images and virtual non-contrast images) is generated and used to evaluate cartilage invasion [9, 10]. While the technical innovations of multidetector CT (MDCT) have led to substantial improvements in image quality in the last decade, the advent of dual-energy CT and its unique post-processing capabilities has now made possible additional tissue characterization and image processing beyond what is possible with conventional, single-energy CT scanners. When dual-source dual-energy CT scans can be applied, the following parameters are applied: 100 and 140 kV tube voltages with a 0.4-mm tin filter (labeled as Sn140 kV). A voltage combination of 100 kV and Sn140 kV, rather than 80 kV and 140 kV, is chosen to minimize noise while maximizing the separation of the X-ray tubes' energy spectra. Two image sets (100 kV and Sn140 kV) are reconstructed with 1-mm slice thickness and a third linearly blended image set (weighted average [WA] images) to obtain a 120-kV equivalent image. WA images are used as diagnostic images since they have equivalent image quality to that of single-energy 120 kV CT images. IO images are generated using three-material decomposition analysis to compute iodine images and virtual non-contrast images [10]. The iodine images and virtual non-contrast or weighted average images can be linearly fused at a ratio of 0.5, creating iodine overlay (IO) images. The spectral attenuation curves generated from dual-energy CT can also be used for evaluation of cartilage invasion [9].

5.4.2 MR Images

MR imaging offers superior soft tissue contrast and is preferred. MRI with morphologic sequences and diffusion-weighted imaging (DWI) provides anatomic, qualitative, and quantitative functional information allowing noninvasive assessment of treatment responses and detection of tumors. MR images are also obtained with the patient supine and during quiet respiration. Typically, axial and coronal T2-weighted, T1-weighted, and DWI (with ADC map) images are obtained with a scan orientation parallel to the true vocal cords with a slice thickness of 3 mm or less. Additional axial fat-saturated T1-weighted images after intravenous administration of gadolinium chelates are obtained routinely. In patients with advanced laryngeal/hypopharyngeal carcinoma, MRI seems to be prone to motion artifacts because of the relatively long scan times, which can render images non-diagnostic [11]. The thin slice 3D sequence reconstruction images are additionally performed within the area from 1 cm above the hyoid bone to the inferior margin of the cricoid cartilage: Images in the coronal or sagittal plane may be obtained to evaluate certain anatomic spaces, such as the preepiglottic space in the sagittal plane or the paraglottic space and ventricle in the coronal plane. Phased-array surface coils can be applied to the neck for reducing motion artifacts and increasing spatial resolution [12], although this technique uses a small field of view, restricting the imaged area to the larynx.

5.4.3 FDG-Pet

FDG-PET/CT is used in the advanced laryngeal and hypopharyngeal cancers for the delineation of the primary tumor, detection of regional nodal metastases, distant metastases, and second primary tumors [13]. FDG-PET is also useful for treatment evaluation and diagnosis of recurrence in follow-up observations [14, 15]. Talking during the FDG uptake phase can cause radiotracer accumulation in the muscles of phonation and vocal cords. These FDG activities can interfere with the interpretation of PET scans in patients with laryngeal and hypopharyngeal cancers [16, 17].

5.5 TNM Classification

The TNM classification of American Joint Committee on Cancer 2018 (AJCC-8th)/Union for International Cancer Control (UICC) for primary laryngeal (glottic, supraglottic, and subglottic) and hypopharyngeal cancers are outlined in Table 5.1 (larynx) and Table 5.2 (hypopharynx) [18]. Clinical staging of the primary site is based on involvement of various subsites of the larynx or adjacent regions of the pharynx and vocal cord mobility. Assessment of the primary tumor is initially accomplished by clinical inspection, using indirect mirror and direct endoscopic examination with fiberscopes. However, these tumors have a tendency to spread submucosally, and this extension into deeply seated tissue planes can be easily missed by clinical examination alone [19–21]. Practically, therefore, clinicians rely on imaging to predict which patients will have T3–4 disease. Even if the primary tumor has been clinically diagnosed as T1–2 disease on the basis of inspection, imaging may be an important adjunct to exclude any T3–4 factor features or the presence of submucosal extension [22, 23]. Therefore, cross-sectional imaging using CT or MRI is mandatory for completing the staging process and should be included in the diagnostic workup.

Table 5.1 Definition of primary tumor of larynx (T)

T category	T criteria
TX	Primary tumor cannot be assessed
Tis	Carcinoma in situ
T1	Tumor limited to one subsite of supraglottis with normal vocal cord mobility
T2	Tumor invades mucosa of more than one adjacent subsite of supraglottis, glottis, or region outside the supraglottis (e.g., mucosa of base of tongue, vallecula, medial wall of pyriform sinus) without fixation of the larynx
T3	Tumor limited to larynx with vocal cord fixation and/or invades any of the following: Postcricoid area, preepiglottic space, paraglottic space, and/or inner cortex of thyroid cartilage
T4a	Tumor invades through the outer cortex of the thyroid cartilage and/or invades extralaryngeal soft tissues[a]
T4b	Tumor invades prevertebral space, encases carotid artery, or invades mediastinal structures
Supraglottis	
T1a	Tumor limited to one vocal cord
T1b	Tumor involves both vocal cords
T2	Tumor extends to supraglottis and/or subglottis and/or with impaired vocal cord mobility
T3	Tumor limited to the larynx with vocal cord fixation and/or invasion of paraglottic space and/or inner cortex of thyroid cartilage
T4a	Tumor invades through the outer cortex of the thyroid cartilage and/or extralaryngeal soft tissues[a]
T4b	Tumor invades prevertebral space, encases carotid artery, or invades mediastinal structures
Subglottis	
T1	Tumor limited to the subglottis
T2	Tumor extends to vocal cord(s) with normal or impaired mobility
T3	Tumor limited to the larynx with vocal cord fixation and/or invasion of paraglottic space and/or inner cortex of thyroid cartilage
T4a	Tumor invades cricoid or thyroid cartilage and/or invades extralaryngeal soft tissues[a]
T4b	Tumor invades prevertebral space, encases carotid artery, or invades mediastinal structures

[a]Note: extralaryngeal soft tissues (e.g., trachea, soft tissues of the neck including deep extrinsic muscles of the tongue, strap muscles, thyroid, or esophagus)

Table 5.2 Definition of primary tumor of hypopharynx (T)

T category	T criteria
TX	Primary tumor cannot be assessed
Tis	Carcinoma in situ
T1	Tumor limited to one subsite of hypopharynx and/or 2 cm or smaller in greatest dimension
T2	Tumor invades more than one subsite of hypopharynx or an adjacent site, or measures larger than 2 cm but not larger than 4 cm in greatest dimension without fixation of hemilarynx
T3	Tumor larger than 4 cm in greatest dimension or with fixation of hemilarynx or extension to esophageal mucosa
T4a	Tumor invades thyroid/cricoid cartilage, hyoid bone, thyroid gland, esophageal muscle, or central compartment soft tissue[a]
T4b	Tumor invades prevertebral fascia, encases carotid artery, or involves mediastinal structures

[a]Note: Central compartment soft tissue includes prelaryngeal strap muscles and subcutaneous fat

5.5.1 Laryngeal Cancer

For laryngeal cancer, the first imaging criterion that defines T3 lesions is extension into the paraglottic and/or preepiglottic space, irrespective of vocal cord mobility. In addition, tumor erosion limited to the inner cortex of the thyroid cartilage indicates a T3 lesion, whereas erosion of the outer cortex of the thyroid cartilage defines a T4a tumor. Arytenoid and epiglottic cartilage involvement does not change the laryngeal tumor stage. Extralaryngeal tumor spread is an important predictor of T4a disease in laryngeal cancer, with or without cartilage invasion.

In the new AJCC-eighth, there are no changes to laryngeal T-category; N-category follows the changes for non-EBV (Epstein-Barr virus) and non-HPV (human papilloma virus) SCCs for the entire head and neck. T0 has been deleted as a new category of unknown primary tumors without EBV and HPV [18].

5.5.2 Hypopharyngeal Cancer

Unlike those for laryngeal cancer, criteria that define T3 lesions for hypopharyngeal cancer are based solely on vocal cord mobility and tumor diameter. Hypopharyngeal cancer with invasion of the thyroid or cricoid cartilage indicates a T4a lesion, even in cases of localized cartilage invasion. In any event, accurate staging requires subtle diagnosis of cartilage invasion. Extralaryngeal tumor spread is also an important predictor of T4a disease, with or without cartilage invasion. In the new AJCC-eighth, there are minor changes to hypopharyngeal T-category [18, 24]. In the T classification, the definition of esophageal extension was as follows: extension to the esophageal mucosa (T3) and esophageal muscle (T4a). T0 has also been deleted as a new category of unknown primary tumors without EBV and HPV.

5.5.3 Nodal Category (N)

The TNM classification of AJCC-eighth for nodal categories of laryngeal and hypopharyngeal cancer is outlined in Table 5.3. Extranodal extension (ENE) of metastatic lymph nodes is a strong factor for poor prognosis. Further, clinical and pathological N classification has changed. This has resulted in a new N3b designation [18, 25]. The term "extracapsular spread" (ECS) has been unified and altered to the term "extranodal extension" (ENE). Currently, the clinical designation of ENE requires overt clinical evidence of ENE on examination, such as skin invasion, infiltration of muscles with tethering or fixation to adjacent structures, or large-nerve invasion with dysfunction such as the brachial plexus, sympathetic trunk, phrenic, or cranial nerves. Therefore, it is necessary to evaluate in detail the presence or absence of ENE as well as the infiltration of surrounding soft tissue by ENE. While indistinct nodal margins and an irregular nodal capsular enhancement suggest ENE [26, 27], the most robust imaging feature supporting the clinical diagnosis of ENE is evident infiltration of perinodal tumors into adjacent fat or muscle, which is most useful for radiologists to describe features indicative of ENE to enable reevaluation of clinical nodal status.

Table 5.3 Definition of regional lymph mode for laryngeal/hypopharyngeal cancer (N)

N category	N criteria
NX	Regional lymph nodes cannot be assessed
N0	No regional lymph node metastasis
N1	Metastasis in a single ipsilateral node ≤3 cm in greatest dimension and ENE(−)
N2a	Metastasis in a single ipsilateral node >3 cm but ≤6 cm in greatest dimension and ENE(−)
N2b	Metastasis in multiple ipsilateral nodes, none >6 cm in greatest dimension and ENE(−)
N2c	Metastases in bilateral or contralateral lymph nodes, none >6 cm in greatest dimension and ENE(−)
N3a	Metastasis in a lymph node >6 cm in greatest dimension and ENE(−)
N3b[a]	Metastasis in any node(s) and clinically overt ENE(+)

Note: Clinical ENE (cENE) indicates the invasion of skin, infiltration of musculature, dense tethering or fixation to adjacent structures, cranial nerve, brachial plexus, sympathetic trunk, or phrenic nerve invasion with dysfunction

[a]The addition of ENE to the staging system, creating a new N3b designation in the eighth edition of the AJCC Cancer Staging Manual. The original source for this material is the AJCC Cancer Staging Manual

5.6 Spread Pattern and Site-Specific Imaging Evaluation

5.6.1 Laryngeal Cancer

Laryngeal cancer is divided into three subsites: supraglottic, glottic, and subglottic. Laryngeal tumor spreads have certain patterns or high-frequency pathways along well-defined routes based on various structures. We have discussed the common and crucial patterns of tumor spread into the deep space and extralaryngeal soft tissue for each site. Laryngeal cartilage invasion, which is extremely important clinically, will be described separately later.

5.6.1.1 Supraglottic Cancer

Supraglottic cancer accounts for approximately 30% of laryngeal cancer. The subsites are divided into the suprahyoid epiglottis (Fig. 5.6) and infrahyoid epiglottis (Fig. 5.7), laryngeal surface of the aryepiglottic fold, and false vocal cords. Since supraglottic SCC is initially clin-

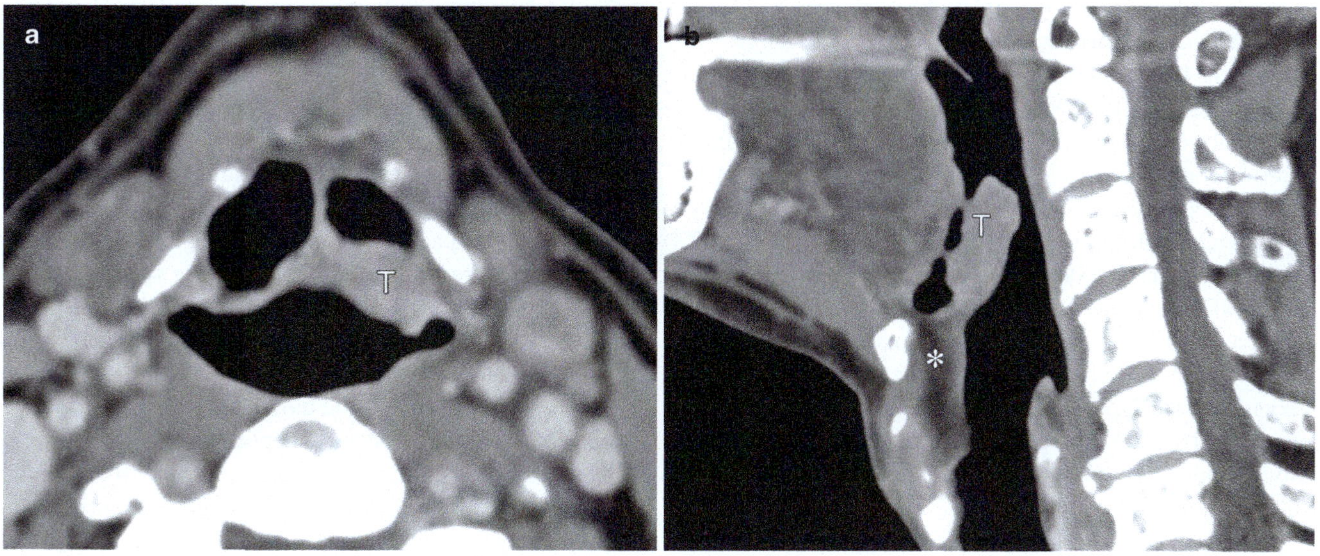

Fig. 5.6 Supraglottic cancer without preepiglottic space invasion. Axial contrast-enhanced CT demonstrated a mass of the left suprahyoid epiglottic (T). On a sagittal image, the tumor was almost limited to the epiglottis, and the fat layer in the preepiglottic space (asterisk) was preserved

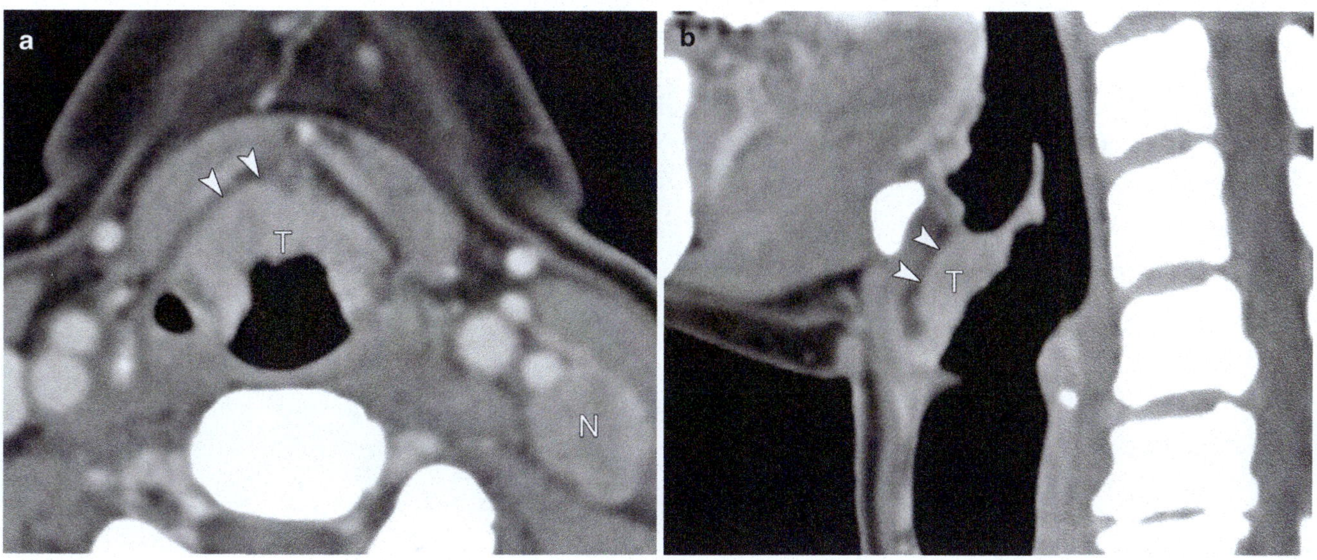

Fig. 5.7 Supralaryngeal cancer of the infrahyoid epiglottis. Axial contrast-enhanced CT (**a**) and sagittal images (**b**) show a mass lesion (T) with an irregular margin on the infrahyoid epiglottis and extending anteriorly to the part of the preepiglottic space (arrowheads). Note the left level III node metastasis (N)

ically occult, supraglottic tumors often present later than glottic tumors and are often large, with poorer prognosis than glottic cancer. The frequency of lymph node metastasis is high (about 50%), and a cervical mass due to lymphadenopathy is often the first symptom [28, 29]. In the case of early lesions (T1, T2), function-preserving treatment such as partial laryngectomy or chemoradiotherapy is performed. For advanced lesions, a multidisciplinary treatment combining radiation therapy, chemotherapy, and surgery is performed, taking into account both the curability and functional prognosis depending on the stage and tumor volume.

5.6.1.2 Glottic Cancer

Among the laryngeal cancers, glottic cancer is the most common, accounting for about 65% of cases. Subsites include the vocal cords (upper surface, free edge, lower surface), anterior commissure, and posterior commissure. There are many cases of hoarse symptoms, which tend to be detected in relatively early lesions. For early lesions (T1, T2, and T3 without vocal cord fixation), (chemo) radiotherapy, laser, or laryngeal preservation surgery is selected (Fig. 5.8). For advanced lesions of T3 or more, a multidisciplinary treatment combining radiation therapy, chemotherapy, and surgery is selected depending on the stage and tumor volume. In recent years, total laryngectomy is increasingly used as a salvage operation for recurrent and residual lesions after chemoradiation.

5.6.1.3 Subglottic Cancer

Primary subglottic cancer is a rare malignant lesion (Fig. 5.9) [30, 31]. Apart from SCCs, adenoid cystic carcinomas are frequently located at the subglottis. Subglottic cancer typically invades the true vocal cords, and it may be difficult to distinguish between cancer originating in the glottis or subglottis. Staging depends on the extent of involvement of the true vocal cords, fixation of the hemilarynx, whether there is invasion of the cricoid or thyroid cartilage, or extralaryngeal spread below the cricoid cartilage into the cervical trachea. Cricoid cartilage invasion and extralaryngeal spread anteriorly through the cricothyroid membrane are commonly present.

Imaging shows a subglottic soft tissue mass (normally no soft tissue is seen between the subglottic air column and the cricoid cartilage) with/without cricoid cartilage alterations (sclerosis, lysis), intratracheal soft tissue thickening, and spreading to the glottic and prelaryngeal soft tissues (Fig. 5.9).

5.6.1.4 Spread Pattern of Laryngeal Cancer (Deep Space)

1. Preepiglottic space involvement (supraglottic, glottic)

   Tumor spreading to the preepiglottic space in laryngeal cancer is considered to be the cause of poor response to radiation therapy, and the frequency of cervical lymph node metastasis is as high as 90% [32]. Both suprahyoid and infrahyoid supraglottic tumors are at risk of involving the preepiglottic space, as the epiglottis lacks a barrier to tumor spread. Infiltration of fat within the preepiglottic space is easy to detect on both CT and MR imaging in both axial and sagittal planes (Figs. 5.6 and 5.7), with a reported sensitivity of 100% [33]. Further, high tumor volume lesions that extensively invade the anterior epiglottis space often involve thyroid cartilage invasion.

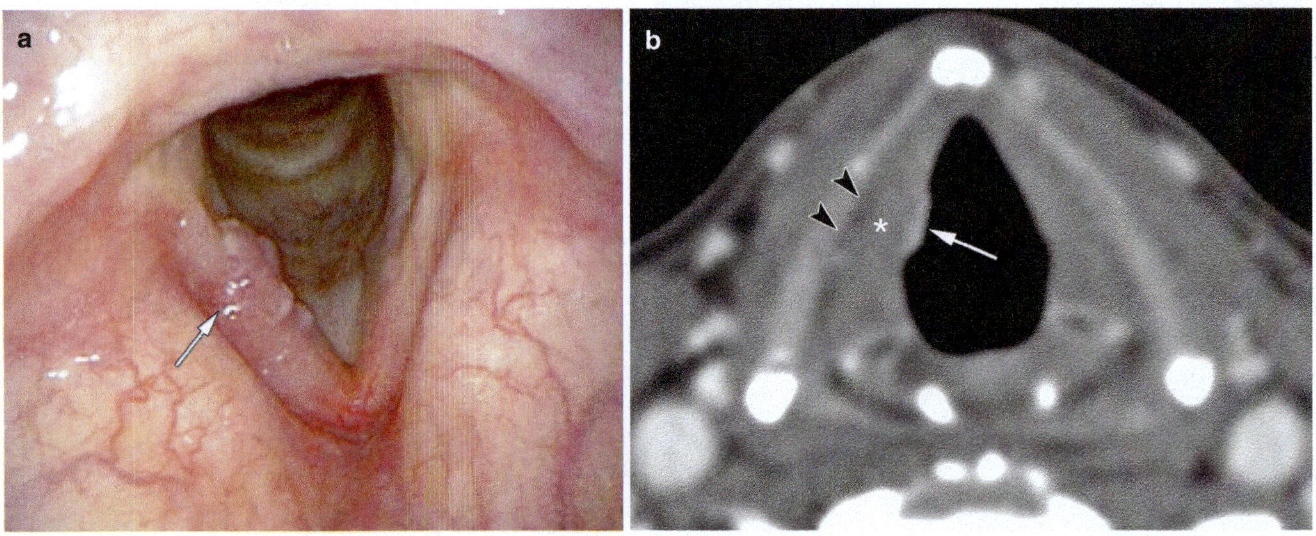

Fig. 5.8 Early glottic cancer (T1a) treated by radiotherapy. (**a**) Small polypoid clinical T1a lesion of the right vocal cord was observed on laryngoscopy. Axial contrast-enhanced CT (**b**) also demonstrated T1a glottic cancer of the right vocal cord (arrow). Note the normal fat layer of the paraglottic space (black arrowheads) and thyroarytenoid muscle (asterisk)

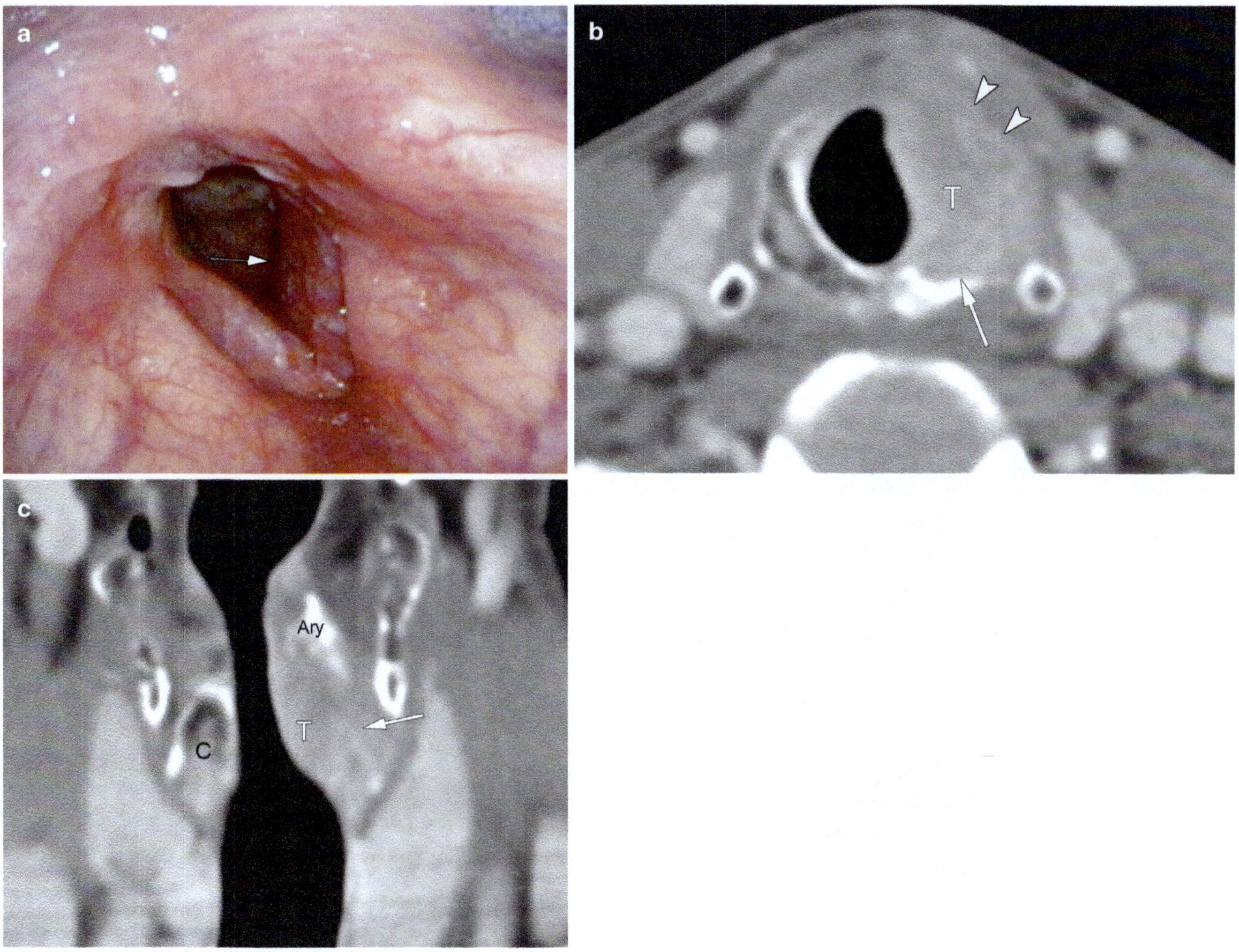

Fig. 5.9 Subglottic carcinoma with cricoid cartilage invasion. Laryngo-fiberscope (**a**) demonstrates a mass lesion (T) mainly at the subglottis. Axial contrast-enhanced CT image (**a**) showing the bulky subglottic tumor (T) with the cricoid cartilage destruction (arrow) and extralaryngeal spread anteriorly thorough the cricothyroid membrane (white arrowheads). *C* cricoid cartilage, *Ary* arytenoid cartilage

2. Paraglottic space involvement (glottic, supraglottic)

   Paraglottic space involvement will also upstage tumors to T3. Due to involvement of the thyroarytenoid muscle, these tumors are often associated with vocal cord paresis or paralysis. Tumor infiltration of the paraglottic space carries a lower response to radiation therapy alone for local control [23, 34]. CT and MRI can confirm early detection of paraglottic space involvement due to obscuration of the lateral thyroarytenoid muscle and disappearance of the thin fat layer along the inner cortex of the thyroid cartilage (Figs. 5.10 and 5.11).

3. Transglottic extension (supraglottic, glottic)

   Supraglottic laryngeal tumors that involved the aryepiglottic folds or false cords may extend inferiorly to cross the laryngeal ventricle, becoming a "transglottic" tumor which is tumor progression across the supraglottic larynx and glottis (Fig. 5.12) [35]. Glottic laryngeal tumors that involved the paraglottic space also extend superiorly to cross the laryngeal deep space as the transglottic cancer (Fig. 5.13).

4. Cricoarytenoid joint and arytenoid area (glottic, supraglottic)

   Imaging findings solely of the posterior extension to the cricoarytenoid joint are insufficient for upstaging tumors to T3, but involvement of the cricoarytenoid joint/muscle is associated with vocal cord paresis or paralysis (clinically T3) and is important as a pathway for subglottic extension (Figs. 5.10 and 5.11) [7].

5. Subglottic extension/cricoid area involvement (glottic, supra glottic)

   Subglottic extension is often much better observed on imaging than via laryngoscopy. When any soft tissue within the airway is observed at the level of the cricoid cartilage, subglottic extension should be of concern (Figs. 5.10 and 5.11). Although the conus elasticus may act as a barrier to subglottic extension of tumors, once the

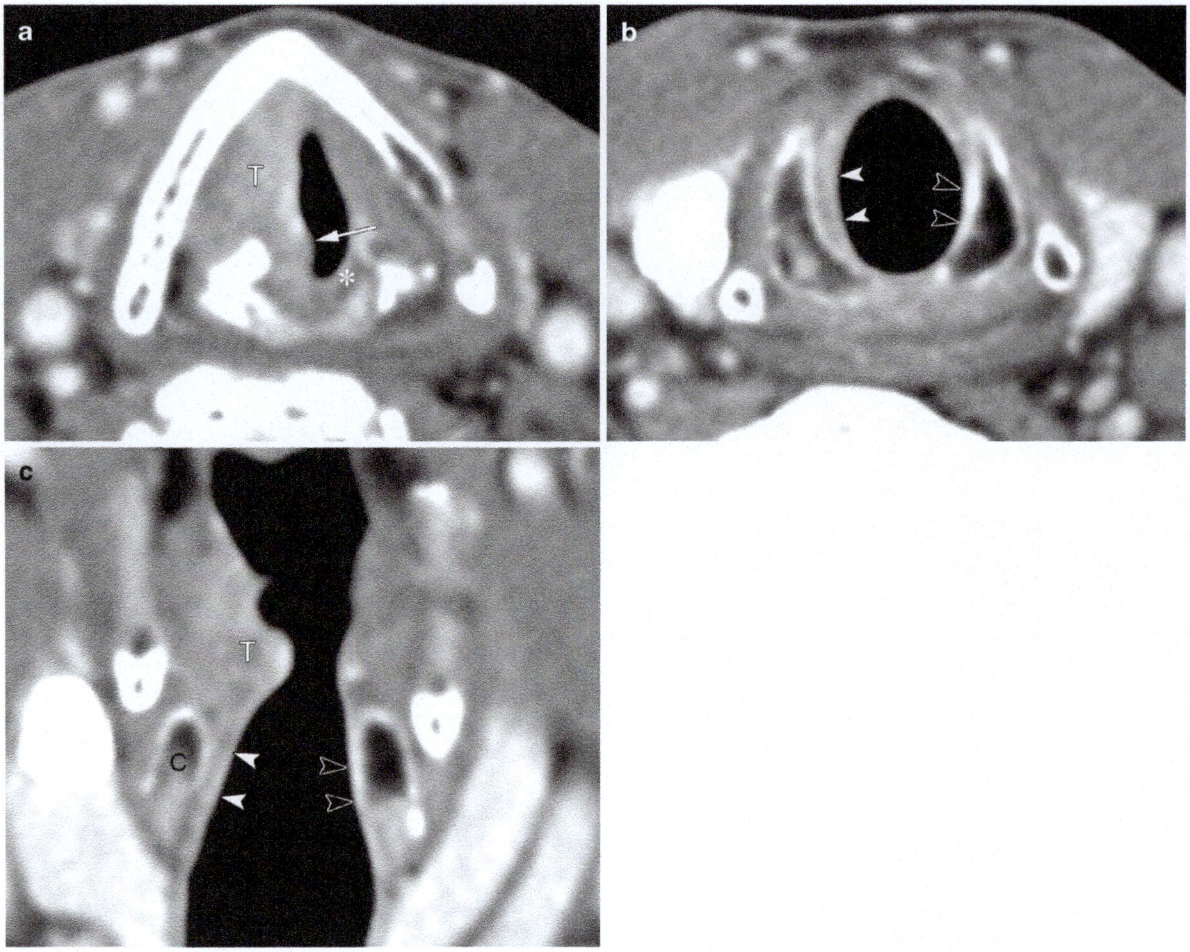

Fig. 5.10 Subglottic extension of a glottic carcinoma (T3). Axial contrast-enhanced CT image (**a**) demonstrates a tumor (T) of the right glottis with infiltration of the paraglottic space, arytenoid area, and cricoid area (arrow). Note the fat tissue of the cricoid area at the normal left side (asterisk). Axial image at the cricoid level (**b**) and coronal image (**c**) show downward tumor extension along the subglottic space (white arrowheads). Note the soft tissue anteriorly at the level of the cricoid cartilage (white arrowheads) but not on the left side (black arrowheads). *C* cricoid cartilage

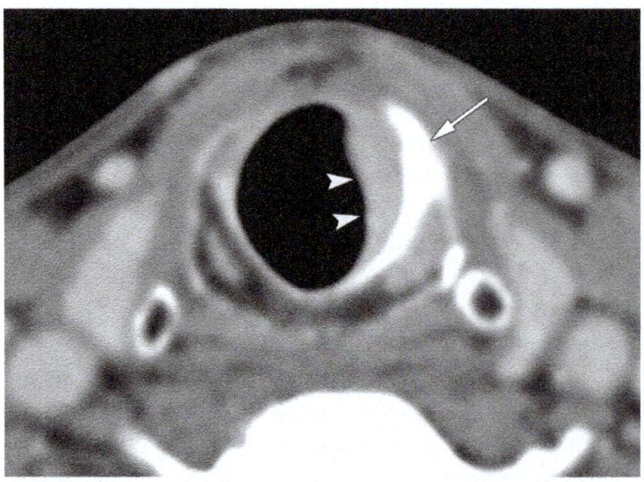

Fig. 5.11 Subglottic infiltration in a glottic carcinoma. Tumor inferiorly within the subglottic space (arrowheads). The cricoid cartilage is sclerotic with erosion due to surrounding tumor (arrows). Histopathological findings confirmed that the tumor cells invaded the cricoid cartilage

tumor extends into the cricoid area (Fig. 5.10) and subglottic space (at the level of the cricoid ring), there is an increased risk of cricoid cartilage invasion (Fig. 5.11) and extralaryngeal spread anteriorly [7]. Coronal images are useful for evaluating the extent of subglottic disease from the level of the true vocal cords.

6. Superior extension into the base of the tongue (supraglottic)

Superior extension with involvement of the vallecula or base of the tongue is important to note because it will likely alter management. Tumors may reach the base of the tongue and even the extrinsic tongue muscles via extension through the preepiglottic space. Spread occurs anteriorly along the glossoepiglottic fold, which overlies the hyoepiglottic ligament, resulting in extension to the vallecula and base of the tongue (Fig. 5.14). Tumors can extend from the suprahyoid epiglottis laterally along the pharyngoepiglottic fold to reach the lateral pharyngeal wall. If there is aggressive involvement of the base of the

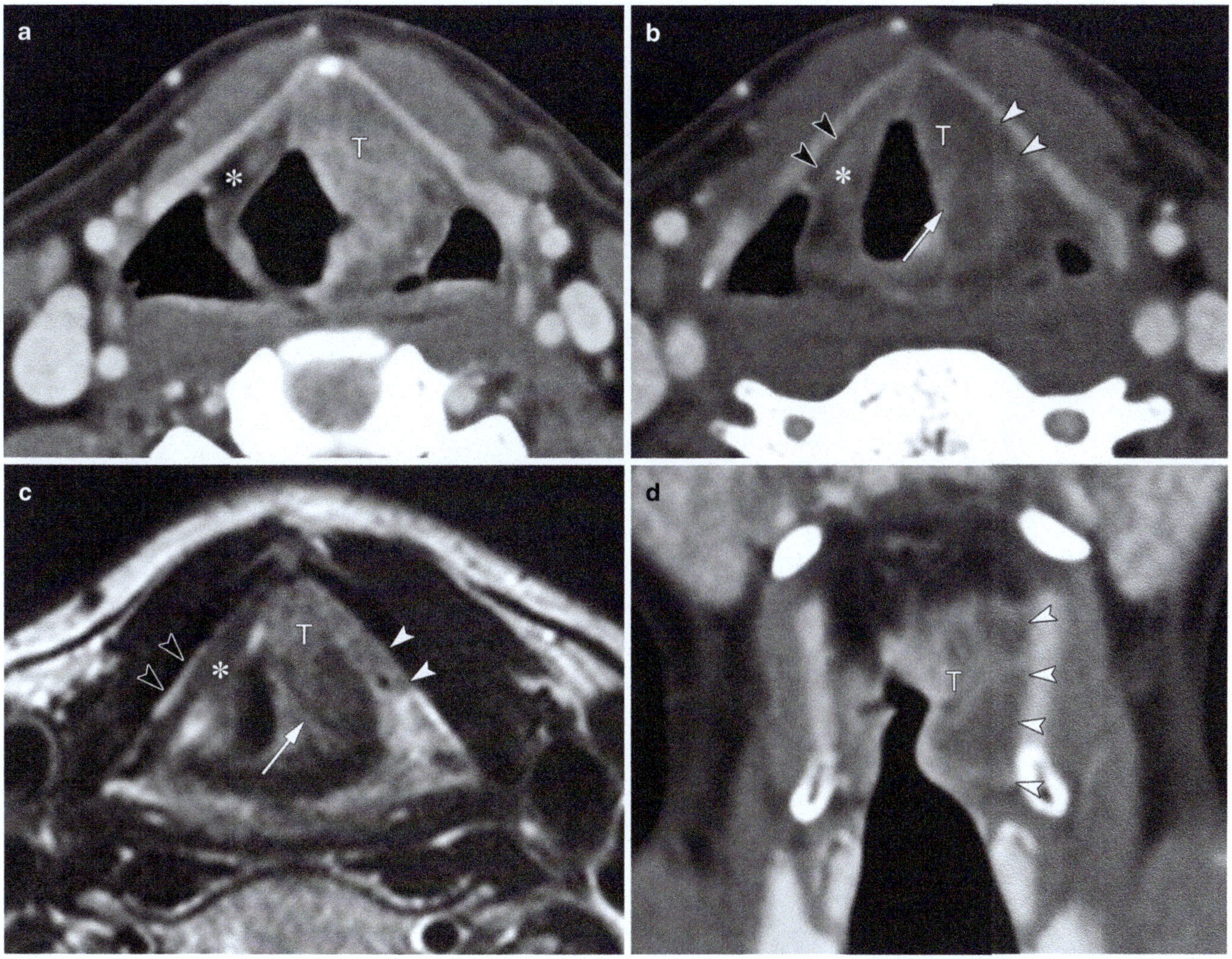

Fig. 5.12 Supraglottic cancer with transglottic spread through the paraglottic space. Axial contrast-enhanced CT images (**a**) demonstrate the tumor (T) of the left infrahyoid epiglottis, with infiltration of the preepiglottic space (the asterisk is normal right preepiglottic space). Axial image, more interiorly (**b**), shows downward tumor extension along with the preepiglottic space and paraglottic space (white arrowheads), as well as posterolateral growth into the thyroarytenoid muscle (arrow). T2-weighted images (**c**) (corresponding the same slice of **b**) reveal tumor spread more clearly through the paraglottic space (white arrowheads) and thyroarytenoid muscle (arrow). Note the thin normal fat signal laterally deep to the thyroid cartilage (**b**, **c**, black arrowheads) and thyroarytenoid muscle (**b**, **c**, asterisk). On the coronal image (**d**), the tumor mass (T) extends throughout the left paraglottic space, abutting and slightly displacing the lower margin of the true vocal cord downward. Note the normal right true vocal cord (**a**–**c**, asterisk) and right laryngeal ventricle (**a**–**c**, arrowhead)

tongue, total laryngectomy, more extensive resection, possible glossectomy, and reconstruction of the neopharynx may be warranted.

5.6.1.5 Extralaryngeal Spread of the Laryngeal Cancer

In this chapter, we would like to emphasize the importance of this tumor spread separately. Extralaryngeal tumor spread is considered to be present when the primary tumor has expanded into extralaryngeal soft tissues, such as cervical soft tissues, infrahyoid muscles, thyroid gland, esophagus, trachea, or deep lingual muscle, with or without cartilage penetration. In clinical practice, patients with T4 disease do not always undergo laryngectomy, and for patients without tumor extension through the cartilage – a diagnosis that is not always straightforward – clinicians rely on imaging for accurate tumor staging, tumor mapping, and detection of possible tumor extension [36–38]. It is then possible to predict which patients may be candidates for function-preserving treatments to a degree, and discussions with patients are part of the treatment decision-making process. According to Beitler et al. [39], extralaryngeal spread without thyroid cartilage penetration was more common than expected in patients with advanced laryngeal and hypopharyngeal cancer. The authors suggested that cartilage invasion was absent in 40% of cases showing extralaryngeal tumor spread. Since extralaryngeal tumor spread is one of the important predictors of T4 disease in laryngeal and hypopharyngeal cancer, the focus of imaging needs to shift from detection of invasion to reliably demonstrating more extensive disease.

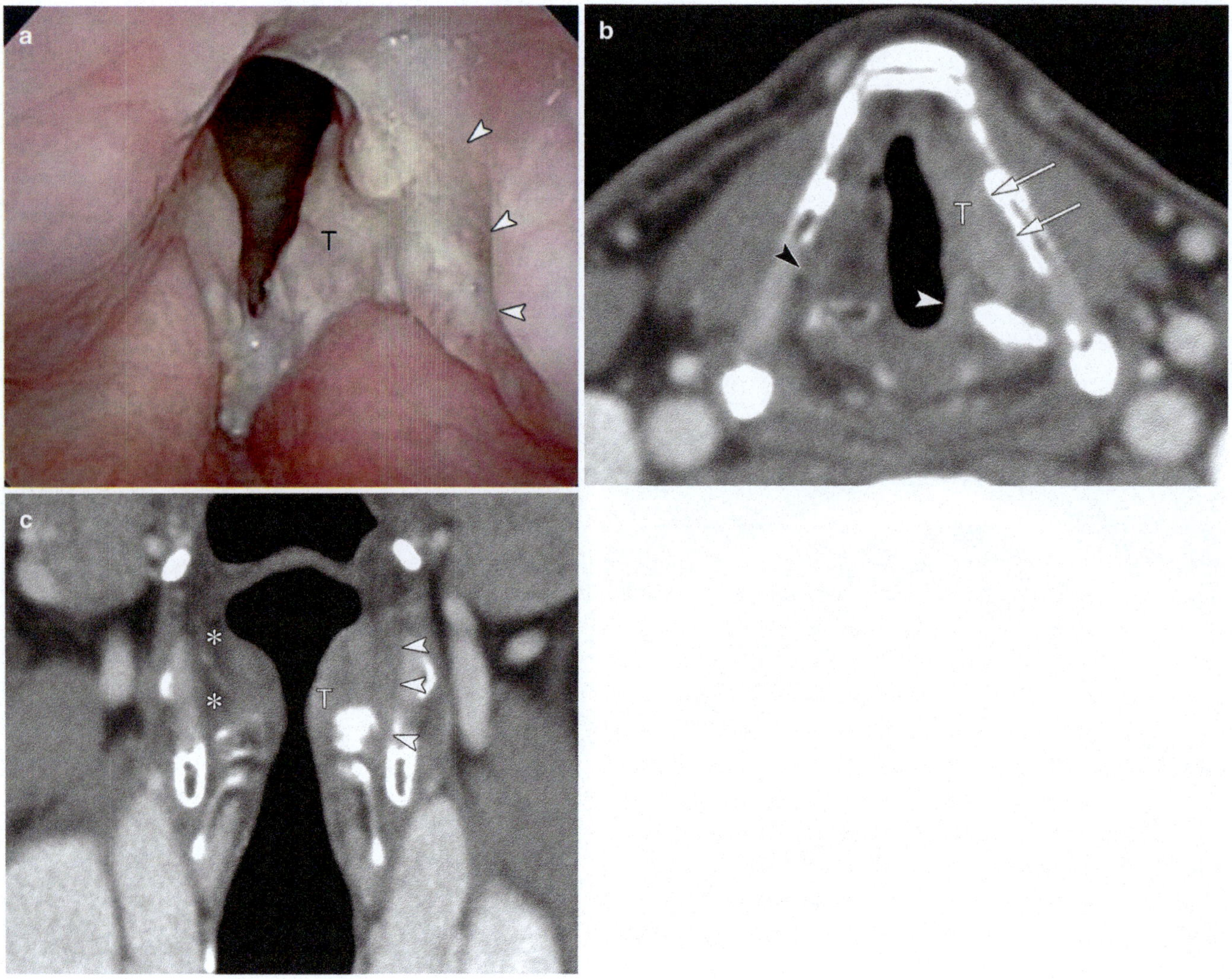

Fig. 5.13 Glottic cancer with radiologic paraglottic space infiltration and superior extension. On the laryngo-fiberscope (**a**), a mass lesion (T) involving the left vocal cord with infiltration into the left supraglottis was observed. The mobility of the vocal cords was clinically favorable. Axial contrast-enhanced CT (**b**) demonstrated an infiltrative tumor (T) involving the paraglottic space. Note the structure of the descending branch of the right superior laryngeal artery maintained on the right side (black arrow) but obscured on the left. The tumor also extended across the posterior arytenoid toward the supraglottic laryngeal direction. Coronal image (**c**) demonstrates the tumor mass (T) extending throughout the left paraglottic space toward the supraglottis. Normal fat density of the paraglottic space is clearly seen on the right side (asterisk)

Extralaryngeal spread is considered if the following features can be identified: substitution by tumor tissue on the outside of the membrane/cartilage or loss of fat attenuation between extralaryngeal structures (such as blood vessels or muscle) and laryngeal components. To detect extralaryngeal spread, it is important to thoroughly understand the complex anatomy in this area and the imaging features of commonly occurring extension patterns [40].

1. Extralaryngeal spread via thyrohyoid membrane (supraglottic)

   One of the most common routes of lesion spread from the larynx through areas of inherent weakness is via the thyrohyoid membrane (Fig. 5.15). The superior laryngeal neurovascular bundle enters the laryngeal component through a posterolateral defect in the thyrohyoid membrane; this defect is known to be the route by which tumors spread [40–42].
2. Extralaryngeal spread via cricothyroid membrane (glottic, supraglottic)

   Another common route of lesion spread from the larynx through areas of inherent weakness is via the cricothyroid membrane (Fig. 5.16) [40]. This extension into deep-seated tissue planes is difficult to evaluate by clinical examination alone. The cricothyroid joint is also an important route of tumor spread toward the extralaryngeal soft tissue such as the thyroid lobe (Fig. 5.17).

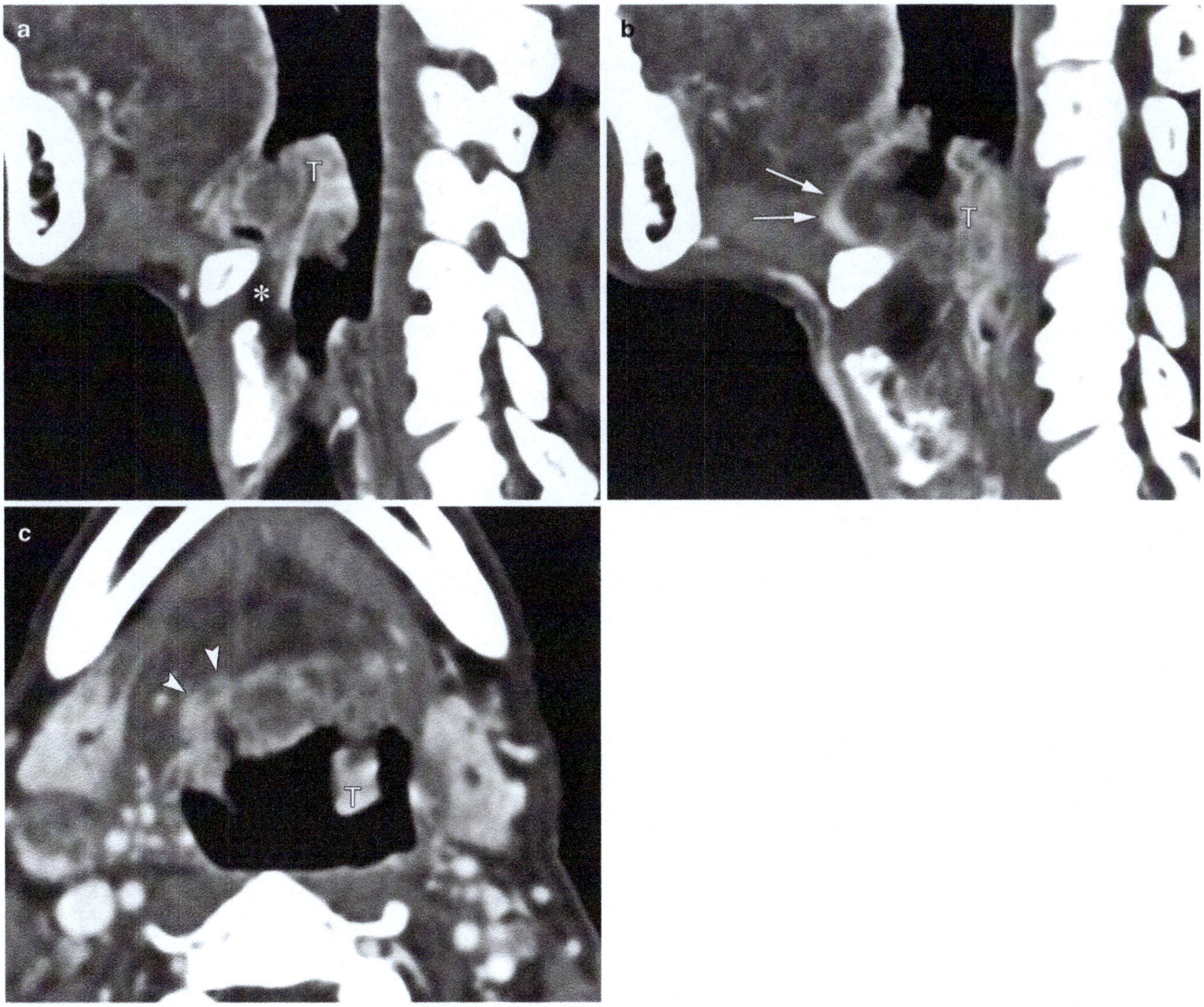

Fig. 5.14 Supraglottic cancer with tumor spreading to the base of tongue. On a sagittal image (**a**), the tumor (T) was almost limited to the epiglottis, and the fat in the preepiglottic space (asterisk) was preserved. However, on the right side, the tumor extended to the epiglottic vallecula (**b**, arrows), reaching the intermuscular fat layer beyond the intrinsic lingual muscle layer of the tongue base (**c**, arrowheads)

5.6.2 Hypopharyngeal Cancer

Hypopharyngeal cancer is divided into three subregions: pyriform sinus (pyriform fossa), pharyngeal posterior wall, and postcricoid. Tumor spreading pattern and treatment strategy for each tumor subsite are different (in particular, laryngeal function preservation treatment is possible). Below, we describe typical tumor spreading patterns for each. Laryngeal cartilage invasion will be also described separately.

5.6.2.1 Pyriform Sinus (PS)

Pyriform sinus SCC accounts for 70–75% of hypopharyngeal cancer subsites. More than 60% of pyriform sinus SCCs tend to be observed initially as T3 or T4 locally advanced lesions, and lymph node metastasis is often visible [2]. In recent years, with the development of endoscopic equipment such as narrow-band imaging (NBI), early superficial lesions are easily detected, and the ratio of T1 or T2 lesions is increasing (Fig. 5.18). The patterns of tumor spread may be mucosal superficial extension and deeper infiltration. Mucosal tumor spreading requires a comprehensive evaluation using both endoscopic and imaging findings. The role of diagnostic imaging is to assess the presence of infiltration in the deep direction and caudal spreading such as the apex of pyriform sinus/postcricoid, which may be difficult to determine with an endoscope. When infiltration that reaches the muscle layer or deep tissue is observed, it may exceed the indication of endoscopic resection. In the case of lesions that extend to the pyriform apex or postcricoid region (Fig. 5.19),

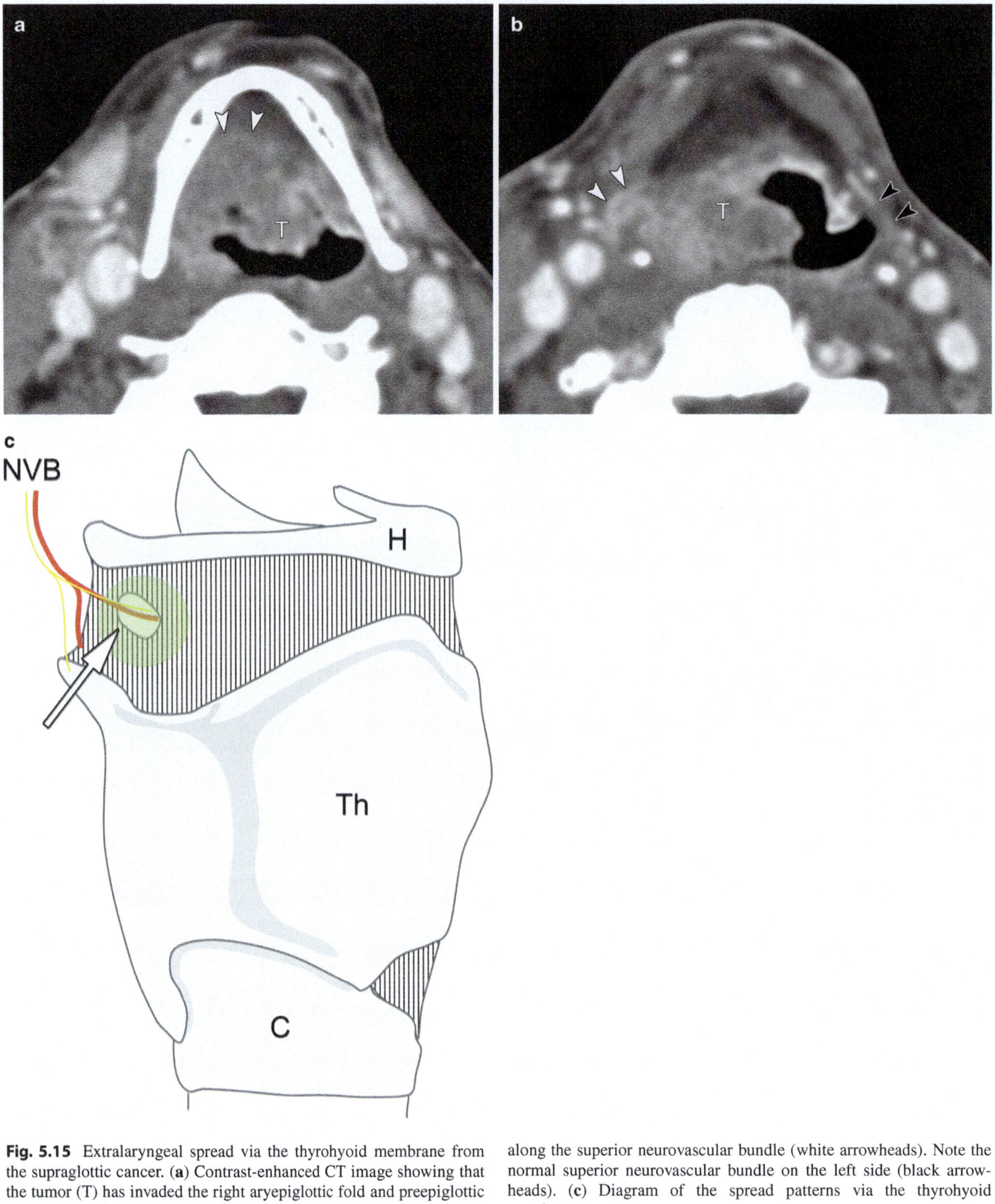

Fig. 5.15 Extralaryngeal spread via the thyrohyoid membrane from the supraglottic cancer. (**a**) Contrast-enhanced CT image showing that the tumor (T) has invaded the right aryepiglottic fold and preepiglottic space. (**b**) Axial image, more inferiorly, showing the tumor (T) extending through the thyrohyoid membrane into the extralaryngeal tissues along the superior neurovascular bundle (white arrowheads). Note the normal superior neurovascular bundle on the left side (black arrowheads). (**c**) Diagram of the spread patterns via the thyrohyoid membrane

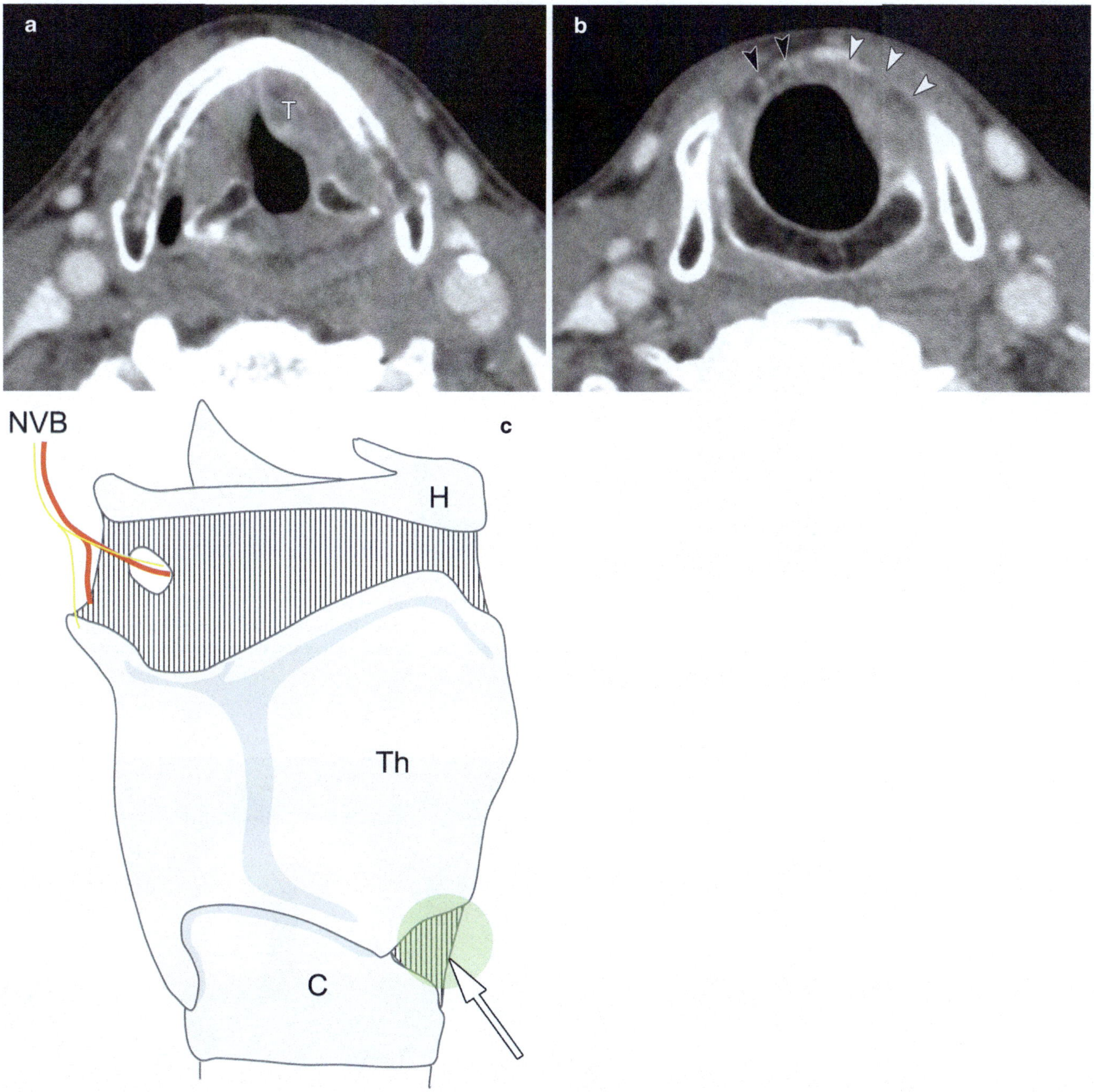

Fig. 5.16 Glottic carcinoma with radiologic extralaryngeal spread (radiologically T4a). Axial contrast-enhanced CT (**a**) demonstrates a tumor (T) involving the paraglottic space. (**b**) On the axial image, more inferiorly, the tumor exhibits submucosal extension to the extralaryngeal soft tissue via the cricothyroid membrane (white arrowheads). Note the normal fat layer and cricothyroid branch of the superior thyroid artery penetrating the cricothyroid ligament (black arrowheads). (**c**) Diagram of the spread patterns via the cricothyroid membrane

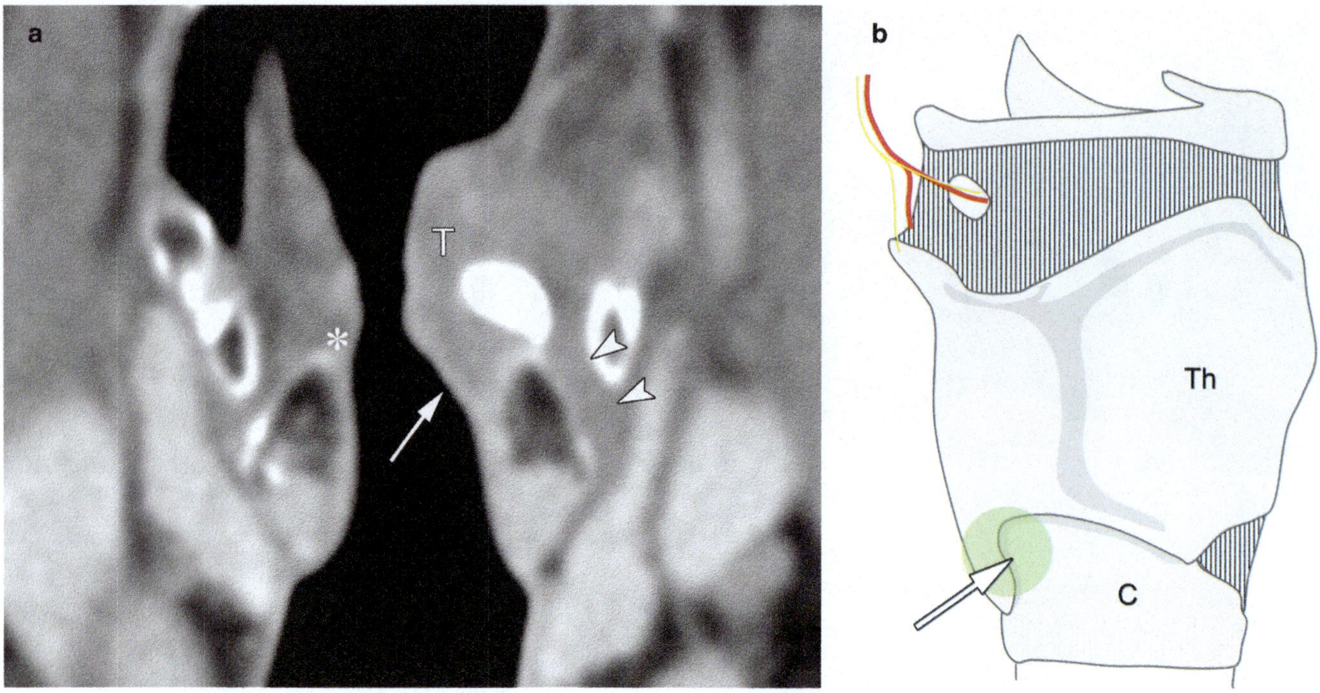

Fig. 5.17 Transglottic carcinoma with extralaryngeal spread through the cricothyroid joint toward the left thyroid lobe. Coronal contrast-enhanced CT images demonstrate a tumor (T) of the left glottis with infiltration of the cricoarytenoid joint and cricoid area (arrow) spreading through the cricothyroid joint toward the left thyroid lobe (white arrowheads). Note the fat tissue of the cricoid area at the normal right side (asterisk). (**b**) Diagram of the spread patterns around the cricothyroid joint

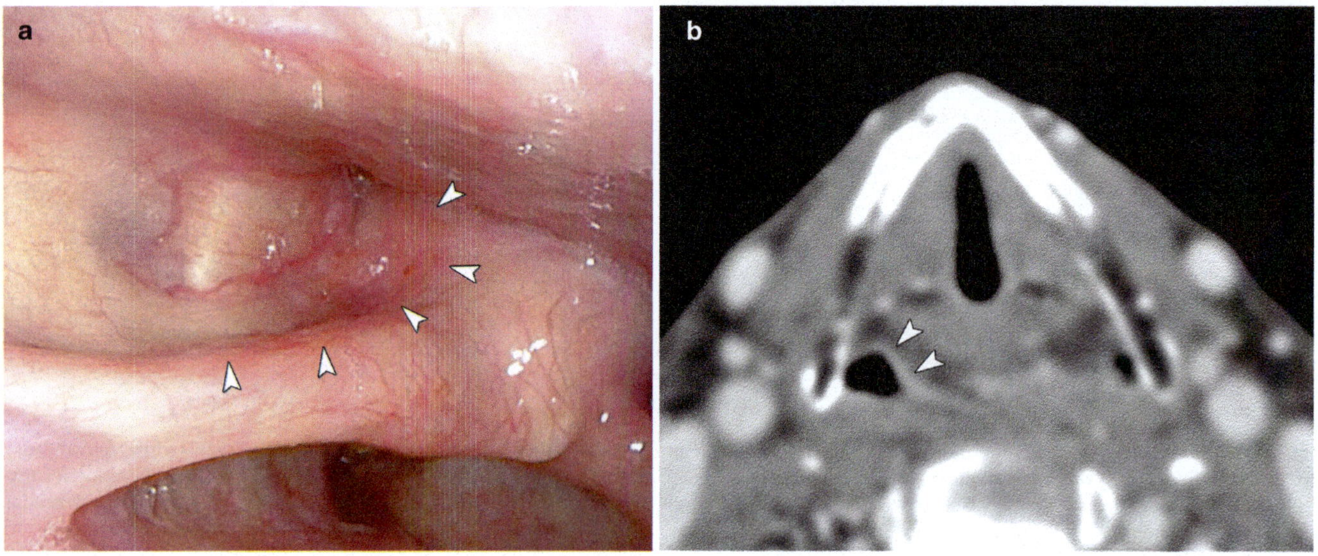

Fig. 5.18 Early pyriform sinus carcinoma treated by endoscopic laryngopharyngeal surgery. (**a**) Nasopharyngeal fiberscopy demonstrated that the mucosa was slightly red at the pyriform sinus with abnormal epithelial lesions in the mucosa of the pharynx with narrow-band imaging. (**b**) Axial contrast-enhanced image showing enhanced mucosal thickness (arrowheads)

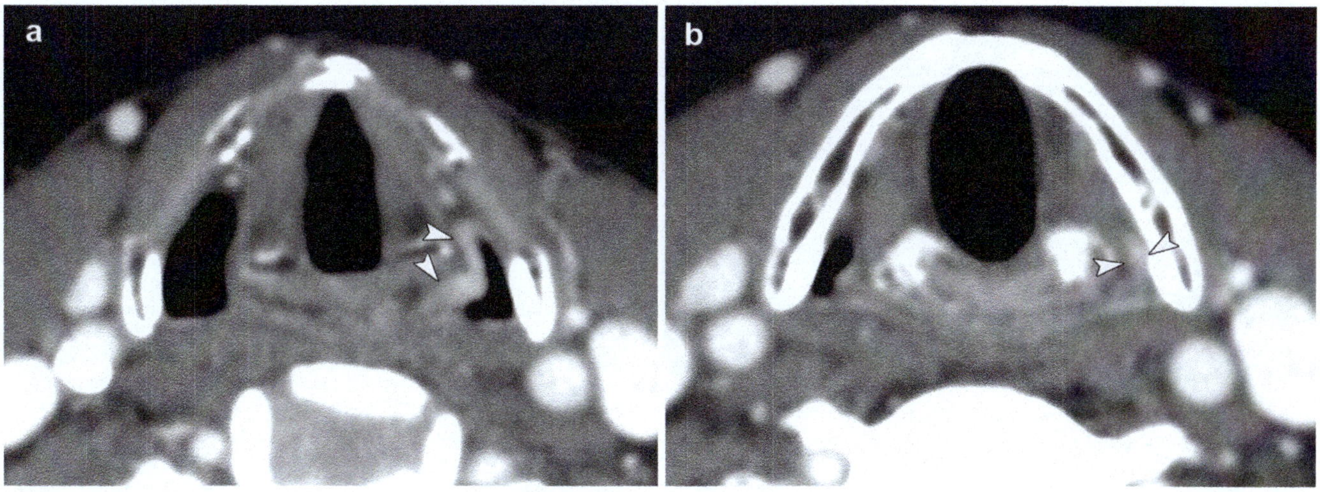

Fig. 5.19 Early hypopharyngeal carcinoma treated by radiation therapy. (**a**) Contrast-enhanced CT exhibits an enhanced tumor of the left medial pyriform sinus to the post arytenoid area (arrowheads). (**b**) Axial CT, more inferiorly, exhibits tumor extension toward the apex of the left pyriform sinus (arrowheads) and part of the postcricoid region

the indication for laryngeal preservation and partial resection may be limited. Moreover, tumor spreading into the pyriform sinus apex has been reported as a significant prognostic factor in radiotherapy [43].

Hypopharyngeal cancer exhibits aggressive local invasion along various routes [21, 43]. This tumor spreading has certain patterns or high-frequency pathways along well-defined routes, which are associated with barriers or weak points based on various lateral, anterior, posterior, cranial, and caudal structures.

5.6.2.2 Postcricoid (PC)

Postcricoid hypopharyngeal carcinoma accounts for 7–10% of hypopharyngeal cancer subsites. PC hypopharyngeal cancer is relatively rare, and many of them spread from pyriform sinus tumors (Fig. 5.20), cervical esophageal cancer, and laryngeal cancer. PC tumors infiltrate into the arytenoid area, arytenoid/cricoid cartilage, and posterior cricoarytenoid muscle from an early stage (Fig. 5.21). It is difficult to determine the extent of tumor spreading with an endoscope, and it is necessary to accurately evaluate the presence or absence of cartilage infiltration, extramural extension, and extension to the esophagus muscle layer. Sagittal imaging is sometime useful in the evaluation of cranial-caudal tumor growth in the hypopharynx and in determining the presence or absence and the extent of infiltration in the postcricoid direction.

5.6.2.3 Posterior Wall (PW)

Posterior wall tumors account for 12–16% of hypopharyngeal cancer subsites. Posterior wall tumors may often be seen continuously with the posterior oropharyngeal wall or cervical esophagus and are sometimes treated as a "posterior wall cancer" lesion. The extent of surgical resection is related to the function of postoperative swallowing. Imaging provides accurate information on tumor extent. In this regard, posterior extension of the retropharyngeal space, anterior vertebral fascia invasion, and anterior vertebral muscle invasion are essential (Fig. 5.22).

5.6.2.4 Spread Pattern of Hypopharyngeal Cancer into the Deep Space and Tissues

1. Paraglottic space extension through the thyroarytenoid gap (PS)

   In the anterior to medial spread (laryngeal direction), paraglottic space extension through the thyroarytenoid gap is important. The thyroarytenoid gap is a potential route of tumor spread between the thyroid and arytenoid cartilages (Fig. 5.23) [44]. Laryngeal and hypopharyngeal cancer extend inferiorly or posteriorly via this gap and the paraglottic space. Upon spreading into the paraglottic space, the tumor presents similarly to advanced glottic cancer. Furthermore, if the tumor invades the cricoarytenoid joint in the arytenoid area and clinically indicates vocal cord fixation, it is classified as T3.

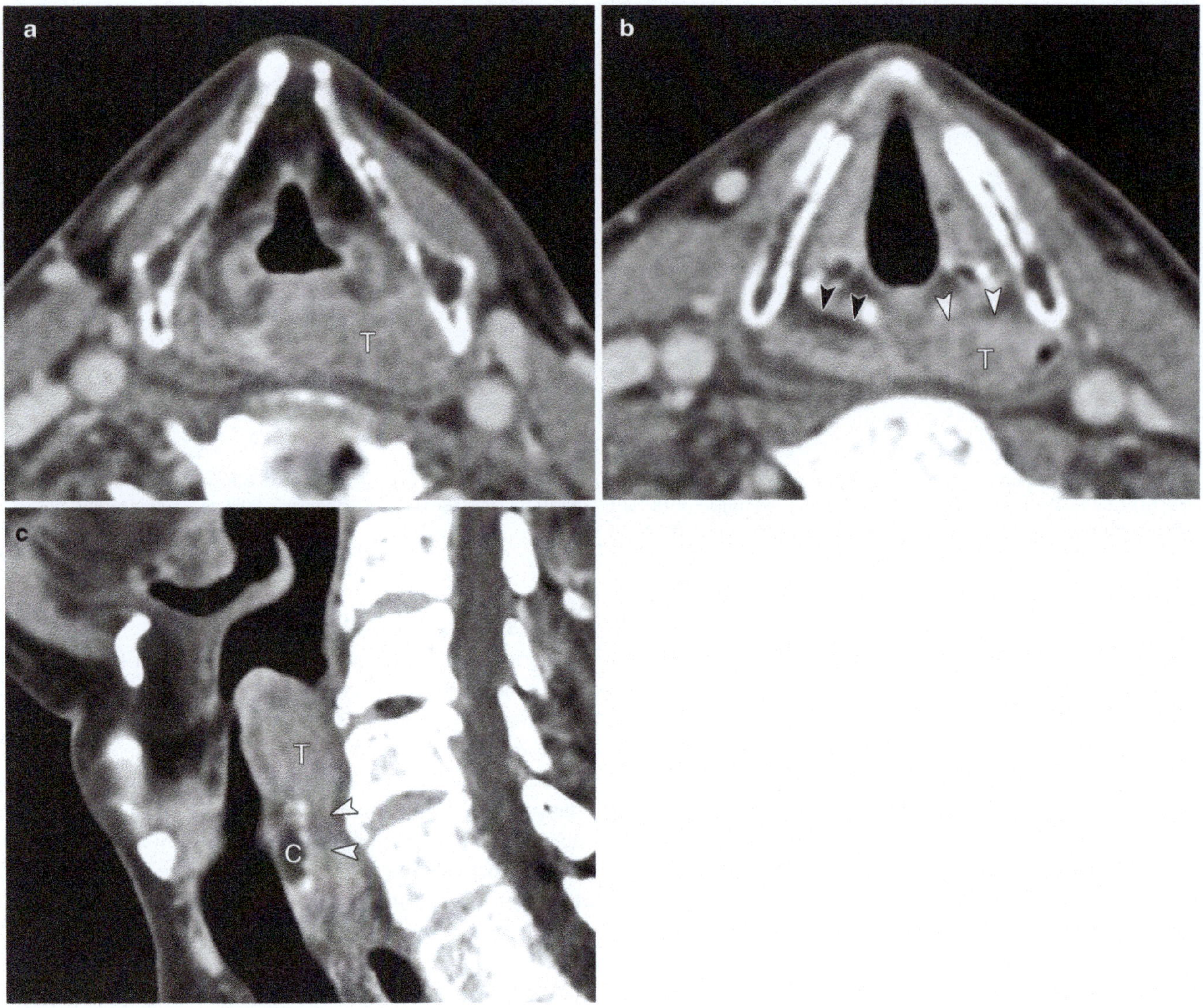

Fig. 5.20 (**a**) Axial contrast-enhanced CT at the false vocal cord level reveals an infiltrative tumor (T) with an irregular surface in the left pyriform sinus and upper postcricoid region. (**b**) A caudal slice shows tumor invasion to the left side of the postcricoid region (white arrowhead). The submucosal fat layer (presented with black arrowheads on the right side) can be confirmed. On the sagittal images (**c**), the tumor (T) is present in the medial pyriform sinus to the postcricoid region (arrowheads). *C* cricoid cartilage

2. Prevertebral muscle infiltration (PS, PW)

   In hypopharyngeal carcinoma, tumors with direct invasion of the prevertebral space or cervical spine are considered challenging for complete resection and are defined as T4b factors. An important imaging finding is to identify the fat layer in the retropharyngeal space with CT and MRI. When the fat of the retropharyngeal space is retained, the negative predictive value for prevertebral muscle infiltration is reported to be 82% (CT) and 97.5% (MRI), and prevertebral muscle infiltration is generally negative [45, 46] (Fig. 5.22). If there is a disruption or obscuring of the pharyngeal constrictor muscle and retropharyngeal space fat layer, it is necessary to evaluate whether contours with the anterior vertebral muscle are maintained (Fig. 5.24). Contrast-enhanced MRI is superior for assessment of vertebral muscle invasion [45–47]. Findings suggestive of vertebral muscle infiltration include irregularities in the contours of prevertebral muscle and replacement of prevertebral muscle with a signal intensity equivalent to that of the tumor; however, the specificity of these imaging findings is low. Ultimately, it is necessary to make a judgment based on intraoperative findings.

3. Postcricoid spreading and extension of the cervical esophagus (PS, PC, PW)

   As for caudal extension, the postcricoid spreading, the cricoid cartilage invasion, and the extension of the cervical esophagus (mucosa and muscle layer) are important

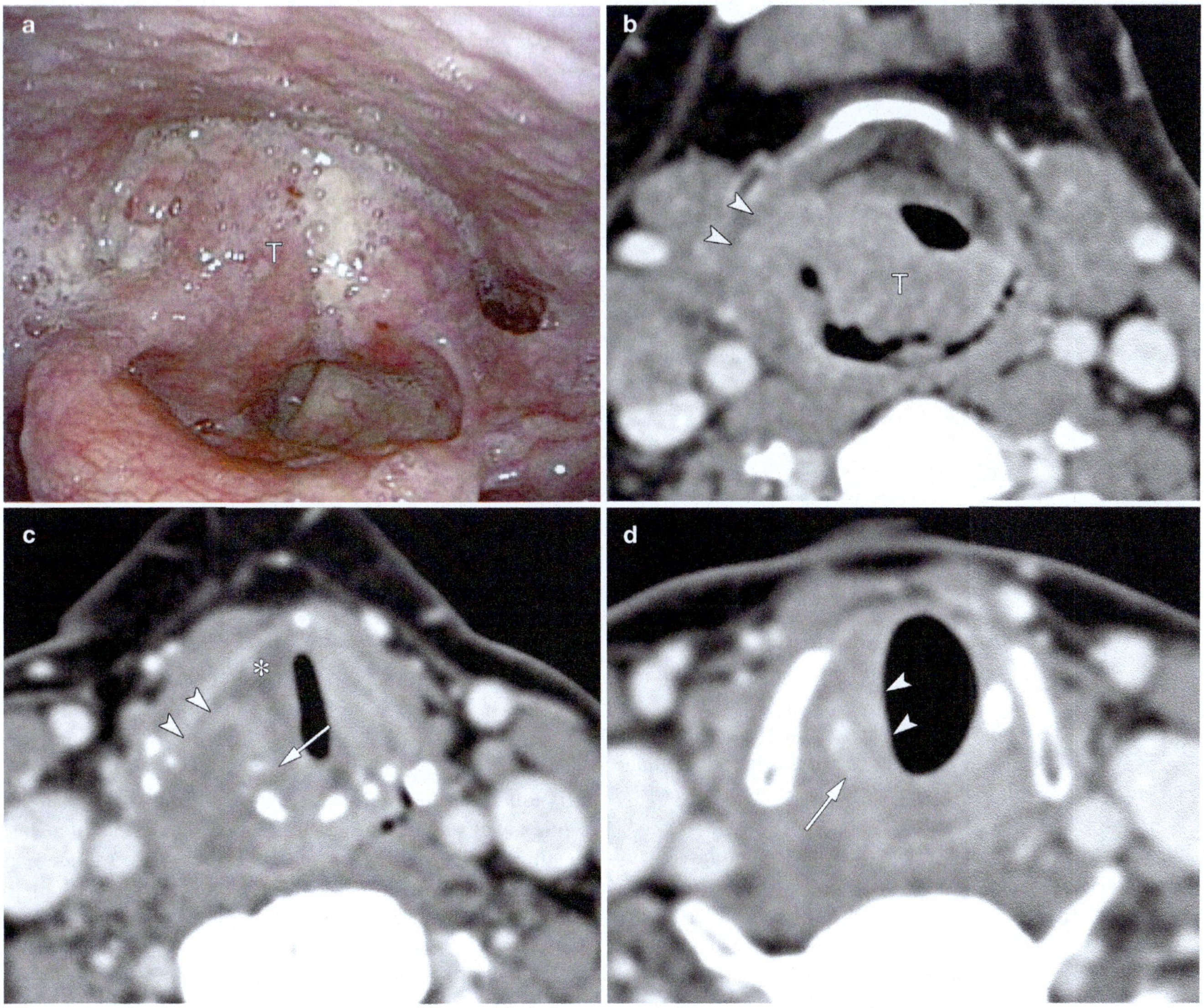

Fig. 5.21 Local advanced hypopharyngeal carcinoma of pyriform sinus and postcricoid. (**a**) Laryngoscopy demonstrates a bulky mass (T) in the arytenoid and postcricoid region. (**b**) Axial contrast-enhanced CT image through the false vocal cord level shows a bulky mass in the bilateral aryepiglottic fold and right pyriform sinus with extension to the thyrohyoid membrane (arrowheads). (**c**) At the true vocal cord level, the tumor of the right pyriform sinus (T) extends through submucosal into the right paraglottic space (asterisk) via the thyroarytenoid gap (arrowheads). The tumor also involves the right cricoarytenoid joint (arrow). (**d**) At the subglottic level, the tumor invades cricoid cartilage (arrow) and subglottic extension (arrowheads)

for staging. In the T classification for hypopharyngeal carcinoma, extension to the esophageal mucosa is T3 disease, and involvement of the esophageal muscle is T4a (Fig. 5.25). It is difficult to determine the muscle layer involvement with an endoscope, and it is necessary to accurately evaluate the extension by CT or MRI.

5.6.2.5 Extralaryngeal Spread of Hypopharyngeal Cancer

1. Extralaryngeal spread via the thyrohyoid membrane (PS)

   As well as supraglottic laryngeal cancer (Fig. 5.15), in lateral extension, extralaryngeal spread via the thyrohyoid membrane (both T4a factor) is also important for pyriform sinus carcinoma. Even in early lesions, the extralaryngeal spread through the supralaryngeal neurovascular bundle via thyrohyoid membrane (Fig. 5.15c) is often seen.

2. Wraparound extralaryngeal spread via the pharyngeal constrictor muscle (PS)

   Another route of extralaryngeal spread, especially in the case of pyriform sinus cancer, is via the inferior pharyngeal constrictor [21, 42] on the basis of its attachment to the lamina of the thyroid cartilage (Fig. 5.26). The wraparound spread that wraps the posterior part of the thyroid cartilage according to adhesion of the pharyngeal constrictor muscle

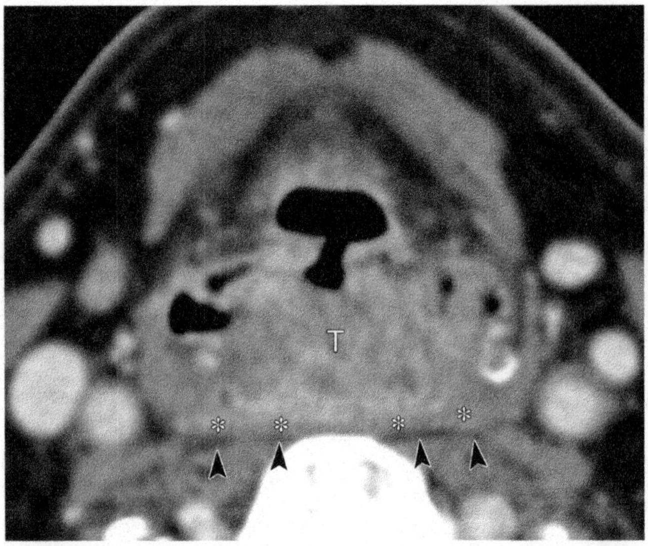

Fig. 5.22 Posterior wall hypopharyngeal carcinoma without retropharyngeal space infiltration. Axial contrast-enhanced CT shows the tumor (T) at the center of the hypopharynx posterior wall. The lesion appears to be limited to the posterior wall of the hypopharynx, not extending to the side wall. In the posterior direction, the inferior pharyngeal constrictor muscle (asterisk) and fat layer of the retropharyngeal space (black arrowheads) are intact

(Fig. 5.26c) is a possible route of extralaryngeal spread and easily invades into the posterior part of the thyroid cartilage (Fig. 5.27). Further, this spreading can be a risk of carotid artery invasion (T4b) (Fig. 5.27).

3. Extralaryngeal spread via cricothyroid membrane and joint (PS, PC)

   The cricothyroid joint is also an important route of tumor spread from hypopharynx toward the extralaryngeal soft tissue such as the thyroid lobe (Fig. 5.28).

5.7 Cartilage Invasion

Determining cartilage invasion is extremely important for treatment decision-making for laryngeal and hypopharyngeal cancer. Patients with laryngeal and hypopharyngeal cancer in whom tumors extend through the cartilage into the soft tissue of the neck generally undergo immediate surgery as the risk of recurrence and cartilage necrosis after radiotherapy alone are high [36, 48, 49]. In clinical practice, patients with T4 disease do not always undergo laryngectomy, and patients without transcartilaginous tumor extension may be potential candidates for function-preserving treatment to a degree. Discussion with patients forms part of the treatment decision-making process. Therefore, it is necessary for imaging to evaluate not just the detection of cartilage invasion but also the degree (depth and range) of cartilage invasion as much as possible. In addition, unnecessary overestimation should be avoided, and denial of cartilage invasion based on appropriate diagnostic imaging is important in laryngeal function preservation.

Both CT and MRI can be used to evaluate cartilage invasion. Each modality has advantages and limitations for the staging of laryngeal and hypopharyngeal cancer. Imaging studies on laryngeal cartilage invasion date back to the 1990s. In studies using single-slice CT in the 1990s, CT had high specificity (96–97%) for cartilage invasion but low sensitivity (50–62%), which was considered inadequate as a preoperative examination. In 1997, Becker et al. reported that CT criteria using a combination of specific diagnostic criteria (sclerosis, erosion, lysis, and transmural extralaryngeal tumor spread) were able to reach an acceptable balance of 71% sensitivity versus 83% specificity for thyroid cartilage [50]. Subsequently, from the late 2000s onwards, evaluation was performed with thin reconstructed images by MDCT. Although the sensitivity increased (85%), the specificity decreased (75%) [51], which is still occasionally overestimated [52, 53]. This arises as CT values of non-ossified cartilage and tumors after iodinated contrast agent injection are similar, and various CT values occur due to ossification of cartilage with aging [8, 50]. Therefore, when the tumor and non-osteogenic cartilage are in contact with each other, it is important to carefully evaluate morphological changes while always taking into consideration the ossification state of thyroid cartilage. Asymmetrical sclerosis (defined as thickening of the cortical margin, increased medullary density, or both) when comparing one arytenoid with the other, or one side of the cricoid or thyroid cartilage with the other side, is a sensitive but nonspecific feature of cartilage invasion on CT [50, 54–56]. For thyroid cartilage especially, asymmetric sclerotic changes (ossification) without erosion or lysis should not be diagnosed as positive (Fig. 5.29a), as these changes can represent reactive changes [40, 50].

MRI is more sensitive than CT for detecting thyroid cartilage invasion (sensitivity up to 96%), as the high-contrast resolution of MR makes it possible to detect small areas of marrow space invasion [57–60] and should be used positively when it is difficult to diagnose by contrast-enhanced CT. When assessing cartilage invasion with MR imaging, T2-weighted and contrast-enhanced T1-weighted signal intensities of cartilage should be compared with the signal intensities of the adjacent tumor [57]. If the cartilage displays signal intensity similar to that of the tumor, cartilage invasion should be suspected (Fig. 5.27). However, MR findings suggestive of cartilage invasion are not specific and may, therefore, lead to false-positive signs. The reason is that

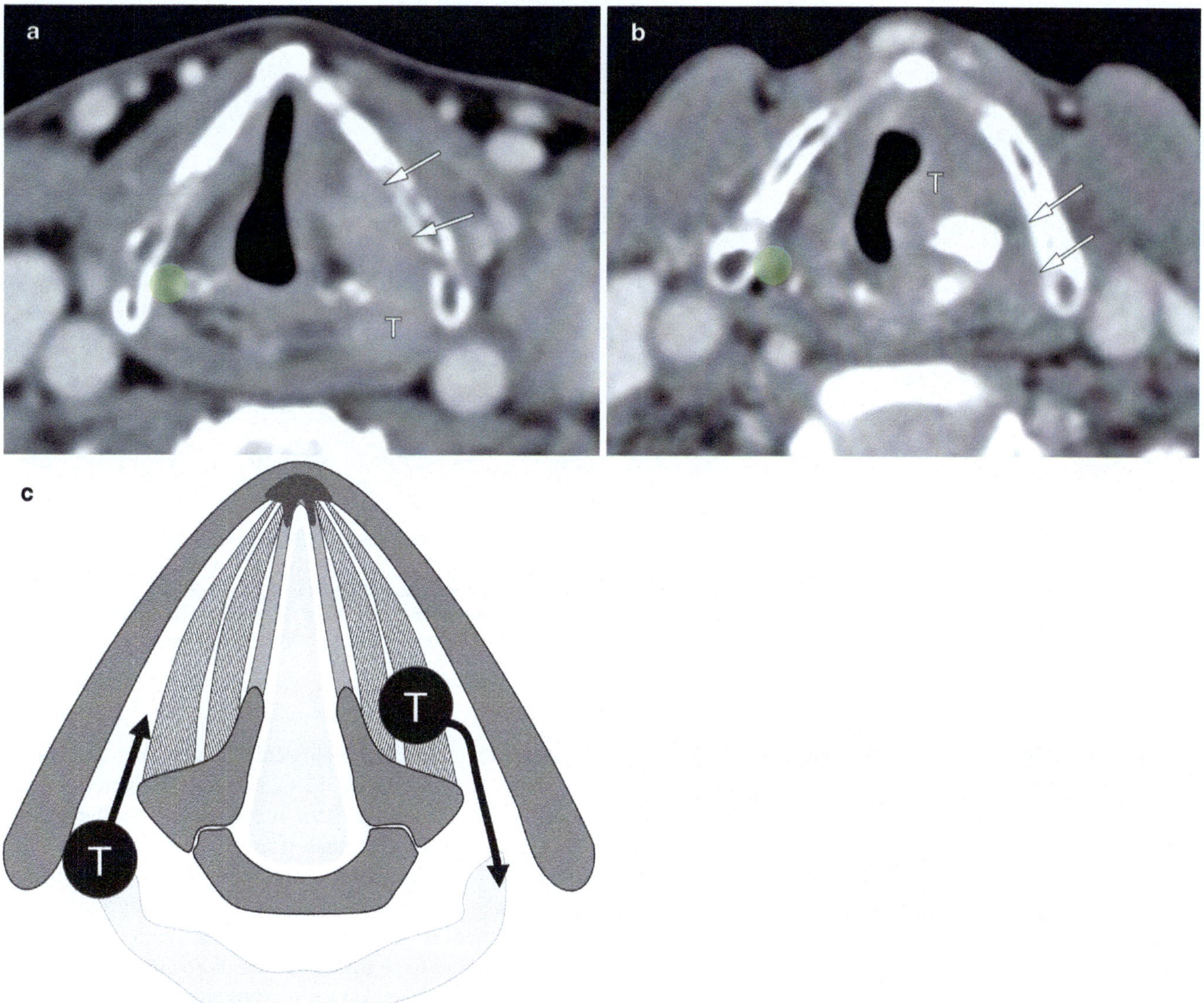

Fig. 5.23 Two-way paths in the thyroarytenoid gap from different primary sites. The thyroarytenoid gap is a potential route of tumor spread between the thyroid and arytenoid cartilages. Hypopharyngeal pyriform sinus carcinoma (**a**) and laryngeal glottic carcinoma (**b**) extend inferiorly or posteriorly via this gap and the paraglottic space. (**c**) Schema diagram of the spread patterns

reactive inflammation, edema, and fibrosis in the vicinity of a tumor may demonstrate diagnostic features similar to those of cartilage invasion; therefore, careful diagnosis should be made considering the possibility of false-positive findings. Inflammatory changes are most common in thyroid ossified cartilage (cortical bone and bone fat marrow). The specificity of MRI for detecting invasion of the thyroid cartilage is 56–65% [57, 58], and the higher sensitivity on MRI may be at the expense of specificity. To avoid overestimation of cartilage invasion using MRI, radiologists should search for areas isointense in signal to the tumor on T1WI, T2WI, and fat-suppressed T2-weighted images (Figs. 5.29 and 5.30). Reactive edema will be T2 hyperintense to the tumor [19].

Dual-energy CT may overcome some of the shortcomings of conventional CT, as iodine contrast may be distributed in tumor tissues but not in normal cartilage. With dual-energy imaging, an iodine-overlay image can be created that distinguishes between an iodine contrast agent (tumor to be imaged), soft tissue, and non-ossified cartilage and can distinguish between tumor-infiltrated and noninvasive areas [10]. The spectral attenuation curves of tumor to non-ossified cartilage can also be used for evaluating cartilage invasion [9]. Even if there is contact between non-osteogenic cartilage and the tumor by conventional CT and the judgment is unclear, if the contrast enhancement of non-osteogenic cartilage is lacking in iodine-overlay images, cartilage infiltration

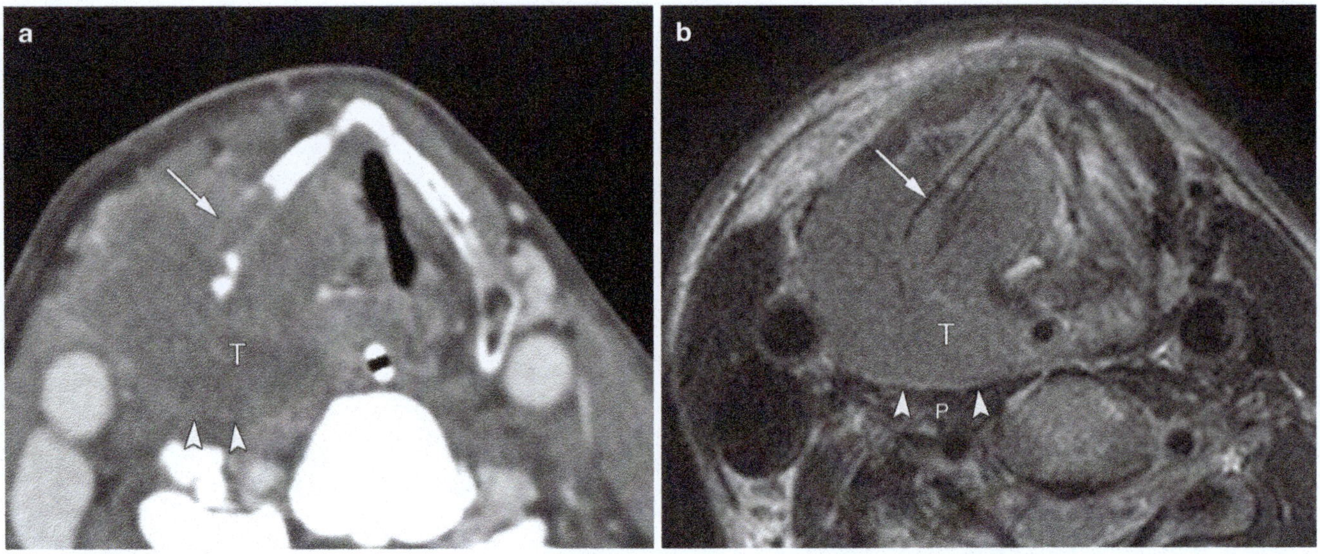

Fig. 5.24 Pyriform sinus carcinoma without prevertebral involvement on MRI. Axial contrast-enhanced CT (**a**) and T2-weighted images (**b**) demonstrate a large tumor mass (T) arising from the right pyriform sinus, spreading into the lateral extralaryngeal soft tissue with thyroid cartilage invasion (arrow). On contrast-enhanced CT (**a**), the large tumor (T) infiltrates posteriorly, and the fatty layer of the retropharyngeal space is unclear. It may be difficult to completely rule out prevertebral muscle infiltration. On T2-weighted image (**b**), the anterior contour of the prevertebral muscle (P) is preserved, and there are no changes in the signal intensity of the prevertebral muscle, suggesting there is no definitive prevertebral fascia infiltration

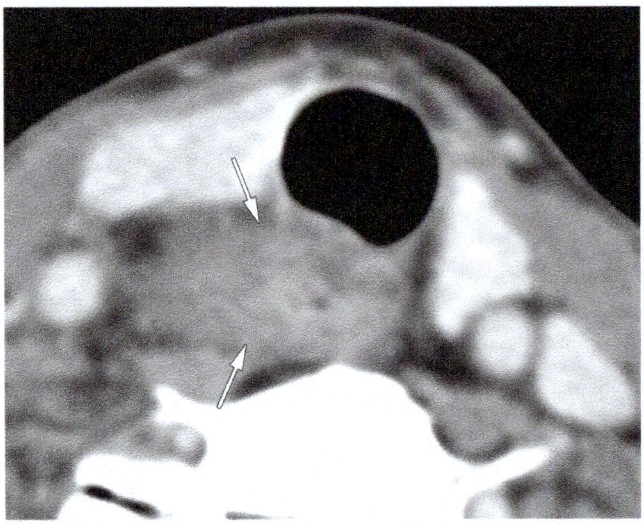

Fig. 5.25 Esophageal extension with hypopharyngeal carcinoma. Note the tumor invades the muscle layer of cervical esophagus (arrows)

is negative (Figs. 5.31 and 5.32). If the cartilage portion has an enhancement effect, it can be judged that the invasion is positive (Fig. 5.33). It is considered that adding an iodine-overlay image to the evaluation significantly increases the specificity (70% → 96%) without degrading the sensitivity (86%), as compared to the usual evaluation of CT alone [10]. In addition, dual-energy CT is less affected by motion artefacts from swallowing motions than is MRI, and it is possible to evaluate minute morphological changes (such as erosion) of bone cortex by virtual 120 kV image (weighted-average image). False positives due to secondary inflammatory changes are less than that from evaluation by contrast-enhanced MRI and significantly improve specificity [11].

Cartilage invasion occurs most frequently in ossified cartilage without perichondrium which can be a natural pathway for the cartilage invasion. The most important sites for cartilage invasion are (1) the thyroid angle at the attachment of the anterior commissure tendon (Fig. 5.33c), (2) the attachments of the cricothyroid membrane to the corresponding cartilage (Fig. 5.28a), (3) the anterior portion of the thyroid lamina near the origin of the thyroarytenoid muscle (Fig. 5.33), (4) the posterior border of the thyroid lamina adjacent to the pyriform sinus (Fig. 5.28a), and (5) the capsule of the cricoarytenoid joint [61]. Diagnostic criteria of cartilage invasion are shown in Table 5.4. For MRI, cartilage invasion can be diagnosed as "positive" in cases where cartilage displayed signals similar to the adjacent tumor on all pre- and post-contrast T1-weighted and T2-weighted images in cortical bone, cartilage, and bone marrow space. When the cartilage had higher signal intensity than the adjacent tumor on T2-weighted images or when stronger enhancement was present on post-contrast T1-weighted images, abnormal signal intensity should be diagnosed as negative because these changes may represent reactive changes. For dual-energy CT, image interpretation always commence with the WA image to evaluate tumor

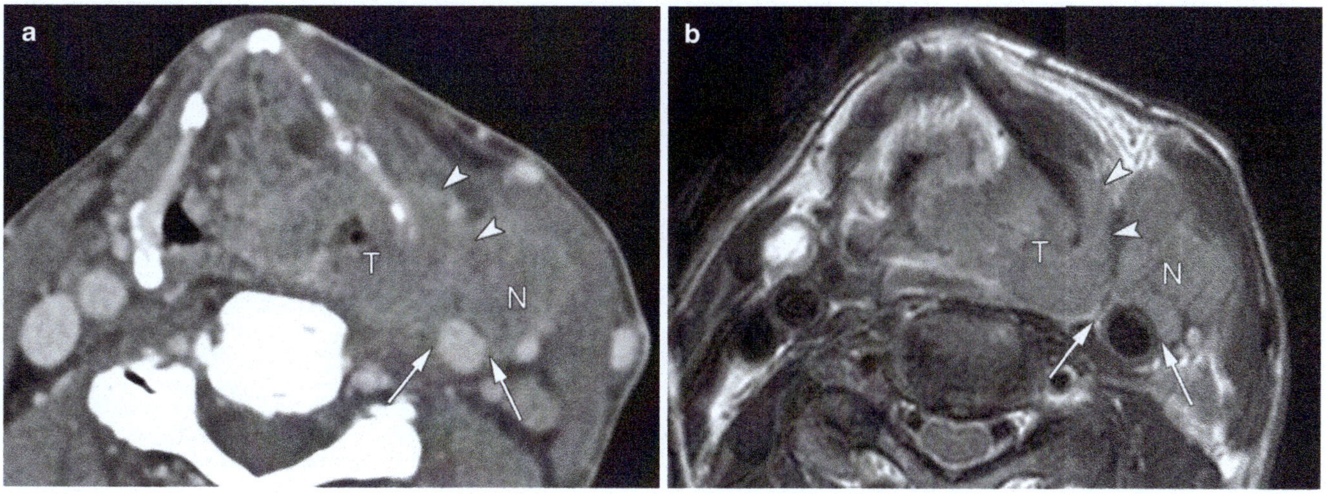

Fig. 5.26 Wraparound spread with advanced pyriform sinus carcinoma with ENE node metastasis. Axial contrast-enhanced CT (**a**) and T2-weighted images (**b**) demonstrate a large tumor mass (T) arising from the left pyriform sinus, spreading into the lateral extralaryngeal soft tissue via the attachment of the inferior pharyngeal constrictor muscle (arrowheads). The tumor also wraps around the posterior border of the thyroid cartilage. Note the level III lymph node metastasis with ENE (N) and in contact with a 90 circumferential area of the common carotid artery (arrows)

location, extension, and invasion [10, 11]. When a lesion was evaluated as having erosion or lysis of ossified cartilage on WA images, the iodine distribution in the remaining non-ossified cartilage should be evaluated on IO images for a final diagnosis of either positive or negative for cartilage invasion. Again, areas of ossified cartilage are thoroughly excluded from evaluation on IO images, because dual-energy algorithms could not distinguish calcium from iodine [10].

5.8 Lymph Node Metastasis

Supralaryngeal cancer frequently shows lymph node metastasis of 50–60%, as there is often significant and bilateral supraglottic lymphatic drainage to the high jugular nodes (levels II and III). Rarely, supraglottic neoplasms can involve submandibular and retropharyngeal nodes. Purely glottic tumors rarely have nodal metastasis, because there is almost no lymphatic drainage of the submucosa of the true vocal cords. However, once the tumor infiltrates the preepiglottic or paraglottic spaces, there is a greater likelihood of nodal disease (level III is typically the most commonly affected level) [62]. Neck adenopathies are uncommonly encountered in small (T1) lesions, but the risk increases to about 8% and 30% in T2 and T3 lesions, respectively. Subglottic tumors including extension from glottic tumor may involve the Delphian nodes (prelaryngeal node) but most frequently involve level VI (paratracheal) lymph nodes. A positive Delphian node is known to predict a poor prognosis in laryngeal and hypopharyngeal cancer [63, 64] (Fig. 5.34). Paratracheal lymph node involvement places the patient at a higher risk for mediastinal nodal and distant metastasis.

Hypopharyngeal cancer is more likely to show lymph node metastasis, even small primary sites, than other sites of head and neck cancer (Fig. 5.35). It is reported that 60–75% of the initial tumor is positive for cervical lymph node metastasis, and 15% are bilateral [28, 29]. This is because hypopharyngeal lymphatic drainage can drain almost all lymph node regions in the neck. Therefore, control of cervical lymph node metastasis is important in hypopharyngeal cancer treatment, and a wide range of neck dissection and radiation must be considered depending on the case. In addition, the frequency of metastasis to the retropharyngeal lymph node is also high at 15% and should be positively included in the radiation field [65]. Again, extranodal extension (ENE) and contralateral nodal disease are negative prognostic indicators and may alter treatment regimens. It is necessary to evaluate the clinical extranodal extension in detail for the presence or absence and also infiltration into adjacent structures (carotid artery, jugular vein, muscle, deep cervical fascia, and/or nerves) (Figs. 5.25 and 5.26).

5.9 Distant Metastasis

Laryngeal cancer has a risk of distant metastasis of approximately 10%. The risk of second primary malignancy in the first 5 years is also high. As HNC patients have common risk behaviors such as smoking, it is known that more than 10% of patients after HNC treatment have second primary lung cancer within 10 years [66]. Compared to other head and neck cancers, hypopharyngeal cancer is considered to have a high frequency of distant metastasis (about 17%), and the need for remote search in pretreatment evaluation and post-

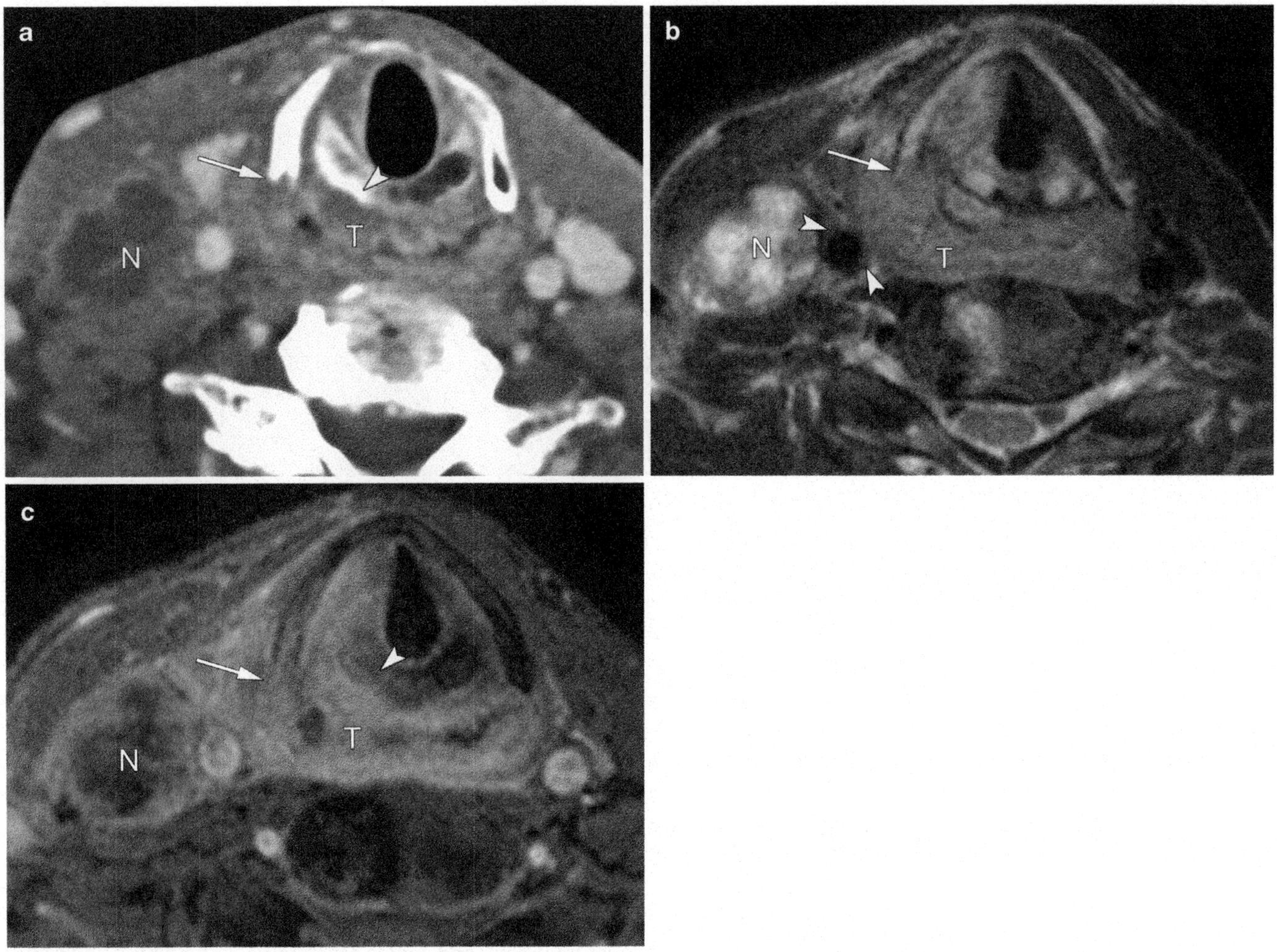

Fig. 5.27 Very advanced hypopharyngeal carcinoma with carotid artery invasion (T4b). Axial contrast-enhanced CT (**a**), T2-weighted images (**b**), and contrast-enhanced fat-suppressed T1-weighted MR image (**c**) demonstrate invasive mass (T) at postcricoid and posterior wall of the hypopharynx. Lysis and erosion of the thyroid (arrow) and cricoid (arrowheads) cartilages and level III lymph node metastasis with ENE (N) are evident. On a T2-weighted image (**b**), the tumor (T) showed tumor extension into the common carotid arteries (arrowheads). ENE lymph node metastasis is also in contact with a 270 circumferential area of the common carotid artery, suggesting carotid artery invasion

treatment follow-up is high. Lung metastases are most common, followed by mediastinal lymph nodes, liver, and bone. Among the mediastinal lymph nodes, level VII is treated as a regional lymph node, and the others are distant metastases.

5.10 Treatment Strategy

Treatments for laryngeal and hypopharyngeal cancer are broadly divided into (chemo)radiotherapy and surgical treatment [49]. Patients with T1, T2, and T3 disease can be considered positively for organ-preserving procedures such as radiation therapy alone, a combination of chemotherapy and radiation therapy, and function-preserving partial laryngectomy or pharyngectomy procedures [37, 38, 67–69]. Patients with T4a disease, particularly when the tumor extends through the cartilage into the soft tissue of the neck, often need aggressive treatments such as total laryngectomy [20, 69, 70], which can have a devastating impact on the quality of life. Since treatment is decided according to the precise extent and invasion pattern of a tumor, imaging plays a crucial role in any multidisciplinary approach for management of laryngeal and hypopharyngeal cancers.

Radiation therapy for early lesions is widely performed (Figs. 5.8 and 5.19), and good local control and laryngeal preservation rates have been reported. However, it must be noted that irradiation of the same site can only be performed once in principle, and salvage surgery for residual cases carries the risk of complications. For advanced cases, total pharyngo-laryngo-esophagectomy (TPLE) is mainly performed. In recent years, combination chemoradiotherapy has been attempted to preserve larynx function. In residual cases,

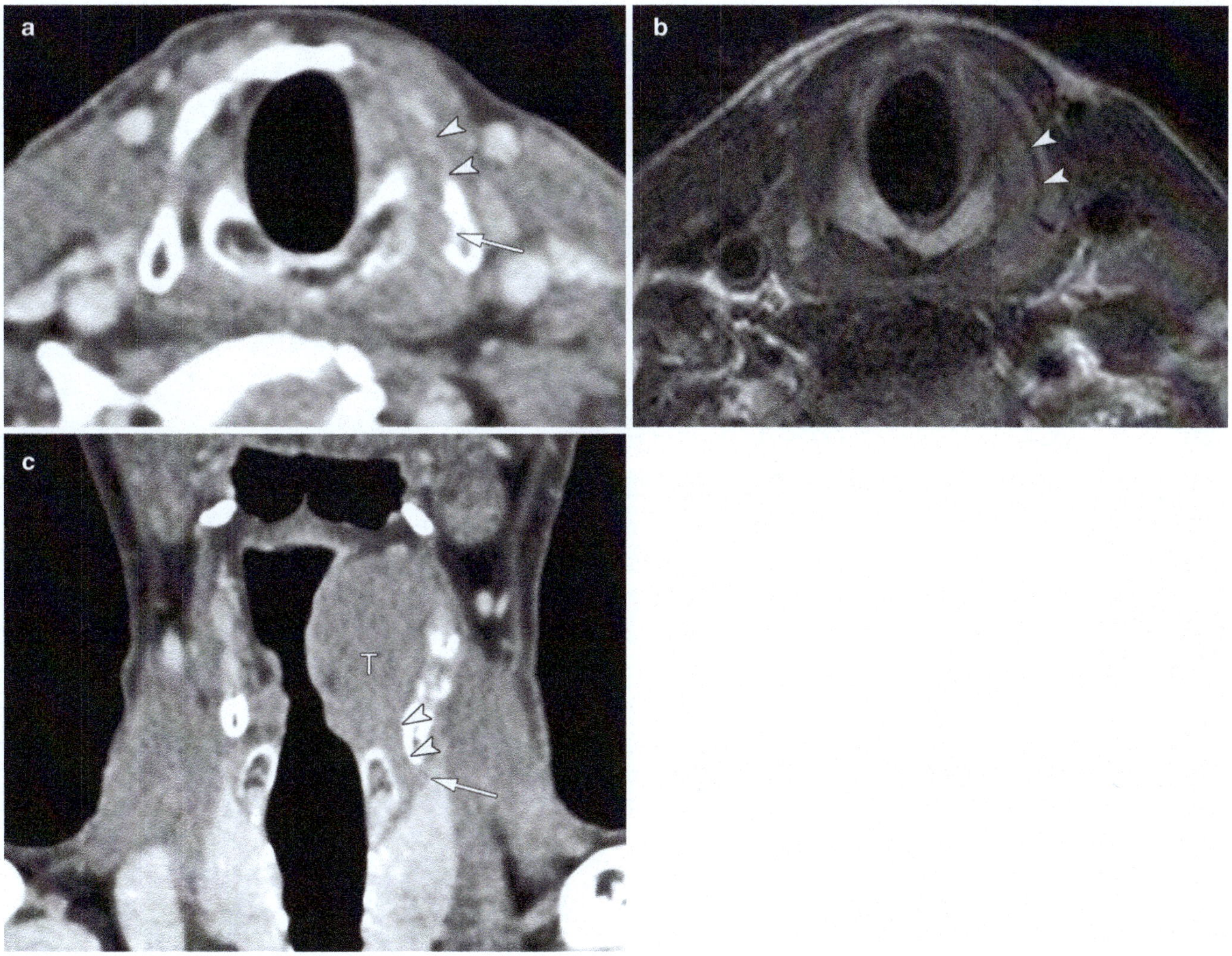

Fig. 5.28 Pyriform sinus carcinoma with extralaryngeal spread through the cricothyroid joint. Axial contrast-enhanced CT (**a**) and T2-weighted MRI image (**b**) demonstrate the extralaryngeal spread through the cricothyroid membrane and joint (arrowheads) with thyroid cartilage erosion (arrow). Coronal contrast-enhanced CT shows the tumor (T) spreading through the cricothyroid joint (arrowheads) toward the left thyroid lobe (arrow)

TPLE is performed after restaging. Determining a treatment plan for laryngeal or hypopharyngeal cancer requires comprehensive judgment based on different information. Ultimately, it is necessary to make decisions via a multidisciplinary tumor board, including head and neck surgeons, oncologists, and radiologists.

For early stages of hypopharyngeal cancer, (chemo)radiotherapy (Fig. 5.19) or laryngeal preservation surgery is selected based on tumor conditions to aim for laryngeal preservation [71–73]. With recent advances in endoscopic diagnosis/treatment, treatment strategies for early (T1–2) hypopharyngeal cancer are changing. Laryngeal preservation surgery (hypopharyngeal partial resection), transoral, or endoscopic resection for superficial lesions of hypopharyngeal cancer, such as endoscopic laryngopharyngeal surgery (ELPS) (Fig. 5.18), transoral laser microsurgery (TLM), transoral video laryngoscopic surgery (TOVS), and transoral robotic surgery (TORS) is indicated [74, 75].

5.11 Posttreatment Imaging

5.11.1 Postoperative Imaging

Various surgical procedures for hypopharyngeal cancer exist, resulting in anatomical changes and deformation after surgery. In partial hypopharyngeal resection, a portion of the cartilage such as the posterior lamina of thyroid cartilage on one side is resected; if necessary, the reconstructed flap tissue is filled (Fig. 5.36). After TPLE, reconstruction using free jejunum (neopharynx) is performed (Fig. 5.37). During follow-up, lymphadenopathy may be observed in the mesen-

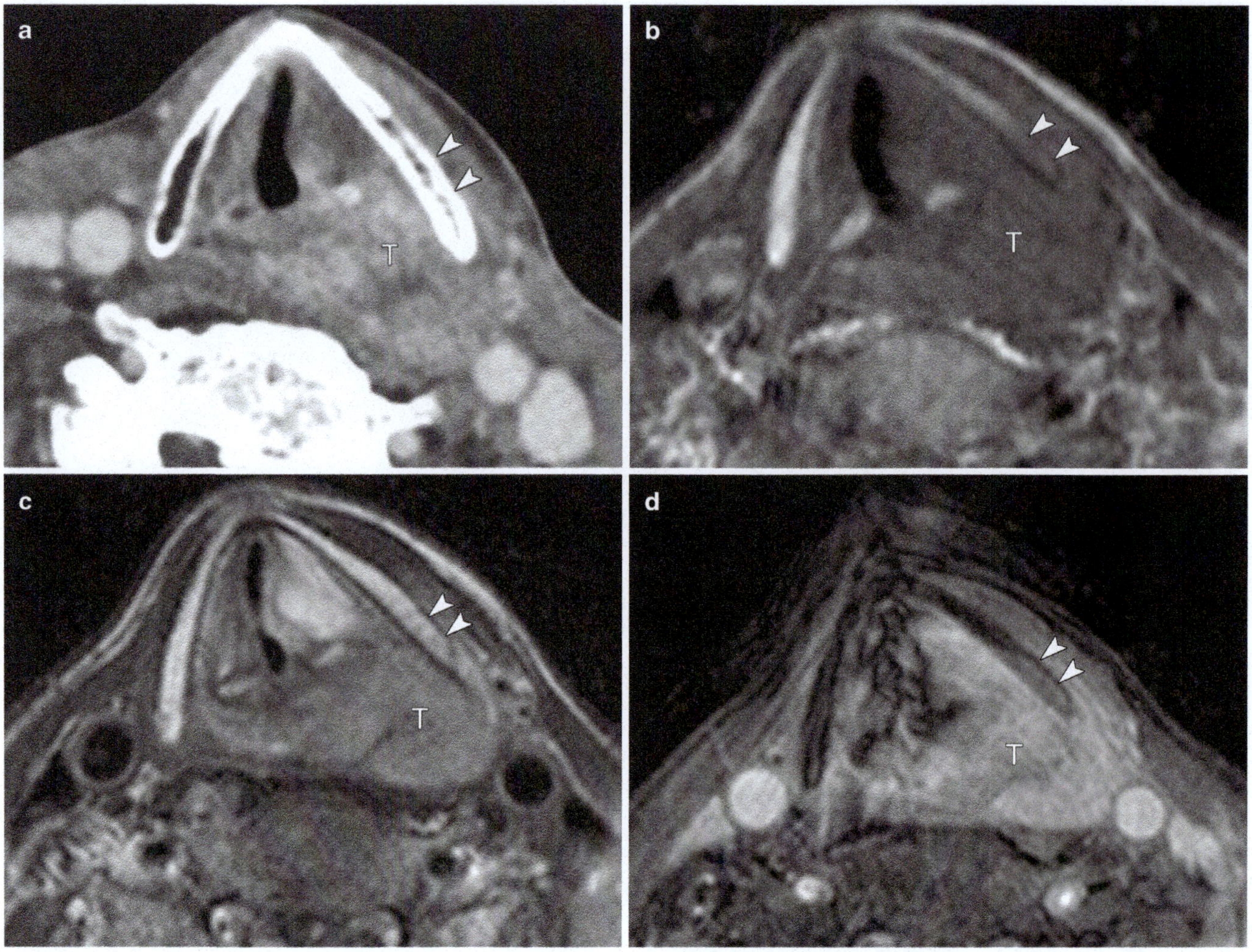

Fig. 5.29 True negative imaging findings for thyroid cartilage invasion with pyriform sinus carcinoma. Contrast-enhanced CT (**a**) images show tumor mass arising from the pyriform sinus. No erosion and lysis are observed at the lamina of the thyroid cartilage although sclerotic changes are observed (arrowheads). T1-weighted image (**b**) shows that adjacent thyroid cartilage has similar low signal intensity to that of the tumor (arrowheads). However, T2-weighted image (**c**) shows that the adjacent left thyroid lamina shows high signal intensity relative to that of the tumor (arrowheads). Contrast-enhanced fat-suppressed T1-weighted MR image (**d**) at the same level shows different contrast enhancement of the tumor (T) and adjacent thyroid cartilage (arrow). These findings suggest inflammation of the thyroid cartilage without neoplastic invasion

tery of the reconstructed neopharynx, and many are reactive enlargements of the mesenteric lymph nodes due to environmental changes [76]. In addition, the residual thyroid sometimes shows a mimic lesion. In follow-up of surgical cases, the area around the reconstructed flap tissue, anastomotic site and wall of the neopharynx, resected margin, and area around the air incisor are the preferred sites of recurrence.

5.11.2 Postradiation Imaging

In hypopharyngeal cancer, radiation therapy affects not only the tumor but also surrounding normal tissues. CT and MR imaging findings of early reactions to radiation therapy are thickening of the skin and platysma, reticulation of subcutaneous fat, edema and fluid in the retropharyngeal space, thickening and increased enhancement of the pharyngeal walls, and thickening of the laryngeal structures [76, 77]. The late reactions to radiation therapy include thickening of the pharyngeal constrictor muscle, platysma, and skin.

After radiation therapy for laryngeal cancer and hypopharyngeal cancer, laryngeal cartilage necrosis occurs at a frequency of about 1% due to endothelial cell injury as well as impaired circulation and lymphatic flow due to fibrosis. CT findings of radiation-induced cartilage necrosis include surrounding soft tissue swelling, segmentalization and collapse of thyroid cartilage, shedding of arytenoid cartilage, and abnormal gas images [78] (Fig. 5.38).

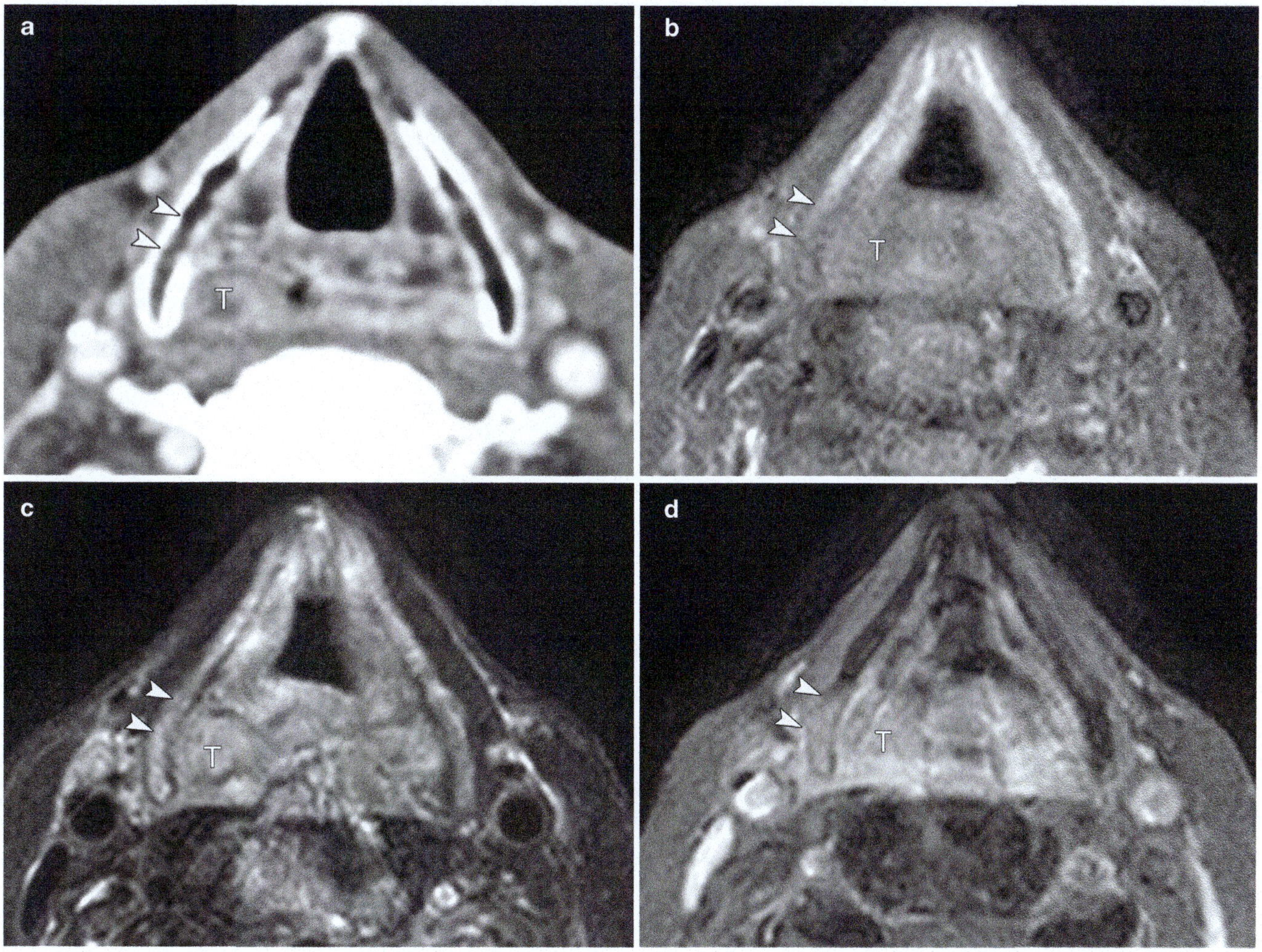

Fig. 5.30 False-positive findings for thyroid cartilage invasion on MR imaging with hypopharyngeal cancer. Contrast-enhanced CT image at the false vocal cord level shows a tumor (T) arising from the right pyriform sinus without erosion or lysis at the thyroid cartilage. T1-weighted image shows that the tumor (T) has low signal intensity, whereas adjacent thyroid cartilage has similar signal intensity (arrowheads). On T2-weighted MR image (**c**), the adjacent posterior right thyroid lamina shows similar high signal intensity to that of the tumor (arrowheads). Contrast-enhanced fat-suppressed T1-weighted MR image (**d**) at the same level shows a similar contrast enhancement of the tumor (T) and adjacent thyroid cartilage (arrowheads). Corresponding surgical specimen confirmed inflammation of the thyroid cartilage without neoplastic invasion

5.11.3 Posttreatment Surveillance Imaging

Tumor recurrence after radiation therapy typically manifests clinically within the first 2 years. The modalities for posttreatment surveillance imaging of patients with head and neck cancer are radiography, endoscopy, US, CT, MR imaging, and FDG PET/CT. Imaging plays an important role in the early detection of recurrence, to allow early intervention of salvage treatment. In locally advanced cancer, even if a good therapeutic effect is obtained, the tumor rarely disappears completely, and it is controlled while maintaining a certain size as soft tissue. In addition, due to changes after radiation treatment, discrimination between recurrent tumors and inflammatory edema, soft tissue necrosis, granulation, and fibrosis can cause issues. Therefore, the combination of precise morphologic CT/MRI imaging and quantitative imaging including MRI (DWI with an ADC value) and FDG-PET is useful for posttreatment evaluation after radiation therapy.

The use of imaging may present formidable challenges in interpreting the post-therapeutic setting due to edema, inflammation, fibrosis, asymmetry, and anatomical distortion. The optimal timing of the first response assessment imaging after definitive (chemo)radiation is not precisely known, but an interval of 6–12 weeks has generally been recommended to balance the drawbacks of imaging too early versus too late by modality. Typically, contrast MRI and FDG-PET will show secondary changes more sensitively

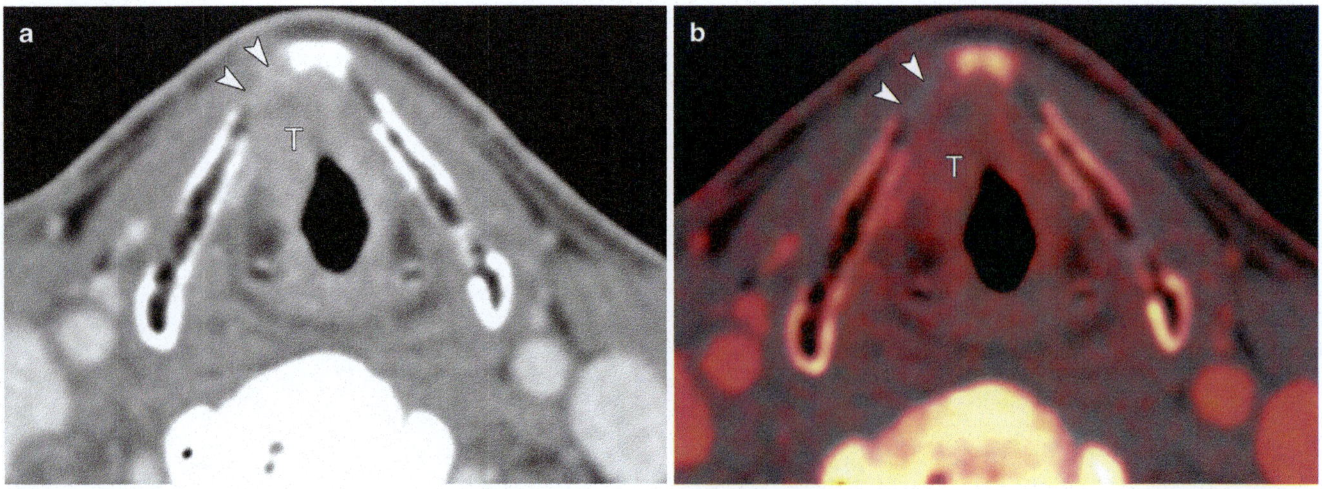

Fig. 5.31 Negative finding for erosion in the thyroid cartilage by dual-energy CT with glottic cancer. WA image (**a**) at the level of the false vocal cords shows a tumor mass (T) that has invaded the paraglottic space and anterior commissure. Non-ossified cartilage of the right thyroid lamina has been substituted by the tumor (arrowheads). IO image (**b**) clearly shows no corresponding enhancement of the thyroid cartilage (arrowheads). The surgical specimen confirmed that the right thyroid cartilage has not been invaded by the tumor cells

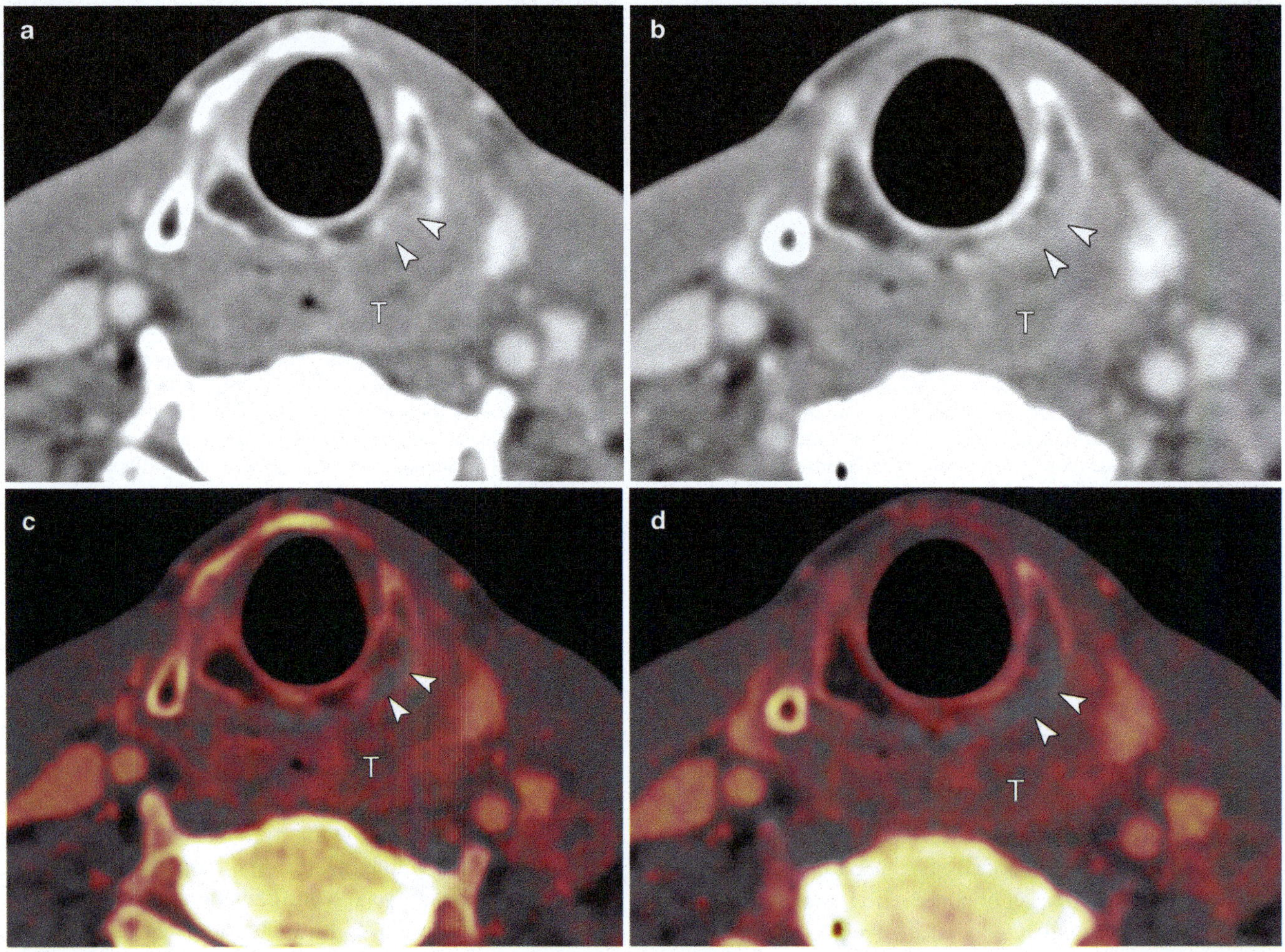

Fig. 5.32 Negative findings for invasion in the cricoid cartilage by dual-energy CT with hypopharyngeal carcinoma. WA image (**a**) shows a large tumor mass (T) in postcricoid area. Left lamina of the cricoid cartilage shows lysis change and has been substituted by the tumor (arrowheads). IO image (**b**) shows no corresponding enhancement of the cricoid cartilage (arrowheads). The surgical specimen confirmed that the cricoid cartilage had not been invaded by the tumor cells

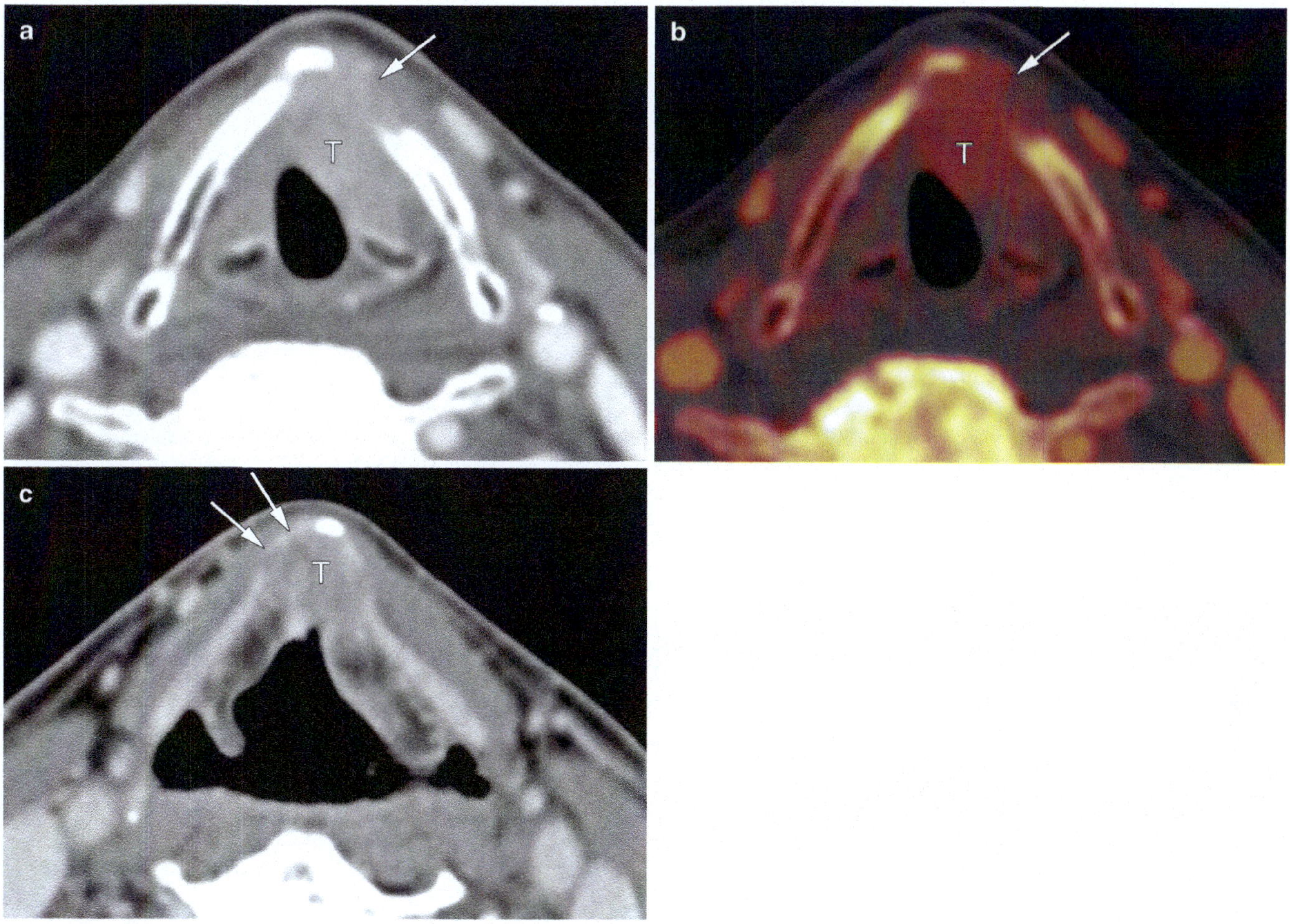

Fig. 5.33 Glottic carcinoma with thyroid cartilage invasion through the outer cortex by dual-energy CT. WA image (**a**) at the glottic level shows tumor (T) invasion into the thyroid cartilage, spreading into the extralaryngeal soft tissue (arrow). On the IO image (**b**), the tumor extent through the thyroid lamina is evident (arrow). Axial image, more superiorly (**c**), shows upward tumor extension along the anterior commissure tendon with thyroid cartilage invasion (arrows)

Table 5.4 Diagnostic criteria of MRI and dual-energy CT (and conventional CT) for detection of cartilage invasion

		Ossified cartilage (cortical bone)	Ossified cartilage (fatty marrow)	Non-ossified cartilage
Normal cartilage				
MRI	T1-weighted	Very low	High	Low
	T2-weighted	Very low	High	Low
	Contrast-enhanced T1-weighted	No enhancement	No enhancement	No enhancement
CT	Conventional image (WA image)	Very high	Low	Intermediate (similar to that of tumor)
	DECT IO image	Could not be evaluated	No enhancement (low)	No enhancement (low)
Positive finding for detecting of cartilage invasion				
MRI[a]	T1-weighted	Similar to that of tumor (low)		
	T2-weighted	Similar to that of tumor (intermediate high)		
	Contrast-enhanced T1-weighted	Similar enhancement to tumor		
CT[b]	Conventional image (WA image)	Erosion, lysis, or transmural extralaryngeal spreading through the cartilage		
	DECT IO image	Positive corresponding enhancement in the region of cartilage indicated in the WA image		

WA image weighted average image, *IO image* iodine overlay image

[a]The cartilage displayed the signal intensity on all the sequences that was needed for "positive" findings

[b]Diagnostic readings always began with the WA image. After a lesion has been evaluated as positive on WA images, the iodine distribution on the IO images is examined to derive a final classification of either positive or negative

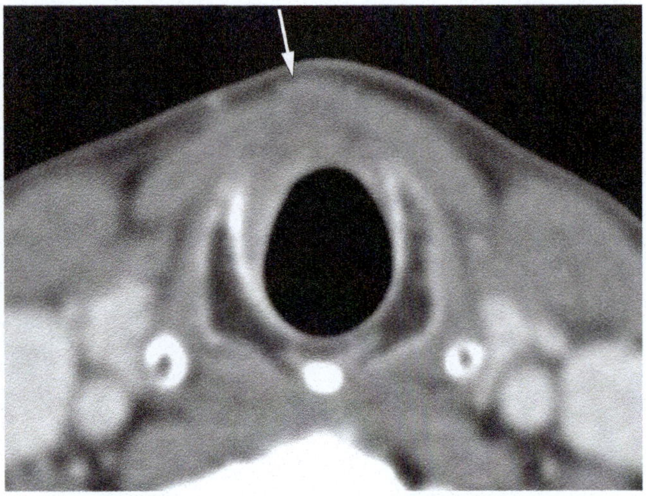

Fig. 5.34 Delphian node metastasis in patients with glottic carcinoma

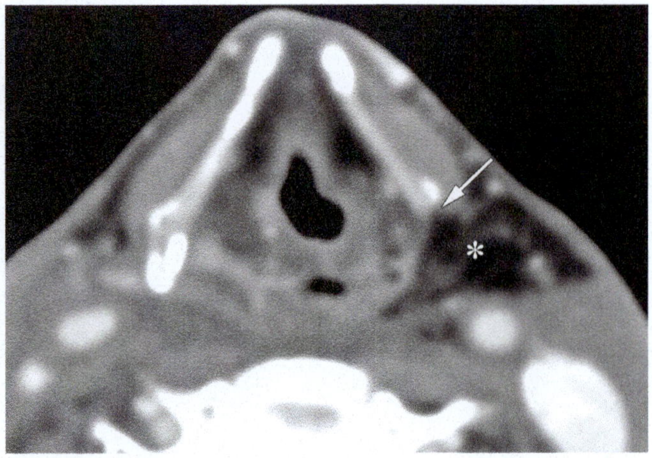

Fig. 5.36 Post partial pharyngectomy. The posterior lamina of thyroid cartilage on the left side is resected (allow) filled with the reconstructed flap tissue (asterisk)

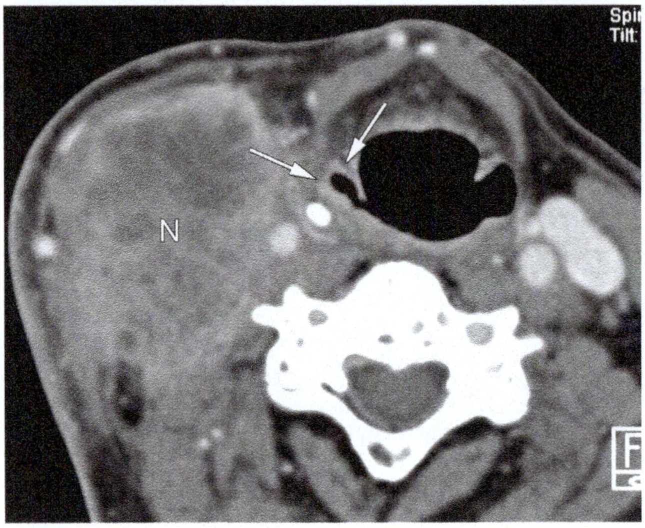

Fig. 5.35 T2N3 hypopharyngeal carcinoma. For hypopharyngeal carcinoma, even if the primary site is small (arrows), lymph node metastasis can often be large (N)

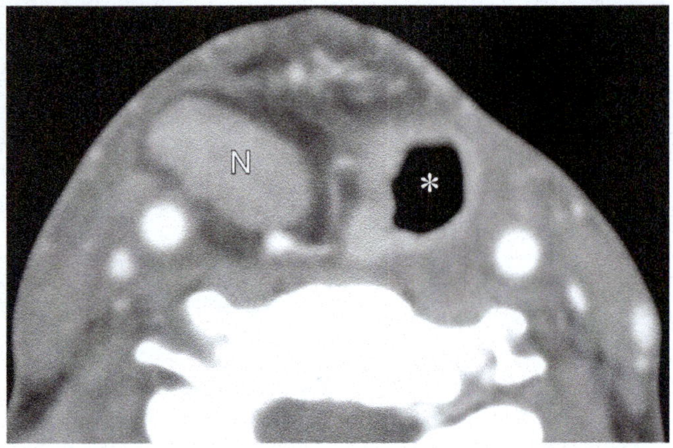

Fig. 5.37 Post TPLE neopharynx. Axial contrast-enhanced CT demonstrates the neopharynx (asterisk). Secondary lymph node swelling is seen at the mesenteric lymph node of the neopharynx. This node was observed to remain the same size for over 3 years after operation

than contrast CT. Therefore, the recommended interval for baseline study would be 4–6 weeks for contrast CT, 6–8 weeks for contrast MRI, and 10–12 weeks for FDG-PET [14]. In follow-up, comparison with baseline study is important.

Contrast-enhanced CT has traditionally been the imaging modality of choice to follow patients with head and neck cancer. In general, the literature suggests that CT has acceptable sensitivity and moderate specificity for assessing tumor response to therapy. MRI is superior to CT in terms of tissue contrast and is useful for treatment evaluation and relapse diagnosis. Diffuse changes in the larynx and hypopharynx should not be regarded as evidence of tumor recurrence. Obvious or subtle focal masses on CT or MRI may alert the radiologist to the possibility of a recurrent tumor. The use of the ADC has been reported to result in high sensitivity and specificity, with nearly no overlap between tumoral and non-tumoral tissue [79–81] (Fig. 5.39). It is important to use a combination of morphologic and quantitative MR imaging including DWI b-value images and ADC images with ADC value for posttreatment evaluation after radiation therapy [80].

The overall diagnostic performance of posttreatment FDG PET (CT) for response assessment and surveillance imaging is excellent, but its positive predictive value is suboptimal (Fig. 5.39). Several systemic reviews and meta-analyses have reported that PET-CT is most accurate at least 2–3 months after (chemo)radiation therapy, and the accuracy increases at 12 weeks or longer [14, 82]. The negative predictive value of PET-CT remains exceptionally high (up to

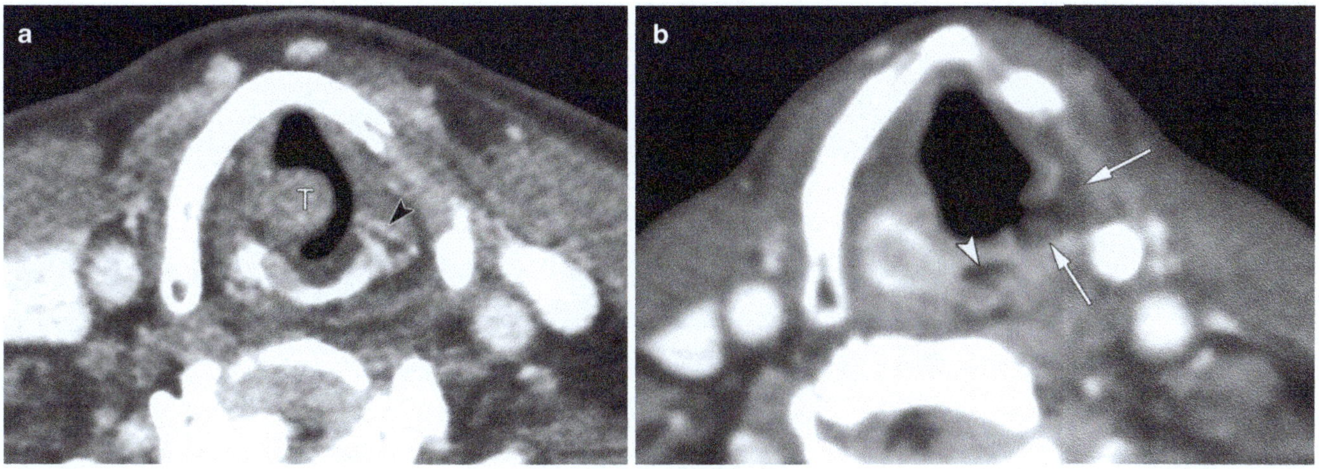

Fig. 5.38 Chondroradionecrosis of the larynx. (**a**) Axial contrast-enhanced CT demonstrated glottic cancer of the right vocal cord (T). Normal left arytenoid cartilage is seen (black arrowhead). (**b**) Contrast-enhanced CT obtained 12 months after RT shows that the left arytenoid has disappeared, leaving a soft-tissue defect (arrow). There is also small air density at the cricoid cartilage (arrowhead)

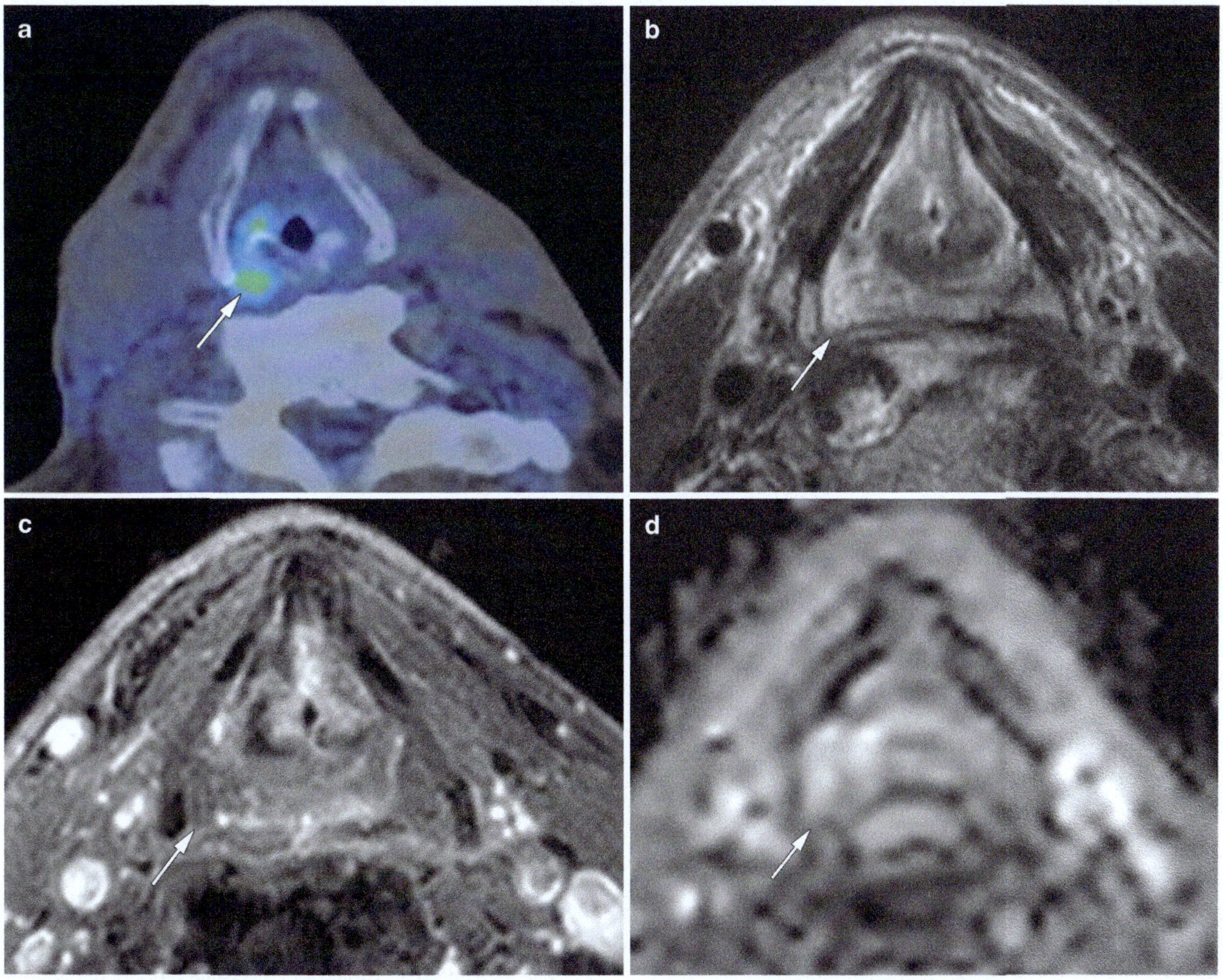

Fig. 5.39 True negative findings for primary site by MRI with hypopharyngeal cancer treated by chemoradiation therapy. On the FDG-PET (**a**) and MRI (**b–d**) obtained 3 months after CRT for pyriform sinus cancer. FDG-PET showed FDG uptake at the primary site. However, axial T2-weighted image (**b**) and contrast-enhanced T1-weighted image (**c**) show a triangular lesion (arrows) in the primary site with high signal intensity on T2 and faint contrast enhancement. The ADC map (**d**) reveals no restricted diffusion in the corresponding area, suggesting post-RT inflammatory edema

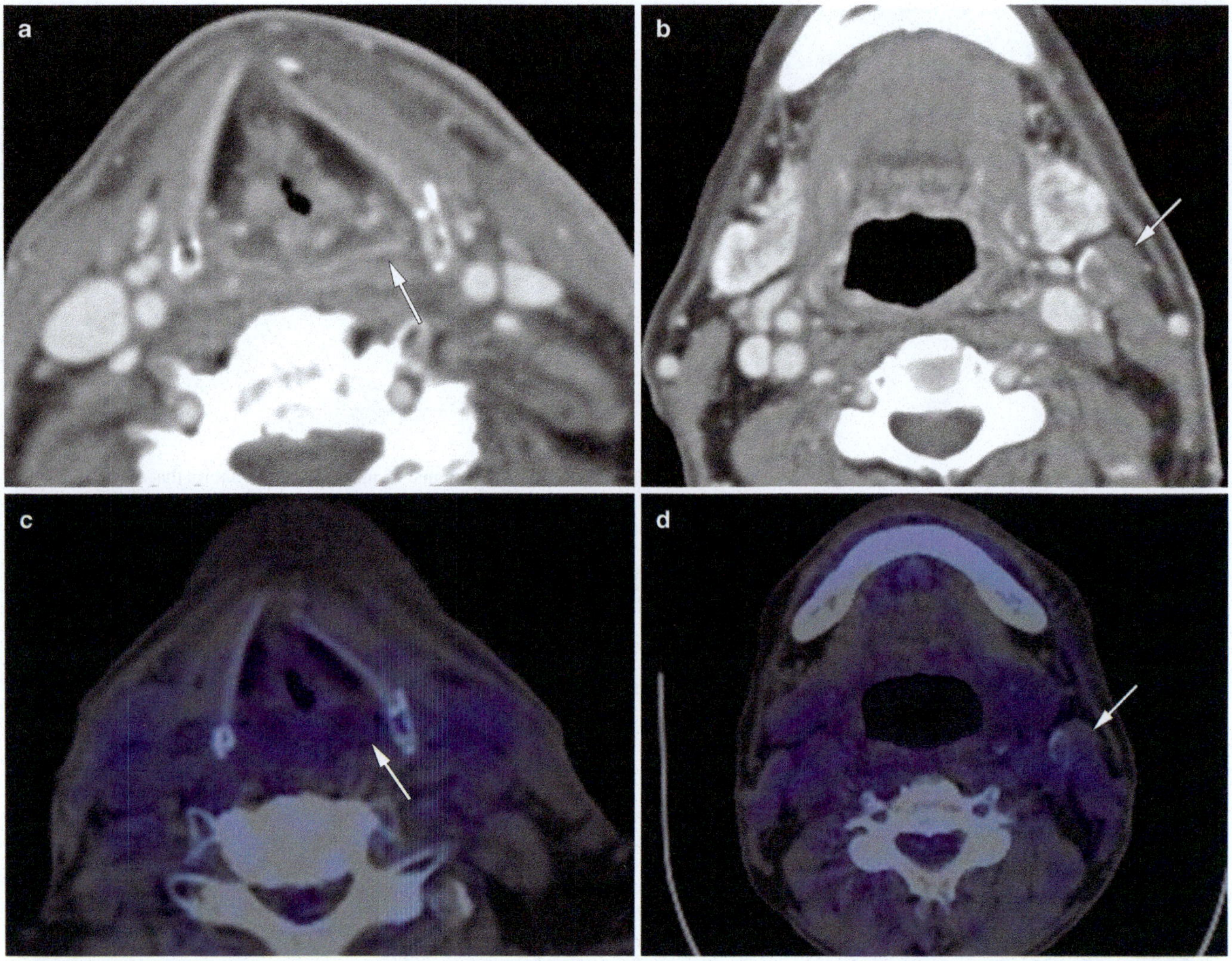

Fig. 5.40 True negative findings for lymph node by FDG-PET/CT with hypopharyngeal cancer treated by chemoradiation therapy. In contrast-enhanced CT obtained 6 months after chemoradiation therapy (**a**, **b**), the remaining lymph node metastasis is observed (**b**, arrow), although the primary tumor has disappeared (**a**, arrow). FDG-PET showed no FDG uptake at the primary site (**c**, arrow) and lymph nodes (**d**, arrow). Biopsy specimens confirmed that the lymph node was negative tumor cells with fibrosis

98%), and specificity at this time excludes residual diseases [83] (Fig. 5.40). Two consecutive PET/CT examinations with negative findings within 6 months posttreatment scan are highly suggestive of the absence of viable disease which could prevent further radiologic imaging in the absence of clinical signs of recurrence [84]. Timing of posttreatment imaging has a moderate but significant impact on diagnostic accuracy.

References

1. Bradley PJ. Epidemiology of hypopharyngeal cancer. Adv Otorhinolaryngol. 2019;83:1–14.
2. Japan Society for Head and Neck Cancer, Cancer Registry Committee. Report of head and neck cancer registry of Japan clinical statistics of registered patients 2014. 2016;40(supplement):52–71.
3. Sato K, Kurita S, Hirano M. Location of the preepiglottic space and its relationship to the paraglottic space. Ann Otol Rhinol Laryngol. 1993;102(12):930–4. https://doi.org/10.1177/000348949310201204.
4. Tucker G Jr, Smith H Jr. A histological demonstration of the development of laryngeal connective tissue compartments. Trans Am Acad Ophthalmol Otolaryngol. 1962;66:308–18.
5. Kutta H, Steven P, Paulsen F. Anatomical definition of the subglottic region. Cells Tissues Organs. 2006;184(3–4):205–14. https://doi.org/10.1159/000099628.
6. Pressman JJ, Simon MB, Monell C. Anatomical studies related to the dissemination of cancer of the larynx. Trans Am Acad Ophthalmol Otolaryngol. 1960;64:628–38. https://www.ncbi.nlm.nih.gov/pubmed/13737879.
7. Sato K, Umeno T, Hirano M, Nakashima T. Cricoid area of the larynx: its physiological and pathological significance. Acta Otolaryngol. 2002;122(8):882–6. https://www.ncbi.nlm.nih.gov/pubmed/12542210.
8. Dadfar N, Seyyedi M, Forghani R, Curtin HD. Computed tomography appearance of normal nonossified thyroid cartilage: implication for

tumor invasion diagnosis. J Comput Assist Tomogr. 2015;39(2):240–3. https://doi.org/10.1097/RCT.0000000000000196.

9. Forghani R, Levental M, Gupta R, Lam S, Dadfar N, Curtin HD. Different spectral hounsfield unit curve and high-energy virtual monochromatic image characteristics of squamous cell carcinoma compared with nonossified thyroid cartilage. AJNR Am J Neuroradiol. 2015;36(6):1194–200. https://doi.org/10.3174/ajnr.A4253.
10. Kuno H, Onaya H, Iwata R, Kobayashi T, Fujii S, Hayashi R, et al. Evaluation of cartilage invasion by laryngeal and hypopharyngeal squamous cell carcinoma with dual-energy CT. Radiology. 2012;265(2):488–96. https://doi.org/10.1148/radiol.12111719.
11. Kuno H, Sakamaki K, Fujii S, Sekiya K, Otani K, Hayashi R, et al. Comparison of MR imaging and dual-energy CT for the evaluation of cartilage invasion by laryngeal and Hypopharyngeal squamous cell carcinoma. AJNR Am J Neuroradiol. 2018;39(3):524–31. https://doi.org/10.3174/ajnr.A5530.
12. Ravanelli M, Farina D, Rizzardi P, Botturi E, Prandolini P, Mangili S, et al. MR with surface coils in the follow-up after endoscopic laser resection for glottic squamous cell carcinoma: feasibility and diagnostic accuracy. Neuroradiology. 2013;55(2):225–32. https://doi.org/10.1007/s00234-012-1128-3.
13. Daisne JF, Duprez T, Weynand B, Lonneux M, Hamoir M, Reychler H, et al. Tumor volume in pharyngolaryngeal squamous cell carcinoma: comparison at CT, MR imaging, and FDG PET and validation with surgical specimen. Radiology. 2004;233(1):93–100. https://doi.org/10.1148/radiol.2331030660.
14. Gupta T, Master Z, Kannan S, Agarwal JP, Ghsoh-Laskar S, Rangarajan V, et al. Diagnostic performance of post-treatment FDG PET or FDG PET/CT imaging in head and neck cancer: a systematic review and meta-analysis. Eur J Nucl Med Mol Imaging. 2011;38(11):2083–95. https://doi.org/10.1007/s00259-011-1893-y.
15. Sheikhbahaei S, Taghipour M, Ahmad R, Fakhry C, Kiess AP, Chung CH, et al. Diagnostic accuracy of follow-up FDG PET or PET/CT in patients with head and neck cancer after definitive treatment: a systematic review and meta-analysis. AJR Am J Roentgenol. 2015;205(3):629–39. https://doi.org/10.2214/AJR.14.14166.
16. Blodgett TM, Fukui MB, Snyderman CH, Branstetter BF, McCook BM, Townsend DW, et al. Combined PET-CT in the head and neck: part 1. Physiologic, altered physiologic, and artifactual FDG uptake. Radiographics. 2005;25(4):897–912. https://doi.org/10.1148/rg.254035156.
17. Purohit BS, Ailianou A, Dulguerov N, Becker CD, Ratib O, Becker M. FDG-PET/CT pitfalls in oncological head and neck imaging. Insights Imaging. 2014;5(5):585–602. https://doi.org/10.1007/s13244-014-0349-x.
18. Amin M, Edge S, Greene F, et al. AJCC cancer staging manual. 8th ed. New York: Springer; 2017.
19. Becker M, Burkhardt K, Dulguerov P, Allal A. Imaging of the larynx and hypopharynx. Eur J Radiol. 2008a;66(3):460–79. https://doi.org/10.1016/j.ejrad.2008.03.027.
20. Hermans R. Staging of laryngeal and hypopharyngeal cancer: value of imaging studies. Eur Radiol. 2006;16(11):2386–400. https://doi.org/10.1007/s00330-006-0301-7.
21. Zbaren P, Egger C. Growth patterns of piriform sinus carcinomas. Laryngoscope. 1997;107(4):511–8. https://www.ncbi.nlm.nih.gov/pubmed/9111382.
22. Mendenhall WM, Morris CG, Amdur RJ, Werning JW, Hinerman RW, Villaret DB. Radiotherapy alone or combined with surgery for adenoid cystic carcinoma of the head and neck. Head Neck. 2004;26(2):154–62. https://doi.org/10.1002/hed.10380.
23. Murakami R, Nishimura R, Baba Y, Furusawa M, Ogata N, Yumoto E, et al. Prognostic factors of glottic carcinomas treated with radiation therapy: value of the adjacent sign on radiological examinations in the sixth edition of the UICC TNM staging system. Int J Radiat Oncol Biol Phys. 2005;61(2):471–5. https://doi.org/10.1016/j.ijrobp.2004.05.024.
24. Amin M, Edge S, Greene F, et al. AJCC updates and corrections. 8th ed. New York: Springer; 2018. https://cancerstaging.org/references-tools/deskreferences/Pages/8EUpdates.aspx.
25. Glastonbury CM, Mukherji SK, O'Sullivan B, Lydiatt WM. Setting the stage for 2018: how the changes in the American Joint Committee on Cancer/Union for International Cancer Control Cancer staging manual eighth edition impact radiologists. AJNR Am J Neuroradiol. 2017;38(12):2231–7. https://doi.org/10.3174/ajnr.A5409.
26. Kimura Y, Sumi M, Sakihama N, Tanaka F, Takahashi H, Nakamura T. MR imaging criteria for the prediction of extranodal spread of metastatic cancer in the neck. AJNR Am J Neuroradiol. 2008;29(7):1355–9. https://doi.org/10.3174/ajnr.A1088.
27. Mermod M, Tolstonog G, Simon C, Monnier Y. Extracapsular spread in head and neck squamous cell carcinoma: a systematic review and meta-analysis. Oral Oncol. 2016;62:60–71. https://doi.org/10.1016/j.oraloncology.2016.10.003.
28. Chung EJ, Kim GW, Cho BK, Park HS, Rho YS. Pattern of lymph node metastasis in hypopharyngeal squamous cell carcinoma and indications for level VI lymph node dissection. Head Neck. 2016;38(Suppl 1):E1969–73. https://doi.org/10.1002/hed.24361.
29. Lindberg R. Distribution of cervical lymph node metastases from squamous cell carcinoma of the upper respiratory and digestive tracts. Cancer. 1972;29(6):1446–9. https://doi.org/10.1002/1097-0142(197206)29:6<1446::aid-cncr2820290604>3.0.co;2-c.
30. Dahm JD, Sessions DG, Paniello RC, Harvey J. Primary subglottic cancer. Laryngoscope. 1998;108(5):741–6. https://doi.org/10.1097/00005537-199805000-00022.
31. Sessions DG, Ogura JH, Fried MP. Carcinoma of the subglottic area. Laryngoscope. 1975;85(9):1417–23. https://doi.org/10.1288/00005537-197509000-00001.
32. Lee WT, Rizzi M, Scharpf J, Lorenz RR, Saxton JP, Adelstein DJ, et al. Impact of preepiglottic space tumor involvement on concurrent chemoradiation therapy. Am J Otolaryngol. 2010;31(3):185–8. https://doi.org/10.1016/j.amjoto.2009.02.001.
33. Loevner LA, Yousem DM, Montone KT, Weber R, Chalian AA, Weinstein GS. Can radiologists accurately predict preepiglottic space invasion with MR imaging? AJR Am J Roentgenol. 1997;169(6):1681–7. https://doi.org/10.2214/ajr.169.6.9393190.
34. Dagan R, Morris CG, Bennett JA, Mancuso AA, Amdur RJ, Hinerman RW, et al. Prognostic significance of paraglottic space invasion in T2N0 glottic carcinoma. Am J Clin Oncol. 2007;30(2):186–90. https://doi.org/10.1097/01.coc.0000251403.54180.df.
35. Mittal B, Marks JE, Ogura JH. Transglottic carcinoma. Cancer. 1984;53(1):151–61. https://doi.org/10.1002/1097-0142(19840101)53:1<151::aid-cncr2820530127>3.0.co;2-x.
36. Forastiere AA, Ismaila N, Lewin JS, Nathan CA, Adelstein DJ, Eisbruch A, et al. Use of larynx-preservation strategies in the treatment of laryngeal cancer: American Society of Clinical Oncology clinical practice guideline update. J Clin Oncol. 2018;36(11):1143–69. https://doi.org/10.1200/JCO.2017.75.7385.
37. Knab BR, Salama JK, Solanki A, Stenson KM, Cohen EE, Witt ME, et al. RG1-functional organ preservation with definitive chemoradiotherapy for T4 laryngeal squamous cell carcinoma (article). Ann Oncol. 2008;19(9):1650–4. https://doi.org/10.1093/annonc/mdn173.
38. Worden FP, Moyer J, Lee JS, Taylor JMG, Urba SG, Eisbruch A, et al. Chemoselection as a strategy for organ preservation in patients with T4 laryngeal squamous cell carcinoma with cartilage invasion (proceedings paper). Laryngoscope. 2009;119(8):1510–7. https://doi.org/10.1002/lary.20294.
39. Beitler JJ, Muller S, Grist WJ, Corey A, Klein AM, Johns MM, et al. Prognostic accuracy of computed tomography findings for patients with laryngeal cancer undergoing laryngectomy (article).

J Clin Oncol. 2010;28(14):2318–22. https://doi.org/10.1200/jco.2009.24.7544.
40. Kuno H, Onaya H, Fujii S, Ojiri H, Otani K, Satake M. Primary staging of laryngeal and hypopharyngeal cancer: CT, MR imaging and dual-energy CT. Eur J Radiol. 2014;83(1):e23–35. https://doi.org/10.1016/j.ejrad.2013.10.022.
41. Mancuso A. Larynx: malignant tumors. In: Mancuso AA, editor. Head and neck radiology. Hanafee, WN: Lippincott Williams & Wilkins; 2010a. p. 1975–2022.
42. Mancuso A. RG10-Hypopharynx: malignant tumors. In: Mancuso AA, editor. Head and neck radiology. Hanafee, WN: Lippincott Williams & Wilkins; 2010b. p. 2147–72.
43. Pameijer FA, Mancuso AA, Mendenhall WM, Parsons JT, Mukherji SK, Hermans R, et al. Evaluation of pretreatment computed tomography as a predictor of local control in T1/T2 pyriform sinus carcinoma treated with definitive radiotherapy. Head Neck. 1998;20(2):159–68.
44. Baugnon KL, Beitler JJ. Pitfalls in the staging of cancer of the laryngeal squamous cell carcinoma. Neuroimaging Clin N Am. 2013;23(1):81–105. https://doi.org/10.1016/j.nic.2012.08.008.
45. Hsu WC, Loevner LA, Karpati R, Ahmed T, Mong A, Battineni ML, et al. Accuracy of magnetic resonance imaging in predicting absence of fixation of head and neck cancer to the prevertebral space (article). Head Neck. 2005;27(2):95–100. https://doi.org/10.1002/hed.20128.
46. Imre A, Pinar E, Erdogan N, Ece AA, Olgun Y, Aladag I, et al. Prevertebral space invasion in head and neck cancer: negative predictive value of imaging techniques. Ann Otol Rhinol Laryngol. 2015;124(5):378–83. https://doi.org/10.1177/0003489414560431.
47. Loevner LA, Ott IL, Yousem DM, Montone KT, Thaler ER, Chalian AA, et al. Neoplastic fixation to the prevertebral compartment by squamous cell carcinoma of the head and neck (article). AJR Am J Roentgenol. 1998;170(5):1389–94. https://doi.org/10.2214/ajr.170.5.9574622.
48. Lefebvre JL, Ang KK. Larynx preservation clinical trial design: key issues and recommendations—a consensus panel summary. Head Neck. 2009;31(4):429–41.
49. NCCN. Guidelines head and neck cancers version 2, 2019. 2019. https://www.nccn.org/professionals/physician_gls/pdf/head-and-neck.pdf.
50. Becker M, Zbaren P, Delavelle J, Kurt AM, Egger C, Rufenacht DA, et al. Neoplastic invasion of the laryngeal cartilage: reassessment of criteria for diagnosis at CT. Radiology. 1997;203(2):521–32. https://doi.org/10.1148/radiology.203.2.9114116.
51. Gilbert K, Dalley RW, Maronian N, Anzai Y. Staging of laryngeal cancer using 64-channel multidetector row CT: comparison of standard neck CT with dedicated breath-maneuver laryngeal CT (article). AJNR Am J Neuroradiol. 2010;31(2):251–6. https://doi.org/10.3174/ajnr.A1796.
52. Hartl DM, Landry G, Hans S, Marandas P, Brasnu DF. Organ preservation surgery for laryngeal squamous cell carcinoma: low incidence of thyroid cartilage invasion. Laryngoscope. 2010;120(6):1173–6. https://doi.org/10.1002/lary.20912.
53. Li B, Bobinski M, Gandour-Edwards R, Farwell DG, Chen AM. Overstaging of cartilage invasion by multidetector CT scan for laryngeal cancer and its potential effect on the use of organ preservation with chemoradiation. Br J Radiol. 2011;84(997):64–9. https://doi.org/10.1259/bjr/66700901.
54. Munoz A, Ramos A, Ferrando J, Gomez B, Escudero L, Relea F, et al. Laryngeal carcinoma: sclerotic appearance of the cricoid and arytenoid cartilage—CT-pathologic correlation. Radiology. 1993;189(2):433–7. https://doi.org/10.1148/radiology.189.2.8210372.
55. Nix PA, Salvage D. Neoplastic invasion of laryngeal cartilage: the significance of cartilage sclerosis on computed tomography images. Clin Otolaryngol Allied Sci. 2004;29(4):372–5. https://doi.org/10.1111/j.1365-2273.2004.00821.x.
56. Schmalfuss IM, Mancuso AA, Tart RP. Arytenoid cartilage sclerosis: normal variations and clinical significance. AJNR Am J Neuroradiol. 1998;19(4):719–22. https://www.ncbi.nlm.nih.gov/pubmed/9576661.
57. Becker M, Zbaren P, Casselman JW, Kohler R, Dulguerov P, Becker CD. Neoplastic invasion of laryngeal cartilage: reassessment of criteria for diagnosis at MR imaging. Radiology. 2008b;249(2):551–9. https://doi.org/10.1148/radiol.2492072183.
58. Becker M, Zbaren P, Laeng H, Stoupis C, Porcellini B, Vock P. Neoplastic invasion of the laryngeal cartilage: comparison of MR imaging and CT with histopathologic correlation. Radiology. 1995;194(3):661–9. https://doi.org/10.1148/radiology.194.3.7862960.
59. Castelijns JA, Gerritsen GJ, Kaiser MC, Valk J, van Zanten TE, Golding RG, et al. Invasion of laryngeal cartilage by cancer: comparison of CT and MR imaging. Radiology. 1988;167(1):199–206. https://doi.org/10.1148/radiology.167.1.3347723.
60. Zbaren P, Becker M, Lang H. Pretherapeutic staging of laryngeal carcinoma. Clinical findings, computed tomography, and magnetic resonance imaging compared with histopathology. Cancer. 1996;77(7):1263–73. https://doi.org/10.1002/(sici)1097-0142(19960401)77:7<1263::aid-cncr6>3.0.co;2-j.
61. Yeager VL, Archer CR. Anatomical routes for cancer invasion of laryngeal cartilages. Laryngoscope. 1982;92(4):449–52. https://www.ncbi.nlm.nih.gov/pubmed/7070185.
62. Joo YH, Park JO, Cho KJ, Kim MS. Relationship between paraglottic space invasion and cervical lymph node metastasis in patients undergoing supracricoid partial laryngectomy. Head Neck. 2012;34(8):1119–22.
63. Nakayama M, Seino Y, Okamoto M, Mikami T, Okamoto T, Miyamoto S. Clinical significance of positive Delphian node in Supracricoid Laryngectomy with Cricohyoidoepiglottopexy. Jpn J Clin Oncol. 2011;41(8):987–91. https://doi.org/10.1093/jjco/hyr091.
64. Olsen KD, Desanto LW, Pearson BW. Positive Delphian lymph node: clinical significance in laryngeal cancer. Laryngoscope. 1987;97(9):1033–7. https://onlinelibrary.wiley.com/doi/pdf/10.1288/00005537-198709000-00007.
65. Amatsu M, Mohri M, Kinishi MJTL. Significance of retropharyngeal node dissection at radical surgery for carcinoma of the hypopharynx and cervical esophagus. Laryngoscope. 2001;111(6):1099–103.
66. Milano MT, Peterson CR 3rd, Zhang H, Singh DP, Chen Y. Second primary lung cancer after head and neck squamous cell cancer: population-based study of risk factors. Head Neck. 2012;34(12):1782–8. https://doi.org/10.1002/hed.22006.
67. Forastiere AA, Goepfert H, Maor M, Pajak TF, Weber R, Morrison W, et al. Concurrent chemotherapy and radiotherapy for organ preservation in advanced laryngeal cancer (article). N Engl J Med. 2003;349(22):2091–8. <go to ISI>://000186779700003.
68. Hoffman HT, Porter K, Karnell LH, Cooper JS, Weber RS, Langer CJ, et al. Laryngeal cancer in the United States: changes in demographics, patterns of care, and survival. Laryngoscope. 2006;116(9 Pt 2 Suppl 111):1–13. https://doi.org/10.1097/01.mlg.0000236095.97947.26.
69. Pfister DG, Laurie SA, Weinstein GS, Mendenhall WM, Adelstein DJ, Ang KK, et al. American Society of Clinical Oncology clinical practice guideline for the use of larynx-preservation strategies in the treatment of laryngeal cancer. J Clin Oncol. 2006;24(22):3693–704. https://doi.org/10.1200/JCO.2006.07.4559.
70. Castelijns JA, Becker M, Hermans R. Impact of cartilage invasion on treatment and prognosis of laryngeal cancer (review). Eur Radiol. 1996;6(2):156–69. https://www.ncbi.nlm.nih.gov/pubmed/8797973
71. Amdur RJ, Mendenhall WM, Stringer SP, Villaret DB, Cassisi NJ. Organ preservation with radiotherapy for T1-T2 carcinoma of

the pyriform sinus. Head Neck. 2001;23(5):353–62. https://www.ncbi.nlm.nih.gov/pubmed/11295808.
72. Rabbani A, Amdur RJ, Mancuso AA, Werning JW, Kirwan J, Morris CG, et al. Definitive radiotherapy for T1-T2 squamous cell carcinoma of pyriform sinus. Int J Radiat Oncol Biol Phys. 2008;72(2):351–5. https://doi.org/10.1016/j.ijrobp.2008.01.003.
73. Yoshimura R, Kagami Y, Ito Y, Asai M, Mayahara H, Sumi M, et al. Outcomes in patients with early-stage hypopharyngeal cancer treated with radiotherapy. Int J Radiat Oncol Biol Phys. 2010;77(4):1017–23. https://doi.org/10.1016/j.ijrobp.2009.06.066.
74. Laccourreye O, Mérite-Drancy A, Brasnu D, Chabardes E, Cauchois R, Ménard M, et al. Supracricoid hemilaryngopharyngectomy in selected pyriform sinus carcinoma staged as T2. Laryngoscope. 1993;103(12):1373–9.
75. Muto M, Nakane M, Katada C, Sano Y, Ohtsu A, Esumi H, et al. Squamous cell carcinoma in situ at oropharyngeal and hypopharyngeal mucosal sites. Cancer. 2004;101(6):1375–81.
76. Saito N, Nadgir RN, Nakahira M, Takahashi M, Uchino A, Kimura F, et al. Posttreatment CT and MR imaging in head and neck cancer: what the radiologist needs to know. Radiographics. 2012;32(5):1261–82; discussion 1282-4. https://doi.org/10.1148/rg.325115160.
77. Mukherji SK, Mancuso AA, Kotzur IM, Mendenhall WM, Kubilis PS, Tart RP, et al. Radiologic appearance of the irradiated larynx. Part I. Expected changes. Radiology. 1994;193(1):141–8. https://doi.org/10.1148/radiology.193.1.8090882.
78. Hermans R, Pameijer FA, Mancuso AA, Parsons JT, Mendenhall WM. CT findings in chondroradionecrosis of the larynx. AJNR Am J Neuroradiol. 1998;19(4):711–8. https://www.ncbi.nlm.nih.gov/pubmed/9576660.
79. Abdel Razek AA, Kandeel AY, Soliman N, El-shenshawy HM, Kamel Y, Nada N, et al. Role of diffusion-weighted echo-planar MR imaging in differentiation of residual or recurrent head and neck tumors and posttreatment changes. AJNR Am J Neuroradiol. 2007;28(6):1146–52. https://doi.org/10.3174/ajnr.A0491.
80. Ailianou A, Mundada P, De Perrot T, Pusztaszieri M, Poletti PA, Becker M. MRI with DWI for the detection of posttreatment head and neck squamous cell carcinoma: why morphologic MRI criteria matter. AJNR Am J Neuroradiol. 2018;39(4):748–55. https://doi.org/10.3174/ajnr.A5548.
81. Vandecaveye V, Dirix P, De Keyzer F, Op de Beeck K, Vander Poorten V, Hauben E, et al. Diffusion-weighted magnetic resonance imaging early after chemoradiotherapy to monitor treatment response in head-and-neck squamous cell carcinoma. Int J Radiat Oncol Biol Phys. 2012;82(3):1098–107. https://doi.org/10.1016/j.ijrobp.2011.02.044.
82. Isles MG, McConkey C, Mehanna HM. A systematic review and meta-analysis of the role of positron emission tomography in the follow up of head and neck squamous cell carcinoma following radiotherapy or chemoradiotherapy. Clin Otolaryngol. 2008;33(3):210–22. https://doi.org/10.1111/j.1749-4486.2008.01688.x.
83. Ong SC, Schoder H, Lee NY, Patel SG, Carlson D, Fury M, et al. Clinical utility of 18F-FDG PET/CT in assessing the neck after concurrent chemoradiotherapy for locoregional advanced head and neck cancer. J Nucl Med. 2008;49(4):532–40. https://doi.org/10.2967/jnumed.107.044792.
84. McDermott M, Hughes M, Rath T, Johnson JT, Heron DE, Kubicek GJ, et al. Negative predictive value of surveillance PET/CT in head and neck squamous cell cancer. AJNR Am J Neuroradiol. 2013;34(8):1632–6. https://doi.org/10.3174/ajnr.A3494.

Diagnostic Imaging of Metastatic Nodal Disease

6

Hiroko Tanaka

Abstract

Knowledge of anatomy, classification, drainage pathways, and morphologic variations of neck lymph node is key to correct interpretation of head and neck imaging. Computed tomography, magnetic resonance imaging, ultrasonography, and PET/CT are complementary imaging modalities that can be used in the evaluation of lymph node metastasis. This chapter discusses the imaging evaluation for metastatic lymph nodes in head and neck squamous cell carcinoma.

Keywords

Head and neck cancer · Neck nodal metastasis · CT · MRI · US · PET/CT

6.1 Introduction

Head and neck squamous cell carcinoma (HNSCC) comprises most common head and neck malignancy. HNSCC generally metastasizes to the cervical lymph nodes, with a frequency of approximately 50%, but the frequency varies depending on the site and stage of the primary tumor. Cervical lymph node metastasis is an important prognostic indicator in HNSCC as it reduces patient survival by 30–50%. Multiple nodes, large size, lower level metastases, and extranodal extension are additional prognostic factors. However, the smoking status and the condition of the primary tumor such as virus (human papilloma virus or Epstein-Barr virus) affect the prognosis. These characteristics and the status of the lymph node metastases influence the treatment options for surgery and/or (chemo)radiotherapy. Therefore, accurate detection of metastasis is essential, and imaging plays an integral role in every stage from initial diagnosis to posttreatment surveillance.

In this chapter, we will review the normal nodal anatomy, classification, and lymphatic drainage in the head and neck region and also will discuss imaging techniques, the imaging criteria, treatment assessment, and post-therapeutic surveillance for metastatic lymph nodes of HNSCC patients.

6.2 Anatomy of Normal Lymph Node

In the head and neck region, there are 150–350 lymph nodes equivalent to one third of the whole body lymph nodes. The lymph nodes are flat lumpy peripheral lymphoid organs.

The afferent lymphatic vessels are on the capsule side of the lymph nodes, and the efferent lymphatic vessels pass through the hilum. The blood supply of the lymph nodes is through the arteries entering from the hilum. The venous blood of the lymph node is collected in the medulla and leaves the lymphatic hilum.

Lymph code is divided into cortex, paracortex, and medulla from the outside. The cortex has numerous lymphoid follicles as B lymphocyte areas. Lymphoid follicles are primary follicles that do not undergo antigen stimulation and secondary follicles that have germinal centers formed by differentiation and proliferation of B lymphocytes under antigen stimulation. The secondary follicle is composed of the germinal center and the mantle zone in which the primary follicle surrounds the germinal center. The paracortex is mostly occupied by T lymphocytes. The medulla exists from the deep paracortex to the hilum, and the small lymphocytes and many plasma cells are distributed in the medulla, resulting in humoral immunity.

The lymph sinus is a lymphatic flow pathway. There are small lymphocytes and sinus histiocytes in the sinus. Lymph fluids draining from the lymphatic vessels that penetrate the lymph node capsule pass through the marginal sinuses, the intermediate sinuses, and the medullary sinuses and are poured from the lymph nodes into the efferent lymphatics.

H. Tanaka (✉)
Department of Diagnostic Imaging, Cancer Institute Hospital, Japanese Foundation for Cancer Research, Koto-ku, Tokyo, Japan
e-mail: hiroko.tanaka@jfcr.or.jp

H. Ojiri (ed.), *Diagnostic Imaging in Head and Neck Cancer*, https://doi.org/10.1007/978-981-15-3188-0_6

The lymph node acts as a filter and plays a role in protecting the body. When antigens, cell fragments, bacteria, and cancer cells are filtered out in the lymph node, the lymphocytes and phagocytes in the lymph node react and the lymph node enlarged. Lymph node metastasis occurs when the filtered cancer cells proliferate in the lymph nodes and often begins in the marginal sinus.

6.3 Lymph Node Classification

The classification of Rouvière in 1938 has been the basis of all the current nodal classification and most commonly used [1]. In 1998, the American Head and Neck Society and American Academy of Otolaryngology-Head and Neck Surgery proposed a new nodal classification with the development of more advanced surgical approaches to head and neck cancer. This system could accurately reflect lymphatic drainage patterns; however, some of the surgical boundaries were difficult to define by imaging. The imaging-based classification by Som et al. in 1999 used well-defined anatomic boundaries that can be easily identified and highly reproducible by both clinicians and radiologists [2]. The imaging-based classification has been widely accepted and applied for initial evaluation and surveillance of HNSCC patients regardless of the method of treatment (Fig. 6.1).

It is important to note that the imaging-based level classification does not include several anatomic groups, such as supraclavicular, retropharyngeal, occipital, parotid, facial, and other superficial nodes discussed in the basic anatomic classification; these groups continue to be referred by their terminology (Fig. 6.2).

6.3.1 Imaging-Based Classification

This classification is intended for lymph nodes for neck dissection of cancer treatment. Cervical lymph nodes can be categorized by imaging-based landmarks. Figure 6.1 summarizes the imaging-based classification except level VII.

Level I is divided into IA and IB. Level IA lymph nodes are submental nodes and found between the anterior bellies of the digastric muscles below the mandible. Level IB nodes are submandibular nodes and found lateral to the anterior bellies of the digastric muscle and anterior to the posterior margin of the submandibular glands within the submandibular space.

Level II, III, and IV nodes extend along the internal jugular vein (IJV) and are deep to the sternocleidomastoid muscle (SCM) and anterior to the posterior edge of the SCM. Level II nodes are the upper portions of the internal jugular chain and spinal accessory chain, extending from the posterior belly of the digastric muscle to the bottom of the hyoid bone. Level IIA nodes are found posterior to the posterior margin of the submandibular gland, and may be anterior, or lateral to the IJV and touching to the posterior wall of the IJV. Level IIB nodes are posterior to the IJV with a fat plane between the node and the IJV. Level III nodes are middle internal jugular chain nodes, extending from below the hyoid bone to the inferior margin of the cricoid cartilage. Level IV nodes are lower internal jugular chain nodes from the inferior margin of the cricoid cartilage to the supraclavicular fossa.

Level V nodes are found in the posterior cervical space corresponding to the spinal accessory chain, lying posterior to the posterior margin of the SCM. Level V nodes are divided into VA and VB. Level VA nodes are from skull base to the inferior of the cricoid cartilage; level VB nodes are from below level VA to the supraclavicular fossa.

Level VI nodes are in the visceral space between the carotid arteries, extending from the bottom of the hyoid bone to the top of the manubrium, including the prelaryngeal, pretracheal, and paratracheal subgroups.

Level VII nodes are the superior mediastinal nodes located between the carotid arteries from the superior margin of the manubrium to the innominate vein.

The supraclavicular nodes lie at or caudal to the level of the clavicle and lateral to the carotid artery on each side of the neck, as seen on each axial scan.

The retropharyngeal nodes lie medial to the internal carotid arteries (ICA) within 2 cm of the skull base.

6.3.2 Basic Anatomic Classification

The supraclavicular nodes are along the transverse cervical artery in the supraclavicular fossa connecting the inferior aspects of internal jugular chain (IJC) and spinal accessory chain (SAC). Although these lymph nodes are not assigned a level in image-based classification, Som et al. distinguish them from levels VB, IV, and VI as indicated in the previous section. The Virchow node is specifically named pathologic node within the left supraclavicular fossa and is clinically significant. If no primary tumor is evident in the neck, this Virchow node is a signal for pulmonary or abdominal primary tumor.

The retropharyngeal nodes (RPN) include both the medial retropharyngeal space (RPS) node found in the paramedian RPS in the suprahyoid neck and the lateral RPS node (Fig. 6.2a) found lateral to the prevertebral muscles and medial to the ICA and IJV. It is important that the RPNs are often subclinical and imaging can be the first indicator of disease.

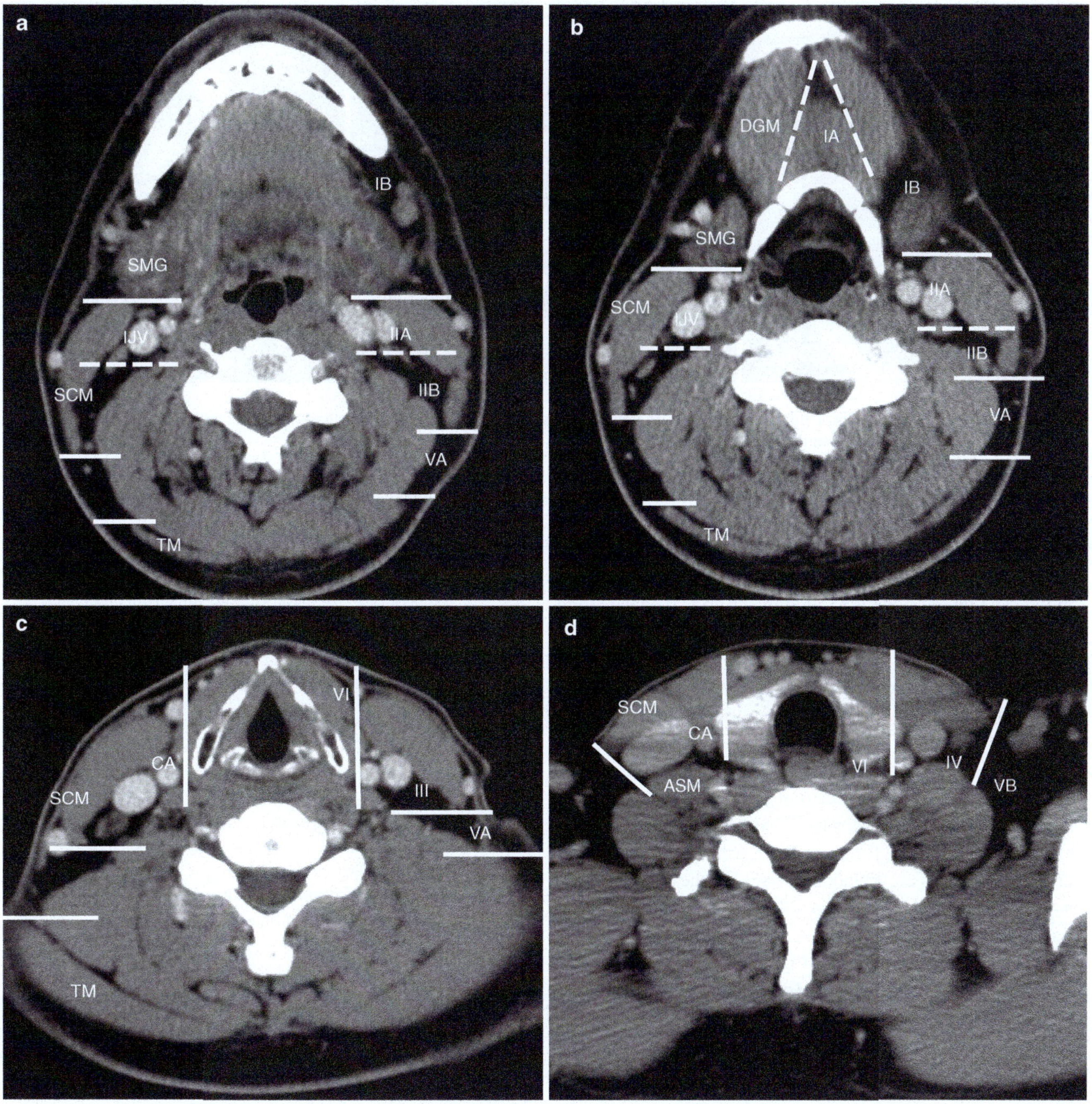

Fig. 6.1 Axial contrast-enhanced computed tomography (CECT) images show distribution of cervical node levels using the imaging-based classification. Solid lines indicate the boundaries of the nodal levels, and dotted lines indicate level subdivisions. (**a**) level IB, IIA, IIB, VA (**b**) level IA, IB, IIA, IIB, VA (**c**) level III, VA, VI (**d**) level IV, VB, VI (*ASM* anterior scalane muscle, *CA* carotid artery, *DGM* anterior belly of the digastric muscle, *IJV* internal jugular vein, *SCM* sternocleidomastoid muscle, *SMG* submandibular gland, *TM* trapezius muscle)

The occipital nodes (Fig. 6.2a) are located within the subcutaneous tissues posterior and inferior to calvarium. These nodes are divided into suprafascial/superficial, subfascial, and submuscular/subsplenius occipital nodes.

The parotid nodes (Fig. 6.2b) are located in the parotid region and are divided into three. The intraglandular nodes are within the fascia circumscribing the parotid space. The preauricular or postauricular nodes are found anterior or posterior to the auricle.

The facial lymph nodes include multiple nodes named for their anatomic location, such as the mandibular nodes superficial to the mandible (Fig. 6.2c), the buccinator nodes within

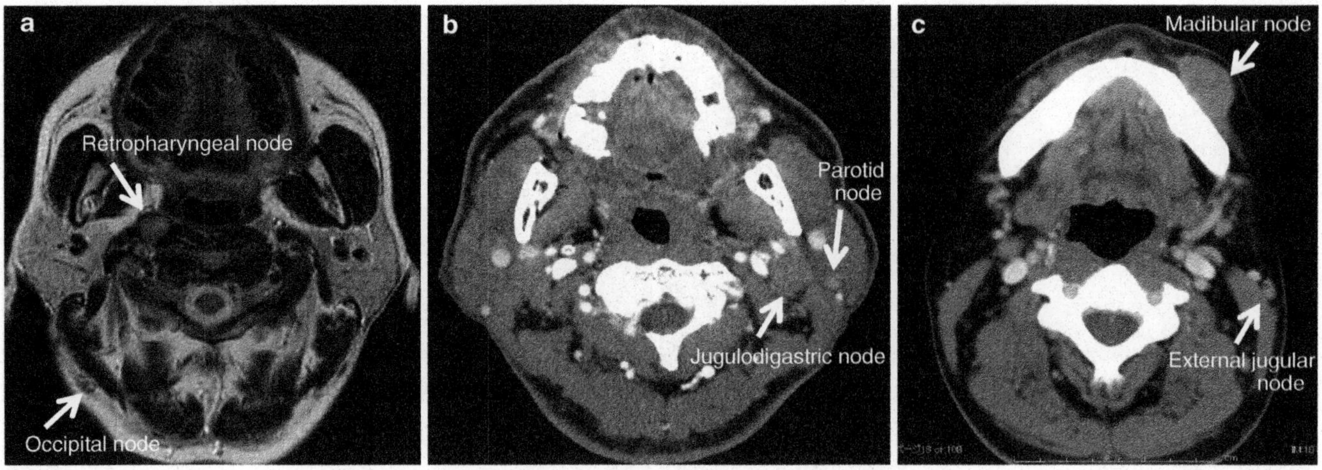

Fig. 6.2 Axial T2WI (**a**) and CECT images (**b**, **c**) show anatomic named nodes. (**a**) Retropharyngeal and occipital nodes, (**b**) jugulodigastric and parotid nodes, (**c**) madibular and external jugular nodes

the subcutaneous tissues of the cheek, the infraorbital nodes below the orbits, the malar nodes along the malar eminence, and the zygomatic nodes superficial to the zygomatic arch.

The lingual/sublingual node is along the lymphatics of the tongue. The lateral node is located in sublingual space along the lingual artery and vein. Lymph nodes between the submandibular gland and the hyoid bone, which are called parahyoid lymph nodes, are classified as lateral lingual lymph nodes. The medial node is located between both genioglossus muscles.

The external jugular node (Fig. 6.2c) is found in the superficial space along the external jugular vein.

The anterior cervical group is located in the infrahyoid anterior neck. Although the prelaryngeal, pretracheal, and paratracheal nodes are included in level VI, the anterior jugular nodes along the anterior jugular vein are not included in imaging-based classification.

The jugulodigastric node (Fig. 6.2b) is a specifically named lymph node and included in the high IJC. This node may normally be larger than other nodes and will quickly enlarge with upper respiratory infections.

6.4 Common Lymphatic Drainage of HNSCC

Lymphatic drainage patterns are important in pathologic processes. HNSCC has a common lymphatic drainage pattern of metastasis. The relationship between primary sites and lymph node metastasis of HNSCC has been well studied [3]. Knowledge of these patterns is essential when evaluating neck lymph nodes in HNSCC patients, and conversely, primary tumors can be suggested from the site of lymph node swelling. Nodal metastases of most HNSCC are present more frequently on the ipsilateral side. Contralateral metastases

Table 6.1 Lymphatic drainage: Main primary sites

Location	Primary site
IA	Lip, tip of tongue, anterior oral floor, skin of face
IB	Tongue, posterior oral floor, buccal mucosa, gingiva, skin of face, paranasal sinuses, submandibular gland
II	Pharynx, oral cavity, supraglottis, paranasal sinuses
III	Pharynx, supraglottis, tongue, base of tongue
IV	Larynx, thyroid, cervical esophagus, infraclavicular primary
V	Pharynx, skin of scalp, thyroid
VI	Larynx, cervical esophagus, thyroid
VII	Subglottis, cervical esophagus, thyroid
SCN	Any HNSCC, cervical esophagus, thyroid, infraclavicular primary
RPN	Nasopharynx, oral cavity, sinonasal, oropharynx, posterior wall of hypopharynx
Parotid	Orbit, nasopharynx, skin, ear, parotid

RPN retropharyngeal node, *SCN* supraclavicular node

can also occur, and the risk increases with the presence of ipsilateral nodal metastases and increased proximity of the primary tumor site to the midline. As a general rule, when contralateral metastasis is present, it often mirrors the nodal distribution of disease in the ipsilateral neck. However, these patterns of lymphatic spread are not defined because of the many lymphatic connections, and skip metastasis to more distal nodal levels without involvement of usual proximal pathways can occur in up to 15% of cases [4]. The common lymphatic drainage pathways are discussed here.

6.4.1 Drainage Patterns to Lymph Nodes

The relationship between nodal classification of neck lymph nodes and primary sites is listed in Table 6.1.

Level I nodes receive lymphatic drainage from the lips, floor of the mouth, and oral tongue. Level IA nodes normally drain into level IB nodes, and level IB nodes usually drain into level II.

Level II, III, and IV nodes typically receive drainage from the pharynx, oral cavity, parotid space, retropharyngeal space, facial nodes, and level I nodes. The usual pattern of lymphatic drainage progresses from level II to level III to level IV and drains into the IJV, the subclavian vein, or the transverse cervical chain.

Levels VA and VB receive drainage from the pharynx; the occipital, or mastoid, or parietal scalp region; and the lateral neck and drain into the transverse cervical chain.

Level VI receives drainage from the visceral space including the larynx, trachea, esophagus, thyroid, and dermal lymphatics of the anterior neck and typically drains into the superior mediastinum and level IV nodes.

The retropharyngeal nodes receive drainage from the sinonasal and pharyngeal mucosal surfaces and usually drain into the high level II.

The intraparotid nodes receive lymphatic drainage from the external auditory canal, the pinna of the ear, the eustachian tube, the skin of the lateral forehead and temporal region, posterior cheek, gums, and buccal mucosa and drain into the high level II.

The transverse chain receives drainage from the internal jugular chain, spinal accessory chain, subclavicular nodes, upper anterior chest wall, and skin of the anterolateral neck.

6.4.2 Drainage Patterns from the Primary Site

The lymphatic drainage pathways from each anatomic area are summarized in Table 6.2.

The anterior nose drains to level IB. The posterior two third nose drains to retropharyngeal nodes, levels IB, II, and III.

Drainage of the tongue is complex. The anterior tongue drains to levels IA and IB. The posterior tongue may drain to level IB or level II. Level III and IV nodes may be involved in advanced disease, or skip metastasis. Midline lesions may have bilateral pathways. Drainage of the other oral cavity may extend from level I to level IV, depending on the location of the primary tumor. Anterior regions drain to level IA nodes, and posterior portions drain preferentially to level II. Oral floor can also have relatively frequent bilateral nodal metastasis [5].

Tumors arising in the pharynx have a higher risk of presenting with nodal metastasis, and midline lesions may result in bilateral drainage patterns. The nasopharynx has rich lymphatic supply and shows one of the highest rates of nodal metastasis when involved with SCC [6]. The nasopharynx also serves as the catchment basin for lymphatic drainage of most of the nasal cavity and paranasal sinuses. The lymphatic drainage is to lateral retropharyngeal nodes and level II nodes,

Table 6.2 Lymphatic drainage: Main drainage routes

Anatomic area	Subdivision	Lymphatic drainage
Nasal cavity	Anterior nose	IB
	Posterior 2/3 nose	RPN, IB, II, III
Paranasal sinus	Paranasal sinus	II, III, IB, RPN
Oral cavity	Tip of tongue	IA
	Tongue	IB, II, III
	Hard palate	II, III
	Upper gingiva	II, III
	Lower gingiva	IB, II
	Lip	IA, IB
	Buccal mucosa	IB, IIA
	Anterior oral floor	IA, II, III
	Posterior oral floor	IB, II, III
	Retromolar trigone	IB, II, III
Pharynx	Nasopharynx	RPN, II, III, IV, V
	Tonsillar fossa	II, III
	Base of tongue	II, III
	Soft palate	II, III, RPN, parotid
	Anterior tonsillar pillar	IB, II, III
	Posterior tonsillar pillar	II, III, IV, V, RPN
	Hypopharynx	II, III, IV, VB, RPN, VI
Larynx	Supraglottis	III, II, IV
	Glottis	III, II
	Subglottis	VI, IV, III
Esophagus	Cervical esophagus	VI, VII, IV, SCN
Scalp	Skin	Parotid, mastoid, occipital, V
Ear	Auricle, EAC	Parotid, mastoid, II, III
Orbit	Orbit	Preauricular, parotid, II
Salivary gland	Parotid	II, III, parotid, V
	Submandibular	IB
	Sublingual	IA, IB

EAC external auricular canal, *RPN* retropharyngeal node, *SCN* supraclavicular node

with drainage to more distal level III, IV, and V nodal groups in more advanced disease and through alternative drainage patterns. The drainage of oropharynx is primarily to level II and III nodal groups, with less common involvement of retropharyngeal and level IV nodes. The hypopharynx has rich lymphatic supply, particularly dense lymphatic drainage in the piriform sinuses. Drainage is similar to that of the oropharynx with predominant involvement of level II to IV and occasionally RPNs from the posterior hypopharyngeal wall. Anterior hypopharyngeal lymphatic channels may directly communicate with laryngeal lymphatics, with eventual involvement of level VI nodes.

Laryngeal drainage patterns are divided into supraglottic, glottic, and subglottic patterns. Supraglottic regions drain primarily to level III, with occasional drainage cephalad to level II. Prominent horizontal drainage patterns lead to an increased risk for bilateral metastasis. Glottic regions have poor lymphatic drainage. More advanced glottic lesions may have involvement of nodal levels II to IV and VI. Subglottic processes have primarily lateral drainage to levels III, IV, and VI.

6.5 Imaging Techniques

The evaluation of the cervical lymph node is an essential part of the management of head and neck cancer. The nodal metastasis in HNSCC patient is a significant negative prognostic factor. Diagnostic accuracy of neck nodal metastasis is improved by the use of imaging rather than clinical palpation alone. Multiple modalities of computed tomography (CT), magnetic resonance imaging (MRI), ultrasonography (US), and fluorodeoxyglucose positron emission tomography (FDG-PET) are currently used for assessment of cervical lymph nodes (Figs. 6.3 and 6.4).

6.5.1 Contrast-Enhanced CT and MRI

CT and MRI are used for staging and surveillance of patients with HNSCC. CT is commonly used for regional nodal staging, because the short examination times reduce motion artifacts and spatial resolution is high compared with MRI [7]. Patients should be positioned with the infraorbitomeatal line, when using CT or MRI to evaluate lymph nodes.

CT is typically obtained helically from above the skull base through the tracheal carina. CT is performed using a contrast agent unless limited. Images with high-resolution CT can be reconstructed and useful for detection of lymph node metastasis.

For MR, T1-weighted images (T1WI), T2-weighted images (T2WI), diffusion-weighted images (DWI), and contrast-enhanced T1WI with fat saturation are recommended (Fig. 6.4b–e). DWI has shown promise in improving detection and characterization of lymph nodes and may be helpful in evaluating the posttreatment neck [8]. Multiple studies demonstrate that malignant nodes tend to have relative diffusion restriction with lower apparent diffusion coefficients. Some studies have shown high sensitivity (84–89%) and specificity (94–97%) for detection of metastatic nodes by DWI, exceeding conventional sequences [9, 10]. However, magnetic field inhomogeneity can reduce the image quality on DWI.

6.5.2 US

US is a convenient way to assess neck lymphadenopathy. US has better spatial resolution in evaluating internal architecture than CT or MRI (Figs. 6.3 and 6.4) [11]. US combined Doppler technique or fine-needle aspiration cytology (FNAC) is useful and improves sensitivity and specificity in diagnosis of metastatic nodes. However, interpretation is observer dependent, and retropharyngeal and mediastinal nodes cannot be assessed with US.

6.5.3 FDG-PET/CT

FDG-PET is an imaging modality that evaluates for metabolically active tissue. Integrated PET-CT units have improved the accuracy of PET image interpretation (Fig. 6.4f) [12]. FDG-PET/PET-CT is used for staging and post-therapeutic surveillance in HNSCC. Several studies have demonstrated higher sensitivity (84–92%) and specificity (95–99%) for PET/CT in the detection of regional lymph node metastases in HNSCC, compared with CT, MRI, or US [12–14]. Although PET-CT has the potential to detect small metastatic deposits in normal-sized nodes, a lower sensitivity for diagnosis of lymph nodes less than 10 mm is limitation. Other limitations are that cystic or necrotic nodes may be false negative while reactive nodes may be false positive (Fig. 6.5) [15].

6.6 Imaging Features of Metastatic Nodes

The primary method of detecting metastatic lymphadenopathy was palpation, and the criteria used were nodal size and fixation. Metastasis was suggested if a palpable node was larger than 1.5 cm in greatest diameter.

The imaging criteria were based on applying the clinical size criteria to CT and scrutinizing the features for evidence of extranodal extension in all size lymph nodes. Imaging criteria for lymph node metastasis have been reported, and the criteria shown below are widely used. However, even with these imaging criteria, occult metastases can be found in several primary lesions such as oral cavity, oropharynx, hypopharynx, and supraglottic cancers.

6.6.1 Size

Size criteria are widely used in evaluating lymph nodes. Nodes measuring greater than 15 mm in maximum diameter in level II and level IB and greater than 10 mm in all other levels are considered abnormal [16]. These criteria correspond to the earlier clinical experience described, and nodes exceeding these dimensions are metastatic by about 80%. Minimum diameter measurements are more accurate, and diameters exceeding 11 mm in level II and 10 mm elsewhere are considered abnormal (Fig. 6.4) [3]. It has been proposed that retropharyngeal nodes should not exceed 8 mm in maximum diameter or 5 mm in minimum short-axis diameter [17, 18]. On US, nodes measuring greater than 7 mm in minimum axial diameter in level II and 6 mm elsewhere are considered abnormal [19]. Although some size criteria for determination of metastatic lymphadenopathy have been proposed, unfortunately none are perfect (Fig. 6.6) [20].

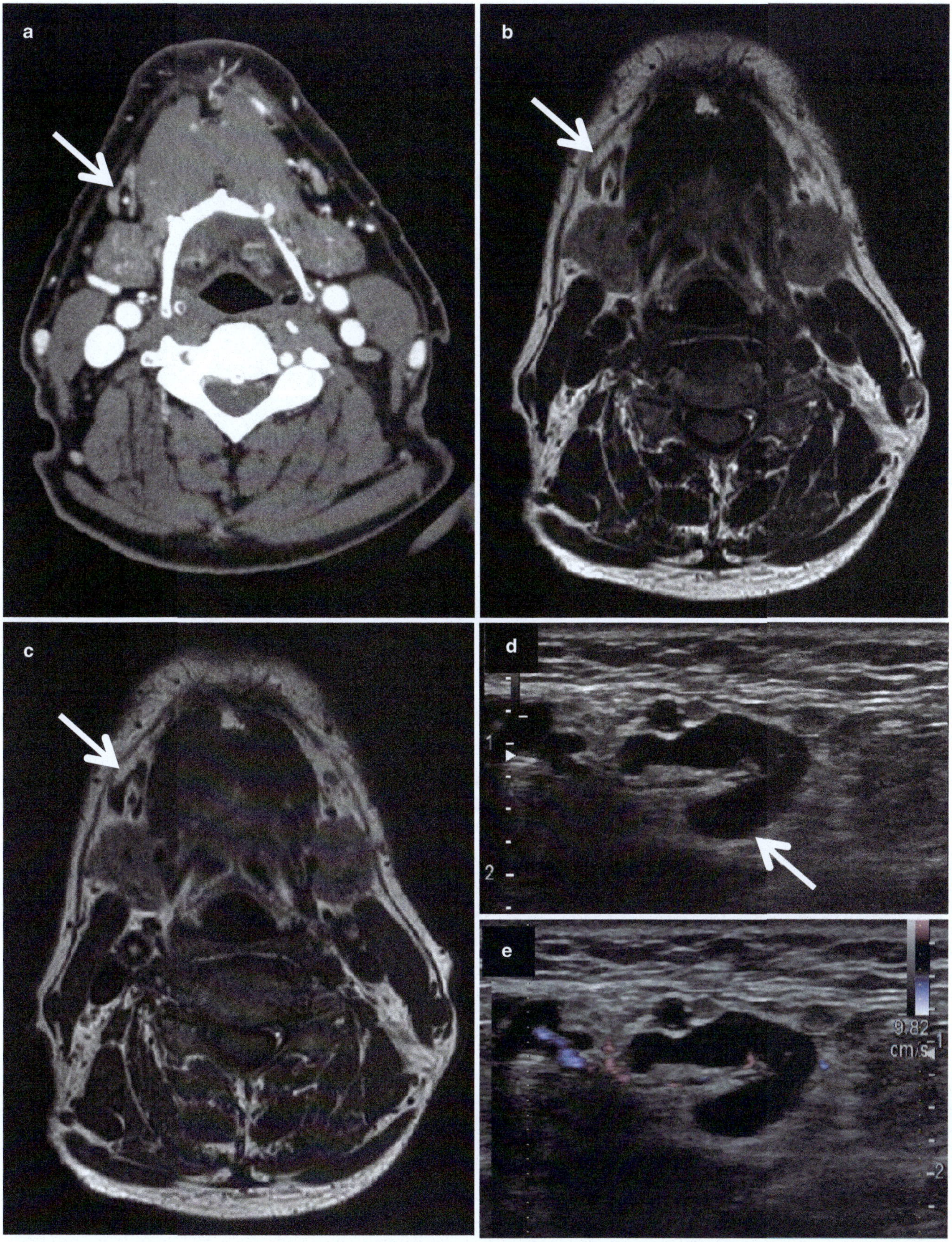

Fig. 6.3 A right level IB lymph node (*arrow*) shows normal size and shape with fatty hilum on axial CECT (**a**), T2WI (**b**), and T1WI (**c**). US shows homogeneous parenchyma (**d**, *arrow*) and echogenic hilum with a hilar vascular pattern on color Doppler (**e**)

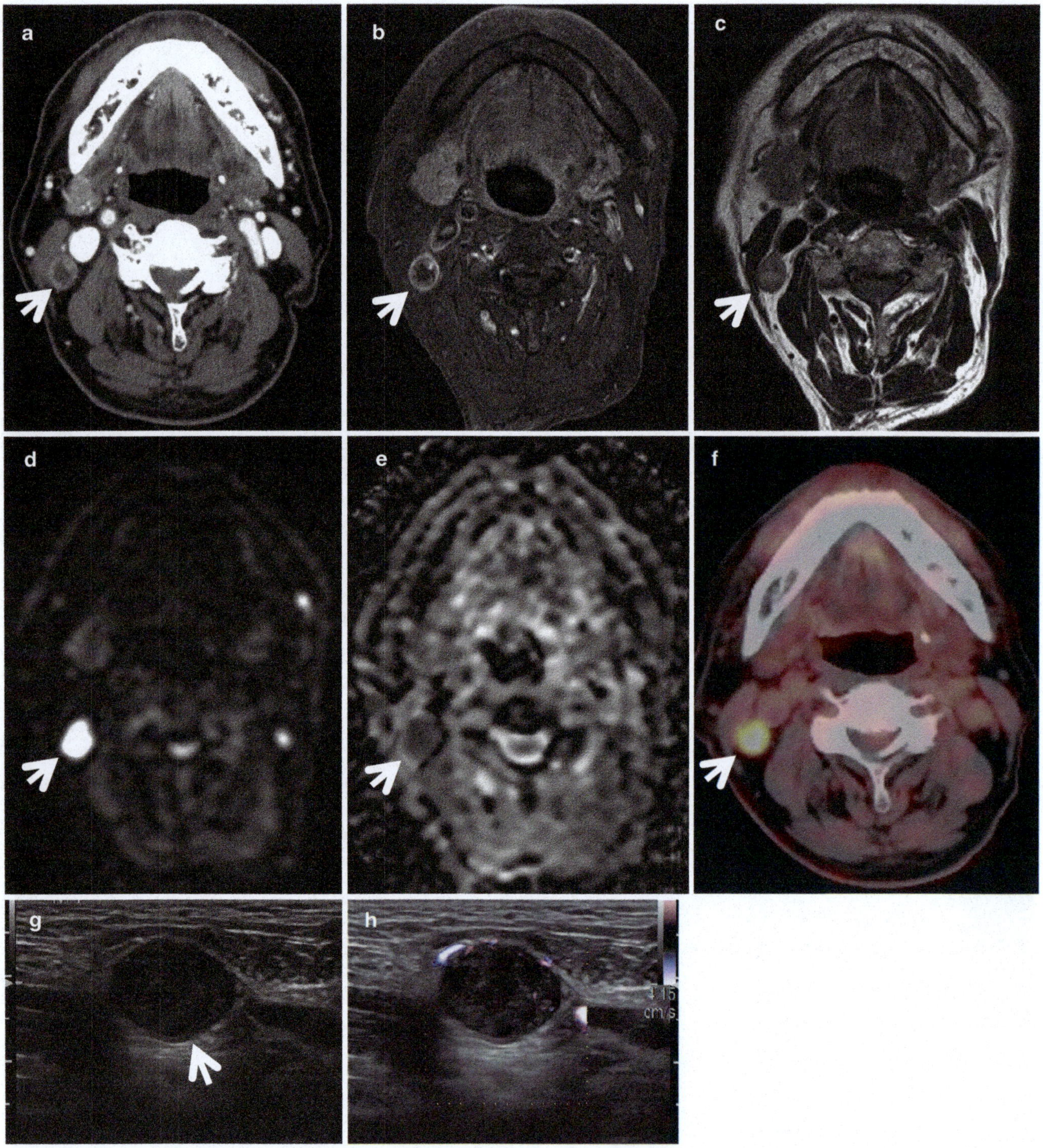

Fig. 6.4 Metastatic right level II node (*arrow*) from hypopharyngeal cancer exceeds 11 mm in minimum diameter with focal inhomogeneity on both enhanced CT (**a**) and T1WI (**b**), intermediate intensity on T2WI (**c**), restricted diffusion on DWI (**b** of 1000 s/mm^2) (**d**), a ADC of 0.74×10^{-3} mm^2/s (**e**), FDG uptake on fused PET/CT (**f**), and absent hilum and a non-hilar vascular pattern on US (**g**, **h**)

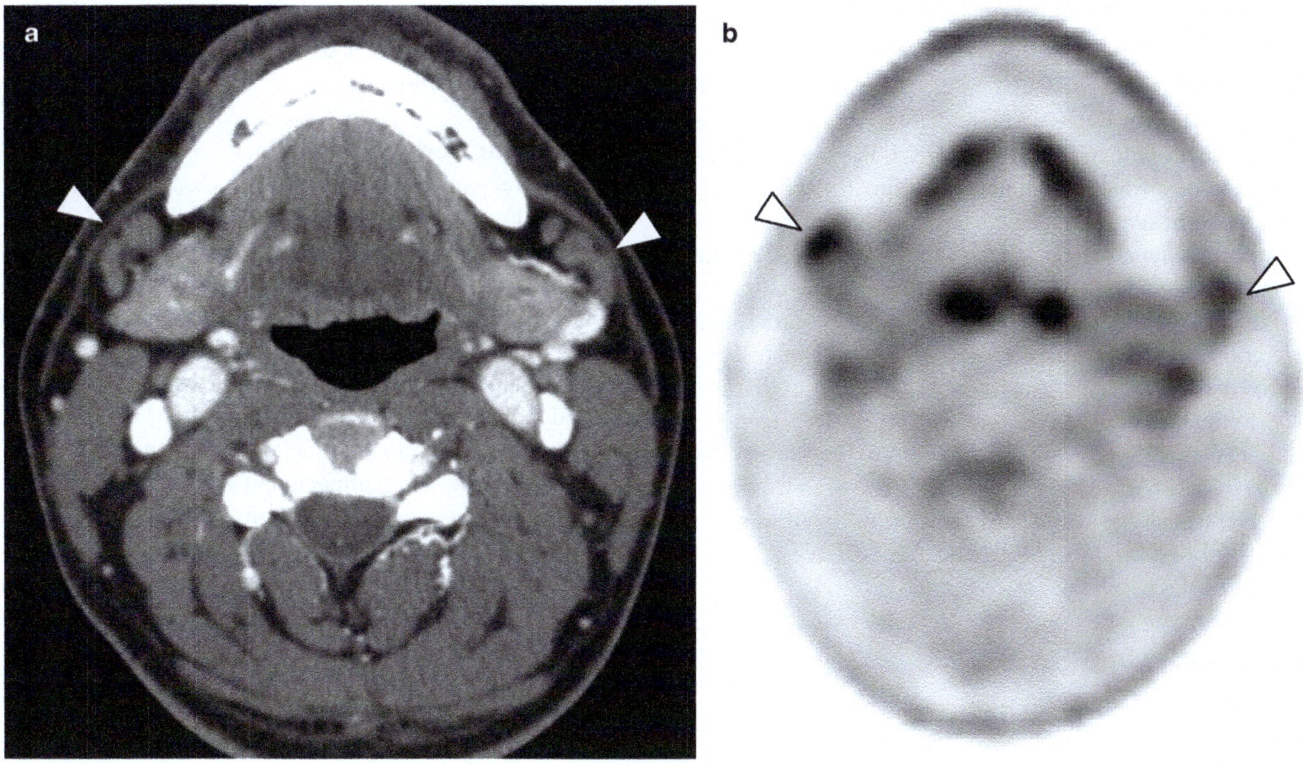

Fig. 6.5 Hyperplastic bilateral level IB nodes (**a**, **b**, *arrowhead*) reveal well-defined margin and lobulated shape on CECT (**a**). FDG-PET shows false-positive uptake (**b**)

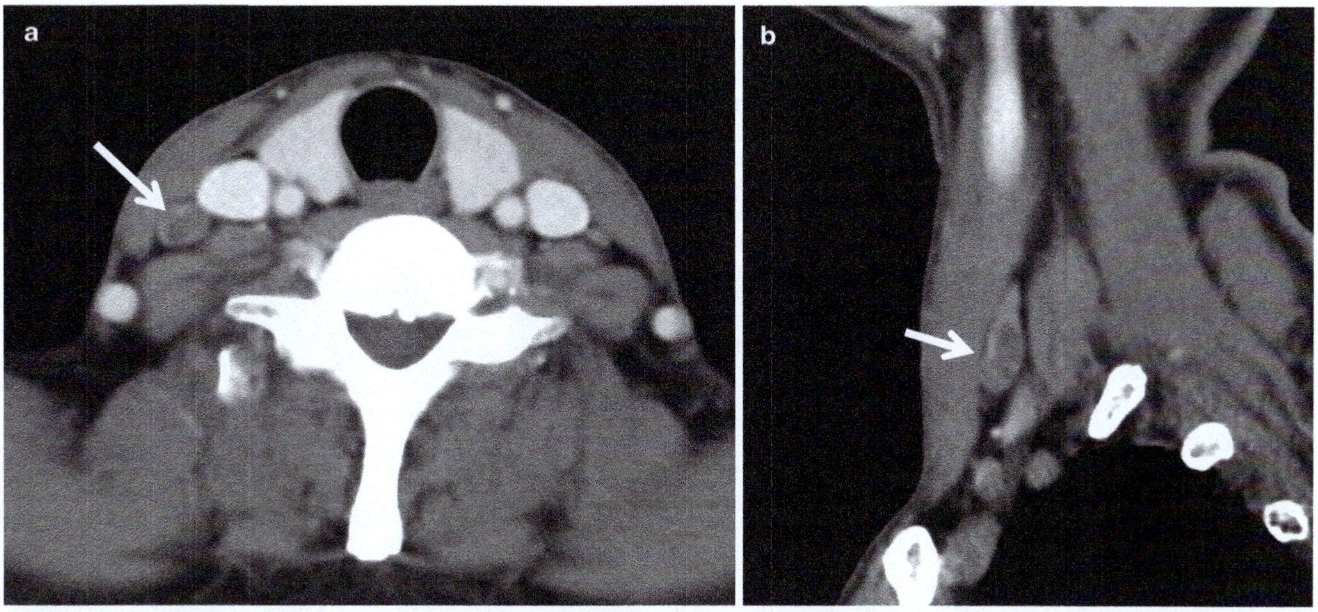

Fig. 6.6 Metastatic right level IV node (**a**, **b**, *arrow*) is less than 10 mm in minimum diameter and, however, has focal inhomogeneity

6.6.2 Shape

Nodal shape criteria are based on the pathologic observation that the normal or hyperplastic node is kidney-bean-shaped, whereas metastatic nodes are rounded. It has been suggested that the ratio of the maximum longitudinal nodal length to the maximum axial nodal length (L/T) should be greater than 2 for normal hyperplastic nodes, whereas a value of less than 2 strongly suggests that the node contains metastatic carcinoma (Fig. 6.4) [3, 16, 17]. If a lymph node is borderline by size criteria, but is round, it is more likely to be metastasis.

Normal nodes have usually well-defined borders and a fatty hilum that may be seen on CT, MRI, and US (Fig. 6.3). Malignant nodes typically show loss of the normal fatty hilum or focal cortical expansion (Figs. 6.4 and 6.6) [21]. However, focal cortical expansion is often found in normal or hyperplastic level IB nodes (Fig. 6.5).

6.6.3 Grouping

Nodal grouping is defined as the presence of three or more confluent lymph nodes with borderline size. Such a grouping along the expected drainage region is highly suggestive of metastasis [3]. When present, the minimal axial size threshold for a metastatic lymph node can be decreased by 1–2 mm, increasing sensitivity, without significantly affecting specificity.

6.6.4 Focal Nodal Inhomogeneity or Central Necrosis

The most reliable imaging criterion for metastatic lymphadenopathy is central necrosis. This term "central necrosis" is a misnomer, and the term "focal nodal inhomogeneity" is more suitable, because the medulla of metastatic nodes contain not only necrosis but also tumor cells [20, 22]. When the tumor metastasizes to the lymph nodes, these internal architecture become heterogeneous. As the majority of tumor cells enter a lymph node via the afferent lymphatics, focal nodal inhomogeneity occurs from the subcapsular region and spreads to the center of the node. If focal nodal inhomogeneity is >3 mm in size, it can frequently be identified on CT and MRI. Focal nodal inhomogeneity shows relatively low attenuation on CT and may appear hypointense on enhanced T1WI and hyperintense on T2WI and STIR images (Figs. 6.4 and 6.6).

The differential diagnosis of focal nodal inhomogeneity is the normal fatty hilum of the node. This hilum can be characterized as fatty attenuation on CT, as high intensity on T1WI and T2WIs, and as hyperechoic area on US (Figs. 6.3 and 6.5). The other differential diagnosis is an intranodal abscess in patients with acute infection and suppurative lymphadenitis. These cases are frequently evident based on the clinical presentation.

6.6.4.1 Cystic Nodal Metastasis

It has been recognized that there is a marked predilection for cystic nodal metastases to be associated with SCC of the tonsils and tongue base, and the incidence of cystic metastases has been reported to be as high as 33–50% [23]. The association between human papilloma virus (HPV) and tonsil and tongue base cancer has been well documented. HPV-related cancer accounts for more than 70% of HNSCC in oropharynx, and most of these cancers have cystic nodal metastases. In the unknown primary HNSCC with cystic nodal metastasis, primary tumors are often found in tonsils and tongue base. The mechanism of cyst formation in cystic nodal metastases has not been fully described. Radiologically, cystic nodes are defined as round or ovoid masses with a thin (<2 mm) enhancing capsule, homogeneous fluid content, and no internal complex, irregular, or solid area (Fig. 6.7). The differential diagnosis includes branchial cleft cyst and nodal metastasis of thyroid cancer.

6.6.5 Extranodal Extension (ENE)

Although terms such as extracapsular extension, extracapsular spread, or extranodal involvement have been used to denote tumor extension outside the capsule of a metastatic

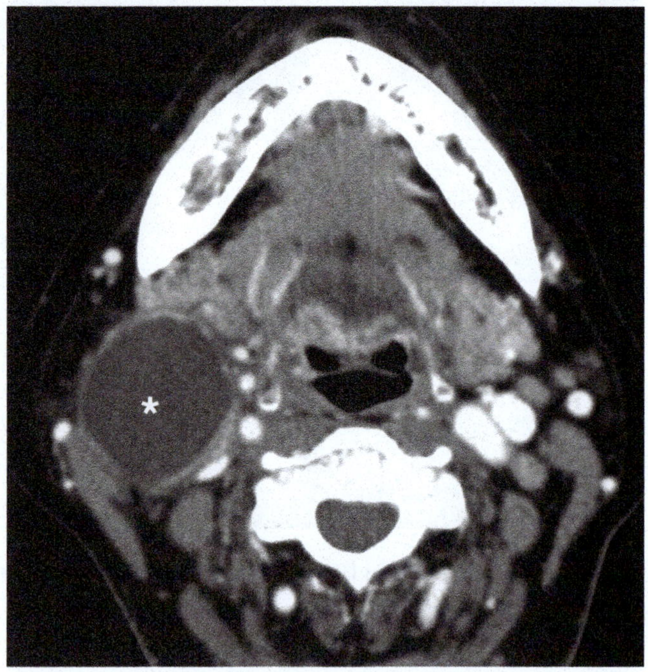

Fig. 6.7 Axial CECT image shows a cystic metastasis (*asterisk*) from HPV-related tongue base cancer. The lesion is similar to a second brachial cleft cyst

node, the American Joint Committee on Cancer (AJCC) and the Union for International Cancer Control (UICC) recommend extranodal extension (ENE) as a preferred wording.

The neck lymph node metastases decrease the overall survival by approximately half, and ENE worsens the prognosis by another 50% [24]. It was initially believed that extranodal extension occurred only in lymph nodes larger than 3 cm in greatest diameter. However, some studies have shown that ENE occurs in 23% on nodes less than 1 cm in greatest diameter, in 53% of nodes 2–3 cm in greatest diameter, and in 74% of nodes greater than 3 cm in greatest diameter. Overall, 60% of nodes with a greatest diameter of less than 3 cm have microscopic or gross extranodal extension [25, 26].

Several CT or MRI features suggest ENE, such as indistinct nodal margins and irregular nodal capsular enhancement; however, the strongest imaging feature supporting the clinical diagnosis for ENE is clear infiltration into the adjacent fat or muscle (Fig. 6.8). CT or MRI generally has low sensitivity (65–80%) but high specificity (86–93%) for the detection of ENE. On US, ENE is suggested by interrupted or undefined nodal contours. US appears to be less accurate in assessment of ENE than CT and MRI.

6.6.5.1 Carotid Arterial Invasion

The common or internal carotid artery is invaded in up to 5–10% of cervical lymph node metastasis of HNSCC [27]. Although it is important to recognize carotid invasion prior to treatment, it is often difficult. The size of metastatic lymph node is not a significant indicator of carotid invasion [28]. Deformity of the contour of carotid artery is a highly indicator of carotid arterial invasion. If the carotid artery is surrounded by a tumor above 270°, no surgical resection is generally attempted. However, it is often difficult to determine resectability by contact angle (Fig. 6.8). Surgical resection of tumor can be performed in cases without adventitial invasion of carotid artery. Because the carotid artery can be dissected from the tumor if the feeding vessels within the adventitia can be detected between the tumor and the carotid artery on enhanced CT, we consider that this finding is important. Even in cases with arterial invasion, resection and reconstruction of the carotid artery may result in better regional control. Therefore, it is important to select a treatment based on the comprehensive consideration including the patient's wishes and condition.

6.6.5.2 Prevertebral Fascia Invasion

The prevertebral fascia is tough and provides a barrier to tumor invasion. There have been previous reports of imaging findings on prevertebral fascia infiltration [29]. Compression and deformity of the fascia and signal changes of the prevertebral muscles on T2WI were considered as useful findings, but their specificities were low. The most reliable finding that indicates there is no invasion is that the fat of the retropharyngeal space is preserved.

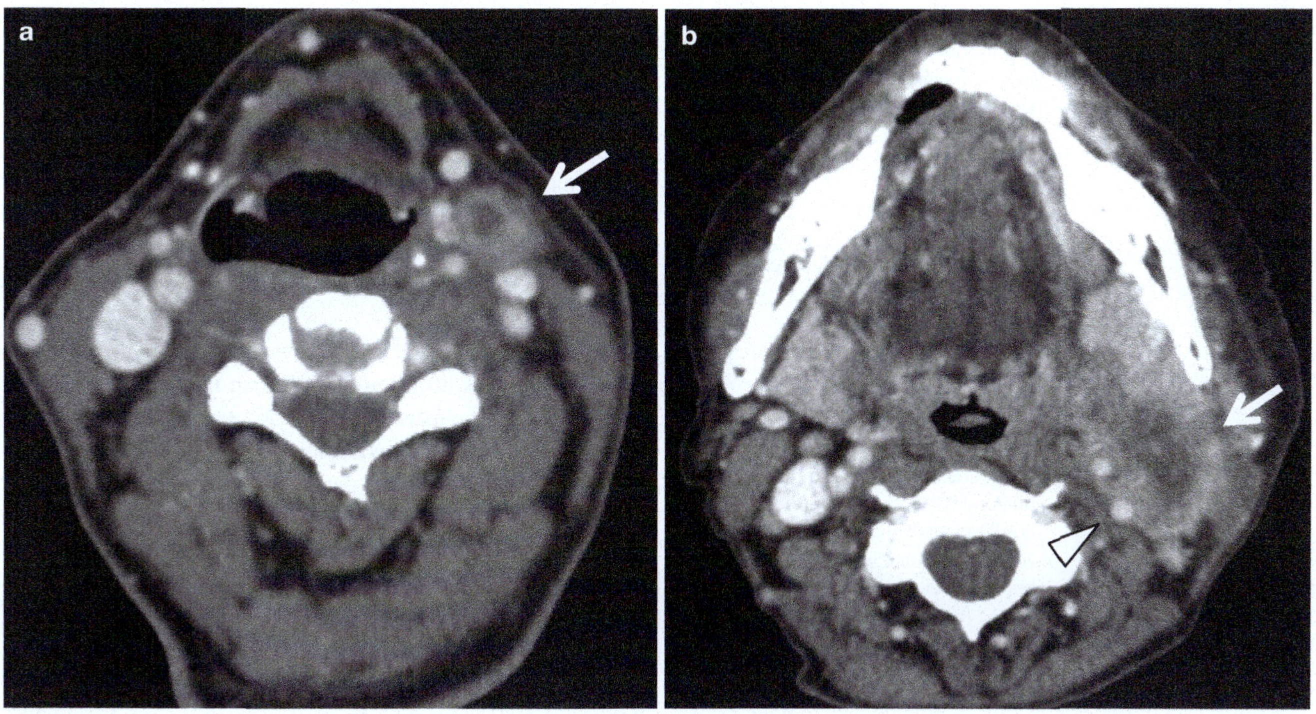

Fig. 6.8 Metastatic nodes reveal radiological ENE, such as enhancement of the nodal periphery, and irregular margins with infiltration to adjacent fat (**a**), or adjacent muscle planes and carotid artery (**b**). In b, the ICA (*arrowhead*) had 180° of contact with the metastatic node; however, adventitial invasion was confirmed at surgery

6.6.6 Vascular Patterns on US

Doppler US is the modality of choice for the assessment of a vascular pattern in neck cervical nodes. A hilar pattern is radiating vessels from the hilum into the node, and this pattern is highly specific for benign lymph nodes (Fig. 6.3) [30]. Non-hilar patterns include vascular displacement due to a focal intranodal lesion and a peripheral pattern due to neovascularization where vessels enter the node via the capsule away from the nodal hilum and are highly specific for metastatic involvement (Fig. 6.4).

6.7 Nodal Staging of HNSCC

TNM classification decided and revised by AJCC and UICC is widely accepted for cancer staging. This system has been classified based on the number, maximum size, and laterality of the affected nodes. After TNM classification seventh edition, HPV-related oropharyngeal cancer has been found to have several different characteristics, such as natural history, response to treatment, and prognosis. Radiation and chemoradiotherapy have been increased in HNSCC treatment. Based on these, the nodal staging of the TNM classification eighth edition instituted two major changes (Tables 6.3 and 6.4) [31, 32].

Table 6.3 Clinical N staging

Primary site	N stage	Definition
Any	NX	Regional nodes cannot be assessed
	N0	No regional nodal metastasis
All excluding p16+ oropharynx, and nasopharynx	N1	Single ipsilateral ≤3 cm ENE(−)
	N2a	Single ipsilateral >3 cm and ≤6 cm ENE(−)
	N2b	Multiple ipsilateral ≤6 cm ENE(−)
	N2c	Bilateral or contralateral ≤6 cm ENE(−)
	N3a	> 6 cm ENE(−)
	N3b	Any node(s) ENE(+)
p16+ oropharynx	N1	Unilateral ≤6 cm
	N2	Contralateral or bilateral ≤6 cm
	N3	>6 cm
Nasopharynx	N1	Unilateral cervical; unilateral or bilateral RPN; above the caudal border of cricoid cartilage ≤6 cm
	N2	Bilateral cervical; above the caudal border of cricoid cartilage ≤6 cm
	N3	Below the caudal border of cricoid cartilage >6 cm

The presence of skin involvement or soft tissue invasion with deep fixation/tethering to underlying muscle or adjacent structures or clinical signs of nerve involvement is classified as clinical ENE
ENE extranodal extension, *RPN* retropharyngeal node

Table 6.4 Pathological N staging

Primary site	N stage	Definition
Any	pNX	Regional lymph nodes cannot be assessed
	pN0	No regional lymph node metastasis
All excluding p16+ oropharynx, and nasopharynx	pN1	Single ipsilateral ≤3 cm ENE(−)
	pN2a	Single ipsilateral ≤3 cm ENE(+); Single ipsilateral >3 cm and ≤6 cm ENE(−)
	pN2b	Multiple ipsilateral ≤6 cm ENE(−)
	pN2c	Bilateral or contralateral ≤6 cm ENE(−)
	pN3a	>6 cm ENE(−)
	pN3b	Single ipsilateral >3 cm ENE(+); Multiple ENE(+)
p16+ oropharynx	pN1	1–4 lymph node(s)
	pN2	5 or more lymph nodes
Nasopharynx		Clinical N staging

ENE detected on histopathologic examination is designated as ENE_{mi} (microscopic ENE ≤2 mm) or EME_{ma} (major ENE >2 mm). Both $ENE_{mi\ and}$ EME_{ma} qualify as ENE(+) for definition of pN
ENE extranodal extension

The first change is that different clinical and pathological N classifications are proposed. Clinical N (cN) classification is required for all patients, and pathological N (pN) classification is only for patient undergoing surgery. Once involved node is identified on histopathological examination for patients undergoing surgery, pN is designated based on measurement of the largest dimension of the metastatic deposit and not of the entire lymph node. Pathological examination is necessary to record the location or level, the number of metastatic lymph nodes, and the presence and extent of ENE. An excisional biopsy of lymph node does not qualify for full evaluation of the pN category and should be assigned cN.

The second change is the use of extranodal extension (ENE). ENE has been known to be an important prognostic factor of nodal metastases in HNSCC, except for HPV-related tumors [33]. The eighth edition introduces ENE in the N category for both clinical and pathologic staging of HNSCC not related to HPV or EBV. Early ENE can only be identified on pathologic examination and cannot be reliably detected on clinical examination or with currently available imaging modality [34]. Therefore, The AJCC/UICC committee has set a high limitation for incorporating ENE into clinical staging. Clinical ENE requires overt clinical signs of gross (macroscopic) ENE supported by imaging findings (Fig. 6.8b). Obvious clinical signs of gross ENE include invasion of skin, infiltration of musculature, dense tethering or fixation to adjacent structures, or cranial nerve, brachial plexus, sympathetic trunk, or phrenic nerve invasion with dysfunction. The presence of clinical ENE migrates them all uniformly to the new subcategory of cN3b (Table 6.3). Pathological ENE also will be clearly defined as extension of metastatic tumor beyond the confines of the lymph node, through the lymph node capsule into the surrounding connective tissue, regardless of the presence of stromal reaction. ENE detected on histopathologic examination is subcategorized as ENE_{mi} (microscopic ENE ≤2 mm from the nodal capsule) or ENE_{ma} (major or macroscopic ENE >2 mm beyond the nodal capsule, or a soft tissue deposit that has completely destroyed nodal architecture). Both ENE_{mi} and ENE_{ma} qualify as ENE-positive for the definition of pN. The presence of ENE in a single ipsilateral lymph node less than 3 cm in maximum dimension migrates that category to pN2a (Table 6.4).

6.7.1 Unknown Primary Tumor

The head and neck region is unique because several different staging classifications are based on anatomic site. The classification of unknown primary site has been improved by understanding the tumorigenesis of head and neck cancer and improvement of histologic methods to identify EBV-related and HPV-related tumors. Patients with EBV-related lymphadenopathy are staged according to nasopharyngeal cancer. Patients with HPV-related lymphadenopathy are staged according to HPV-related oropharyngeal cancer. All other patients with EBV-unrelated and HPV-unrelated lymphadenopathy are staged according to the N category of unknown primary tumor.

6.8 Treatment Assessment

6.8.1 Prediction of Treatment Response to (Chemo)Radiotherapy

Several findings that predict treatment effects and prognosis are obtained from functional imaging techniques performed before treatment or early in treatment. Regional control is more likely to occur in nodes with higher vascularity, as shown by higher K trans in dynamic MRI [35]. Tumor control is also seen in lymph nodes with lower pretreatment ADC and higher rise of ADC early in treatment (Fig. 6.9) [36, 37]. Using FDG-PET, primary tumors with lower SUV are more likely to show an overall response in the neck [38]. In addition, high FDG uptake before treatment in lymph node metastasis of HNSCC may be a risk factor for distant metastasis [39].

6.8.2 Assessment for Post (Chemo) Radiotherapy

Most HNSCC lymph node metastases respond completely to radiation or chemoradiotherapy (CRT). Previously, planned neck dissection was done after radiation or CRT. Fortunately, with the development of an effective chemotherapy regimen, neck dissection has only been performed in patients who have clinical evidence of residual disease after radiation or CRT. The selection of patients with posttreatment residual disease requiring early salvage surgery has become an important part of imaging.

The changes after radiation or CRT occur within 2 weeks of therapy and are initially an acute inflammatory response, which ultimately result in scar at 6 weeks to 1 year after treatment.

CT and MRI both have a high negative predictive value (94–97%) for residual nodal disease if the nodal metastases have essentially disappeared. However, lymph node metastases are often poorly regressive, leaving varying amounts of scar tissue. In CT-based studies, it has been reported that residual nodes of 15 mm or less without focal inhomogeneity or nodes with a reduction in size greater than 90% were associated with tumor control. However, even if the remaining lymph nodes exceed 15 mm, there may be no residual cancer. Therefore, focusing on the scar that occurred after treatment improves the accuracy of diagnosis. Scar tissue shows faint or absent enhancement and lower attenuation than surrounding muscles on contrast-enhanced CT. MRI is more useful than CT; scar tissue shows low signal intensity on T2WI, low signal intensity on DWI obtained with b of 0 s/mm^2 and b of 1000 s/mm^2 and low ADC value [40]. This low signal intensity is characteristic of benign scar tissue, indicating hyalinization, and should be differentiated from intermediate T2 signal intensity encountered in persistent lymph nodes at 6–8 weeks after treatment (Fig. 6.10).

FDG-PET/CT is increasing to assess lymph nodes after treatment and is performed at 10–12 weeks after treatment to prevent false positives or false negatives. FDG-PET/CT shows a high negative predictive value (96%) and is more accurate than CT and MRI, although the positive predictive value is low (49%) [41].

6.8.3 Posttreatment Surveillance

Because most recurrences occur within the first 2 years of treatment, close clinical and imaging surveillance is important for the detection of relapses (Fig. 6.11). Post-therapeutic baseline images are performed within

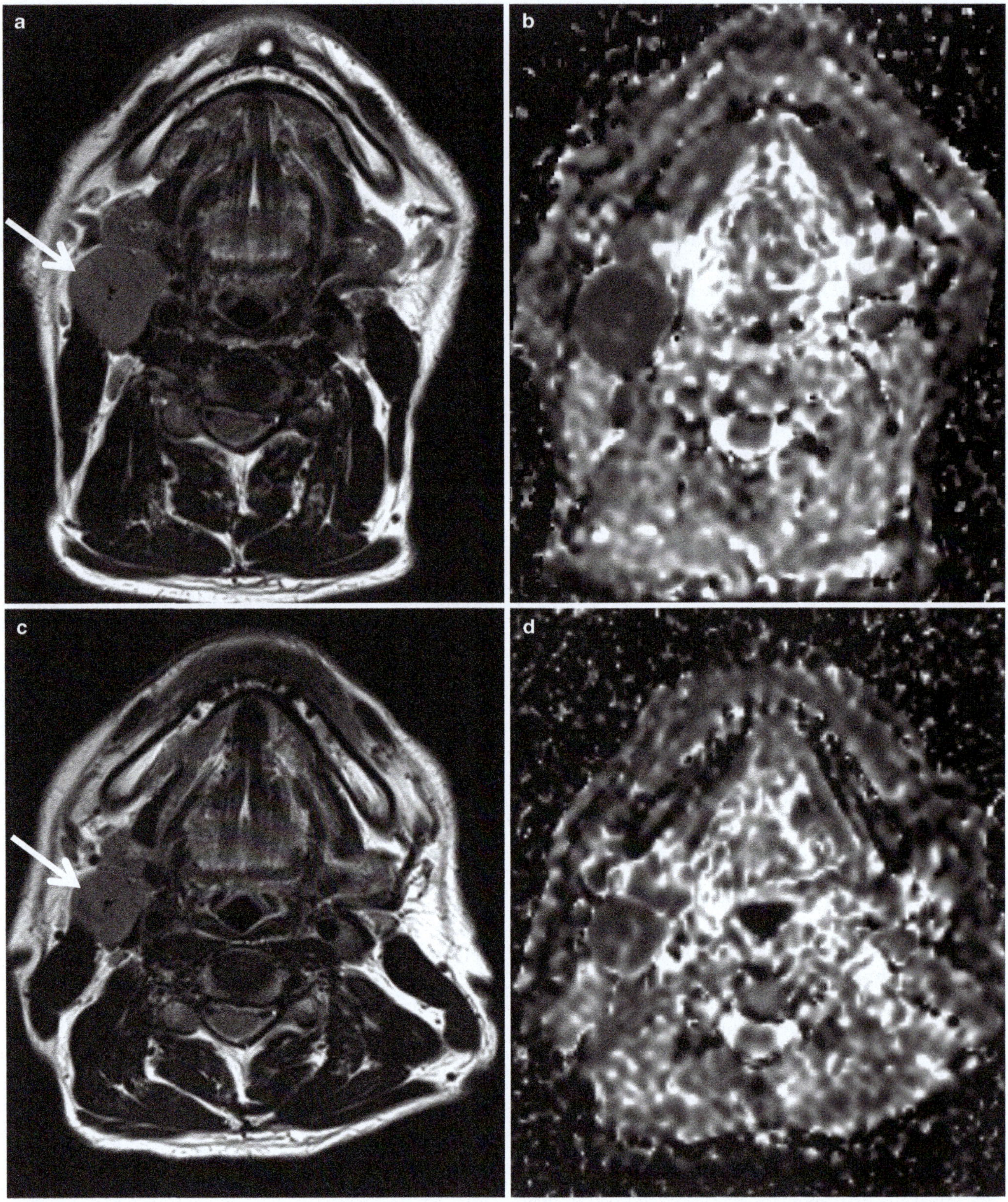

Fig. 6.9 Comparing the metastatic right level II lymph node before treatment (*top row*) and at 2 weeks with concomitant chemoradiotherapy (*bottom row*), the size of the node decreased and the ADC value increased 0.7×10^{-3} mm^2/s pretreatment to 1.1×10^{-3} mm^2/s at 2 weeks intra-treatment. This indicates increased diffusion, which favors a treatment response

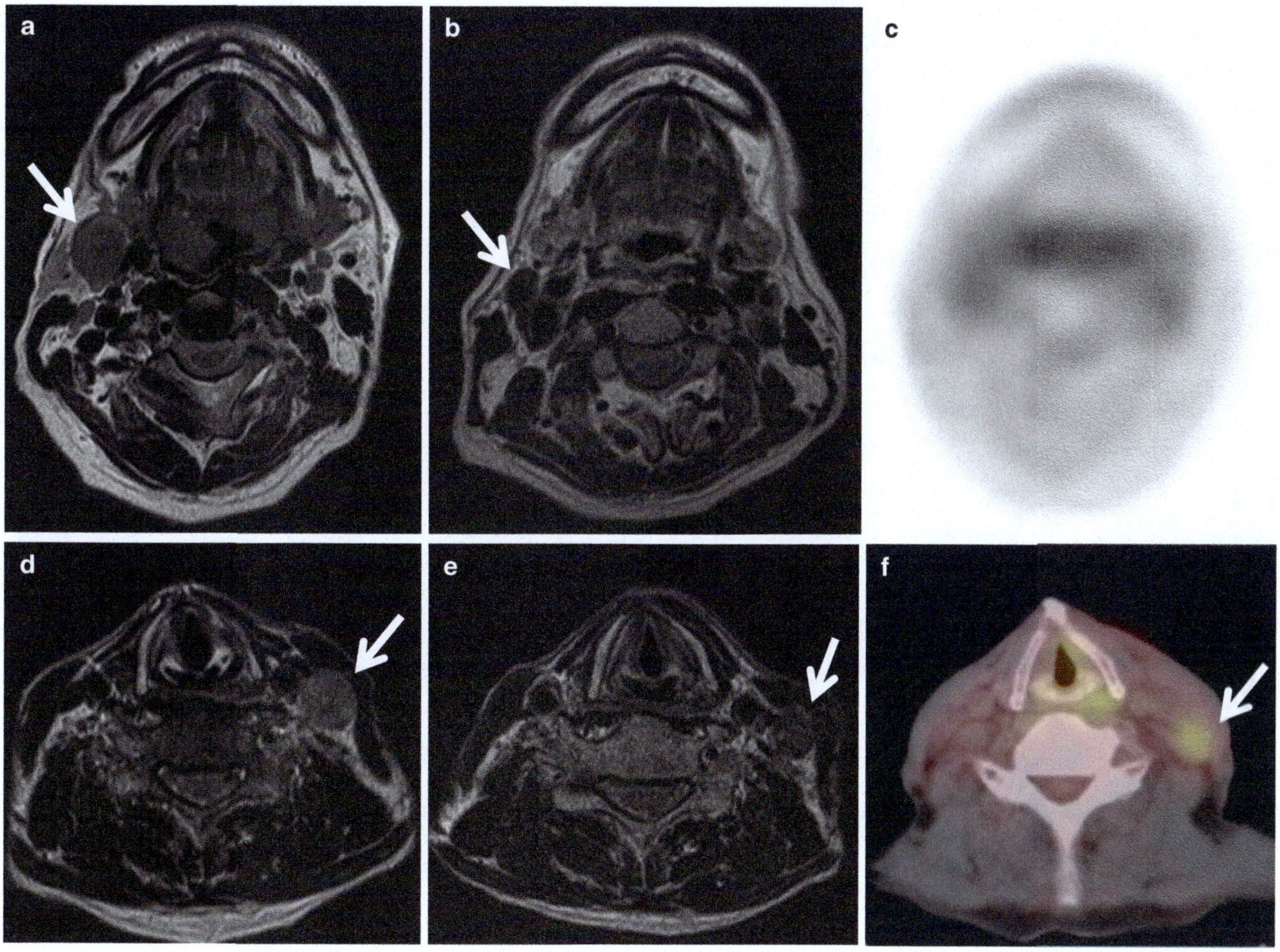

Fig. 6.10 Metastatic lymph node showing intermediate intensity before treatment has low intensity on T2WI and no FDG accumulation in CR case (*top row*). However, in non-CR case (*bottom row*), a metastatic node still shows intermediate intensity on T2WI and FDG accumulation after treatment

4–8 weeks after treatment, and the patients generally undergo imaging every 3–6 months for 2–3 years, being more frequent in the earlier posttreatment period.

The effects of surgery, radiation, and chemotherapy can drastically alter the normal anatomy [42, 43]. Altered tissue after treatment and recurrent nodes may show mimic findings. Lymph node metastasis may occur in unexpected areas, as lymphatics also changes after treatment. Some relapses may occur from occult metastasis. Therefore, it is important to compare the baseline image and the follow-up image to obtain valuable information in the interpretation.

Although the imaging modality used to monitor HNSCC patients is variable, CT or MRI is generally performed. CT has a high sensitivity and moderate specificity for differentiating recurrence from posttreatment changes. If it is difficult to distinguish recurrence from posttreatment changes on CT, DWI may be useful as recurrent nodal diseases show restricted diffusion with low ADCs. US-FNAC also plays a role in posttreatment surveillance and early detection of potential lymph node metastases, increasing the possibility of performing salvage surgery with US follow-up. Now, there are also institutions that perform FDG-PET routinely as a posttreatment baseline or for patients with suspected recurrent disease on conventional imaging. Inflammatory or infectious conditions can lead to false-positive PET finding; no FDG-PET/CT should be performed without knowledge of clinical findings.

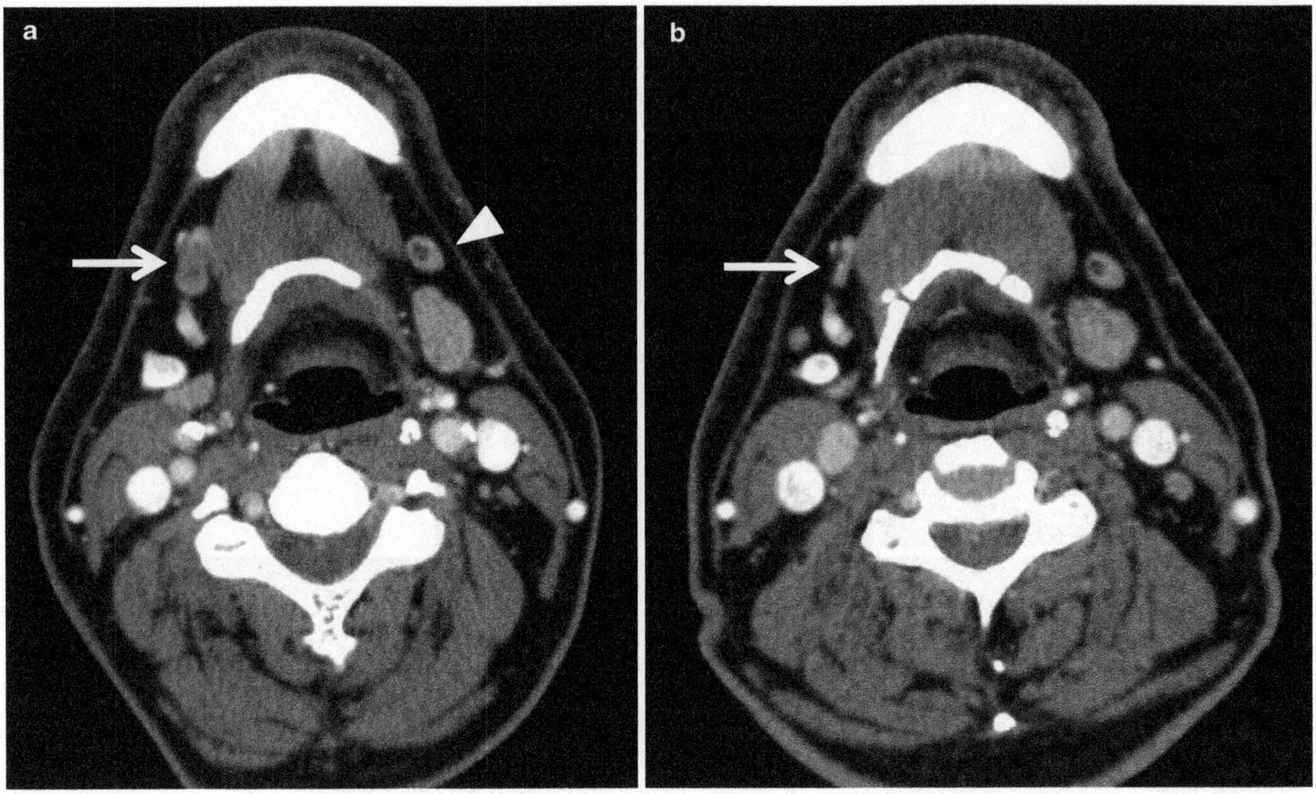

Fig. 6.11 Axial follow-up CECT 6 months after surgery of tongue cancer (**a**) shows a metastatic lymph node (*arrow*) with focal inhomogeneity in right level IB. Before treatment (**b**), this node (*arrow*) is in normal size and attenuation. Left level IB lymph node (**a**, *arrowhead)* shows no change in morphology before and after treatment

References

1. Rouvière H. Lymphatic system of the head and neck. Ann Arbor, MI: Edwards Brothers; 1938. p. 5–28.
2. Som PM, Curtin HD, Mancuso AA. An imaging-based classification for the cervical nodes designed as an adjunct to recent clinically based nodal classifications. Arch Otolaryngol Head Neck Surg. 1999;125:388–96.
3. van den Brekel M, Stel H, Castelijns J, Nauta JJ, Van der Waal I, Valk J, et al. Cervical lymph node metastasis: assessment of radiologic criteria. Radiology. 1990;177:379–84.
4. Byers RM, Weber RS, Andrews T, McGill D, Kare R, Wolf P. Frequency and therapeutic implications of "skip metastases" in the neck from squamous carcinoma of the oral tongue. Head Neck. 1997;19:14–9.
5. Melkane AE, Mamelle G, Wycisk G, Temam S, Janot F, Casiraghi O, et al. Sentinel node biopsy in early oral squamous cell carcinomas: a 10-year experience. Laryngoscope. 2012;122:1782–8.
6. Wang Y, Ow TJ, Myers JN. Pathways for cervical metastasis in malignant neoplasms of the head and neck region. Clin Anat. 2012;25:54–71.
7. Sumi M, Ohki M, Nakamura T. Comparison of sonography and CT for differentiating benign from malignant cervical lymph nodes in patients with squamous cell carcinoma of the head and neck. Am J Roentgenol. 2001;176:1019–24.
8. Curtin HD, Ishwaran H, Mancuso AA, Dalley RW, Caudry DJ, McNeil BJ. Comparison of CT and MR imaging in staging of neck metastases. Radiology. 1998;207:123–30.
9. Thoeny HC, De Keyzer F, Kinf AD. Diffusion-weighted MR imaging in the head and neck. Radiology. 2012;263:19–32.
10. Vandecaveye V, Keyzer FD, Pooten VV, Dirix P, Verbeken E, Nuyts S, et al. Head and neck squamous cell carcinoma: value of diffusion-weighted MR imaging for nodal staging. Radiology. 2009;251:134–46.
11. Dirix P, Vandecaveye V, De Keyzer F, de Beeck KO, Pooten VV, Delaere P, et al. Diffusion-weighted MRI for nodal staging of head and neck squamous cell carcinoma: impact on radiotherapy planning. Int J Radiat Oncol Biol Phys. 2010;76:761–6.
12. Jeong HS, Baek CH, Son YI, Chung MK, Lee DK, Choi JY, et al. Use of integrated 18F-FDG PET/CT to improve the accuracy of initial cervical nodal evaluation in patients with head and neck squamous cell carcinoma. Head Neck. 2007;29:203–10.
13. Gordin A, Golz A, Keidar Z, Daltzchman M, Shalom RB, Israel O. The role of FDG-PET/CT imaging in head and neck malignant conditions: impact on diagnostic accuracy and patient care. Otolaryngol Head Neck Surg. 2007;137:130–7.
14. Adams S, Baum RP, Stuckensen T. Prospective comparison of 18F-FDG PET with conventional imaging modalities (CT, MRI, US) in lymph node staging of head and neck cancer. Eur J Nucl Med. 1998;25:1255–60.
15. Stoeckli SJ, Steiner H, Pfaltz M, Schmid S. Is there a role for positron emission tomography with 18F-fluorodeoxyglucose in the initial staging of nodal negative oral and oropharyngeal squamous cell carcinoma. Head Neck. 2002;24:345–9.
16. Snow GB, Annyas AA, Van Slooten EA, Bartelink H, Hart AA. Prognostic factors of neck node metastasis. Clin Otolaryngol. 1982;7:185–92.

17. Som PM. Detection of metastasis in cervical lymph nodes: CT and MR criteria and differential diagnosis. Am J Roentgenol. 1992;158:961–9.
18. Mancuso A, Harnsberger H, Muraki Am Stevens M. Computed tomography of cervical and retropharyngeal lymph nodes: normal anatomy, variants of normal, and application in staging head and neck cancer. Part II. Radiology. 1983;148:715–23.
19. Mizowaki T, Nishimura Y, Shimada Y, Nakano Y, Imamura M, Konishi J, et al. Optimal size criteria of malignant lymph nodes in the treament planning of radiotherapy for esophageal cancer; evaluation by computed tomography and magnetic resonance imaging. Int J Radiat Oncol Biol Oncol Biol Phys. 1996;36:1091–8.
20. van den Brekel MW, Castelijins JA, Snow GB. The size of lymph nodes in the neck on sonograms as a radiologic criterion for metastasis: how reliable is it? Am J Neuroradiol. 1998;19:695–700.
21. Forghani R, Curtin HD. Imaging evaluation of cervical lymph nodes. In: Yu E, Shankar L, editors. Introductory head and neck imaging. New Delhi: Jaypee Brochers Medical Publishers; 2014. p. 421–504.
22. Rubaltelli L, Proto E, Salmaso R, Bortoletto P, Candiani F, Cagol P. Sonography of abnormal lymph nodes in vitro; correlation of sonographic and histologic findings. Am J Roentgenol. 1990;155:1241–4.
23. Som PM, Brandwein-Gensler MS. Lymph nodes of the neck. In: Som PM, Curtin HD, editors. Head and neck imaging. St. Louis: Mosby; 2011. p. 2287–383.
24. Regauer S, Mannweiler S, Anderhuber W, Gotschuli A, Berghold A, Schachenreiter J, et al. Cystic lymph node metastases of squamous cell carcinoma of Waldeyer's ring origin. Br J Cancer. 1999;79:1437–42.
25. Bataskis JG. Squamoud cell carcinoma of the oral cavity and the oropharynx. In: Tumor of the head and neck: clinical and pathological considerations. 2nd ed. Baltimore: Williams & Wilkins; 1979. p. 144–76.
26. Chong V. Cervical lymphadenoathy: what radiologists need to know. Cancer Imaging. 2004;4:116–20.
27. Nemeth Z, Domotor G, Talos M. Resection and head and neck cancer. Int J Oral Maxillofac Surg. 2003;32:645–50.
28. Pons Y, Ukkola-Pons E, Clement P, Gauthler J, Conessa C. Relevance of 5 different imaging signs in the evaluation of carotid artery invasion by cervical lymphadenopathy in head and neck squamous cell carcinoma. Oral Surg Oral Med Oral Pathol Oral Radiol Endod. 2010;109:775–8.
29. Loevner LA, Ott IL, Yousem SM, Montone KT, Thaler ER, Chalian AA, et al. Neoplastic fixation to the prevertebral compartment by squamous cell carcinoma of the head and neck. Am J Roentogenol. 1998;170:1389–94.
30. Ahuja A, Ying M. Sonographic evaluation of cervical lymphadenopathy: is power Doppler sonography routinely indicated? Ultrasound Med Biol. 2003;29:353–9.
31. Amin MB, Edge SB, Greene FL, Byrd DR, Brookland RK, Washington MK, et al. American Joint Committee on Cancer manual for staging of cancer. 8th ed. New York: Springer; 2017.
32. Brierley JD, Gospodarowicz MK, Wittekind C. Union for International Cancer Control TNM classification of malignant tumours. 8th ed. New York: Wiley; 2017.
33. Liu JT, Kann BH, De B, Buckstein M, Bakst RL, Genden EM, et al. Prognostic value of radiographic extracapsular extension in locally advanced head and neck squamous cell cancers. Oral Oncol. 2016;52:52–7.
34. Prabhu RS, Magliocca KR, Hanasoge S, Aiken AH, Hudgins PA, Hall WA, et al. Accuracy of computed tomography for predicting pathologic nodal extracapsular extension in patients with head-and-neck cancer undergoing initial surgical resection. Int J Radiat Oncol Biol Phys. 2014;88:122–9.
35. Kim S, Loevner LA, Quon H, Kilger A, Sherman E, Weinstein G, et al. Prediction of response to chemoradiation therapy in squamous cell carcinomas of the head and neck using dynamic contrast-enhanced MR imaging. Am J Neuroradiol. 2010;31:262–8.
36. Vandecaveye V, Dirix P, De Keyzer F, de Beeck KO, Poorten VV, Roebben I, et al. Predictive value of diffusion-weighted magnetic resonance imaging during chemoradiotherapy for head and neck squamous cell carcinoma. Eur Radiol. 2010;20:1703–14.
37. Noji DP, Martens RM, Marcus JT, de Bree R, Leemans R, Castelijns JA, et al. Intravoxel incoherent motion magnetic resonance imaging in head and neck cancer: a systematic review of the diagnostic and prognostic value. Oral Oncol. 2017;68:81–91.
38. Schwartz DL, Rajendran J, Yueh B, Coltrera M, Anzai Y, Krohn K, et al. Staging of head and neck squamous cell cancer with extended-field FDG-PET. Arch Otolaryngol Head Neck Surg. 2003;129:1173–8.
39. Kubicek GJ, Champ C, Fogh S, Wang F, Reddy E, Intenzo C, et al. FDG-PET staging and importance of lymph node SUV in head and neck cancer. Head Neck Oncol. 2010;2:19–25.
40. King AD, Keung CK, Yu KH, Mo FKF, Bhatia KS, Yeung DKW, et al. T2-weighted MR imaging early after chemoradiotherapy to evaluate treatment response in head and neck squamous cell carcinoma. Am J Neuroradiol. 2013;34:1237–41.
41. Isles MG, McConkey C, Mehanna HM. A systematic review and meta-analysis of the role of positron emission tomography in the follow up of head and neck squamous cell carcinoma following radiotherapy or chemoradiotherapy. Clin Otolaryngol. 2008;33:210–22.
42. Hadgins PA. Flap reconstruction in the head and neck: expected appearance, complications, and recurrent disease. Eur J Radiol. 2002;44:130–8.
43. Offiah C, Hall E. Post-treatment imaging appearances in head and neck cancer patients. Clin Radiol. 2011;66:13–24.

7 Diagnostic Imaging of Sinonasal Tumors

Keiko Toyoda

Abstract

The sinonasal tract is the site of origin for an enormous variety of neoplasms. Sinonasal neoplasms are broadly classified as either epithelial or mesenchymal. Among sinonasal malignancies, squamous cell carcinoma (SCC) accounts for approximately 80%.

Approximately 25–60% of these carcinomas involve the maxillary antrum; however, the maxillary sinus is secondarily involved by direct extension in 80% of patients.

These cancers of the paranasal sinuses are clinically silent without apparent symptoms when small and, in nearly all cases, have already become large with invasion of surrounding organs at the time of the initial examination.

Diagnostic imaging is necessary for evaluating tumor location and extension. CT and MRI play complementary roles especially in the assessment and staging of these sinonasal malignancies. CT is superior to MR imaging for identifying bone involvement of thin walls and septa of the paranasal sinuses using multiplanar reconstruction. MR imaging offers soft tissue resolution, contrast, and multiplanar capabilities. In addition, MRI is helpful for tumor mapping and for distinguishing between tumor extension and obstruction. From these imaging findings, appropriate treatment planning including curability and functionality can be considered.

As other nonepithelial tumors, malignant lymphoma, mucosal malignant melanoma, and inverted papilloma also occur in the sinonasal cavities, and these tumors are differentiated from these carcinomas by diagnostic imaging.

K. Toyoda (✉)
Department of Radiology, The Jikei University Daisan Hospital, Tokyo, Japan

Keywords

Squamous cell carcinoma · Adenoid cystic carcinoma · Malignant lymphoma · Malignant melanoma

Abbreviations

ADC Apparent diffusion coefficient
SCC Squamous cell carcinoma

7.1 Introduction

The sinonasal tract is the site of origin for an enormous variety of neoplasms. Sinonasal neoplasms are broadly classified as either epithelial or mesenchymal. Among sinonasal malignancies, squamous cell carcinoma (SCC) accounts for 80% of sinonasal malignancies [1–4].

Approximately 25–60% of these carcinomas involve the maxillary antrum; however, the maxillary sinus is secondarily involved by direct extension in 80% of patients and followed by the nasal cavity (25–35%) and ethmoid sinus (1–15%) [3, 5]. The carcinogenic process for SCC occurs together with metaplasia of pseudostratified epithelium in the stratified squamous epithelium within the sinus. Chronic inflammation is heavily involved. SCCs are classified as keratinizing type and non-keratinizing type. Other rare carcinomas of the sinonasal cavities include spindle cell (sarcomatoid) SCC, lymphoepithelial carcinoma, sinonasal undifferentiated carcinoma, NUT (nuclear protein in testis) carcinoma, intestinal-type adenocarcinoma, and non-intestinal-type adenocarcinoma. Other cancers include carcinomas originating in the minor salivary glands (adenoid cystic carcinoma, undifferentiated carcinoma, mucoepidermoid carcinoma).

H. Ojiri (ed.), *Diagnostic Imaging in Head and Neck Cancer*, https://doi.org/10.1007/978-981-15-3188-0_7

SCC of the nasal cavity and paranasal sinuses has a sex difference, with more cases seen in middle-aged and older men. It appears to have a higher prevalence in people whose work involves nickel exposure, wood furniture, chrome, isopropyl alcohol, radium, mustard gas, and other substances [6].

These cancers of the paranasal sinuses are clinically silent without apparent symptoms when they are small and, in nearly all cases, have already become large with invasion to surrounding organs at the time of the initial examination.

Diagnostic imaging is necessary for evaluating tumor location and extension, and from these imaging findings, the treatment planning regarding curability and functionality can be considered.

The staging system of sinonasal cancer is most commonly based on the American Joint Committee on Cancer (AJCC). The tumor node metastasis (TNM) classification was created in a joint effort between the AJCC and UICC (Union for International Cancer Control) committees. The staging guidelines are applicable to all forms of carcinoma, including those arising from the minor salivary glands.

As other sinonasal tumors, malignant lymphoma, mucosal malignant melanoma, and inverted papilloma occur, and these tumors have characteristic imaging features and should be differentiated from carcinomas. Those are also additionally mentioned in this chapter.

7.2 Sinonasal SCC

7.2.1 General Knowledge

The carcinogenic process for SCC occurs together with metaplasia of pseudostratified epithelium in the stratified squamous epithelium within the paranasal sinus. Chronic inflammation is deeply implicated. Previously, maxillary sinus carcinoma accounted for a high proportion of head and neck cancers, namely about 30% of all of these cancers. Recently, however, the predisposing risk factor of chronic inflammation has been decreasing with the spread of endoscopic endonasal surgery. Sinonasal tract malignancies have been found to comprise only 3.6% of upper aerodigestive tract ones [7].

SCCs are classified as keratinizing type and nonkeratinizing type. Other rare carcinomas of the sinonasal cavities include spindle cell (sarcomatoid) SCC, lymphoepithelial carcinoma, sinonasal undifferentiated carcinoma, NUT (nuclear protein in testis) carcinoma, intestinal-type adenocarcinoma, and non-intestinal-type adenocarcinoma [8]. Other cancers include carcinomas originating in the minor salivary glands (adenoid cystic carcinoma, undifferentiated carcinoma, mucoepidermoid carcinoma).

These cancers of the paranasal sinuses are clinically silent without apparent symptoms when small and, in nearly all cases, have already become large with invasion of surrounding organs at the time of the initial examination. Diagnostic imaging such as CT and MRI is necessary for evaluating tumor location and extension and for differentiation from benign tumors or inflammation. From these imaging findings, tumor staging is classified, and the treatment planning including curability and functionality can be considered, although the imaging findings of sinonasal cancer are somewhat nonspecific regardless of the histologic type.

AJCC/UICC TNM staging system is periodically updated, with the most recent eighth edition published in 2017 [9, 10]. The staging guidelines are applicable to all forms of carcinoma, including those arising from the minor salivary glands. Other nonepithelial tumors such as those of lymphoid tissue, soft tissue, bone, and cartilage (i.e., lymphoma and sarcoma) are not included [11]. Among other enormous variety of tumors in the sinonasal cavities, malignant lymphoma, mucosal malignant melanoma, and inverted papilloma are not relatively rare as nonepithelial malignancies or epithelial borderline tumor. Those tumors should be differentiated from carcinomas with CT and MRI.

7.2.2 Maxillary Sinus

When maxillary sinus cancers are small, they generally do not present apparent symptoms; thus, in nearly all cases, the tumor has already become large at the time of the initial examination (Figs. 7.1, 7.2 and 7.3). Of 650 patients with maxillary sinus cancer extracted from the Surveillance, Epidemiology, and End Results database for the time period 1988 to 1998, 77.5% of patients presented with advanced (T3/T4) disease [12]. The specific site of origin of maxillary sinus carcinomas is thought to have prognostic significance. Maxillary sinus cancers spread to all directions with bony destruction. Posteriorly, the carcinoma tends to spread to the masticator space, or else into the cranium in the superior direction, resulting in advanced stage.

Ohngren divided the maxillary antrum into posterosuperior and anteroinferior segments, drawing a line on a lateral view of the face from the medial canthus of the eye to the angle of the mandible (Ohngren's line). It separates the posterosuperior and anteroinferior parts. The superior part includes the posterior half of the posterior and superior bone walls. Other bony parts are included in the inferior portion. SCC of the anteroinferior part is thought to have a relatively better prognosis. The staging system of maxillary sinus neoplasm historically involved the use of Ohngren's line [6].

Lymphatic drainage from the nasal cavity and paranasal sinus occurs in two directions, anterior and posterior. The anterior mucosal and antral skin drainage is by way of

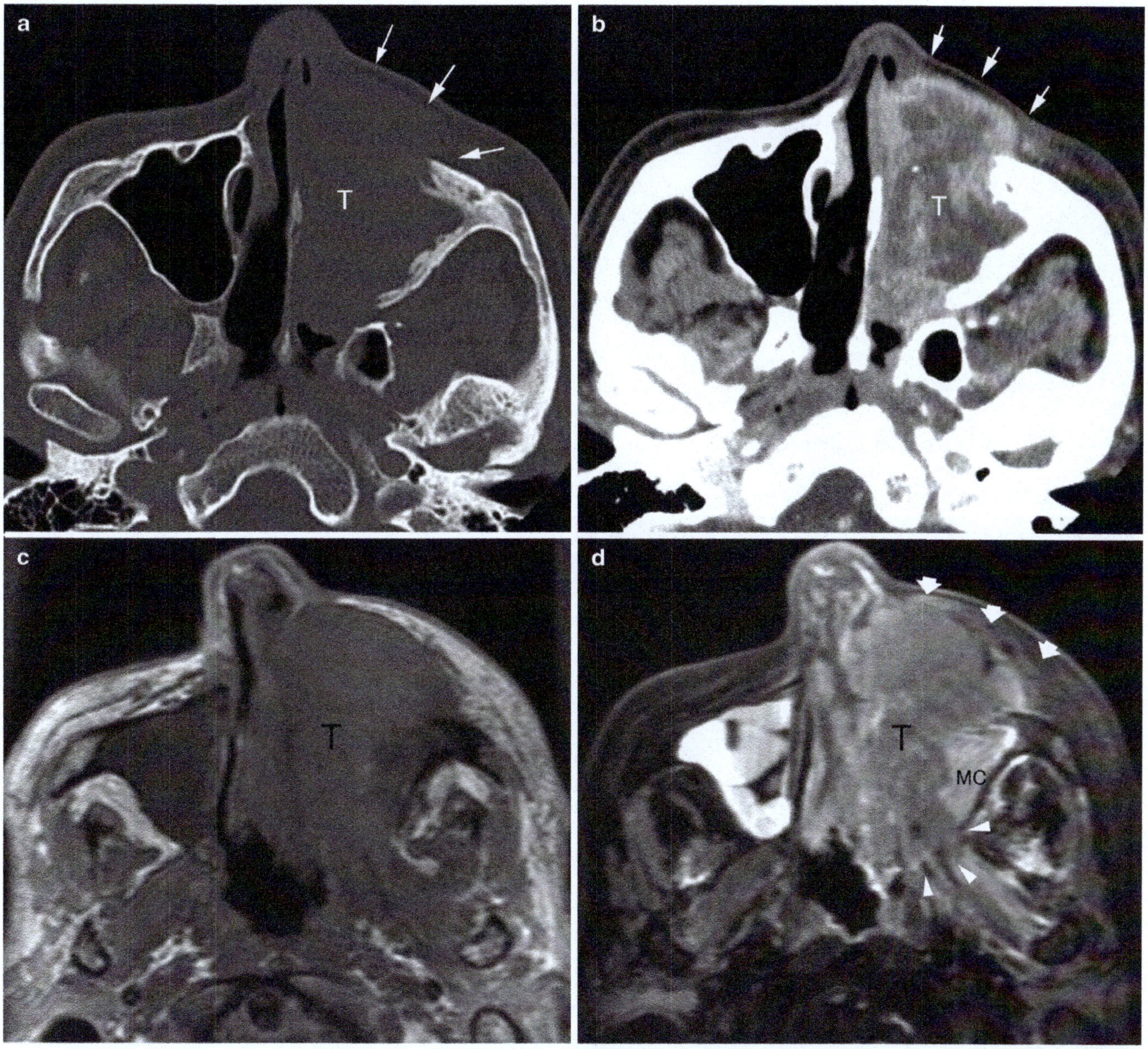

Fig. 7.1 Squamous cell carcinoma of the maxillary sinus. (**a**) Bone algorithm CT. (**b**) Enhanced CT. (**c**) Axial T1-weighted image. (**d**) Axial T2-weighted image. (**e**) Axial Gd-enhanced T1-weighted image. (**f**) Axial Gd-enhanced T1-weighted image (cranial to **b**). (**g**) Coronal Gd-enhanced T1-weighted image. Contrast-enhanced (**a**) and bone algorithm (**b**) CT scans show an enhancing mass (T) in the left maxillary sinus massively destroying anterior bony wall (arrows). The medial wall is also destroyed. Axial T1-weighted (**c**), T2-weighted (**d**), and contrast-enhanced T1-weighted (**e**) images demonstrate a mass (T) in the left maxillary sinus. T2-weighted image allows separation of the neoplasm from trapped mucous collection (MC). Gd-enhanced T1-weighted image shows inhomogeneous enhancement of the tumor, indicating viable and necrotic (*) components. Also, contrast-enhanced T1-weighted (**e**) image reveals invasion to the premaxillary fat (thick arrows). Posteriorly, tumor invades pterygopalatine fossa and pterygoid palate (**f**, arrowheads) with T2 hyperintensity of the pterygoid muscle bundles indicating secondary denervation (**d**). Gd-enhanced T1-weighted coronal image shows perineural spread of maxillary nerve (V2) and cavernous sinus (**g**, open arrows). The patient has squamous cell carcinoma. *T* tumor, *MC* mucous collection. *: necrotic component

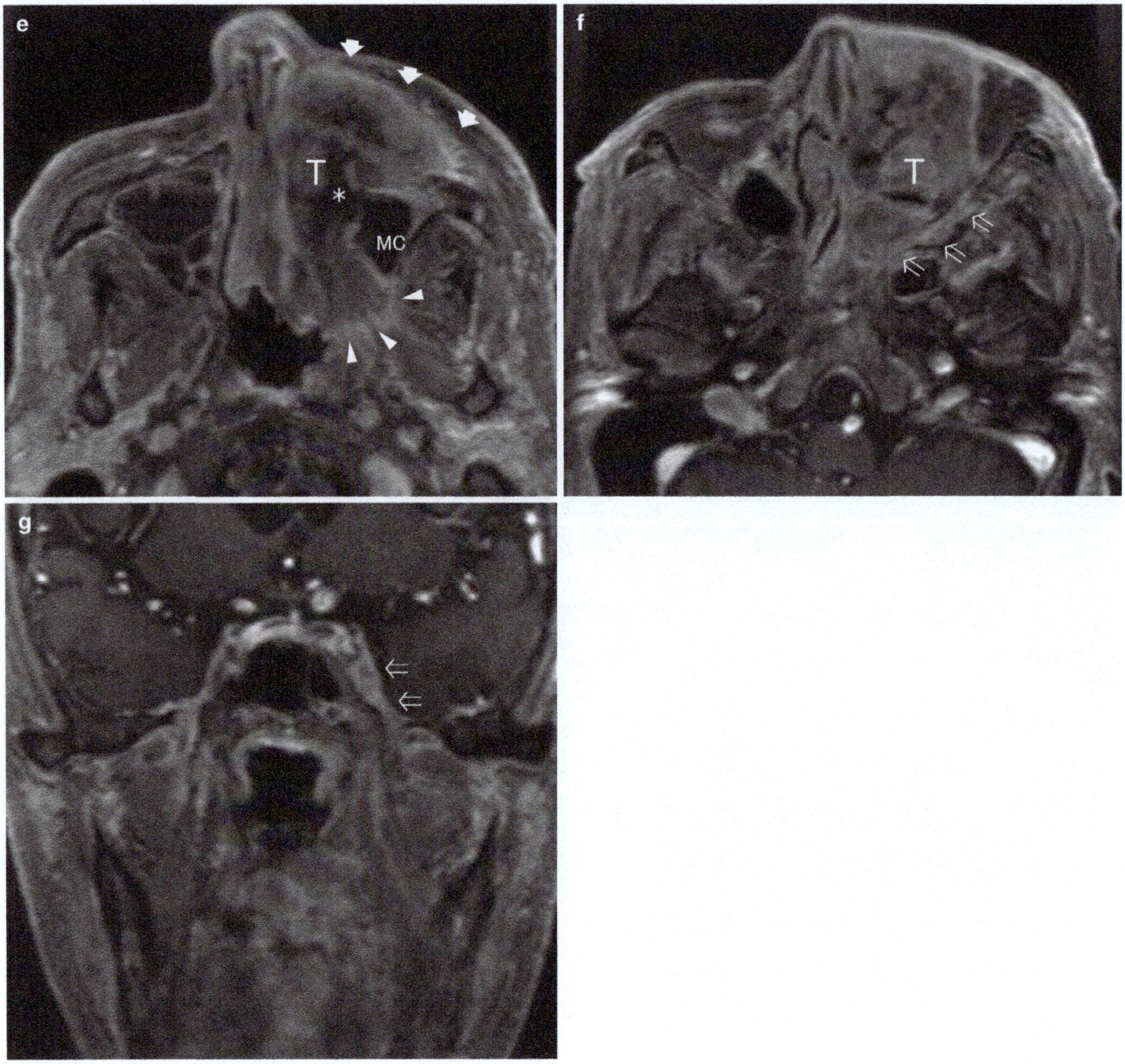

Fig. 7.1 (continued)

lymphatic channels traveling to the facial, parotid, or submandibular nodes (level I) and then to the superior internal jugular chain, primarily level II. The posterior lymphatics course posteriorly to a plexus anterior to the torus tubarius, posterior to the retropharyngeal nodes, and inferior to the superior internal jugular chain (level II).

The retropharyngeal nodes are frequently obliterated by repeated childhood infections, and so sinonasal malignancies often metastasize to the secondary nodes in levels I and II [6].

On AJCC/UICC TNM staging, T definitions of maxillary sinus tumor are as follows: T0, NO evidence of primary tumor; Tis, carcinoma in situ; T1, tumor limited to the mucosa with no erosion or destruction of bone; T2, tumor causing bone erosion or destruction, including extension into the hard palate and/or middle nasal meatus, except extension to the posterior wall of the maxillary sinus and pterygoid plates; T3, tumor invades any of the following: bone of posterior wall of maxillary sinus, subcutaneous tissues, floor, or medial wall of orbit, pterygoid fossa or ethmoid sinuses; T4a, tumor invades any of the following: anterior orbital contents, skin of cheek, pterygoid plates, infratemporal fossa, cribriform plate, sphenoid, or frontal sinuses; and T4b, tumor invades any of the following: orbital apex, dura, brain,

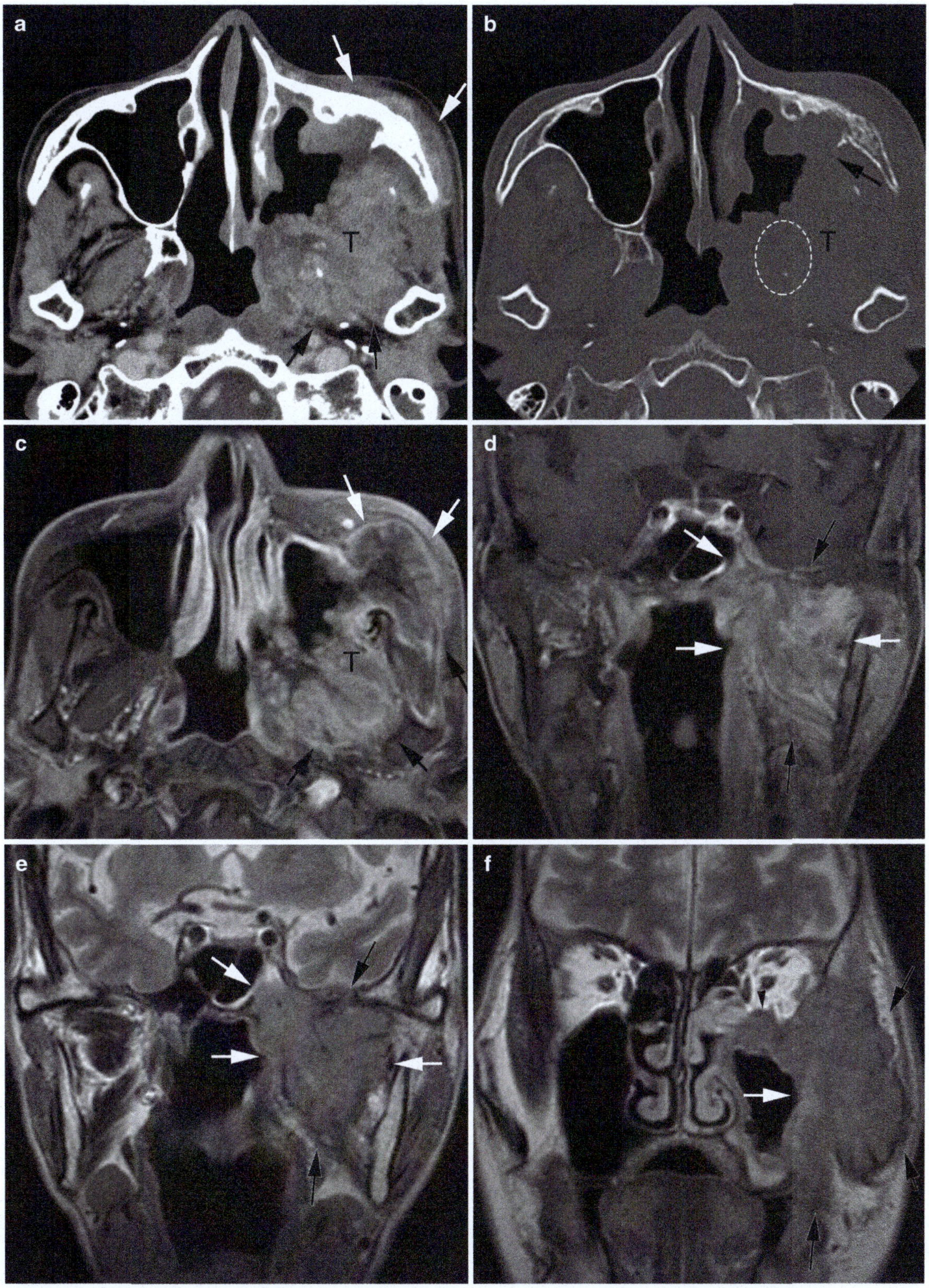

Fig. 7.2 Squamous cell carcinoma of the maxillary sinus. (**a**) Enhanced CT. (**b**) Bone algorithm CT. (**c**) Axial Gd-enhanced T1-weighted image. (**d**) Coronal Gd-enhanced T1-weighted image. (**e**) Coronal T2-weighted image. (**f**) Coronal T2-weighted image (anterior to **e**). Axial CT scans (**a** and **b**) show a mass (T) in the left maxillary sinus massively invading the masticator space with destruction of posterior and lateral walls (arrows). The pterygoid palate is also destroyed (dotted circle). Axial (**c**) and coronal (**d**) Gd-enhanced T1-weighted and T2-weighted (**e**) images show a large mass occupying the lateral and medial pterygoid muscles which originate from the left maxillary sinus. The mass invades the pterygoid plate and sphenoid bone. Anteriorly, the mass extends to the upper wall and invades the orbit on T2-weighted image (**f**, arrowhead). The patient has squamous cell carcinoma. *T* tumor

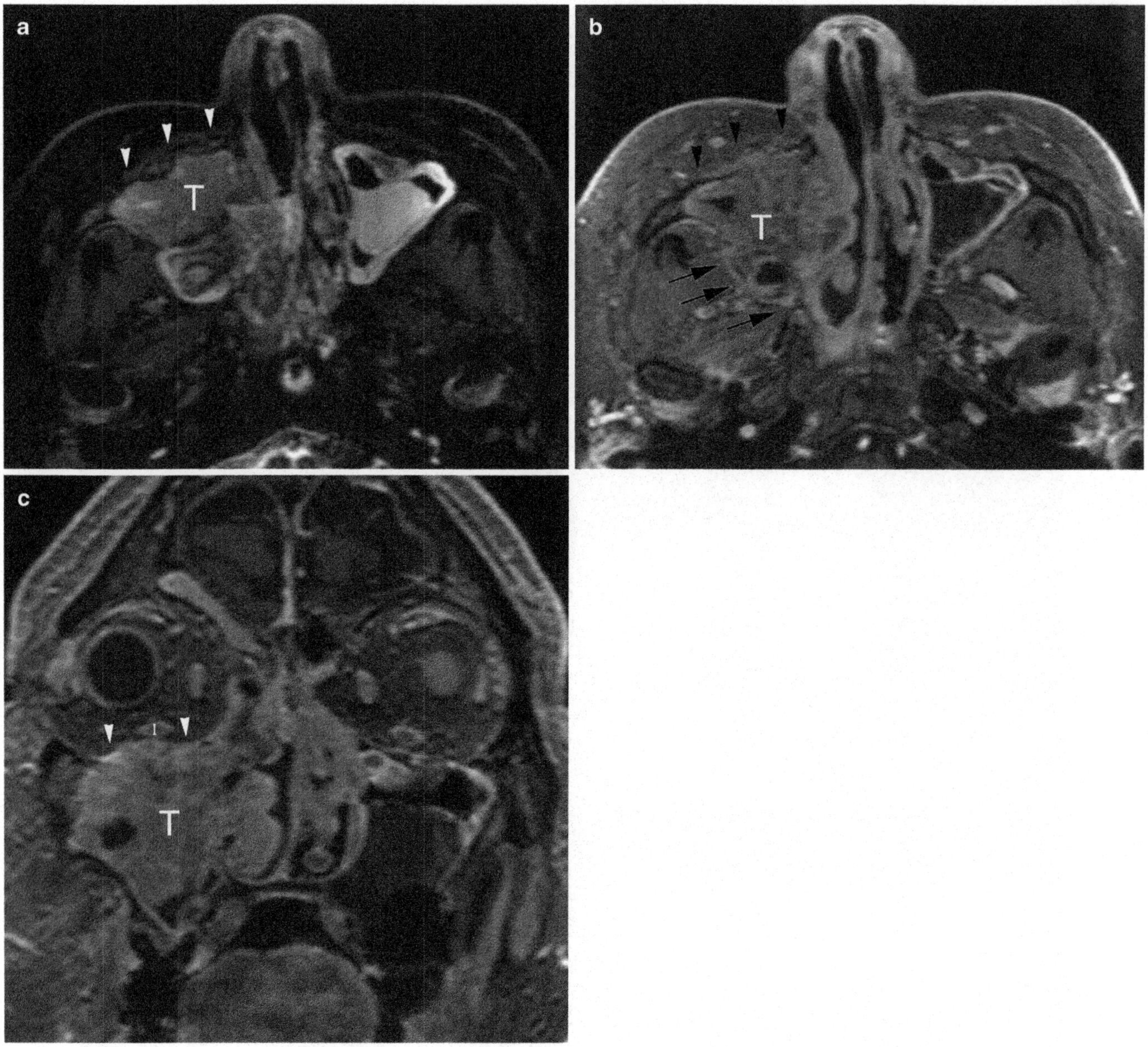

Fig. 7.3 Squamous cell carcinoma of the maxillary sinus. (**a**) Axial T2-weighted image. (**b**) Axial Gd-enhanced T1-weighted image. (**c**) Coronal Gd-enhanced T1-weighted image. Axial T2-weighted (**a**) and postcontrast T1-weighted (**b**) images demonstrate a solid mass (T) that nearly fills the right maxillary sinus, with slight invasion to anterior subcutaneous fat (arrowheads). The axial contrast-enhanced T1-weighted image reveals inhomogeneous enhancement of the tumor and posterior invasion of the pterygopalatine fossa extension to posterior alveolar nerve (arrows). Coronal postcontrast T1-weighted image (**c**) demonstrates tumor invasion of the orbital floor and medial wall (arrowheads) without invasion of the inferior rectus muscle (I). The patient has squamous cell carcinoma. *T* tumor, *I* inferior rectus muscle

middle cranial fossa, cranial nerve other than maxillary division of trigeminal nerve (V2), nasopharynx, or clivus (Fig. 7.4).

Meanwhile, in reported investigations of lymph node metastasis, at the time of diagnosis, metastasis to retropharyngeal lymph nodes (MRI evaluation: positive ≥5 mm) was seen in about 18.6% of sinonasal SCCs, namely, a higher frequency than previously recognized [13].

Cervical lymph node metastasis is seen in 23% of patients with infiltration of the posterior wall. There are reports of posterior wall infiltration in all cases of cervical lymph node metastasis, and so in cases with posterior wall infiltration, attention needs to be directed to the cervical lymph nodes, particularly the retropharyngeal lymph nodes.

N definition of regional lymph nodes is as follows: N0, No regional lymph node metastasis; N1, Metastasis in a single ipsilateral lymph node, 3 cm or less in greatest dimension without extranodal extension; N2a, Metastasis in a single ipsilateral lymph node, more than 3 cm but not more than 6 cm in greatest dimension without extranodal extension;

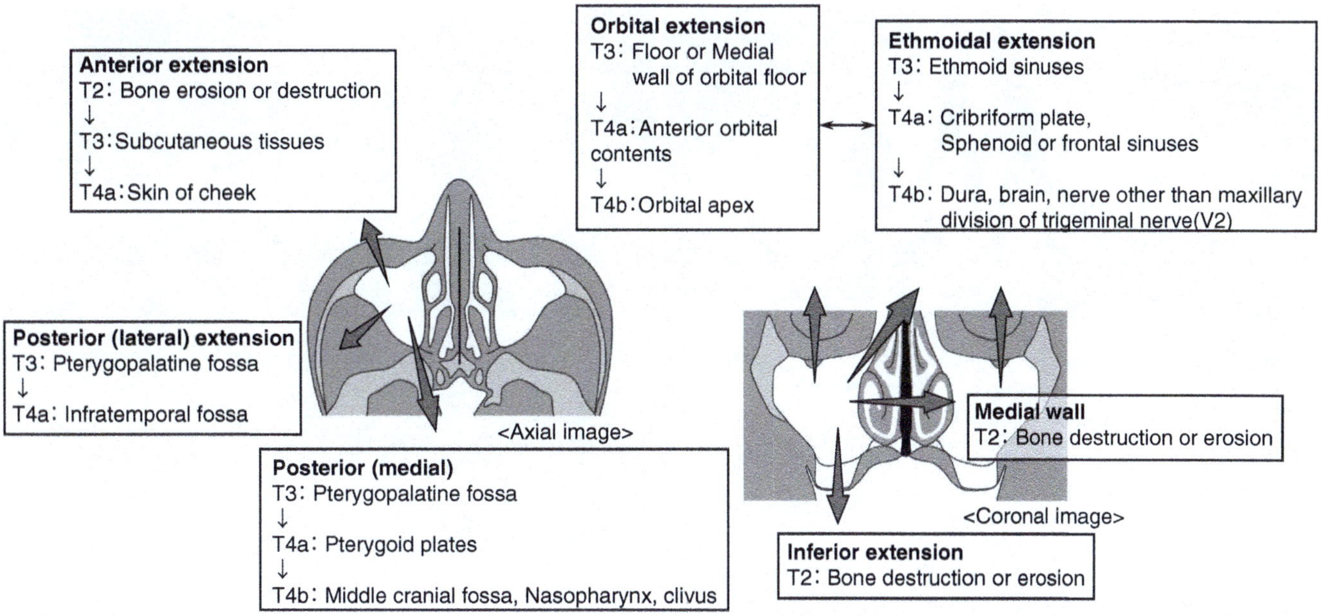

Fig. 7.4 Tumor extension and T classification. (Modified and Permission from Kuno H, Sekiya K, Kobayashi T, et al. Sinonasal malignant tumor: squamous cell carcinomas. Jpn J Diagn Imaging 2015;35:75–85)

N2b, Metastasis in multiple ipsilateral lymph nodes, none more than 6 cm in greatest dimension, without extranodal extension; N2c, Metastasis in bilateral or contralateral lymph nodes, none more than 6 cm in greatest dimension, without extranodal extension; N3a, Metastasis in a lymph node more than 6 cm in greatest dimension without extranodal extension N3b, Metastasis in a single or multiple lymph nodes with clinical extranodal extension [11]. The AJCC 8th edition introduces the use of extranodal extension (ENE) in categorizing the N category for metastatic cancer to neck nodes.

7.2.3 Nasal Cavity

Nasal cancer is the second most common malignancy in the sinonasal cavity after maxillary sinus cancer. It is most frequently seen in patients aged 60–79 years, and the male/female ratio is 3:1. SCC occurs most often (37%) (Fig. 7.5), followed by malignant melanoma, olfactory neuroblastoma, and adenoid cystic carcinoma. Nasal cavity cancer often starts to form on the outer wall of the nasal cavity, and about 50% of the cases start from the turbinate. Prognosis is more strongly related to the T stage than the site of formation.

In the TNM classification [11], nasal cavity cancers have been grouped with ethmoid sinus cancers, and T factors are classified as follows: T1, tumors restricted to one subtype of nasal cavity, or ethmoid sinus, with or without bony destruction; T2, tumors involve two subsites in a single site or extend to involve an adjacent site within the nasoethmoidal complex, with or without bony invasion; T3, tumors extend to invade the medial wall or floor of the orbit, maxillary sinus, palate, or cribriform plate; T4a, tumor invades any of the following: anterior orbital contents, skin of nose or cheek, minimal extension to anterior cranial fossa, pterygoid palate, sphenoid or frontal sinuses; and T4b, tumor invades any of the following: orbital apex, dura, brain, middle cranial fossa, cranial nerves other than V2, nasopharynx or clivus. Prognosis is strongly correlated to the T stage rather than the occurrence site.

Imaging features. On diagnostic imaging, it is essential to evaluate cancer invasion to the anterior skull base when it has advanced into the superior nasal meatus or ethmoid sinus. This is shown by osteolytic damage of the cribriform plate of the ethmoid bone and thickening of the dura mater of the anterior skull base. SCC is often accompanied by osteolytic damage.

7.2.4 Ethmoid Sinus and Frontal Sinus

Cancer of the ethmoid sinus is rare and accounts for about 10–15% of all paranasal sinus cancers. Most are SCCs (55.8–27.8%) (Fig. 7.6), but adenocarcinomas, undifferentiated carcinomas, and adenoid cystic carcinomas also occur [14]. Primary ethmoid carcinoma is often difficult to distinguish from secondary extension from other sites. Sarcomas, malignant lymphoma, and various other malignancies also occur. Among them, sinonasal intestinal-type adenocarcinoma (ITAC) was recognized in workers in the hardwood and shoe industries [15]. Workers exposed to wood dust have an extremely high risk of developing adenocarcinoma. The many mucous glands in the middle concha are related to the

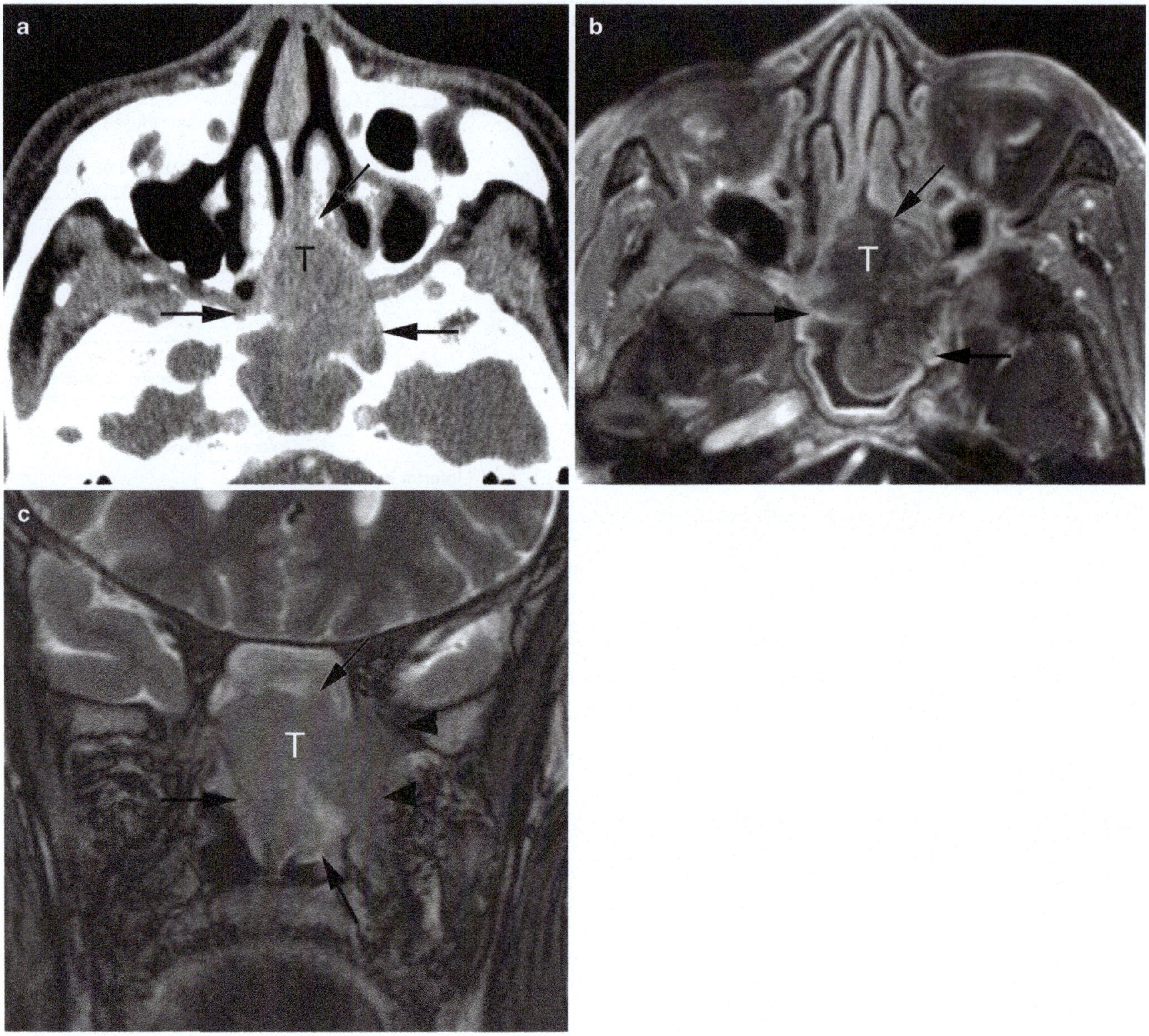

Fig. 7.5 Squamous cell carcinoma of the nasal cavity. (**a**) Enhanced CT. (**b**) Axial Gd-enhanced T1-weighted image. (**c**) Coronal T2-weighted image. CT (**a**), axial contrast-enhanced T1-weighed (**b**), and coronal T2-weighted (**c**) images demonstrate an ill-defined mass lesion (T) in the nasal cavity, extending to the nasopharynx (arrows). Trapped secretion is noted in the sphenoid sinus. Invasion of the pterygopalatine fossa and pterygoid palate and perineural spread along the V2 branch (posterior alveolar nerve) are evident (**c**, arrowheads). *T* tumor

development of adenocarcinoma, and stimulation of the mucosa from continuous, long-term inhalation of sawdust, leather dust, and particulates is thought to be a possible trigger.

Pathological assessment of ethmoid cancer by diagnostic imaging is difficult, as was mentioned also in the section on maxillary sinus cancer. The arteries that feed ethmoid sinus cancers are the sphenopalatine artery, anterior deep temporal arteries, and infraorbital artery. All are branches of the maxillary artery, making arterial infusion of anticancer agents possible. However, ethmoid sinus cancers easily infiltrate the base of the cranium, and advanced cancers are fed from the posterior and anterior ethmoid arteries, which branch from the internal carotid artery.

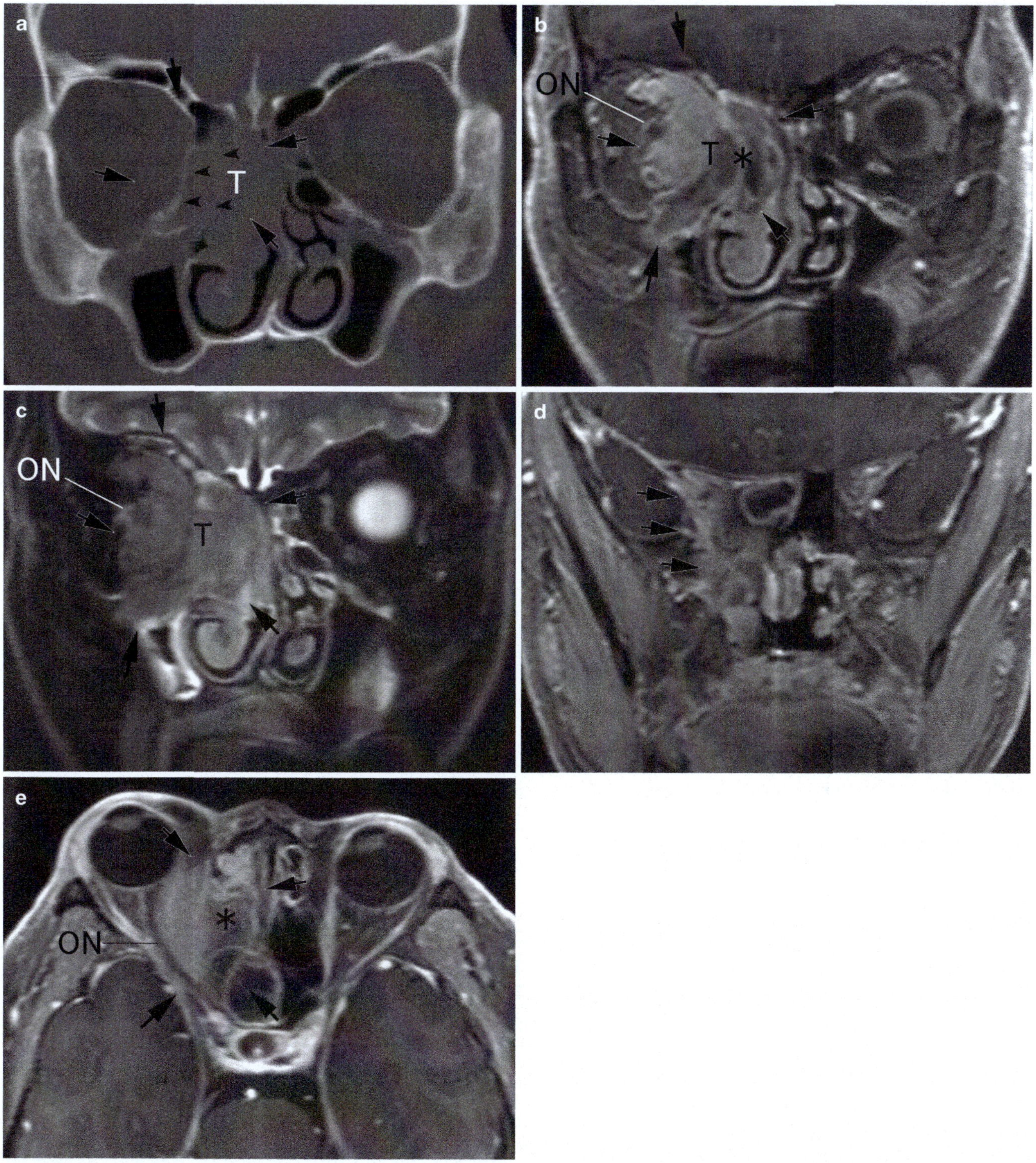

Fig. 7.6 Squamous cell carcinoma of the ethmoid sinus. (**a**) CT bone algorithm. (**b**) Coronal Gd-enhanced T1-weighted image. (**c**) Coronal fat-suppressed T2-weighted image. (**d**) Coronal Gd-enhanced T1-weighted image. (**e**) Axial Gd-enhanced T1-weighted image. A tumorous lesion (T) is found extending from the right ethmoid sinus to the orbit and destroying the lamina papyracea (arrows). The medial walls of both the infraorbital and maxillary sinuses show osteolytic changes (**a**, arrowheads). With contrast, the tumorous component in the ethmoid sinus of the tumor shows weak enhancement, thought to reflect a necrotic component (**b**, **e**, *). On the other hand, the tumor component extending into the orbit is a solid component, and the optic nerve is displaced laterally (**b**, **c**, **e**). The tumor extends to the orbital apex and inferior orbital fissure (arrowheads), but no infiltration into the skull base is evident (**d**). *T* tumor, *ON* optic nerve. *: necrotic component

Frontal sinus carcinoma is also rare. In cases with frontal sinus carcinoma, the presenting symptoms are similar to those of acute frontal sinusitis such as frontal pain and swelling; however, the frontal bone erosion is rapidly progressive.

7.2.5 Symptoms

In nearly all cases, the tumor has already become large at the time of the initial examination. Symptoms such as buccal pain, buccal protrusion, or exophthalmos occur when these carcinomas spread to the anterior, and the main effects are nasal obstruction, nasal bleeding, rhinorrhea, and extension of the anterior or superior nasal wall. Patients with antral and ethmoidal cancers have an average delay of 6 months between the onset of symptoms and the establishment of a final diagnosis. Pain secondary to malignancy usually signifies an advanced tumor stage and possible perineural tumor invasion, especially in adenoid cystic carcinoma [16].

7.2.6 Extension

Maxillary sinus cancers spread medially, superiorly, inferiorly, anteriorly, laterally, and posteriorly. Especially in squamous cell carcinoma, aggressive bony destruction can occur [6]. Posteriorly, the carcinoma tends to spread to the masticator space, or else into the cranium in the superior direction. This includes cases of direct infiltration and cases in which perineural spread occurs, especially along the second branch of trigeminal nerve (maxillary nerve). The infratemporal fossa is adjacent to the posterior wall of the maxillary sinus, and the pterygopalatine fossa is adjacent to the medial side.

Anteriorly, the tumor extends to the buccal space with destruction of the anterior bony wall, inferiorly to the alveolar region, medially to the nasal cavity, and superiorly to the orbit and ethmoid sinuses.

With regard to ethmoid sinus malignancies, tumors spread readily into the cranium due to the structure of the ethmoid ceiling. Because of this, the prognosis is poorer than with maxillary sinus cancer. Inferiorly, the tumor spreads toward the nasal cavity, while anteriorly it spreads to the frontal sinus. Laterally, it spreads to the orbit.

From the nasal septum tumor spreads to the contralateral ethmoid sinus, breaks down the cribriform plate and fovea ethmoidalis, and spreads intracranially.

7.2.7 Diagnostic Imaging

Both CT and MRI play complementary roles in the diagnosis of paranasal sinus tumors.

CT is more sensitive and accurate in assessing the osseous margins of the sinonasal cavity, osseous floor of the anterior cranial fossa, and walls of the orbit. CT may also detect early erosive or sclerotic changes of the cortical skull base. Reconstructed coronal and sagittal images are useful for these purposes. MR imaging offers soft tissue resolution, contrast, and multiplanar capabilities. Thin-section T1-weighted images, T2-weighted images, and contrast-enhanced T1-weighted images are valuable for assessment of deep extension of the mass into the orbit, skull base, and adjacent intracranial compartment and for perineural spread.

3D volume (1 mm thickness) acquisition and fat suppression techniques are also of value.

Imaging findings of maxillary sinus cancer are somewhat nonspecific regardless of the histologic type. The roles of diagnostic imaging are accurate staging and the proper assessment of locoregional invasion and extension to surrounding structures.

On CT, carcinoma is depicted as a soft tissue mass with irregular destruction of the maxillary bone. The pattern of bony changes on CT can be useful to establish the differential diagnosis for radiologists, although the bony pattern is not sufficiently specific to predict histology. Especially in SCC, aggressive bony destruction can occur (Figs. 7.1a, b and 7.2a, b). In other sarcomas, as well as lymphomas, bony destruction may occur but is less common [6]; sarcoma, malignant lymphoma, olfactory neuroblastoma, minor salivary gland tumor, plasmacytoma, inverted papilloma, and schwannoma are associated with bone remodeling. Breast cancer metastasis is an osteoblastic tumor. Calcification is rare in paranasal sinus tumors (especially SCC), but is sometimes seen with olfactory neuroblastoma and inverted papilloma. Tumoral calcifications and/or tumoral bone have been reported with diffuse bone lesions or calcification, sarcomas (osteosarcoma, chondrosarcoma, undifferentiated sarcoma) [6]. Usually, sclerotic bony change is not seen with neoplastic processes.

On MRI, the tumor shows moderate signal intensity on T2-weighted and T1-weighted images and enhancement effect with contrast material. The tumor shows a uniform signal intensity, but when it becomes larger, there is accompanying necrosis or hemorrhagic content (Figs. 7.1c–f, 7.2c–f, 7.3 and 7.7). Carcinomas also enhance with contrast. Gd contrast T1-weighted imaging is useful in addition to T2-weighted imaging. It is also useful for dividing the tumorous and non-tumorous changes. The latter of these are secondary mucinous collections caused by occlusion of the drainage pathway (Fig. 7.1d–e) [17, 18]. The forms of spread outside the paranasal sinus are direct spread and perineural spread. Adjacent spread causes bone destruction, and so the low signal intensity indicating bone disappears. Disappearance of subcutaneous fat toward the retroantral fat pad of the infratemporal fossa and the preantral fat pad of subcutaneous fat in the buccal region is seen. Fat suppression

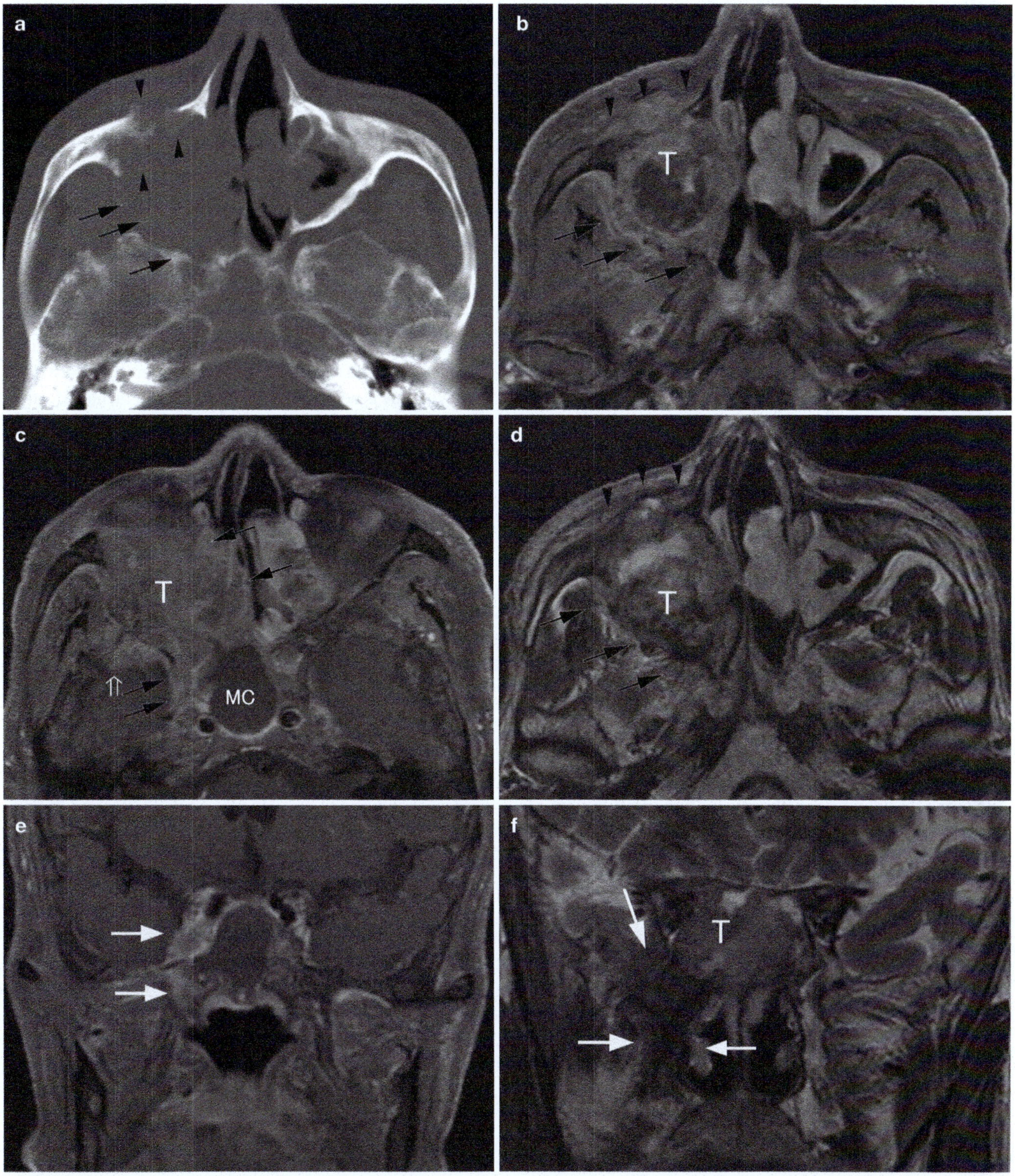

Fig. 7.7 Adenoid cystic carcinoma of the maxillary sinus. (**a**) CT bone. (**b**) Axial Gd-enhanced T1-weighted image. (**c**) Axial Gd-enhanced T1-weighted image (cranial to **b**). (**d**) Axial T2-weighted image. (**e**) Coronal Gd-enhanced T1-weighted image. (**f**) Coronal T2-weighted image. Bone algorithm CT (**a**), axial contrast-enhanced T1-weighted (**b**, **c**), and T2-weighted images (**d**) demonstrate an ill-demarcated, bulky mass lesion (T) occupying the right maxillary sinus with extension through anterior (arrowheads), medial, and posterior bony walls (arrows). Note the trapped mucous collection in the sphenoid sinus. In **d**, areas of T2-hypointensity without contrast enhancement reflect the hemorrhagic contents. In **b** and **c**, enhancement of the tumor and several areas of perineural spread are seen. There is spread along the infraorbital nerve (**a**), posterior superior alveolar nerves, main trunk of the maxillary nerve within the pterygopalatine fossa (**b**–**c**, arrows), and foramen rotundum to cavernous sinus (**d**, arrows). Dural invasion is recognized (**d**, open arrow). Coronal image shows perineural spread involving V2 (second branch of the trigeminal nerve) and cavernous sinus (**e**, arrow). Invasion of the pterygoid plate is also noted, showing diffuse hypointensity on T2-weighted image (**f**, arrows). *T* tumor, *MC* trapped mucous collection

is useful for this and to see any spread into the orbital region, and it is used together with T2-weighted imaging and contrast-enhanced T1-weighted imaging. With maxillary sinus carcinoma, it is important for the prognosis to determine whether there is any spread, especially in the cranial (orbit and ethmoid air cells, ethmoid cribriform plate) or dorsal (pterygoid plates and pterygopalatine fossa) directions.

Therefore, the carcinoma spreads to these structures when there is infiltration of the posterior wall (Fig. 7.2). When the posterior wall breaks down and the carcinoma spreads posteriorly and cranially, MRI is essential because of its superior resolution of the soft tissue. The pterygopalatine nerve, a branch of V2, runs in the pterygopalatine fossa, as well as in the infratemporal fossa, and this nerve should be checked for perineural spread (Fig. 7.1f). If the spread is superior to that, attention should be paid to any spread to V2 itself, as well as the maxillary nerve and cavernous sinus (Figs. 7.1g and 7.7c–e]. The pterygoid process of the sphenoid bone is dorsal to the pterygopalatine fossa, and infiltration of it is assessed by changes in bone marrow signal intensity (Fig. 7.7f). The pterygoid process has masticatory muscle attachments, and infiltration to it causes signal intensity changes in the medial and lateral pterygoid muscles (Fig. 7.1d). The mandibular nerve runs between these muscles and needs to be examined to determine whether there is perineural spread.

Imaging findings of perineural spread include nerve thickening, widening of the neural foramen, loss of the fat surrounding the nerve, and abnormal perineural contrast enhancement. Tumors of the nasal and paranasal sinus region often occur at the maxillary nerve V2 of the trigeminal nerve, but they are also seen at mandibular nerve V3 and ophthalmic nerve V1, which are pathways for tumor infiltration into the cranium. From V3, there are also cases of spread to the auriculotemporal nerve via a transportation route.

Since there are few lymph channels in the paranasal sinuses, lymph node or distant metastasis is uncommon. Thus, the factor that most determines the prognosis is the T factor, and local control is important for the prognosis. With T1 and T2, lymph node metastasis is almost never seen, while with T3, metastasis is seen in about 14% of cases and with T4 in about 25% of cases [19]. Nodal metastases occur in progressive cases and are associated with tumor extension to the skin, buccal sulcus, or pterygoid musculature, often as demonstrated on CT or MRI. Attention should be paid to whether there is enlargement of the retropharyngeal, submandibular, or jugular nodes on these images. The presence of cervical node metastasis is predictive of distant metastases.

7.2.8 Perineural Spread

Proximal perineural spread is seen in many cases, with tumor or mass infiltration along the outer membranes of neurons, but it is also seen distally. Symptoms sometimes appear several months after perineural spread is detected on imaging. Perineural spread tends to occur with adenoid cystic carcinoma, but it may also occur with squamous cell carcinoma. Perineural spread also occurs with malignant lymphoma, malignant melanoma, IgG4-related disease, and invasive fungal sinusitis.

7.2.9 Treatment

Recommended treatments for locally advanced maxillary cancer in the Practice Guidelines in Oncology dv.1.2016 of the National Comprehensive Cancer Network (NCCN) are surgical resection followed by postoperative radiotherapy (RT; T3 and T4a) or chemoradiation therapy (T4b) [20]. However, this is accompanied by changes in facial deformity and dysfunction, such as dysarthria or dysphagia. To overcome such problems, highly selective arterial infusion therapy is also indicated. Radiotherapy and concomitant intra-arterial cisplatin (RADPLAT), combining highly selective arterial infusion of large doses of cisplatin simultaneously with radiotherapy, is becoming increasingly resorted to [21, 22] for T3, T4a, and T4b patients and reported to achieve a favorable survival rate. With RADPLAT, the 5-year local progression-free survival rate was 78.4% for all patients (T3, T4a, T4b), 69.0% for patients with T4b disease, and 83.2% for patients with <T4b disease. The 5-year overall survival rate was 69.3% for all patients, 61.1% for patients with T4b disease, and 71.1% for patients with <T4b disease [23]. Another report described 5-year progression-free survival and overall survival rates of patients with T3, T4a, or T4b disease as being 72.2%, 46.6%, and 33.3% and 83.3%, 51.6%, and 33.3%, respectively [20].

Regarding ethmoid cancers, transcranial en bloc resection has become possible in recent years, making local control achievable in an increasing number of patients. Surgeries indicated for ethmoid sinus cancer are surgery in the anterior base of the cranium in cases in which the carcinoma touches the ethmoid ceiling and transfacial resection of the tumor when it is not. Surgery is indicated for the anterior base of the cranium when there is no infiltration of the cerebral parenchyma superiorly, there is infiltration to the orbital periosteum on the unaffected side laterally, and there is no infiltration to the cavernous sinus posteriorly. The dura mater is a powerful barrier to tumor infiltration, and so radical resection is possible if the dura mater is resected in one piece together with the tumor. If radical resection is possible, postoperative radiation is performed after the resection. If radical resection is not possible, combined modality therapy with chemotherapy, including selective arterial infusion chemotherapy, and radiotherapy is performed. For glandular carcinomas other than SCCs, combined modality therapy is said to be a useful therapeutic strategy.

7.3 Other Tumors: Non-SCCs and Nonepithelial Tumors

7.3.1 Adenoid Cystic Carcinoma

This is one type of cancer originating in the small salivary glands and is the most common of the small salivary gland carcinomas that occur in the nasal cavity and paranasal sinuses. Other cancers originating in the small salivary glands are mucoepidermoid carcinoma, unclassified carcinoma, acinar cell carcinoma, and malignant pleomorphic adenoma. In the sinonasal region, the age of onset is most commonly from the 30s through the 60s, but these carcinomas can occur at any age. In order of frequency, they develop in the maxillary sinus (47%), nasal cavity (32%), and ethmoid sinus (7%). Of the primary sinonasal lesions, 47% arise in the maxillary sinuses, 32% involve the nasal fossae, 7% reside in the ethmoidal sinuses, 3% occur in the sphenoidal sinuses, and 2% are found in the frontal sinuses [6].

Pathologically, adenoid cystic carcinomas have variable patterns (cribriform or tubular). They have a relatively high incidence of perineural spread including skip lesions along nerves, with secondary extension into the orbit and intracranial compartment.

Symptoms persist for 5 years on average, including symptoms attributable to the tumor itself and those related to perineural spread. Dull pain is characteristic of these tumors. In some cases, the course is long, and there have been recurrences after more than 20 years. Distant metastasis is seen in about one half of cases, occurring in the lungs, brain, lymph nodes, and bone. In this regard as well, they tend to differ from SCC. CT examinations of the chest and abdomen should be included in the routine evaluation of these patients [24].

Regarding treatment, most studies describe a combination of primary surgery followed by adjuvant radiotherapy as the recommended reference treatment [25]. Local recurrence is seen in more than one half of patients at 1-year follow-up and 75% of patients at 5 years [5]. The 5-, 10-, 15-, and 20-year actuarial survival for patients with sinonasal adenoid cystic carcinoma was 73%, 60%, 32%, and 20%, respectively [26]. Similar survival figures were reported by Wiseman et al. in patients with adenoid cystic carcinoma of the paranasal sinuses, with 5-year, 10-year, and 15-year overall survival rates of 65%, 55%, and 28%, respectively [27].

7.3.1.1 Imaging Features

On imaging, adenoid cystic carcinoma presents a bloated morphology (Fig. 7.7), and the formation of a cystic component caused by T1 shortening is characteristic. The growth pattern of maxillary sinus adenoid cystic carcinomas can be classified into an expansile type with minimal bony defects and a destructive type with extensive bony defects [28].

7.3.2 Sinonasal Undifferentiated Carcinoma

Sinonasal undifferentiated carcinoma (SNUC) is a highly malignant, aggressive neoplasm. It is of neuroendocrine origin along the spectrum of esthesioneuroblastoma.

7.3.2.1 Imaging Features

There are no characteristic imaging findings of SNUC that are usually indistinguishable from those of SCC: an aggressive soft-tissue mass (Fig. 7.8) that erodes and invades adjacent bone rather than remodeling it [6]. There is frequent involvement of adjacent structures, including orbit, skin, and skull base. Up to 30% of persons will have nodal disease on presentation [29].

7.3.3 Olfactory Neuroblastoma

Olfactory neuroblastoma is a malignant tumor of neuroendocrine origin arising from the olfactory neuroepithelium. There is no sex predilection, and it has a bimodal incidence of occurrence in the second and sixth decades of life.

The clinical staging system most frequently used is the classification proposed by Kadish et al. [30], with Hyams histological grading system. Kadish stage A tumors are limited to the nasal cavity, stage B tumors are limited to the nasal cavity and paranasal sinuses, and stage C lesions extend beyond the nasal cavity and paranasal sinuses. Morita published a revised Kadish system including a stage D indicating distant metastases [31].

7.3.3.1 Imaging Features

On imaging, a heterogeneous mass is seen to be centered high in the nasal vault near the cribriform plate. The lesion is hypointense on T1-weighted images, intermediate to hyperintense on T2-weighted images, and enhanced by contrast material. It may cross the cribriform plate with intracranial extension. It tends to assume a dumbbell-shaped form based on the anatomical features from the site of occurrence (Fig. 7.9). Peripheral cyst of the intracranial portion is a finding highly suggestive of olfactory neuroblastoma [32].

7.3.4 Mucosal Malignant Melanoma

Primary sinonasal mucosal melanoma is considered to arise from aberrant melanocytes that have migrated during embryologic development from the neural crest to the sinonasal cavity. Mucosal malignant melanoma of the head and neck is

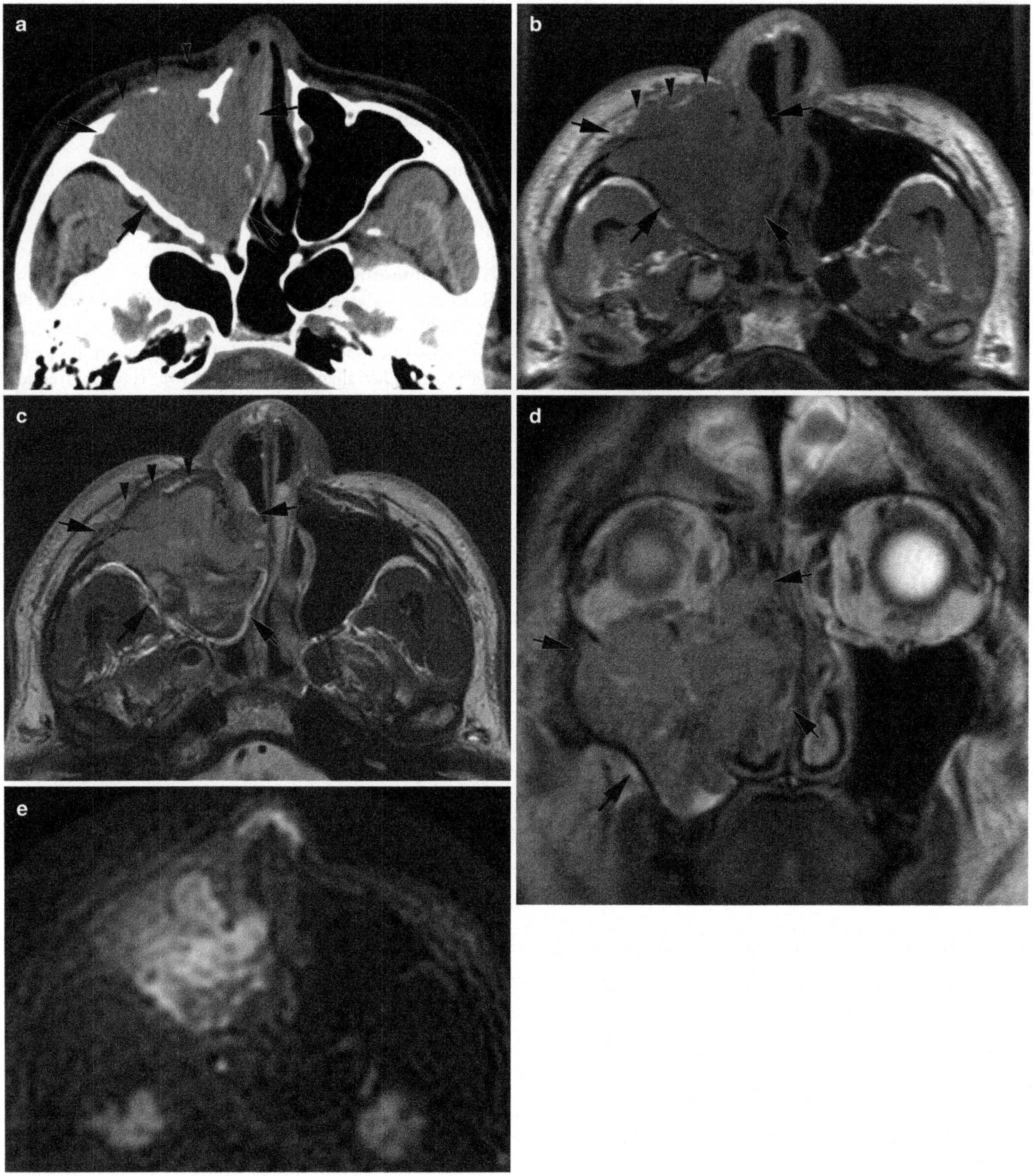

Fig. 7.8 Undifferentiated carcinoma of the maxillary sinus. (**a**) Bone CT. (**b**) Axial T1-weighted image. (**c**) Axial Gd-enhanced T1-weighted image. (**d**) Coronal T2-weighted image (Posterior to **b**). (**e**) Diffusion-weighted image. CT (**a**), T1-weighted (**b**), and contrast enhanced T1-weighted (**c**) images show a solid mass occupying the right maxillary sinus, with destruction of the anterior wall bone (arrowheads). Coronal T2-weighted image (**d**) shows an inhomogeneously hypointense, solid mass in the right maxillary sinus with invasion of the medial wall (arrows). Coronal postcontrast T1-weighted image (**c**) demonstrates tumor invasion of the orbital floor and medial wall. Diffusion-weighted image shows inhomogeneous hyperintensity of the tumor (**e**). The patient has an undifferentiated carcinoma

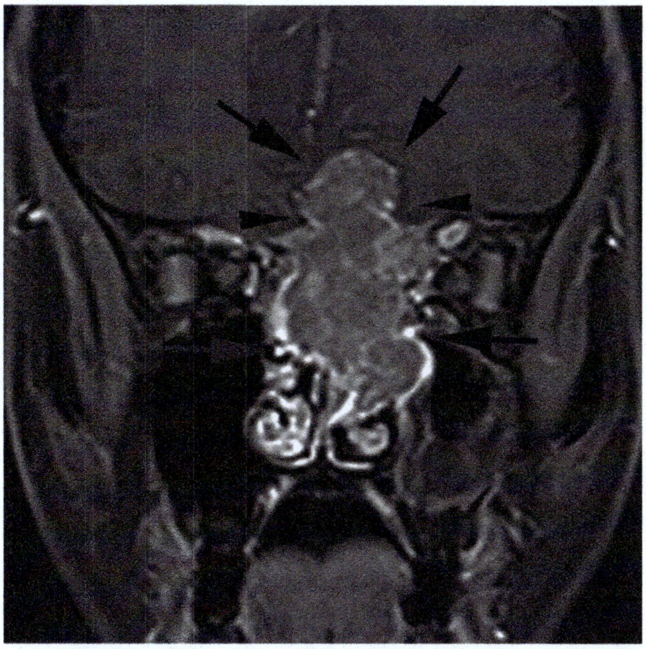

Fig. 7.9 Olfactory neuroblastoma. Coronal Gd-enhanced T1-weighted image. An enhanced tumorous lesion (arrows) is found to extend intracranially from the nasal cavity sandwiching the cribriform plate of ethmoid bone with dumbbell-shaped configuration (arrowheads)

said to account for 1–2% of all malignant melanomas in Western countries, but many more, 17.9–23%, in Japan. This is attributed to the lower frequency of occurrence in the skin in Japan than in Western countries, resulting in a relatively higher proportion of primary mucosal cancers developing in the head and neck.

Of mucosal melanomas of the head and neck, a high proportion approximately two thirds of these lesions arise in the nasal cavity and paranasal sinuses [33]. Within the sinonasal cavity, about 70% are said to be of nasal origin, followed by those originating in the maxillary sinus (80% of paranasal sinuses). Within the nasal cavity, the most common sites of melanomas are the anterior nasal septum, lateral nasal wall, and the inferior turbinates [34]. Rarely, they develop in the ethmoid sinus or sphenoid sinus. The mean age of patients is 60. There is no relationship with viruses.

Mucosal melanoma of the sinonasal cavity accounts for fewer than 5% of all sinonasal cavity tumors [35]. Symptoms are a feeling of nasal obstruction, nasal bleeding, nasal polyps, and brown nasal discharge. Nasal pain is rare.

Pathologically, tumors appear ash, brown, or black lumpy or polypoid that bleed easily, with occasional ulcer formation. At sizes of 2–3 cm or more, there is invasion to the paranasal sinuses. Microscopically, melanoma cells are large to medium size, with high nuclear to cytoplasmic ratios with basophilic nuclei and intranuclear inclusions. Melanin pigment may also be present within cells. Most sinonasal melanomas are melanotic; 10–30% are amelanotic [36]. Tumor-like hyperplasia around blood vessels is characteristic, and vessel invasion is seen. Immunologically, they are positive for S100 protein, Melan A, HMB45, tyrosinase, and vimentin, which are useful in making the definitive diagnosis.

Seventy to eighty percent of mucosal melanomas of the sinonasal cavity are localized, and there is enlargement of regional lymph nodes in 10–20% of cases. As many as 40% present with cervical nodal metastases.

The TNM staging of mucosal malignant melanoma of the head and neck is as follows: T3, tumors limited to the mucosa and immediately underlying soft tissue, regardless of thickness or greatest dimension; T4, moderately advanced or very advanced; T4a, moderately advanced disease tumor involving deep soft tissue, cartilage, bone, or overlying skin; and T4b, very advanced disease tumor involving the brain, dura, skull base, lower cranial nerves (IX, X, XI, XII), masticator space, carotid artery, prevertebral space, or mediastinal structures [33].

Treatment is surgery, pre- or postoperative radiation therapy, and chemotherapy. The 5-year local control rate for mucosal malignant melanomas of the head and neck is 46–71%, and the 5-year crude survival rate is about 50%.

Hematogenous metastases occur in the lungs, brain, liver, and skin. Neurotrophic spread is not uncommon.

7.3.4.1 Diagnostic Imaging

With malignant melanoma, a lumpy mass is seen in the nasal cavity. As the tumor grows, it tends to remodel bone, although elements of frank bone erosion may also be present. Because of their rich vascular network, melanomas enhance well on contrast-enhanced CT and MR scans, and their MR imaging appearance is usually that of a homogeneous mass of intermediate signal intensity on all imaging sequences. On MR images, in pigmented tumors with a high melanin content, high signal intensity is seen on T1-weighted images, and areas with low signal intensity are seen on T2-weighted images (Fig. 7.10). These signal changes correspond to the intratumoral bleeding that is often seen with these tumors [37]. Melanin is thought to be reflected more by the high signal intensity on T1-weighted images than the low signal intensity on T2-weighted images [36]. As mentioned earlier, about 30% of these tumors are amelanotic, and heterogeneous, with moderate-intensity signals seen on both T1-weighted and T2-weighted images. This makes differentiation from other tumors somewhat difficult. With both, these tumors show a rich vasculature, and strong enhancement after contrast is added. The apparent diffusion coefficient (ADC) of diffusion-weighted images is reported to be useful in determining prognosis.

18F-FDG/PET CT is useful in determining the focus and whether there are metastases.

Malignant melanoma is included among the small round cell tumors, and undifferentiated carcinoma, malignant

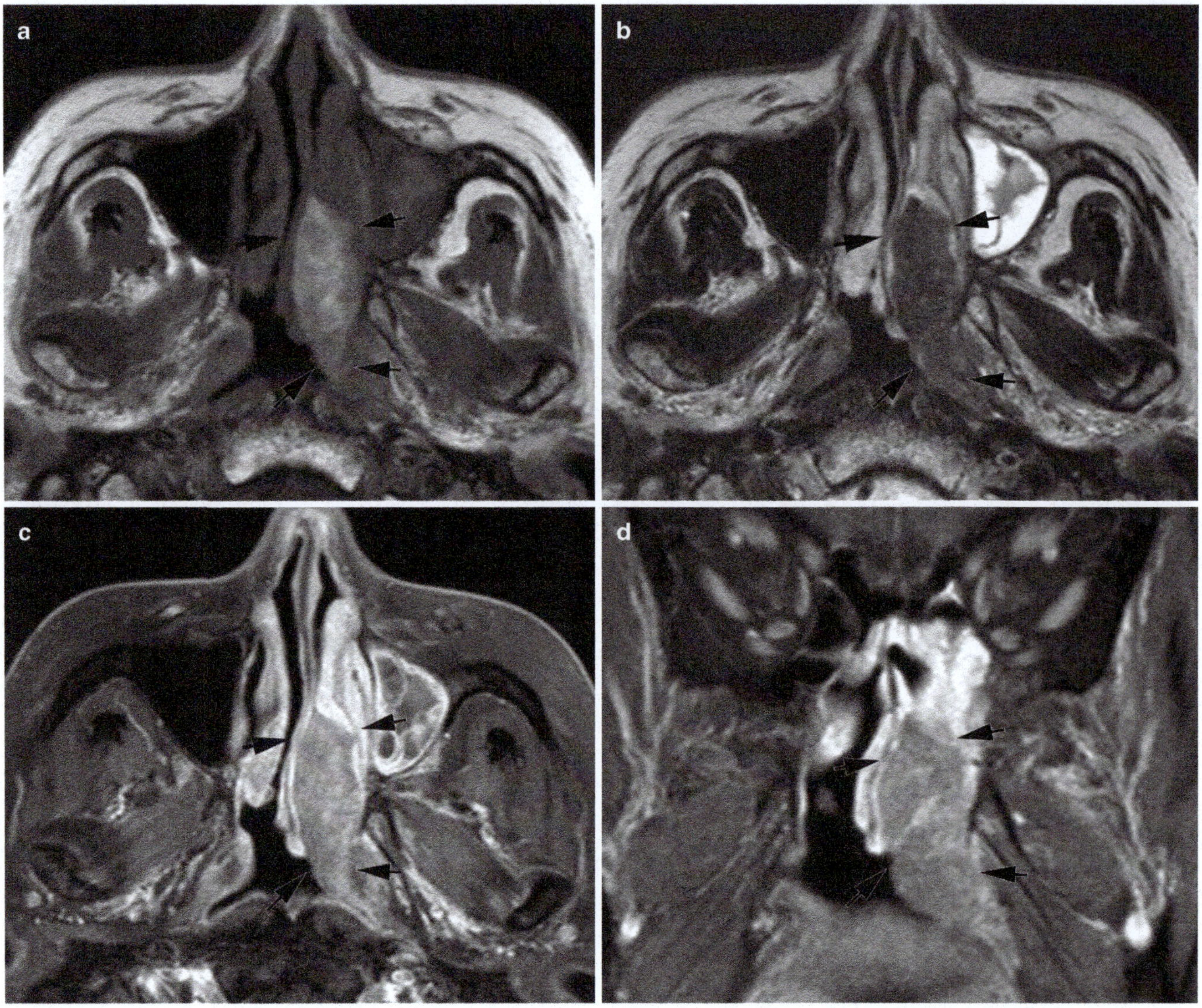

Fig. 7.10 Malignant melanoma. (**a**) Axial T1-weighted image. (**b**) Axial T2-weighted image. (**c**) Axial Gd-enhanced T1-weighted image. (**d**) Coronal Gd-enhanced T1-weighted image. Axial T1-weighted (**a**), T2-weighted (**b**), and contrast-enhanced fat-suppressed weighted (**c**) images demonstrate a polypoid mass in the left nasal cavity with a moderately high T1-weighted signal intensity and a lower T2-weighted signal intensity, consistent with melanotic melanoma (arrows). There is moderate enhancement of the tumor. This patient has a mucosal malignant melanoma

lymphoma, plasmacytoma, and olfactory neuroblastoma are considered in the differential diagnosis.

7.3.5 Non-Hodgkin's Lymphomas of the Sinonasal Cavity

Non-Hodgkin's lymphomas of the sinonasal cavity are classified as diffuse B-cell malignant lymphomas and extranodal natural killer (NK)/T-cell lymphomas (ENKTLs).

Sinonasal lymphoma accounts for 12–15% of all head and neck cancers. It is the third most common sinonasal malignancy, after squamous cell carcinoma and adenocarcinoma [38]. In the nasal cavity, nasal-type ENKTL is the most common in Asians. Diffuse large B-cell lymphoma (DLBCL) is more common from the paranasal sinuses, but may arise from the nasal cavity [38]. Other neoplasms that develop in the sinonasal cavity are Burkitt's lymphoma, follicular lymphoma, lymphoma of mucosa-associated lymphoid tissue, and peripheral T-cell lymphoma, and these are rare.

In Asia, B-cell lymphomas and NK/T or T-cell lymphomas make up 82% and 18% of primary neoplasms in the paranasal sinuses, respectively, whereas in the nasal cavity, the former make up 71% and the latter 29%.

7.3.5.1 Diffuse Large B-Cell Lymphoma

In DLBCLs, pathologically, diffuse infiltration of large- or medium-sized cells is seen. They have round nuclei or nuclei curved by the cell membrane. They fall into the category of small round cell tumors. Polyp-like or aggregated smooth-surface masses are formed, and unlike SCC, there is no accompanying ulcer or necrosis. In reported cases, in these tumors bleeding does not readily occur. The tumor cells express pan B-cell markers (CD20, CD79a). In the paranasal sinuses, they most often develop in the maxillary sinus.

The treatment is radiation therapy and/or systemic chemotherapy for localized lesions. The therapeutic strategy for diffuse large B-cell tumors of the sinonasal cavity is the same protocol as for such tumors arising in other locations. CHOP therapy and other chemotherapies are often used together with Rituximab. The prognosis is somewhat better than with NK/T-cell lymphoma, and the likelihood of cure with standard therapy can be predicted using the International Prognostic Index.

Diagnostic Imaging

The N/C ratio of tumor cells is high, and on magnetic resonance imaging (MRI), moderately uniform signal intensity is seen on T1- and T2-weighted images. It commonly shows relatively low signal intensity and contrast enhancement that are uniform on T2-weighted images, and it forms a lump-like mass, filling in the paranasal sinuses (Figs. 7.11 and 7.12). Bone remodeling or frank erosion may be present. It is accompanied by infiltration of the soft tissue on the ventral side of the maxillary sinus and thickening of the maxillary sinus mucosa, which may indicate the possibility of early-stage lymphoma [39]. Posteriorly, it also sometimes infiltrates the adipose tissue adjacent to the sinus without destruction of bone. Contrast enhancement is moderate (Figs. 7.11c and 7.12b), but in some cases, no enhancement is seen. On diffusion-weighted images, there is high signal intensity reflecting the high cell density (Figs. 7.11e and 7.12d), and the apparent diffusion coefficient is decreased (Fig. 7.12e).

In the differential diagnosis, SCC is the most common histological type of paranasal sinus cancer, and it is considered in the differential, but with DLBCL, there is little necrosis or bleeding, and relatively uniform signal intensity and density are seen on imaging.

7.3.5.2 Extranodal Natural Killer/T-Cell Lymphoma

Among ENKTLs, tumors with the primary lesion in the nasal cavity and surrounding tissue are called nasal NK/T-cell lymphomas. In addition to the sinonasal cavity, they develop in the skin, upper airway, lungs, digestive tract, testicles, soft tissue, spleen, and other organs.

Nasal NK/T-cell lymphoma is more common in East Asian countries, such as Japan, South Korea, and Taiwan, Mexico, and Central and South America than in western countries. About 75% of all are said to be the NK cell type, and the remainder are T-cell type, but clinically there are cases in which it is difficult to distinguish between the two.

It occurs most commonly in persons in their 50s, with a male-to-female ratio of 3:1. Symptoms include nasal congestion, nasal discharge, nasal bleeding, and nasal swelling.

Pathologic examination shows necrotic granuloma-like lesions covered with crust in the nasal cavity or ulcer or edema of the inferior turbinate. Perforation of the nasal septum and extensive destruction centered on the face may also occur. Histological features of the lymphoma include angiocentric and polymorphous lymphoreticular infiltrates, called polymorphic reticulosis. Clinically, the lymphoma is characterized by progressive unrelenting ulceration and necrosis of the nasal cavity and midline facial tissues [40]. There is diffuse tumor infiltration with intravascular invasiveness and often extensive necrosis that looks similar to inflammation, making diagnosis difficult. The tumor cells are positive for CD56, CD2, and CD3ε+, and more than 95% are positive for Epstein-Barr virus [41].

Treatment is with chemotherapy and radiation. With nasal NK/T-cell lymphoma, multidrug-resistant genes are expressed, and the prognosis is poor with the regimens that are normally used for malignant lymphomas. In stages I and II, the lesions are localized, and long-term survival is possible in about 40% of cases, but in stages III and IV, the prognosis is very poor. The recurrence rate is high, at above 50%.

Diagnostic Imaging

On CT, contrast enhancement is irregular, and in 40–75% of cases, there is bone destruction in the paranasal sinuses or turbinates.

On MRI (Fig. 7.13), the solid portions of tumors show signal intensity equivalent to or slightly higher than that of muscle on T1-weighted images and signal intensity that is higher than that of muscle and lower than that of nasal mucosa on T2-weighted images. Contrast enhancement is stronger than that of muscle and weaker than that of nasal mucosa. Imaging findings are nonspecific, and differentiation is difficult, but in cases in which there is diffuse infiltration in the nasal cavity, necrosis, destruction of midline structures (turbinates, nasal septum, palate, orbit), and spread to nasopharyngeal, subcutaneous, and nose and lip soft tissues, extranasal NK/T-cell lymphoma is a possibility.

In the differential diagnosis, diseases associated with destruction of the bone and cartilage of the nasal cavity are considered, including granulomatosis polyangiitis in the first place, followed by other conditions such as SCC, undifferentiated carcinoma, malignant melanoma, and olfactory neuroblastoma.

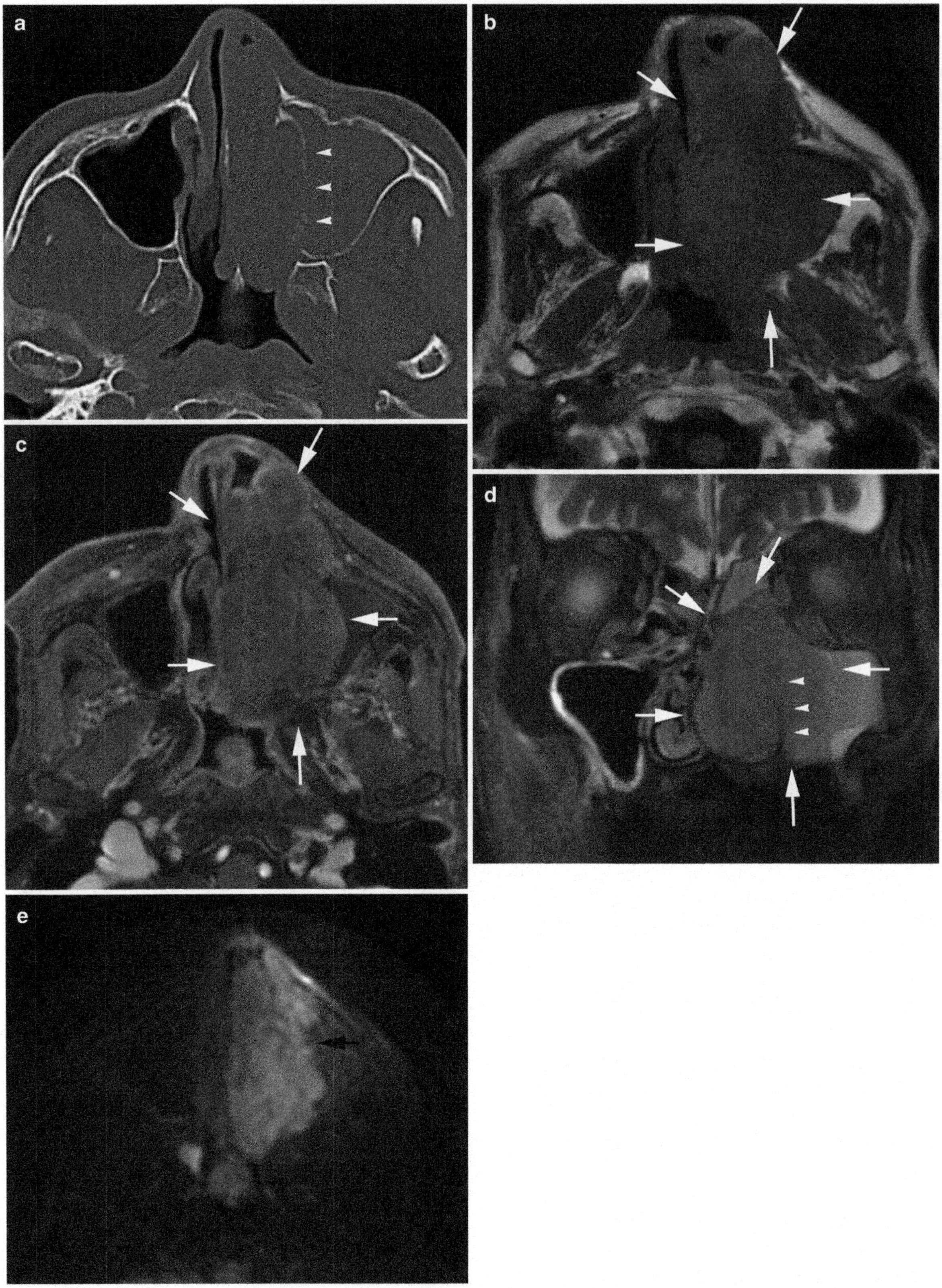

Fig. 7.11 Diffuse large B-cell lymphoma involving nasal cavity and maxillary sinus. (**a**) Bone CT. (**b**) Axial T1-weighted image. (**c**) Axial Gd-enhanced T1-weighted image. (**d**) Coronal T2-weighted image. (**e**) Diffusion-weighted image. CT (**a**), T1-weighted (**b**), contrast-enhanced T1-weighted (**c**), and T2-weighted (**d**) images demonstrate a bulky soft tissue mass in the left nasal cavity extending to the maxillary sinus with homogeneous intensity (arrows). In **a**, the mass permeative bony change is noted at the medial wall bone (arrowheads). In **b**, tumor is enhanced intermediately homogeneously, and in **c**, homogeneous enhancement is noted

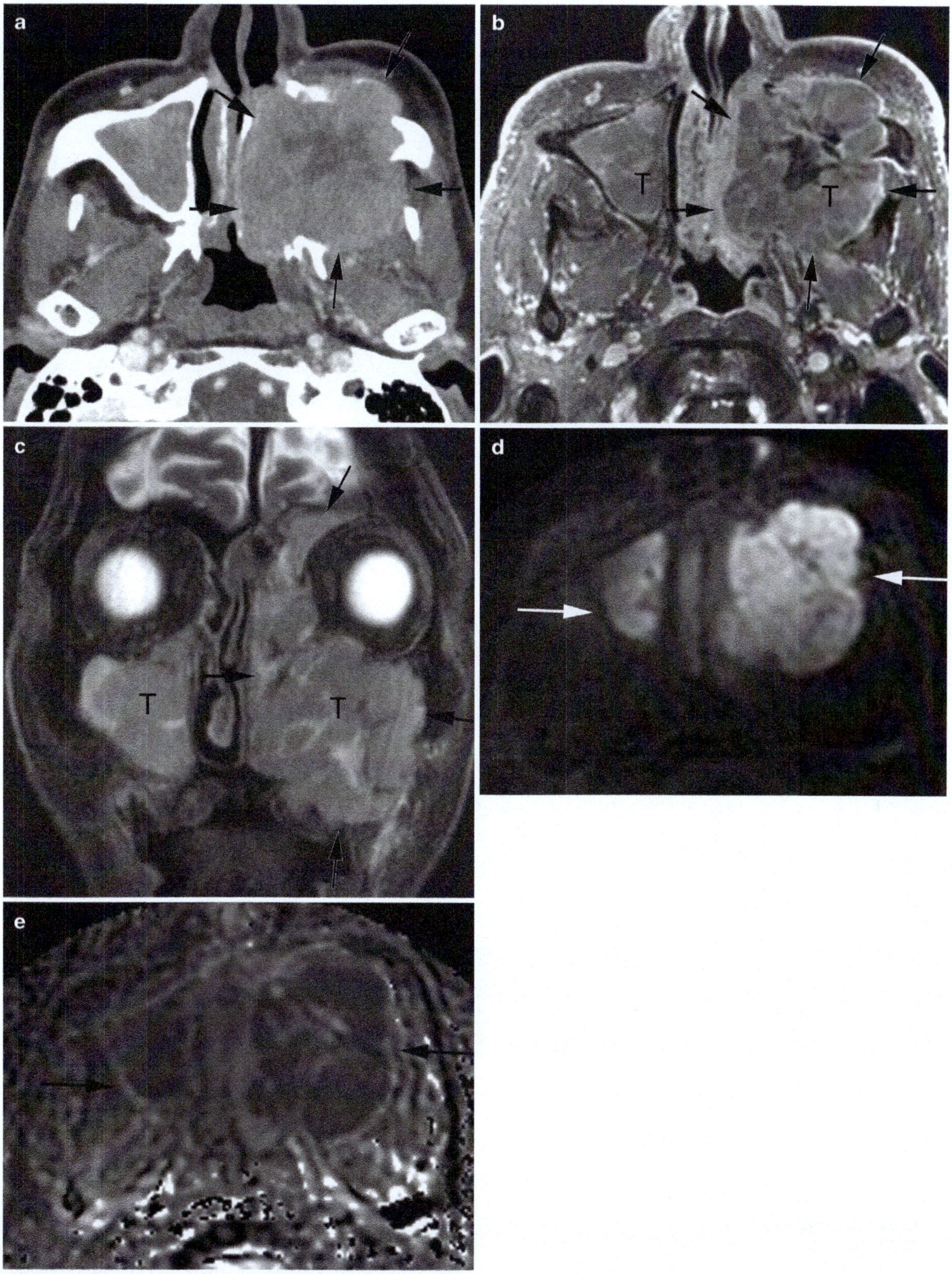

Fig. 7.12 Diffuse large B-cell lymphoma involving bilateral maxillary sinuses. (**a**) Enhanced CT. (**b**) Axial Gd-enhanced T1-weighted image. (**c**) Coronal T2-weighted image. (**d**) Diffusion-weighted image. (**e**) ADC. In the bilateral maxillary sinuses, tumorous lesions are found, being more prominent in the left maxillary sinus (arrows and T). The tumors occupy the cavity and infiltrate out of it anteriorly posteriorly, inferiorly, and medially (**a**, **b**). On T2-weighted images, the tumor is hypointense (**c**).With contrast most of the tumor was seen to be a heterogeneously moderately enhanced solid tumor, but in its central part, a non-enhanced component reflecting necrosis is found (**b**). The masses are hyperintense on diffusion-weighted image (**d**) and hypointense on ADC image (**e**)

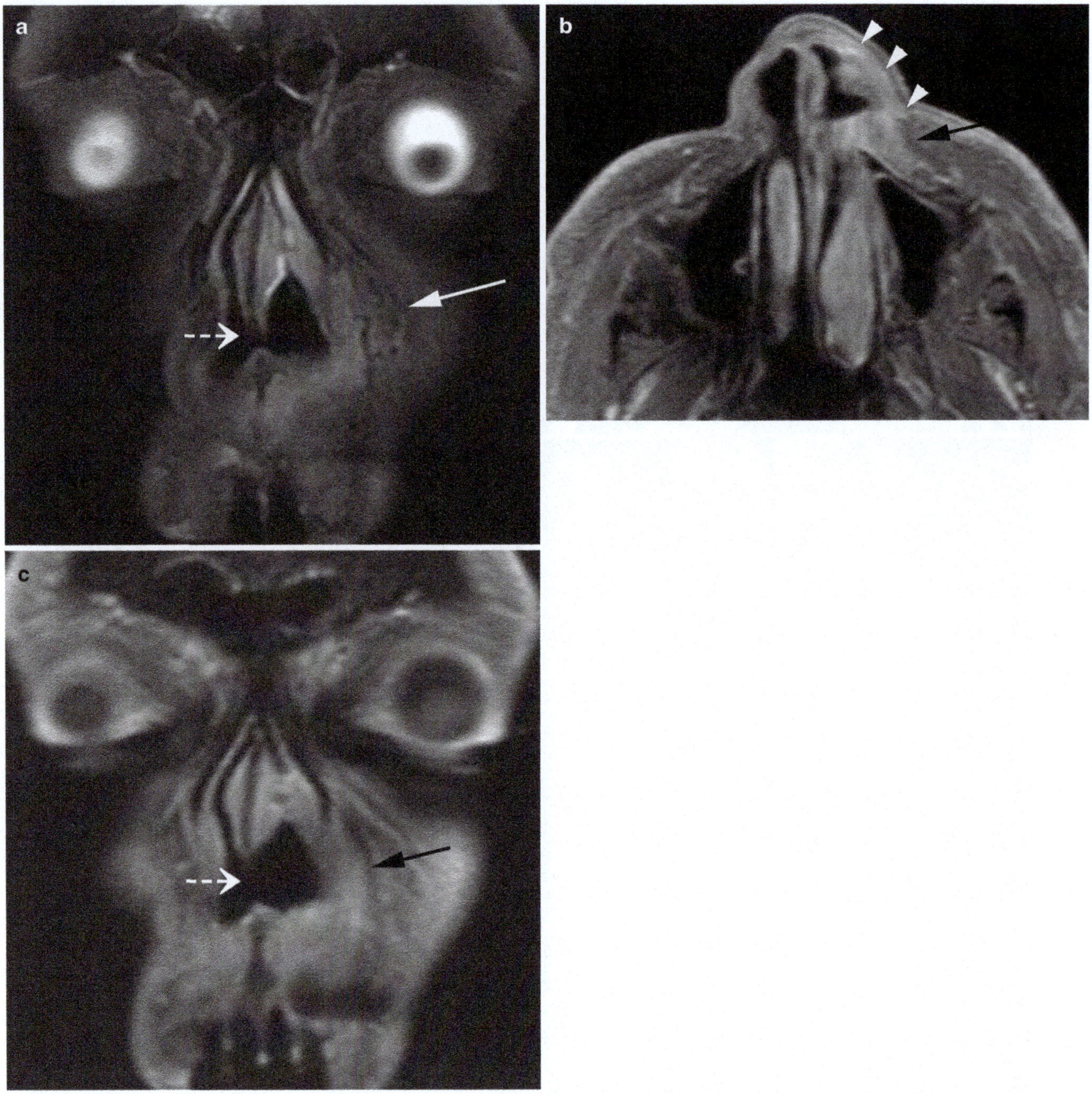

Fig. 7.13 Natural killer/T-cell lymphoma of the nasal cavity. (a) Coronal fat-suppressed T2-weighted image. (**b**) Axial Gd-enhanced T1-weighted image. (**c**) Coronal Gd-enhanced T1-weighted image. On coronal fat-suppressed T2-weighted image (**a**), infiltration of a poorly demarcated tumorous lesion from the left nasal vestibular mucosa (arrowheads) to the subcutaneous layer of the buccal region (arrow) is observed. On post-contrast T1-weighted images, the tumor is enhanced and causes nasal septum perforation (**b**, **c** dotted arrow)

7.3.6 Inverted Papilloma

Transitional cell papillomas are an intermediate group that develop from Schneiderian mucosa originating in the ectoderm, and they are characterized by squamous cell differentiation. They are relatively rare tumors, accounting for 0.5–4% of nasal tumors. They are classified into the following three types based on their development pattern. The inverted type is the most common, with a frequency of about 61%. The exophytic or fungiform type (34%) tends to occur in the nasal septum and is histologically squamous. The oncocytic type (5%) develops in the lateral wall of the nasal cavity, and there is an underlying SCC in 4–17% of cases [42].

Inverted papillomas, the most common type, occur with a frequency that is 2–5 times higher in males than in females, and the age of predilection is 40–70 years. They arise around the natural ostium of the maxillary sinus on the lateral wall and spread in the nasal cavity and maxillary sinus. In the maxillary sinus, they are often associated with chronic sinusitis. Rarely, they also arise in the frontal sinus or sphenoid sinus as solitary lesions not in the nasal cavity. For solitary sphenoid sinus lesions, there are reports of only about 60 cases in the English language literature [43]. They only rarely develop in the nasal septum, in 8% of cases.

Human papilloma virus infection is implicated in the development of these tumors, but there are also reports of Epstein-Barr virus involvement. Pathologically, they are thought to occur as a result of the release of cytokines in the tissue where the tumor develops, and inflammatory infiltration is also involved. Osteitis or neo-osteogenesis is also thought to occur [44].

Unilateral nasal obstruction is about the only subjective symptom, although nasal bleeding or discharge is also seen in some cases. Depending on the direction of the tumor progression, complaints may also include lacrimation, exophthalmos, swelling of the cheek, double vision, or headache. The duration of symptoms is relatively long, and it is not uncommon for symptoms to be felt over several months. There are also a fair number of cases in which there is a history of removal of nasal polyps from the nasal cavity and, thus, recurrence at the time the patient presents to the hospital.

The classification of Krouse et al. is commonly used in tumor staging. T1 is tumor restricted to the nasal cavity; T2 is tumor in the medial or superior wall of the maxillary sinus or in the ethmoid sinus; T3 is tumor involving the lateral, inferior, anterior, or posterior maxillary sinus and/or the ethmoid sinus and/or the frontal sinus; and T4 is tumor developing beyond the paranasal sinuses. When there is spread to the base of the skull, it is T4. Other staging systems that consider the operative procedure or recurrence have been proposed by Furuta, Citardi, and others in recent years [45].

Inverted papillomas also very rarely occur in the middle ear, and these have higher recurrence and carcinogenesis rates than those originating in the paranasal sinuses.

7.3.6.1 Diagnostic Imaging

On CT scans, unilateral masses with superficial lobular shapes are seen in the nasal cavity or the paranasal sinuses [46]. Also, as mentioned previously, osteitis and neo-osteogenesis are seen in the tissue where the tumor arises, and it is reported that hyperostosis is identified in about 90% of these tissues on CT [47].

Identification of attachments is important in surgical tumor removal. In rare cases, calcification is seen in these tumors. On MRI, convoluted cerebriform appearance on T2-weighted images or Gd contrast-enhanced T1-weighted images strongly suggests the diagnosis of inverted papilloma (Fig. 7.14) [48]. Contrast enhancement extends to the entire tumor. A columnar pattern, as if swept by a brush, is also seen in some cases [49]. Though MRI is more useful in the qualitative diagnosis, CT with the bone setting is needed to identify the abovementioned site of occurrence. There are also many cases with secondary mucus retention/sinusitis due to obstruction of the natural ostium, and in actual diagnostic imaging, it is often a struggle to determine the extent of tumor spread.

In a recent imaging report, dynamic contrast-enhanced MR imaging was said to be useful in differentiating between inverted papilloma and lobular capillary hemangioma (also called pyogenic granuloma, eruptive hemangioma, and pregnancy tumor) [50].

Inverted papillomas commonly recur (10–70%), but the recurrence rate decreases with endoscopic endonasal surgery (0–33%, mean 13.4%). Complete removal is the most effective and necessary in preventing recurrence, and efforts are made to accurately diagnose the extent of the cancer spread with preoperative endoscopy or imaging.

Associated cancers occur in 2–27% of cases. In a review of 2684 patients, the rate was 8.9–11%, of which 67.3–61% were said to be simultaneous cancers, and the remaining 32.6–39% cases subsequently developed cancer [51]. With these tumors, follow-up observation is important. Cancers inside papillomas include those that arise from the papilloma and those that simply develop within the papilloma. Associated cancers are suspected to occur with infiltration of neighboring bone, destructive changes, and extensive necrosis within the tumor on diagnostic imaging. In addition to squamous cell carcinoma, cancers of other histologic types also occur. There are also imaging reports of associated cancers that retain a convolutional pattern without central necrosis. As differential diagnosis, nasal cavity cancers, expanding hematoma, and pyogenic granuloma are considered. The cancers perforate the nasal septum and spread to the contralateral side or infiltrate subcutaneous tissues. Expanding hematomas occur near the natural ostium of the maxillary sinus. They have a low-intensity component on MRI T2-weighted images and uneven contrast enhancement. Pyogenic granulomas show high intensity with marginal hypointensity on T2-weighted images. There is marked enhancement with contrast agents.

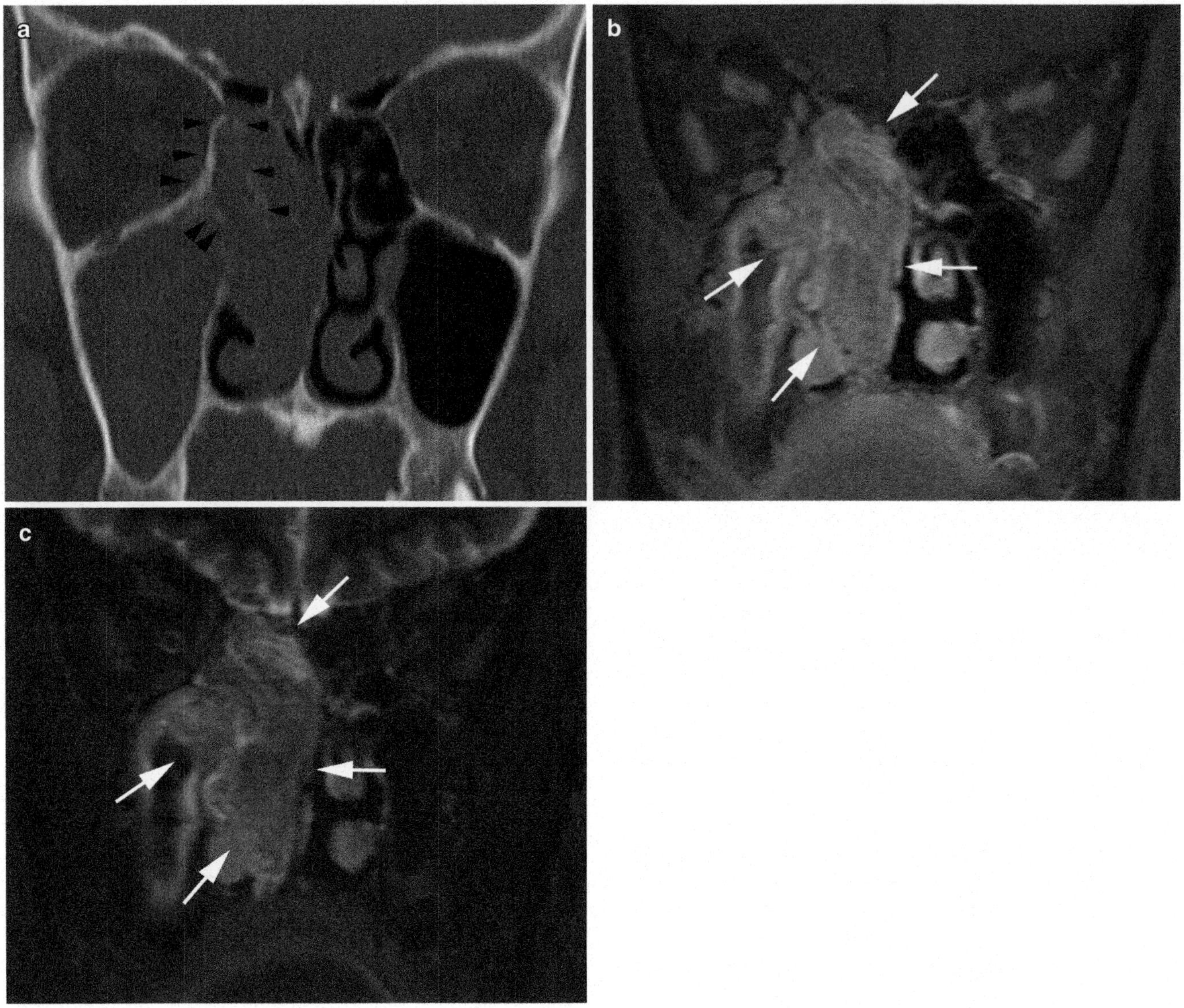

Fig. 7.14 Inverted papilloma. (**a**) Bone CT. (**b**) Coronal Gd-enhanced T1-weighted image. (**c**) Coronal T2-weighted fat-suppressed image. A tumorous lesion is found in the right nasal cavity. Gd contrast T1-weighted (**b**) and T2-weighted (**c**) images show convoluted cerebriform appearance, with striping present centered on the lamina papyracea (arrows). The nasal septum is compressed by the tumor and deviates to the left. The inferior nasal turbinate shows lateral deviation. The maxillary sinus is obstructed by the tumor, which also causes thickening of the maxillary sinus wall and mucus retention. On CT from approximately the lamina papyracea to maxillary sinus wall, sclerotic change is seen (**a**, arrowheads), suggesting papilloma attachment. No clear bone destruction is noted

Acknowledgment I would like to express my gratitude to Dr. Hiroshi Oba, Dr. Hiroya Ojiri, Dr. Masato Mochiki, and Dr. Ken Ito for their support from radiological and otolaryngological aspects.

Also, I am very grateful to Mr. Jonn Gelblum for his help with the translation and Ms. Yukiko Ishii for helping in the preparation of the manuscript.

References

1. Goldenberg D, Golz A, Fradis M, Martu D, Netzer A, Joachims HZ. Malignant tumors of the nose and paranasal sinuses: a retrospective review of 291 cases. Ear Nose Throat J. 2001;80:272–7. https://doi.org/10.1177/014556130108000417.
2. Goepfert H, Luna MA, Lindberg RD, White AK. Malignant salivary gland tumors of the paranasal sinuses and nasal cavity. Arch Otolaryngol. 1983;109:662–8. https://doi.org/10.1001/archotol.1983.00800240028005.
3. Rao VM, el-Noueam KI. Sinonasal imaging: anatomy and pathology. Radiol Clin North Am. 1998;36:921–39, vi.
4. Loevner LA, Sonners AI. Imaging of neoplasms of the paranasal sinuses. Magn Reson Imaging Clin N Am. 2002;10:467–93.
5. Barnes L, Verbin RS, Gnepp DR. Diseases of the nose, paranasal sinuses, and nasopharynx. In: Barnes L, editor. Surgical pathology of the head and neck, vol. 1. New York: Marcel Dekker; 1985. p. 403–51.
6. Som PM, Brandwein-Gensler MS, Kassel EE, Gendon EM. Tumors and tumor-like conditions of sinonasal cavities. In: Som PM, Curtin H, editors. Head and neck imaging. 5th ed. St Louis: Mosby Elsevier; 2011. p. 9878–14882.

7. Murir C, Weland L. Upper aerodigestive tract cancers. Cancer. 1995;75(Suppl):147–53.
8. El-Naggar AK, Chan JKC, Grandis JR, Takata T. In: Slootweg PJ, editor. WHO classification of head and neck tumours. 4th ed. Lyon: IARC; 2017.
9. Amin MB, Edge SB, Greene FL, et al., editors. AJCC cancer staging manual. 8th ed. Berlin: Springer; 2017.
10. Brierley J, Gospodarowicz M, Wittekind C. UICC TNM classification of malignant tumours. 8th ed. Chichester: Wiley; 2017.
11. Kraus DH, Lydiatt WM, Patel SG, O'Sullivan B, Ghossein RA, Mukherji SK, et al. Nasal cavity and paranasal sinuses. In: Amin MB, Edge SB, Greene FL, Byrd DR, Brookland RK, Washington MK, et al., editors. AJCC cancer staging manual. 8th ed. Chicago, IL: American College of Surgeons, Springer; 2017. p. 137–47.
12. Bhattacharyya N. Factors affecting survival in maxillary sinus cancer. J Oral Maxillofac Surg. 2003;61:1016–21.
13. Guan X, Wang X, Liu Y, Hu C, Zhu G. Lymph node metastasis in sinonasal squamous cell carcinoma treated with IMRT/3D-CRT. Oral Oncol. 2013;49:60–5. https://doi.org/10.1016/j.oraloncology.2012.07.009.
14. Bhattacharyya N. Factors predicting survival for cancer of the ethmoid sinus. Am J Rhinol. 2002;16:281–6.
15. Choussy O, Ferron C, Védrine PO, Toussaint B, Liétin B, Marandas P, et al. Adenocarcinoma of Ethmoid: a GETTEC retrospective multicenter study of 418 cases. Laryngoscope. 2008;118:437–43. https://doi.org/10.1097/MLG.0b013e31815b48e3.
16. Harrison D. The management of malignant tumors of the nasal sinuses. Otolaryngol Clin North Am. 1971;4:159–77.
17. Mossa-Basha M, Blitz AM. Imaging of the paranasal sinuses. Semin Roentgenol. 2013;48:14–34. https://doi.org/10.1053/j.ro.2012.09.006.
18. Maroldi R, Ravenelli M, Borghesi A, Farina D. Paranasal sinus imaging. Eur J Radiol. 2008;66:372–86. https://doi.org/10.1016/j.ejrad.2008.01.059.
19. Maeda A, Chijiwa H, Sakamoto K, Miyajima Y, Umeno H, Nakashima T. Clinical study of cervical lymph node metastasis in maxillary cancer patients. Nippon Jibiinkoka Gakkai Kaiho. 2008;111:486–9. https://doi.org/10.3950/jibiinkoka.111.486.
20. Ono T, Tanaka N, Umeno H, Chitose SI, Shin B, Aso T, et al. Treatment outcomes of locally advanced squamous cell carcinoma of the maxillary sinus treated with chemoradioselection using superselective intra-arterial cisplatin and concomitant radiation: Implications for prognostic factors. J Craniomaxillofac Surg. 2017;45:2128–34. https://doi.org/10.1016/j.jcms.2017.10.003.
21. Robbins KT. The evolving role of combined modality therapy in head and neck cancer. Arch Otolaryngol Head Neck Surg. 2000;126:265–9.
22. Rabbani A, Hinerman RW, Schmalfuss IM, Amdur RJ, Morris CG, Peters KR, et al. Radiotherapy and concomitant intraarterial cisplatin (RADPLAT) for advanced squamous cell carcinomas of the head and neck. Am J Clin Oncol. 2007;30:283–6. https://doi.org/10.1097/01.coc.0000258118.38177.74.
23. Homma A, Oridate N, Suzuki F, Taki S, Asano T, Yoshida D, et al. Superselective high-dose cisplatin infusion with concomitant radiotherapy in patients with advanced cancer of the nasal cavity and paranasal sinuses: a single institution experience. Cancer. 2009;115:4705–14. https://doi.org/10.1002/cncr.24515.
24. Loevner LA, Sonners AI. Imaging of neoplasms of the paranasal sinuses. Neuroimaging Clin N Am. 2004;14:625–46. https://doi.org/10.1016/j.nic.2004.07.005.
25. Michel G, Joubert M, Delemazure AS, Espitalier F, Durand N, Malard O. Adenoid cystic carcinoma of the paranasal sinuses: retrospective series and review of the literature. Eur Ann Otorhinolaryngol Head Neck Dis. 2013;130(5):257–62.
26. Tran L, Sidrys J, Horton D, Sadeghi A, Parker RG. Malignant salivary gland tumors of the paranasal sinuses and nasal cavity. The UCLA experience. Am J Clin Oncol. 1989;12:387–92.
27. Wiseman SM, Popat SR, Rigual NR, Hicks WL Jr, Orner JB, Wein RO, et al. Adenoid cystic carcinoma of the paranasal sinuses or nasal cavity: a 40-year review of 35 cases. Ear Nose Throat J. 2002;81:510–4, 516-7. Epub 2013 Jun 6. https://doi.org/10.1016/j.anorl.2012.09.010.
28. Kato H, Kanematsu M, Sakurai K, Mizuta K, Aoki M, Hirose Y, et al. Adenoid cystic carcinoma of the maxillary sinus: CT and MR imaging findings. Jpn J Radiol. 2013;31:744–9. https://doi.org/10.1007/s11604-013-0247-z.
29. Tanzler ED, Morris CG, Orland CA, Werning JW, Mendenhall WM. Management of sinonasal undifferentiated carcinoma. Head Neck. 2008;30:595–9. https://doi.org/10.1002/hed.20748.
30. Kadish S, Goodman M, Wang CC. Olfactory neuroblastoma. A clinical analysis of 17 cases. Cancer. 1976;37:1571–6. https://doi.org/10.1002/1097-0142(197603)37:3<1571::aid-cncr2820370347>3.0.co;2-l.
31. Morita A, Ebersold MJ, Olsen KD, Foote RL, Lewis JE, Quast LM. Esthesioneuroblastoma: prognosis and management. Neurosurgery. 1993;32:706–14; discussion 714–705. https://doi.org/10.1227/00006123-199305000-00002.
32. Som PM, Lidov M, Brandwein M, Catalano P, Biller HF. Sinonasal esthesioneuroblastoma with intracranial extension: marginal tumor cysts as a diagnostic MR finding. Am J Neuroradiol. 1994;15:1259–62.
33. Lydiatt WM, Brandwein-Weber M, Kraus DH, Mukherji SK, Ridge JA, Shah JP. Mucosal melanoma of the head and neck. In: Amin MB, Edge SB, Greene FL, Byrd DR, Brookland RK, Washington MK, et al., editors. AJCC cancer staging manual. 8th ed. Chicago, IL: American College of Surgeons, Springer; 2017. p. 163–9.
34. Barnes L, Peel RL. Head and neck pathology: a text/atlas of differential diagnosis. New York: Igaku-Shoin; 1990. p. 122–3.
35. Mihajlovic M, Vlajkovic S, Jovanovic P, Stefanovic V. Primary mucosal melanomas: a comprehensive review. Int J Clin Exp Pathol. 2012;5:739–53.
36. Yousem DM, Li C, Montone KT, Montgomery L, Loevner LA, Rao V, et al. Primary malignant melanoma of the sinonasal cavity: MR evaluation. Radiographics. 1996;16:1101–10. https://doi.org/10.1148/radiographics.16.5.8888393.
37. Kim SS, Han MH, Kim JE, Lee CH, Chung HW, Lee JS, et al. Malignant melanoma of the sinonasal cavity: explanation of magnetic resonance signal intensities with histopathologic characteristics. Am J Otolaryngol. 2000;21:366–78. https://doi.org/10.1053/ajot.2000.18865.
38. Chuang SS, Ferry JA. Hematolymphoid tumors overview. In: El-Naggar AK, JKC C, Grandis JR, Takata T, Slootweg PJ, editors. WHO classification of head and neck tumours. 4th ed. Lyon: IARC; 2017. p. 52.
39. Yasumoto M, Taura S, Shibuya H, Honda M. Primary malignant lymphoma of the maxillary sinus: CT and MRI. Neuroradiology. 2000;42:285–9. https://doi.org/10.1007/s002340050887.
40. Chuang SS, Gaulard P, Jaffe ES, Ko YH. Extranodal NK/T-cell lymphoma. In: El-Naggar AK, Chan JKC, Grandis JR, Takata T, Slootweg PJ, editors. WHO classification of head and neck tumours. 4th ed. Lyon: IARC; 2017. p. 52–5.
41. Harabuchi Y, Takahara M, Kishibe K, Moriai S, Nagato T, Ishii H. Nasal natural killer (NK)/T-cell lymphoma: clinical, histological, virological, and genetic features. Int J Clin Oncol. 2009;14:181–90. https://doi.org/10.1007/s10147-009-0882-7.
42. Barnes L. Schneiderian papillom as and nonsalivary glandular neoplasms of the head and neck. Mod Pathol. 2002;15:279–97. https://doi.org/10.1038/modpathol.3880524.
43. Cheng K, Chen H, Zhou S, Wang S, Zhong B. Isolated inverting papilloma of the sphenoid sinus: clinical presentations, imaging manifestations, and therapeutic strategies. Craniofac Surg. 2012;23:1109–14. https://doi.org/10.1097/SCS.0b013e31825434fc.

44. Bhalla RK, Wright ED. Predicting the site of attachment of sinonasal inverted papilloma. Rhinology. 2009;47:345–8. https://doi.org/10.4193/Rhin08.229.
45. Kim DY, Hong SL, Lee CH, Jin HR, Kang JM, Lee BJ, et al. Inverted papilloma of the nasal cavity and paranasal sinuses: a Korean multicenter study. Laryngoscope. 2012;122:487–94. https://doi.org/10.1002/lary.22495.
46. Petit P, Vivarrat-Perrin L, Champsaur P, Juhan V, Chagnaud C, Vidal V, et al. Radiological follow -up of inverted papilloma. Eur Radiol. 2000;10:1184–9. https://doi.org/10.1007/s003309900292.
47. Lee DK, Chung SK, Dhong HJ, Kim HY, Kim HJ, Bok KH. Focal hyperostosis on CT of sinonasal inverted papilloma as a predictor of tumor origin. Am J Neuroradiol. 2007;28:618–21.
48. Ojiri H, Ujita M, Tada S, Fukuda K. Potentially distinctive features of sinonasal inverted papilloma on MR imaging. Am J Roentgenol. 2000;175:465–8. https://doi.org/10.2214/ajr.175.2.1750465.
49. Maroldi R, Farina D, Palvarini L, Lombardi D, Tomenzoli D, Nicolai P. Magnetic resonance imaging findings of inverted papilloma: differential diagnosis with malignant sinonasal tumors. Am J Rhinol. 2004;18:305–10.
50. Yang BT, Li SP, Wang YZ, Dong JY, Wang ZC. Routine and dynamic MR imaging study of lobular capillary hemangioma of the nasal cavity with comparison to inverting papilloma. Am J Neuroradiol. 2013;34:2202–7. https://doi.org/10.3174/ajnr.A3523.
51. Lawson W, Kaufman MR, Biller HF. Treatment outcomes in the management of inverted papilloma: an analysis of 160 cases. Laryngoscope. 2003;113:1548–56. https://doi.org/10.1097/00005537-200309000-00026.

8 Diagnostic Imaging of Salivary Gland Tumors

Hiroki Kato

Abstract

Salivary gland cancers are rare malignancies that can involve any of the major and minor salivary glands. The 4th edition of the World Health Organization (WHO) classification of head and neck tumors, published in 2017, identified 20 different histological subtypes of salivary gland malignancies. There exists a considerable diagnostic difficulty owing to their diverse histological features in individual lesions and the presence of a number of types and variants, in addition to overlapping histological patterns similar to those observed in different tumor entities. However, CT and MRI can play an important role for the evaluation of tumor differentiation and tumor extension. In this chapter, clinical features, histopathology, staging, and radiological imaging of salivary gland cancers are reviewed. Subsequently, clinical, histological, and radiological features of each subtype of salivary gland cancer are specifically described.

Keywords

Salivary gland cancer · Major salivary gland · Parotid gland · Submandibular gland · Sublingual gland · Minor salivary gland · CT · MRI

8.1 Introduction

Tumors of the salivary gland account for approximately 3% of all head and neck tumors and 0.6% of all neoplasms of the human body in general. Salivary gland tumors affect both major and minor salivary glands, affecting the parotid gland in the majority (64–84%) of cases, followed by the minor salivary glands in 9–23% of cases, submandibular gland in 7–11% of cases, and sublingual gland in fewer than 1% of cases [1]. The most common site for minor salivary gland tumors is the palate, followed by the buccal mucosa and the lip. Eighty percent of the parotid gland parenchyma lies lateral to the facial nerve, in the superficial lobe; 80–90% of parotid gland neoplasms exist in this superficial lobe. The most common subtype of salivary gland tumor is the pleomorphic adenoma, which accounts for 60–70% of all parotid tumors, followed by Warthin tumor.

Salivary gland cancers are uncommon, with annual incidences ranging from 0.5 to 3 per 100,000 depending on location. The peak incidence of salivary gland cancers is observed between the fifth and seventh decades of life. The sex distribution for salivary gland cancers is equal between men and women; however, incidence at older ages is higher in men than in women. Generally speaking, in clinical practice, the smaller the salivary gland, the higher the rate of malignancy. Approximately 15–32% of parotid tumors, 41–45% of submandibular tumors, 50% of minor salivary gland tumors, and 70–90% of sublingual gland tumors are malignant [1]. Although most salivary gland cancers arise in excretory or intercalated duct reserve cells, etiological agents behind salivary gland cancers remain unclear. Genetic alterations, including allelic loss, chromosomal translocation, and the absence or addition of chromosomes, may be risk factors for these diseases. Additionally, environmental risk factors include exposure to ionizing radiation, prior radiotherapy, occupational exposure during rubber manufacture and woodworking, and employment in hairdressers and beauticians. History of previous cancers related to Epstein-Barr virus, immunosuppression, and radiation are also associated with an increased risk of salivary gland cancer. Patients who develop benign salivary gland tumors (e.g., pleomorphic adenoma) at a young age have a higher risk of developing malignant salivary gland cancers, as these tumors have the potential for malignant transformation.

The purpose of the general statement in this chapter is to review clinical features, histopathology, staging, and radiological imaging of salivary gland cancers. In addition,

H. Kato (✉)
Department of Radiology, Gifu University School of Medicine, Gifu, Japan
e-mail: hkato@gifu-u.ac.jp

H. Ojiri (ed.), *Diagnostic Imaging in Head and Neck Cancer*, https://doi.org/10.1007/978-981-15-3188-0_8

clinical, histological, and radiological features of each subtype of salivary gland cancer are specifically described.

8.2 Clinical Features

Salivary gland tumors of the parotid and submandibular glands usually present as growing masses, whereas tumors of minor salivary glands present as submucosal intraoral masses which subsequently ulcerate. Initial presentation of the tumor depends on the anatomical location and site of involvement. Salivary gland cancers generally present as painless, slow-growing masses which are indistinguishable from benign tumors. Concerning clinical features for suspected salivary gland cancers include rapid tumor growth, facial nerve palsy, palpable cervical lymph nodes, localized pain, hard consistency, and tumor fixation to overlying skin or underlying muscle. Overall detection rates for salivary gland malignancies based on these clinical features are approximately 30% [2], although only 10% of patients with parotid cancers present with facial paralysis, which is associated with poor prognosis [3]. Patients with deep lobe parotid tumors may present with distortion of the lateral pharyngeal wall on intraoral examination [3]. The occurrence of trismus may indicate infratemporal fossa involvement. Finally, skin ulceration and fistulas may also be present in advanced cancers.

8.3 Histopathology

The 4th edition of the World Health Organization (WHO) classification of head and neck tumors, published in 2017, identified 20 different histological subtypes of salivary gland malignancies (Table 8.1) [4]. This classification includes several new entities, for instance, secretory carcinomas, and modifies several carcinomas, including polymorphous adenocarcinomas, clear cell carcinomas, and intraductal carcinomas. Histological classification of salivary gland tumors is an evolving field, and the importance of tumor grading has become widely accepted, although this may be difficult even for experienced pathologists. Common histological subtypes of such cancers include mucoepidermoid carcinomas, adenoid cystic carcinomas, "adenocarcinomas, NOS (not otherwise specified)," and salivary duct carcinomas. Mucoepidermoid carcinoma is the most common cancer of the parotid gland, while adenoid cystic carcinoma is the most common in the submandibular and minor salivary glands. These cancers are typically divided into those arising from major salivary glands (commonly occurring major salivary gland cancers include acinic cell carcinoma, basal cell adenocarcinoma, salivary duct carcinoma, epithelial-myoepithelial carcinoma, and oncocytic carcinoma) and those arising from minor salivary glands (commonly occurring minor salivary gland cancers include polymorphous adenocarcinoma and clear cell carcinoma). Histological tumor grading is intended to reflect the inherent biological nature of tumors. A diverse spectrum of biological behaviors is expressed, ranging from indolent, low-grade tumors which almost mimic benign processes to aggressive, high-risk lesions with a propensity for early disseminated metastasis. Some tumors are known to be low grade (acinic cell carcinoma, polymorphous adenocarcinoma, basal cell adenocarcinoma, and epithelial-myoepithelial carcinoma), whereas others are generally high grade (salivary duct carcinoma, carcinoma ex pleomorphic adenoma, poorly differentiated carcinoma, and squamous cell carcinoma). Mucoepidermoid carcinoma, adenoid cystic carcinoma, and "adenocarcinoma, NOS" can be histologically classified into three categories: low, intermediate, and high grade.

Table 8.1 WHO classification of tumors of malignant salivary glands

Malignant tumors
Mucoepidermoid carcinoma
Adenoid cystic carcinoma
Acinic cell carcinoma
Polymorphous adenocarcinoma
Clear cell carcinoma
Basal cell adenocarcinoma
Intraductal carcinoma
Adenocarcinoma, NOS
Salivary duct carcinoma
Myoepithelial carcinoma
Epithelial-myoepithelial carcinoma
Carcinoma ex pleomorphic adenoma
Secretory carcinoma
Sebaceous adenocarcinoma
Carcinosarcoma
Poorly differentiated carcinoma
Undifferentiated carcinoma
Large cell neuroendocrine carcinoma
Small cell neuroendocrine carcinoma
Lymphoepithelial carcinoma
Squamous cell carcinoma
Oncocytic carcinoma
Sialoblastoma (*Uncertain malignant potential*)
Hematolymphoid tumors
Extranodal marginal zone lymphoma of mucosa-associated lymphoid tissue (MALT lymphoma)

8.4 Staging

The staging system for major salivary gland cancers is based on an extensive retrospective review of the existing literature worldwide; this system is important for predicting patient prognosis. Numerous factors have an impact on patient survival, including histological diagnosis, cellular differentiation (grade), site, size, the degree of fixation or local extension, facial nerve involvement, and status of regional lymph nodes, as well as distant metastases. From 2017 onward, all major salivary gland cancers are staged accord-

Table 8.2 Definitions of AJCC TNM: Definition of primary tumor (T)

T category	T criteria
TX	Primary tumor cannot be assessed
T0	No evidence of primary tumor
Tis	Carcinoma *in situ*
T1	Tumor 2 cm or smaller in greatest dimension without extraparenchymal extension[a]
T2	Tumor larger than 2 cm but not larger than 4 cm in greatest dimension without extraparenchymal extension[a]
T3	Tumor larger than 4 cm and/or tumor having extraparenchymal extension[a]
T4	Moderately advanced or very advanced disease
T4a	Moderately advanced disease Tumor invades skin, mandible, ear canal, and/or facial nerve
T4b	Very advanced disease Tumor invades skull base and/or pterygoid plates and/or encases carotid artery

[a]Extraparenchymal extension is clinical or macroscopic evidence of invasion of soft tissues. Microscopic evidence alone does not constitute extraparenchymal extension for classification purposes

Table 8.3 Definitions of AJCC TNM: Definition of regional lymph node (N)—Clinical N (cN)

N category	N criteria
NX	Regional lymph nodes cannot be assessed
N0	No regional lymph node metastasis
N1	Metastasis in a single ipsilateral lymph node, 3 cm or smaller in greatest dimension and ENE(−)
N2	Metastasis in a single ipsilateral node larger than 3 cm but not larger than 6 cm in greatest dimension and ENE(−); *or* metastases in multiple ipsilateral lymph nodes, none larger than 6 cm in greatest dimension and ENE(−); *or* in bilateral or contralateral lymph nodes, none larger than 6 cm in greatest dimension and ENE(−)
N2a	Metastasis in a single ipsilateral node larger than 3 cm but not larger than 6 cm in greatest dimension and ENE(−)
N2b	Metastases in multiple ipsilateral lymph nodes, none larger than 6 cm in greatest dimension and ENE(−)
N2c	Metastasis in bilateral or contralateral lymph nodes, none larger than 6 cm in greatest dimension and ENE(−)
N3	Metastasis in a lymph node larger than 6 cm in greatest dimension and ENE(−); *or* metastasis in any node(s) with clinically overt ENE(−)
N3a	Metastasis in a lymph node larger than 6 cm in greatest dimension and ENE(−)
N3b	Metastasis in any node(s) with clinically overt ENE(+)

Note: A designation of "U" or "L" may be used for any N category to indicate metastasis above the lower border of the cricoid (U) or below the lower border of the cricoid (L)
Similarly, clinical and pathological ENE should be recorded as ENE(−) or ENE(+)

Table 8.4 Definitions of AJCC TNM: Definition of regional lymph node (N)—Pathological N (pN)

N category	N criteria
NX	Regional lymph nodes cannot be assessed
N0	No regional lymph node metastasis
N1	Metastasis in a single ipsilateral lymph node, 3 cm or smaller in greatest dimension and ENE(−)
N2	Metastasis in a single ipsilateral lymph node, 3 cm or smaller in greatest dimension and ENE(+); *or* larger than 3 cm but not larger than 6 cm in greatest dimension and ENE(−); *or* metastases in multiple ipsilateral lymph nodes, none larger than 6 cm in greatest dimension and ENE(−); *or* in bilateral or contralateral lymph nodes, none larger than 6 cm in greatest dimension and ENE(−)
N2a	Metastasis in single ipsilateral or contralateral node 3 cm or smaller in greatest dimension and ENE(+); *or* a single ipsilateral lymph node larger than 3 cm but not larger than 6cm in greatest dimension and ENE(−)
N2b	Metastasis in multiple ipsilateral nodes, none larger than 6 cm in greatest dimension and ENE(−)
N2c	Metastasis in bilateral or contralateral lymph nodes, none larger than 6 cm in greatest dimension and ENE(−)
N3	Metastasis in a lymph node larger than 6 cm in greatest dimension and ENE(−); *or* in a single ipsilateral node larger than 3 cm in greatest dimension and ENE(+); *or* multiple ipsilateral, contralateral, or bilateral nodes any with ENE(+)
N3a	Metastasis in a lymph node larger than 6 cm in greatest dimension and ENE(−)
N3b	Metastasis in a single ipsilateral node larger than 3 cm in greatest dimension and ENE(+); *or* multiple ipsilateral, contralateral, or bilateral nodes any with ENE(+)

Note: A designation of "U" or "L" may be used for any N category to indicate metastasis above the lower border of the cricoid (U) or below the lower border of the cricoid (L)
Similarly, clinical and pathological ENE should be recorded as ENE(−) or ENE(+)

ing to the 8th Edition of the American Joint Committee on Cancer (AJCC) Cancer Staging Manual [5]. In contrast, minor salivary gland cancers are staged similarly to squamous cell carcinoma, according to sites in which they arise.

Primary tumors (T) are staged according to size, extraparenchymal extension, and direct invasion into the skin, mandible, ear canal, facial nerve, the base of the skull, pterygoid plates, and carotid artery (Table 8.2). Although histological subtype of the primary salivary gland cancer is an important prognostic factor, T stage is based on general principles, due to the relative rarity and wide histological variety of salivary gland cancers.

Regional lymph node (N) staging is dependent on size, location, and extranodal extension (ENE) of metastatic lymph nodes (Tables 8.3 and 8.4). The TNM system has been revised and has been a strong predictor of disease prognosis over the years. Currently, the new ENE parameter of metastatic lymph nodes is proving to be an important prognostic factor; thus ENE of nodal metastases is considered in the 8th Edition of the AJCC, including major salivary gland cancers.

Detection of distant metastasis is designated as M1, with the lung being the most frequently involved site of distant metastasis (Table 8.5). The overall cancer stage is derived from the combination of T (primary tumor), N (regional lymph nodes), and M (distant metastasis) scores (Table 8.6).

Table 8.5 Definitions of AJCC TNM: Definition of distant metastasis (M)

M category	M criteria
T0	No distant metastasis
T1	Distant metastasis

Table 8.6 AJCC prognostic stage groups

When T is...	And N is...	And M is...	Then the stage group is...
Tis	N0	M0	0
T1	N0	M0	I
T2	N0	M0	II
T3	N0	M0	III
T0, T1, T2, T3	N1	M0	III
T4a	N0, N1	M0	IVA
T0, T1, T2, T3, T4a	N2	M0	IVA
Any T	N3	M0	IVB
T4b	Any N	M0	IVB
Any T	Any N	M1	IVC

8.5 Radiological Imaging

A number of cross-sectional imaging modalities, including ultrasonography (US), computed tomography (CT), and magnetic resonance imaging (MRI), are employed for the evaluation of salivary gland tumors. These modalities can be used to delineate tumor locations, such as intraglandular or extraglandular positions, determine the presence in the superficial or deep lobe of the parotid gland, detect malignant features, define local extension and invasion of surrounding tissues, and detect regional nodal and distant metastases.

US is the preferred technique for the initial assessment of salivary gland tumors, due to low cost, ease of accessibility, and high sensitivity using high-resolution US, which provides excellent resolution and tissue characterization without any risk of radiation exposure. Particularly for superficial parotid and submandibular gland tumors, US is an ideal tool for initial assessment due to their relatively superficial locations. It can be used to distinguish focal from diffuse disease, assess adjacent vascular structures and vascularity, distinguish between solid and cystic tumors, guide fine needle aspiration biopsy, and perform nodal staging. However, US allows only limited visualization of the deep parotid or deep extensions, which are obscured by the mandible, and minor salivary glands are also not accessible using the conventional US. In addition, the utility of US depends on the skill and experience of the operator, which are both affected by the availability of training and the performance of ultrasound devices.

Particularly for tumors located in the deep parotid or minor salivary glands, CT and MRI are the first-choice imaging modalities and are optimal for delineating complete tumor extent and regional lymphadenopathy. CT is the method of choice for patients with suspected inflammatory diseases associated with sialolithiasis, or in patients for whom MRI is contraindicated. Although CT is useful for the evaluation of cortical bone involvement and identification of intratumoral calcification, beam hardening artifacts arising from metallic dental implants often degrade CT images. Despite dental fillings potentially causing susceptibility artifacts in MRI, they are generally located far from major salivary glands and, therefore, do not degrade MRIs of major salivary glands. If salivary gland cancer is strongly suspected, MRI is a particularly useful technique for evaluating tumor extension, including bone marrow infiltration, skull base invasion, meningeal invasion, facial nerve involvement, and perineural spread. This is due to the excellent soft tissue contrast resolution of the MRI technique. Because T1-weighted images give an excellent assessment of tumor margins, infiltrative growth patterns and deep extension, suggestive of malignancy, are well demonstrated on T1-weighted images. In addition, fat-suppressed contrast-enhanced T1-weighted images are required for the detection of bone invasion, meningeal invasion, and perineural spread along the facial nerve and auriculotemporal nerve (at the third division of the trigeminal nerve). While hyperintense masses on T2-weighted images are generally benign, hypointense or isointense masses tend to be malignant. Exceptions exist; low-grade malignancy often shows hyperintensity, while Warthin tumor usually shows hypointensity on T2-weighted images; however, T2-weighted imaging has been shown as a reasonably reliable predictor of whether salivary gland tumors are benign or malignant. MRI can discriminate between benign and malignant tumors as certain imaging findings, including T2 hypointensity, ill-defined tumor margins, diffuse growth patterns, and invasion of subcutaneous tissue, are all strongly indicative of malignant processes.

The usefulness of dynamic contrast-enhanced MRI parameters and time signal intensity curves (or contrast index curve) for differential diagnosis of salivary gland tumors have been reported previously [6]. Time of peak enhancement (T_{peak}) with a cutoff point of 120s is capable of differentiating between pleomorphic adenomas and malignant tumors, although assessment of T_{peak} of 120s alone is not sufficient to differentiate Warthin tumors from malignant tumors [6]. Washout ratio with a cutoff value of 30% is capable of differentiating between malignant and Warthin tumors [6]. Time signal intensity curves based on a combined assessment of T_{peak} of 120s and washout ratio of 30% possess high sensitivity (91%) and specificity (91%) for differentiating between benign and malignant salivary gland tumors [6].

The apparent diffusion coefficient (ADC) value is a quantitative parameter of diffusion-weighted imaging (DWI), which reflects the diffusion movement of water molecules in various tissues. There is a strong negative correlation between ADC and tumor cellularity. ADC is significantly smaller in lymphomas than in all other salivary gland tumors, and the mean ADC of salivary gland cancers is significantly smaller than in pleomorphic adenomas [7], whereas the mean ADC of Warthin tumors is smaller than that of malignant tumors [8]. This characteristic finding of Warthin tumors could be attributed to intense lymphoid accumulation in the stroma and proliferation of the epithelial component, leading to a decrease in extracellular extravascular space and, therefore, a decrease in ADC [9]. However, overlap in ADC exists between cellular pleomorphic adenomas and intermediate-grade malignant tumors and between Warthin tumors and high-grade malignant tumors [7, 8, 10].

8.6 Mucoepidermoid Carcinoma

Mucoepidermoid carcinoma (MEC) is the most common salivary gland cancer, accounting for approximately 30% of all salivary gland malignancies [11]. The incidence of MEC is rare in the pediatric population compared to adults; however, it accounts for 50% of salivary gland malignancies in children and adolescents. In adults, MECs most commonly occur in the fourth to sixth decades, with the highest prevalence noted during the fifth decade. A slight female predilection is observed, with a female-to-male ratio of 3:2 [11]. MEC is also the most common malignant neoplasm of the parotid gland. Approximately 60% of cases occur in the major salivary glands, with 35% occurring in the minor glands [11]. The parotid gland is the predominant site of tumors, representing 48% of cases, with 11% in the submandibular gland and 1% in the sublingual gland [11]. The palate and buccal mucosa are the most frequently affected sites in the minor salivary glands, followed by the antrum, tongue, gingiva, floor of the mouth, and nasal cavity [11]. Clinical presentation varies depending on tumor location, size, and histological grade. MECs usually present as slow-growing, long-standing, painless masses. Regardless of the location, the presenting symptom is an asymptomatic mass in 75% of cases. Although low-grade and intermediate-grade MECs may present as slow-growing masses, high-grade MECs generally grow rapidly. Fixation on the skin or deeper tissue, partial or complete facial nerve palsy, and ulceration, which are rarely observed, are signs of high-grade MECs. These can recur and metastasize to regional lymph nodes or distant viscera. Although overall disease prognosis is favorable, this is largely based on age, clinical stage, and histological grade.

Grossly, some MECs appear well-circumscribed and may be partially encapsulated, whereas others are poorly defined and infiltrative. Cut surfaces of tumors show solid or cystic appearances, often with abundant mucus. The microscopic appearance of MECs greatly depends on their histological grade of differentiation. Prominent cystic structures are hallmarks of low-grade MEC: multiple well-developed cystic or microcystic structures are lined by mature mucin-producing, intermediate, or epidermoid (squamous) cells. Intermediate-grade MECs have fewer and smaller cysts than low-grade MECs, in which intermediate cells predominate and form solid islands. High-grade MECs are characterized predominantly by solid cellular proliferation of squamous and intermediate cells, with higher degrees of atypia, anaplasia, multiple mitoses, and necrosis. Considering MECs, the 4th edition of the WHO classification of head and neck tumors is less dogmatic with regard to the application of grading and does not endorse a specific grading scheme [12]. Several grading schemes have been devised in the literature, each with advantages and limitations, particularly with respect to intermediate-grade tumors.

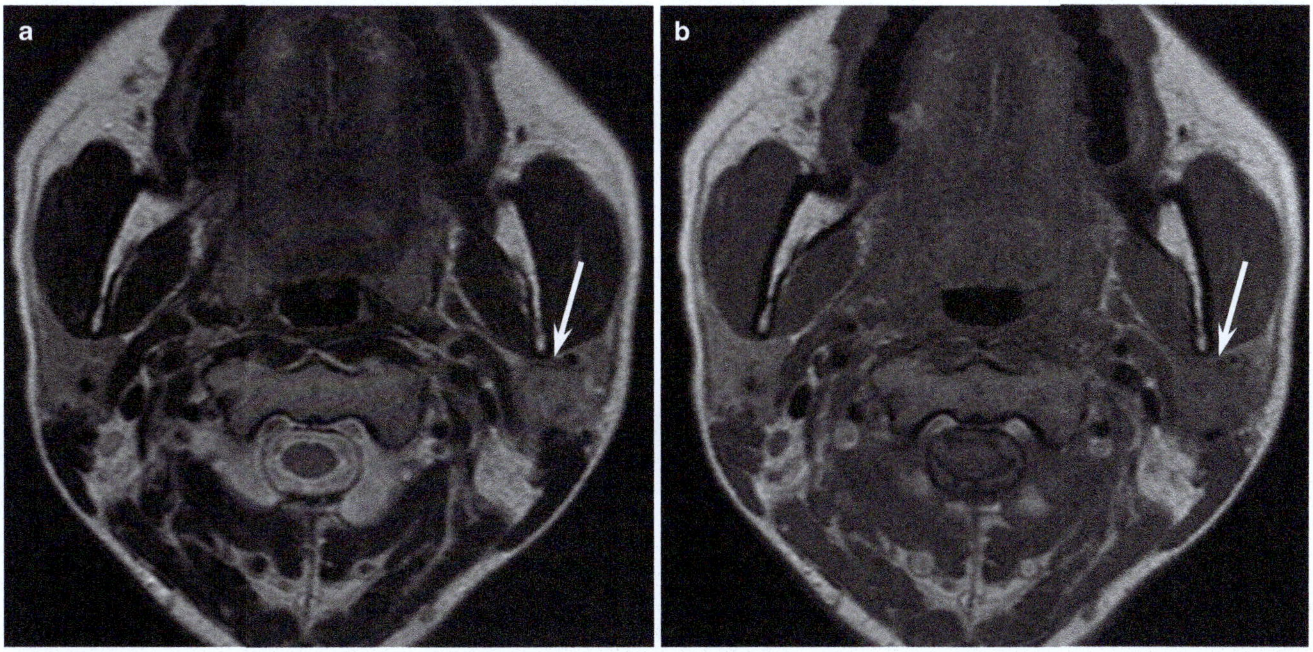

Fig. 8.1 A 47-year-old woman with low-grade mucoepidermoid carcinoma of the left parotid gland. (**a**) T2-weighted image shows an ill-defined, heterogeneously hyper- to isointense lesion (arrow). (**b**) T1-weighted image shows an ill-defined, hypointense lesion (arrow)

On MRI, low-grade MECs are well-circumscribed and characterized by cysts containing mucin, appearing as hyperintense spots within the tumor on both T1- and T2-weighted images; high-grade MECs are more solid and tend to infiltrate surrounding tissues (Figs. 8.1, 8.2 and 8.3) [13]. However, low-grade MECs often have ill-defined margins, reflecting peritumoral inflammatory changes rather than invasive tumor growth (Figs. 8.1 and 8.3) [14]. Generally, most solid components within tumors show hypointensity on T2-weighted images, possibly representing abundant fibrous tissue (Figs. 8.2 and 8.3). However, with regard to solid components on T2-weighted images, low-grade MECs may have hyperintense areas because of the presence of abundant mucin-secreting cells, whereas high-grade MECs show heterogeneous, low to intermediate signal intensities, reflecting high tumor cellularity (Figs. 8.1 and 8.2) [14].

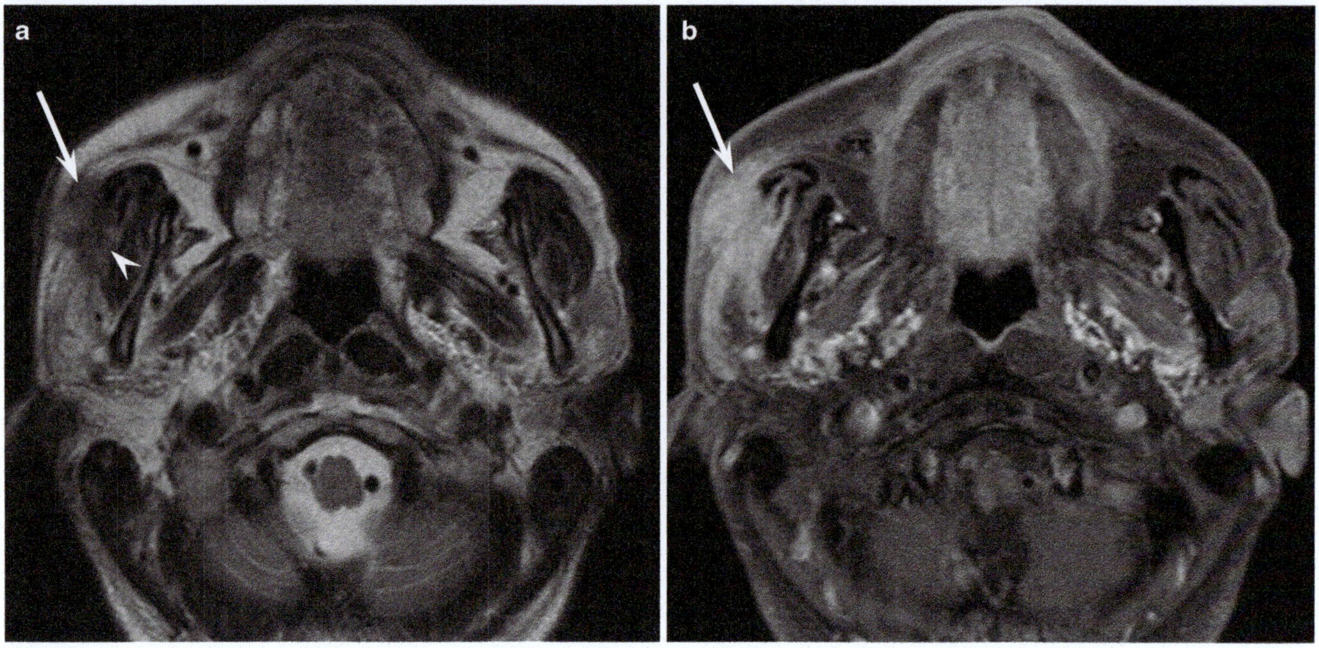

Fig. 8.2 A 79-year-old man with high-grade mucoepidermoid carcinoma of the right parotid gland. (**a**) T2-weighted image shows an ill-defined, heterogeneously hypo- to isointense lesion (arrow) with invasion of the masseter muscle (arrow head). (**b**) Fat-suppressed gadolinium-enhanced T1-weighted image shows an infiltrative lesion (arrow) with extensive invasion of surrounding tissues

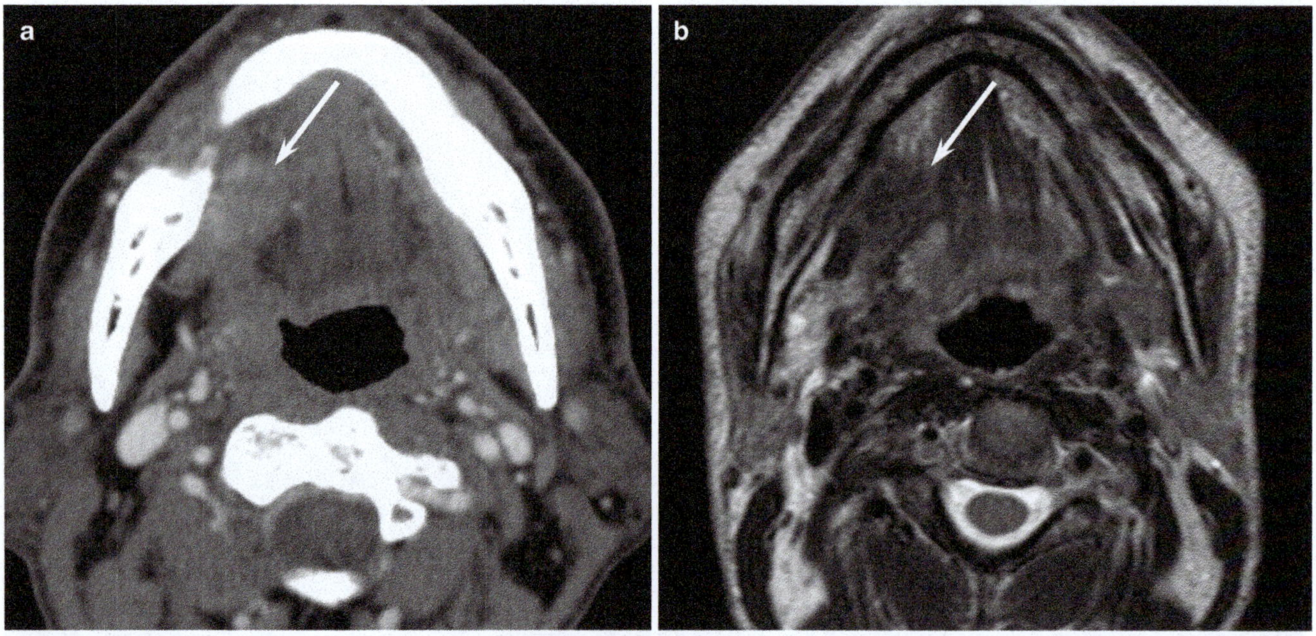

Fig. 8.3 A 74-year-old man with low-grade mucoepidermoid carcinoma of the right sublingual gland. (**a**) Contrast-enhanced CT image shows an ill-defined, heterogeneously enhanced lesion (arrow). (**b**) T2-weighted image shows an ill-defined, heterogeneously hypointense lesion (arrow)

8.7 Adenoid Cystic Carcinoma

Adenoid cystic carcinoma (AdCC) is a slow-growing and relentless salivary gland cancer, characterized by wide local infiltration, perineural spread, propensity for local recurrence, and late onset of distant metastasis. AdCC is the second most common salivary gland cancer, representing approximately 22% of all salivary gland malignancies. The age distribution is wide, with a peak incidence between the fifth and sixth decades. AdCC is more frequent in females, with a female-to-male ratio of 3:2. AdCC is considered the most common malignant neoplasm of the submandibular and minor salivary glands. AdCCs arise from minor salivary glands in 65% of cases, the parotid gland in 19% of cases, and submandibular gland in 16% of cases [15]. Among those which originate in the minor salivary glands, AdCC most frequently occurs in the palate, followed by the paranasal sinuses and other oral cavity sites. Tumor location in minor salivary glands is associated with a higher risk of recurrence and worse prognosis. AdCCs usually do not show any specific signs and symptoms; classical presentation is an asymptomatic mass with long-term clinical course. Over time, as the tumor grows, it has a propensity to invade nerves, causing pain and numbness as the lesion advances. There is a strong correlation between pain and perineural invasion, and the histological pattern and clinical stage are major prognostic factors for the disease. The 5-year overall survival rate can be as high as 90%, but 15-year survival is less than 70%. This poor long-term prognosis is caused by failure to control late-onset distant metastases, most commonly to the lungs, followed by the bone, liver, and brain. Regional nodal involvement is uncommon but is more frequent in the solid variants of the disease.

Typical gross appearance is well-defined but not encapsulated, as it can be seen infiltrating surrounding normal tissue. The rare finding of necrosis and/or hemorrhage may indicate the presence of a high-grade tumor. Microscopically, AdCC consists of a characteristic infiltrative proliferation of luminal ducts and abluminal myoepithelial cells arranged in three histological patterns: cribriform, tubular, and solid. The cribriform subtype is the most common and easily recognized pattern, characterized by nests of tumor cells interrupted by sharply punched-out spaces filled with basophilic matrix. The tubular subtype represents more apparent ductal spaces and is also the most differentiated microscopic pattern of AdCC. The solid subtype usually contains nonexistent or occasional cyst-like spaces and a much greater degree of nuclear and cellular pleomorphism and mitotic activity. As polymorphism is common in AdCC, all three subtypes may be observed in a single specimen. Based on the percentage of solid components, a proposed pathological grading system is widely used: Grade I, tubular and cribriform pattern without solid component; Grade II, mostly cribriform but less than 30% solid component; and Grade III, predominantly solid component [16].

On MRI, AdCC appears both as a well-defined and ill-defined mass. Tumors with ill-defined margins often show diffuse infiltration into surrounding structures. AdCCs with hyperintensity on T2-weighted images correspond to less cellular tumors (cribriform or tubular subtype) with better prognosis, whereas those with hypointensity on T2-weighted images correspond to highly cellular tumors (solid subtype) with poor prognosis (Figs. 8.4, 8.5 and 8.6) [17]. Retrograde tumor extension to the base of the

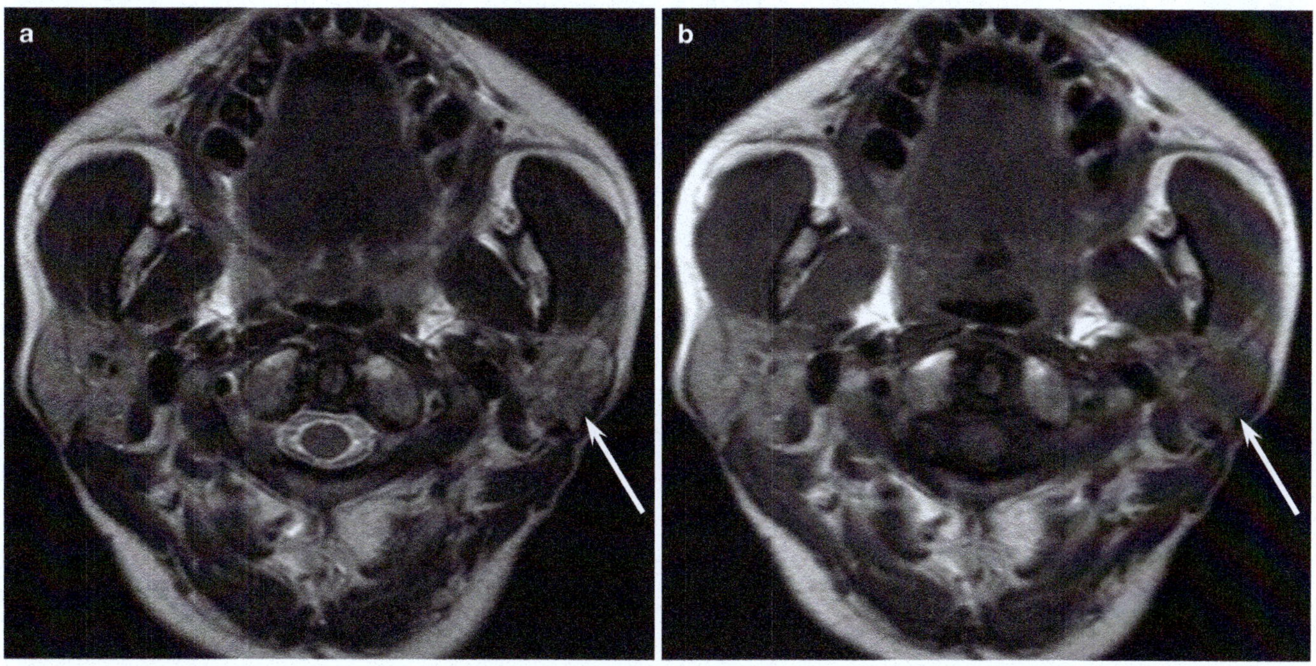

Fig. 8.4 A 54-year-old woman with adenoid cystic carcinoma of the left parotid gland. (**a**) T2-weighted image shows an ill-defined, heterogeneously iso- to hyperintense lesion (arrow). (**b**) T1-weighted image shows an ill-defined, hypointense lesion (arrow)

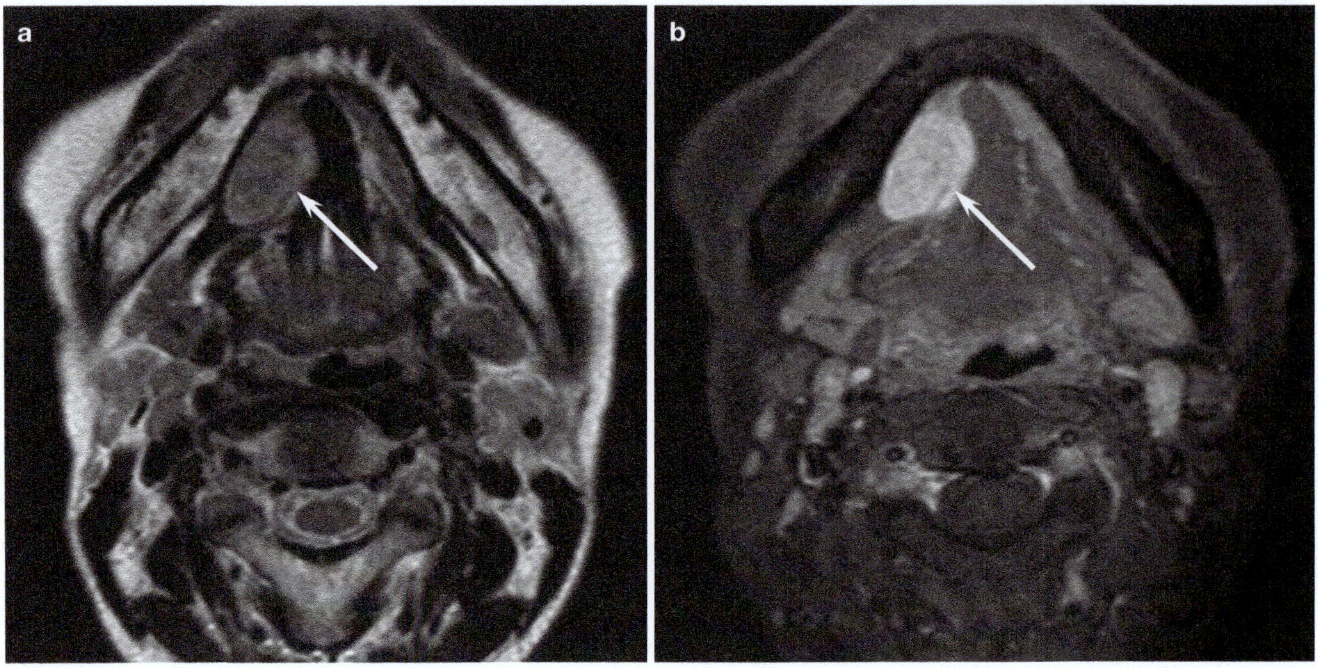

Fig. 8.5 A 55-year-old woman with adenoid cystic carcinoma of the right sublingual gland. (**a**) T2-weighted image shows a well-demarcated, homogeneously hyperintense lesion (arrow). (**b**) Fat-suppressed gadolinium-enhanced T1-weighted image shows a homogeneously enhanced lesion (arrow) with well-delineated tumor borders

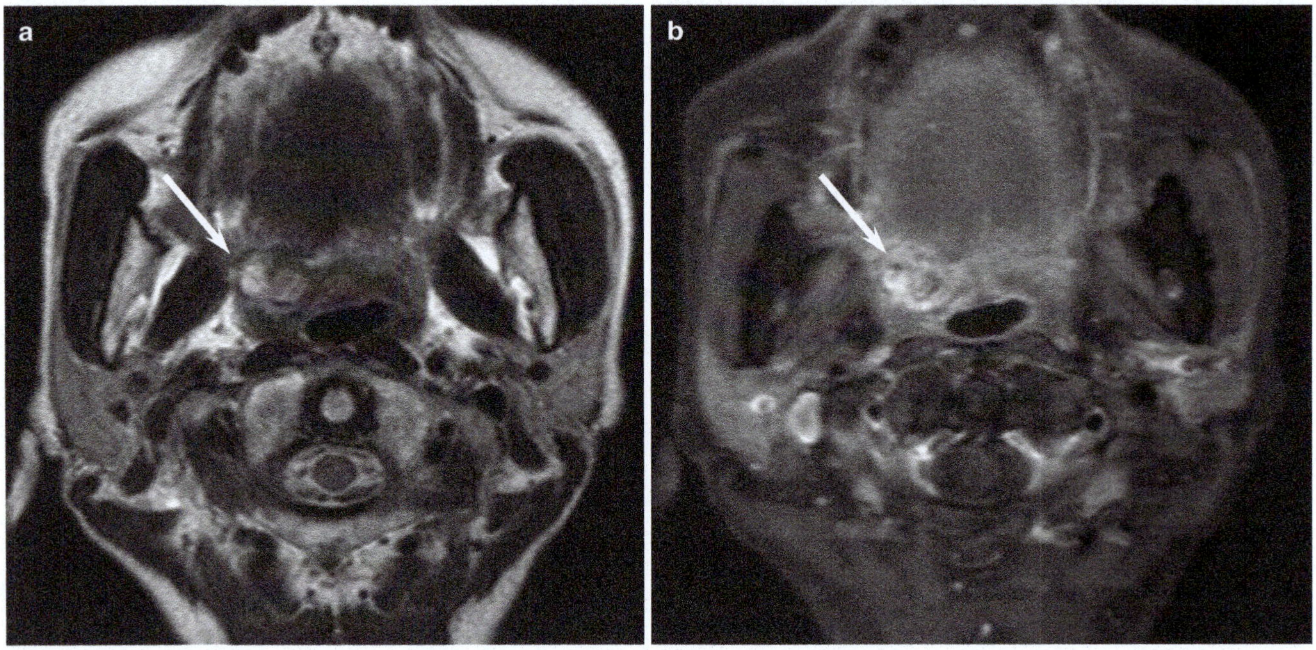

Fig. 8.6 A 70-year-old woman with adenoid cystic carcinoma of the right soft palate. (**a**) T2-weighted image shows a well-demarcated, heterogeneously hyperintense lesion (arrow). (**b**) Fat-suppressed gadolinium-enhanced T1-weighted image shows a heterogeneously enhanced lesion (arrow) without invasive growth

skull often occurs via the facial nerve or the mandibular nerve; imaging characteristics of the perineural tumor spread include (a) foraminal enlargement, (b) foraminal destruction, (c) obliteration of fat planes, (d) nerve enlargement, (e) nerve enhancement, (f) neuropathic atrophy, (g) convexity of the lateral cavernous sinus wall, and (h) replacement of the trigeminal subarachnoid cistern with soft tissue [18].

8.8 Acinic Cell Carcinoma

Acinic cell carcinoma (AcCC) is a low-grade malignant neoplasm. It constitutes approximately 17% of all salivary gland malignancies, representing the third most common epithelial malignancy of salivary glands in adults, following MEC and AdCC [19]. In the pediatric age group, AcCC is the second most common epithelial malignancy, following MEC. Mean patient age at presentation is approximately 50 years old and tends to be younger than for other salivary gland cancers. AcCC shows a slight female predilection, with a female-to-male ratio of 3:2. More than 80% of AcCCs occur in the parotid, and approximately 10% occur in the minor salivary glands, most commonly in the palate. Less than 1% of AcCCs arise in the sublingual gland [19]. Bilateral tumors are unusual but can occur [20]. AcCCs typically present with slowly growing, solitary, unfixed masses, but a few are multinodular and/or fixed to the skin or muscle. One-third of patients experience pain, which is often vague and intermittent, and 5–10% develop facial paralysis. Although AcCC is generally not aggressive, with a 5-year overall survival rate of 90%, it has a significant tendency to recur and produce metastases to the cervical nodes and lungs. Multiple recurrence, cervical nodal metastases, and distant metastases predict poor prognosis.

Gross appearance includes well-circumscribed mass but lacking a true capsule. The cut surface usually displays both solid and cystic areas; however, these can be homogeneously solid or extensively cystic. While AcCC is defined as serous acinar cell differentiation, several cell types and histomorphologic growth patterns are recognized. Variable cell types include uniform acinar (serous) type cells with basophilic granular cytoplasm, clear cells (hypernephroid pattern, contains glycogen or mucin), vacuolated, intercalated duct, and nonspecific glandular cells (smaller, syncytial). Variable patterns include solid, microcystic, papillary cystic (associated with hemorrhage), and follicular growth patterns.

Typical imaging features of AcCC are well-circumscribed, solid, or partially cystic lesions with thin or incomplete capsules (Fig. 8.7). AcCC can be classified into three categories depending on the morphological appearance: solid mass, cystic mass, and cystic mass with a mural nodule. The most frequently observed solid masses usually include focal hypodense portions, which correspond to microcyst, hemorrhage, or necrosis on pathologic examination. On T1-weighted images, cystic components can appear hyperintense due to hemorrhage. The signal intensity of solid components on T2-weighted images varies, reflecting various pathologic conditions. These imaging characteristics are nonspecific and quite like benign salivary gland tumors, such as pleomorphic adenoma, Warthin tumors, basal cell adenoma, and myoepithelioma.

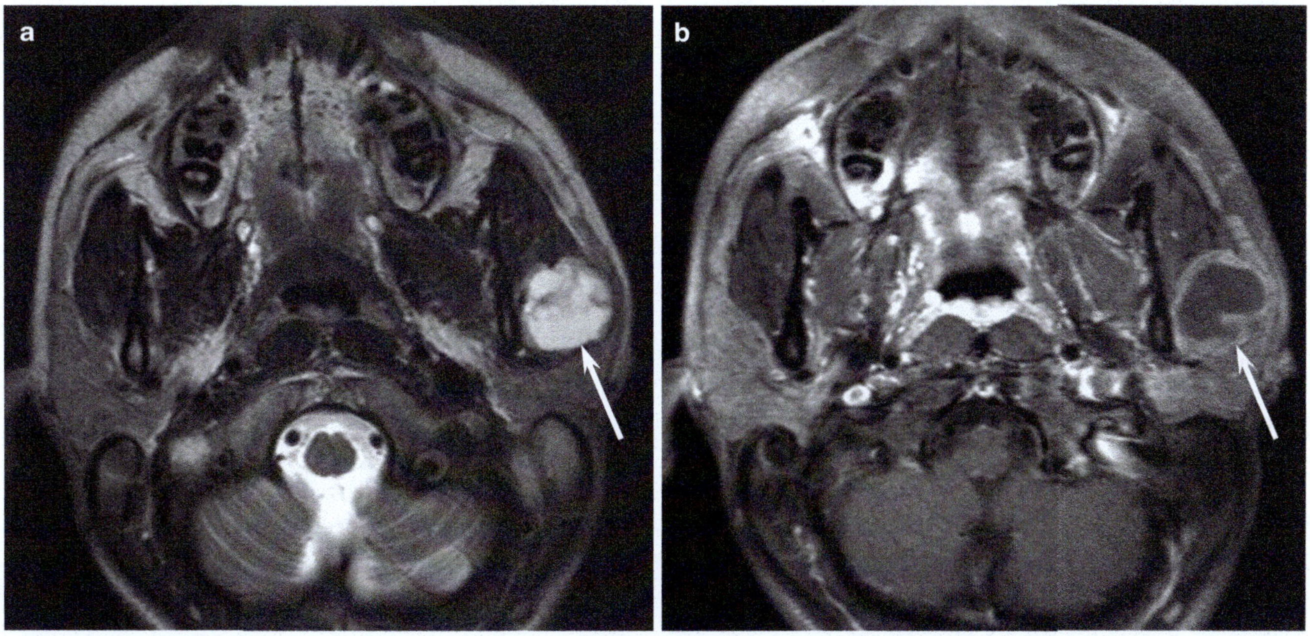

Fig. 8.7 A 19-year-old man with acinic cell carcinoma of the left parotid gland. (**a**) T2-weighted image shows a predominantly cystic lesion (arrow). (**b**) Fat-suppressed gadolinium-enhanced T1-weighted image shows a well-demarcated lesion (arrow) with extensive unenhanced areas

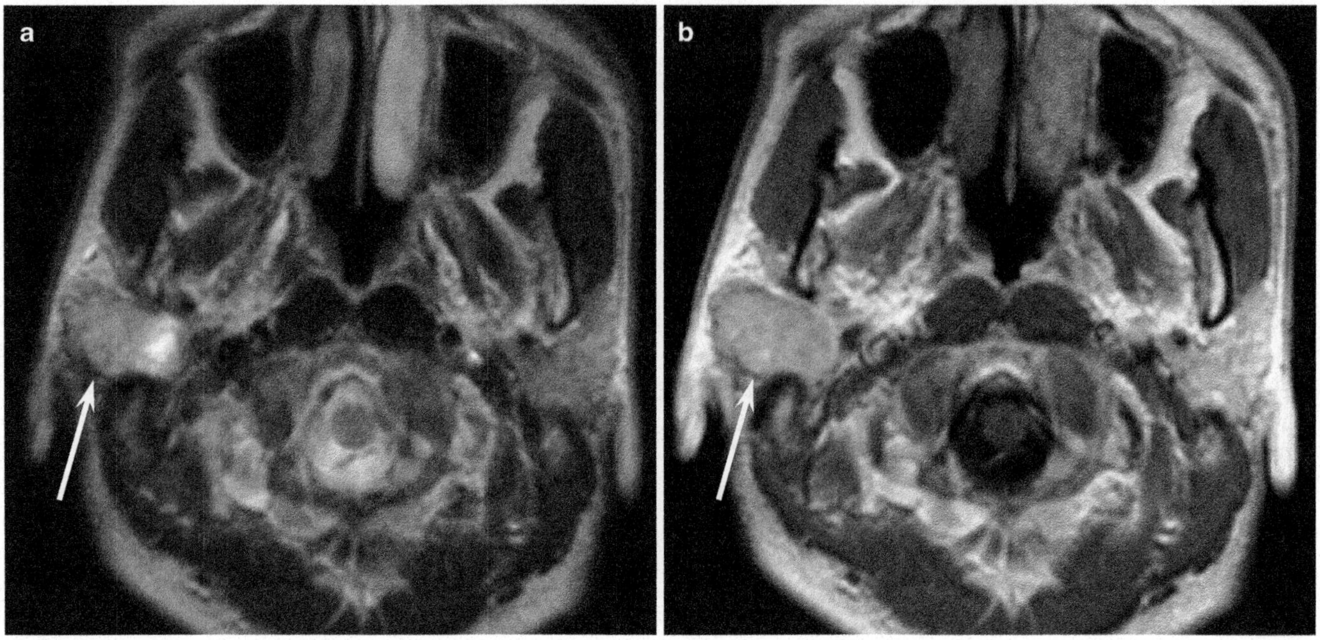

Fig. 8.8 A 44-year-old man with secretory carcinoma of the right parotid gland. (**a**) T2-weighted image shows a well-demarcated, hyperintense lesion (arrow). (**b**) Gadolinium-enhanced T1-weighted image shows a homogeneously enhanced lesion (arrow) with well-delineated tumor borders

8.9 Secretory Carcinoma

Secretory carcinoma (SC), also known as mammary analog secretory carcinoma, is a newly described entity based on its resemblance to breast secretory carcinoma. Most cases can be discovered in archived cases, which had previously been classified as AcCC or "adenocarcinomas NOS." It is named for recapitulation of breast SC, along with shared *ETV6-NTRK3* gene fusion [12]. Given this similarity and in an effort to standardize nomenclature across organ sites, the official designation for this entity is now simply "secretory carcinoma" [12]. SC usually presents in adults and frequently occurs in the fifth to sixth decades. There is no gender predilection, in contrast with the female predilection in AcCC [21]. Sites of incidence, in descending order, are the parotid gland (68%), buccal mucosa (9%), submandibular gland (8%), lower lip (5%), upper lip (4%), and hard palate (4%) [21]. Although parotid gland is still the most common site, SC arises in minor salivary sites more frequently than AcCC [22]. Most cases present as slow-growing, painless, nontender masses. SC is typically indolent, like AcCC, but it may show a higher nodal metastatic rate than true AcCC. Distant metastases are rare. High clinical stage and high-grade transformation are the main adverse prognostic factors.

Gross appearance is of a poorly circumscribed solid mass, occasionally with cyst formation. Microscopically, SC has a lobulated growth pattern, composed of microcystic and glandular spaces with abundant eosinophilic homogeneous or bubbly secretory material. They share nearly identical growth patterns with AcCC, but instead are characterized by the multivacuolated eosinophilic cytoplasm, often with luminal and intracytoplasmic mucin and no true zymogen granules. Papillary cystic architecture is now considered rare in true AcCC, being far more common in SC.

As with pathological findings, imaging features of SC are similar to those of AcCC (Fig. 8.8). SC has well-defined margins and presents as a predominantly cystic mass with the papillary projection of solid components [23]. Signal intensity of the cystic components on T1-weighted images is usually hyperintensity with or without fluid-fluid level formation [23]. Signal intensity of the solid components on T2-weighted images is variable, appearing to reflect varying degrees of microcyst formation in tumor cells, desmoplastic stromal reaction, and cellularity [23].

8.10 Polymorphous Adenocarcinoma

Polymorphous low-grade adenocarcinoma (PLGA), shortened to polymorphous adenocarcinoma (PAC), has been the most contentious entity over the past decade. The term PLGA was first used to describe an infiltrative salivary gland tumor with various growth patterns but bland nuclei [24]. The growth pattern and stromal characteristics mimic those of AcCC and have been histologically challenging to differentiate [12]. Age at presentation typically peaks in the sixth and seventh decades. Incidence shows a female predilection with a female-to-male ratio of 2:1 [25]. PACs almost exclusively involve the palate, mainly occurring in the posterior hard and soft palate. Other intraoral sites include the buccal mucosa, retromolar region, upper lip, and the base of the tongue. Up to 9% of PACs have been reported to originate from major salivary glands [25]. PACs typically present as asymptomatic, slow-growing, intraoral masses with various durations, ranging from a few weeks to 40 years. Bleeding, telangiectasia, and ulceration of the overlying mucosa may occasionally be found. Most PACs are indolent, and the 5-year overall survival rate can be as high as nearly 90%; however, local recurrence rates can reach 10–30% and regional metastases can reach up to 15%. Distant metastases have seldom been reported for this condition.

Grossly, this tumor is well-circumscribed but unencapsulated. The presence of central tumor necrosis and hemorrhage is rare. Tumor histology is characterized by cytological uniformity, histological diversity, and an infiltrative growth pattern. Growth patterns include solid, trabecular, tubular, cribriform, fascicular, and papillary and are arranged in fascicles with targetoid neurotropism. Tumor cells are monomorphic and monotypic with a (terminal) ductal phenotype, consisting of uniform ovoid vesicular nuclei and scant-to-moderate eosinophilic cytoplasm.

Although no case series regarding PAC imaging findings can be found, heterogeneous signal intensity on T2-weighted images and heterogeneous enhancement on contrast-enhanced images are usually observed, reflecting histological diversity (Fig. 8.9). Pathological growth pattern is infiltrative, but PAC may appear as a well-circumscribed

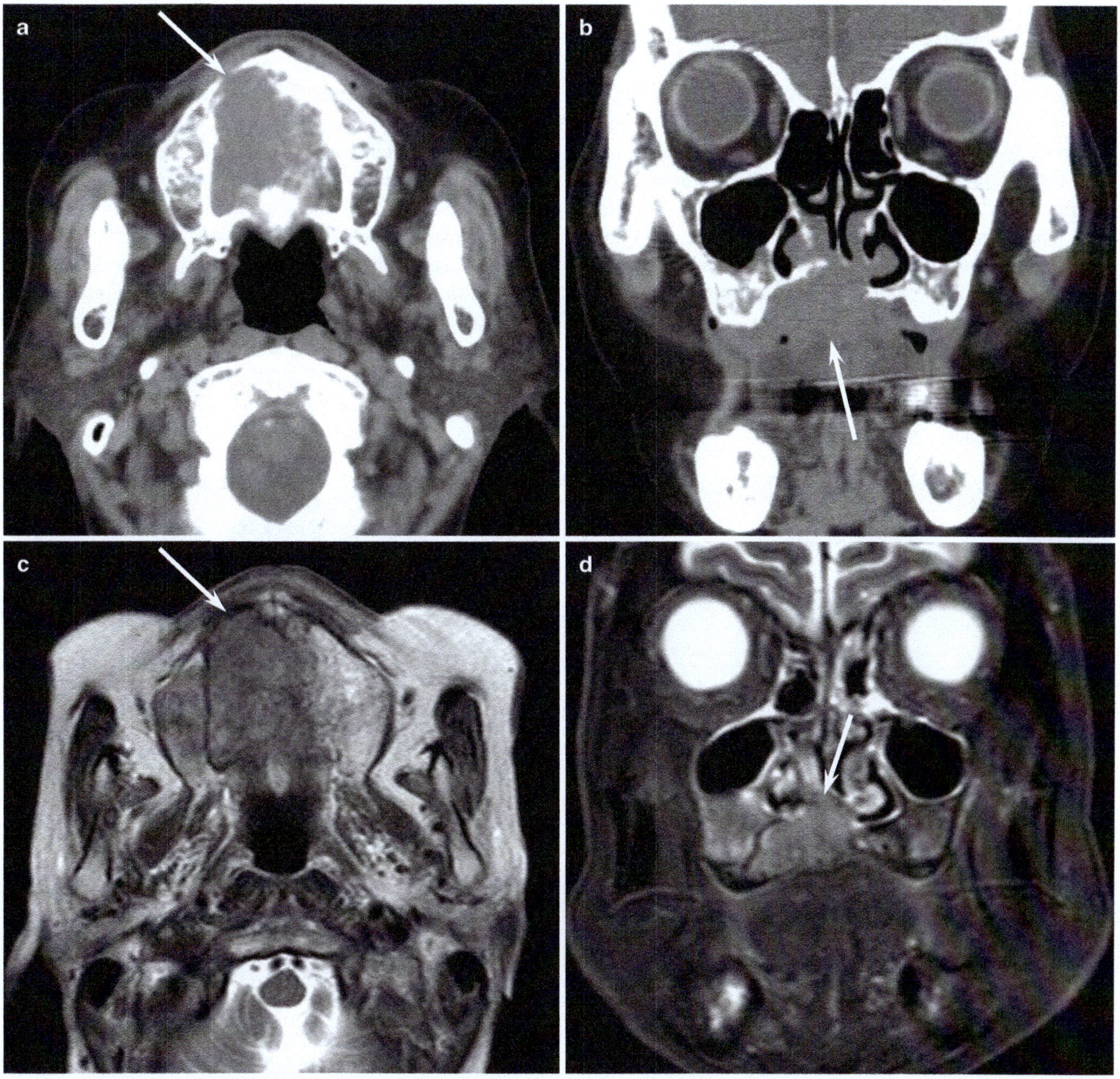

Fig. 8.9 A 90-year-old woman with polymorphous adenocarcinoma of the right palate. (**a**, **b**) Unenhanced CT images show an ill-defined, invasive lesion (arrow) with destruction of palatine bone. (**c**) T2-weighted image shows an ill-defined, heterogeneously isointense lesion (arrow). (**d**) Coronal fat-suppressed T2-weighted image shows invasion of nasal cavity (arrow)

mass because of its slow-growing nature over a long time [26]. As such tumors grow, pressure erosion at the adjacent palatine bone and extension into the nasal cavity and maxillary sinus can be observed (Fig. 8.9) [27].

8.11 Adenocarcinoma NOS

Adenocarcinoma NOS (ANOS) is a malignant epithelial salivary gland tumor with ductal or glandular differentiation, lacking sufficient histological features of currently recognized salivary gland cancers to allow for a more specific diagnosis. ANOS is usually listed as the fourth or fifth most common salivary gland cancer, accounting for approximately 10–15% of all salivary gland malignancies. Peak incidence is observed between the sixth and the seventh decades. ANOS shows a clear female predilection with a female-to-male ratio of 4:1 [28]. More than 50% of ANOS arise in the parotid gland; 40% arise in minor salivary glands, occurring most often in the hard palate, buccal mucosa, and lips. ANOS in the parotid gland usually presents as an asymptomatic firm or cystic mass, occasionally associated with pain. Tumor location, histological grade, and clinical stage are important prognostic factors. Cervical nodal metastases develop in 23% of cases and distant metastases in 37% of cases.

Gross pathology reveals an irregular and infiltrative growth pattern with or without areas of necrosis and hemorrhage. Microscopically, tumor cells can be cuboidal, columnar, polygonal, clear, mucinous, oncocytoid, and/or plasmacytoid in morphology and arranged in a variety of growth patterns with areas of glandular or ductal proliferation, not resembling any named salivary malignancy [28]. For pathological diagnosis of ANOS, salivary duct carcinoma, high-grade MEC, PAC, and metastatic adenocarcinoma should be carefully excluded.

In cross-sectional imaging, ANOS is identified as an ill-demarcated, invasive, infiltrative mass, reflecting high-grade malignancies (Figs. 8.10 and 8.11). Cystic components and non-enhancing areas within the tumor, which are frequently observed, correspond to necrosis and/or hemorrhage (Fig. 8.10). Due to high cellularity, the solid components of ANOS usually show low to intermediate signal intensity on T2-weighted images (Fig. 8.11).

8.12 Salivary Duct Carcinoma

Salivary duct carcinoma (SDC) is an aggressive and infiltrative epithelial salivary gland malignancy microscopically resembling high-grade ductal carcinoma of the breast, representing approximately 10% of all salivary gland malignancies. SDC generally affects the elderly, with a peak incidence in the sixth and seventh decades There is a male predilection, with a male-to-female ratio of 2:1. Most SDCs arise from the parotid gland (83%), and the second most frequent site is the submandibular gland (12%) [29]. Although a common presenting symptom is a painless mass, SDC exhibits rapid

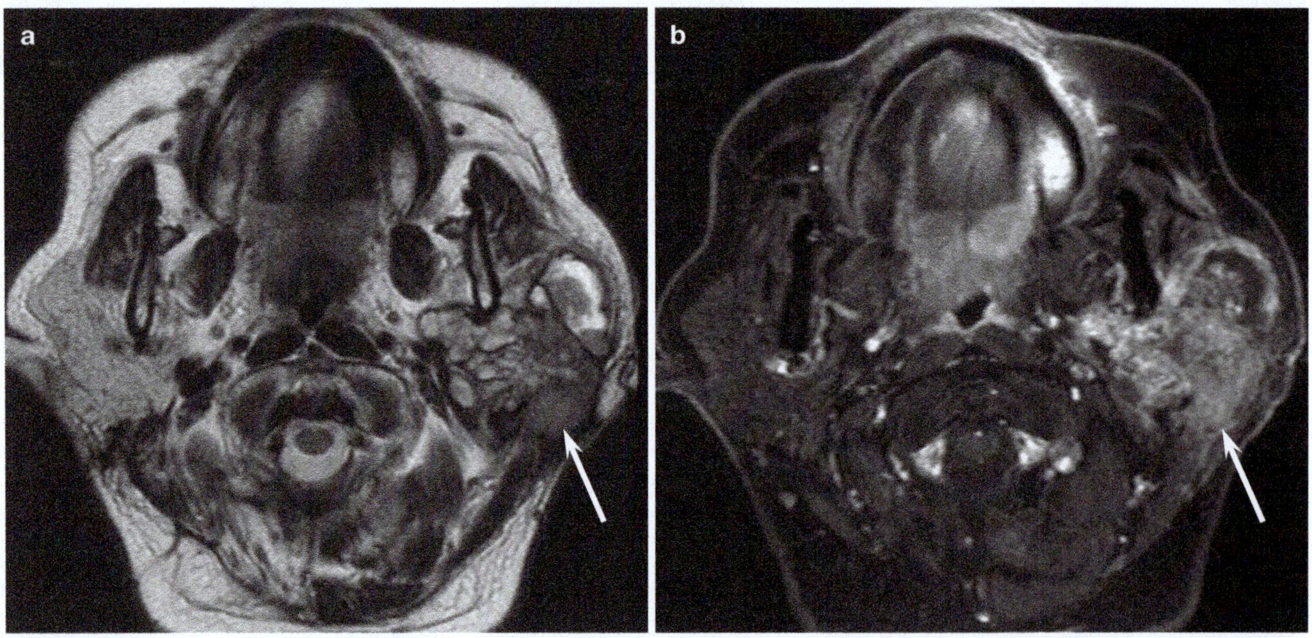

Fig. 8.10 A 61-year-old woman with adenocarcinoma NOS of the left parotid gland. (**a**) T2-weighted image shows a considerably heterogeneous lesion (arrow) with a mixture of solid and cystic components. (**b**) Fat-suppressed gadolinium-enhanced T1-weighted image shows a heterogeneously enhanced lesion (arrow) with partially ill-delineated tumor borders

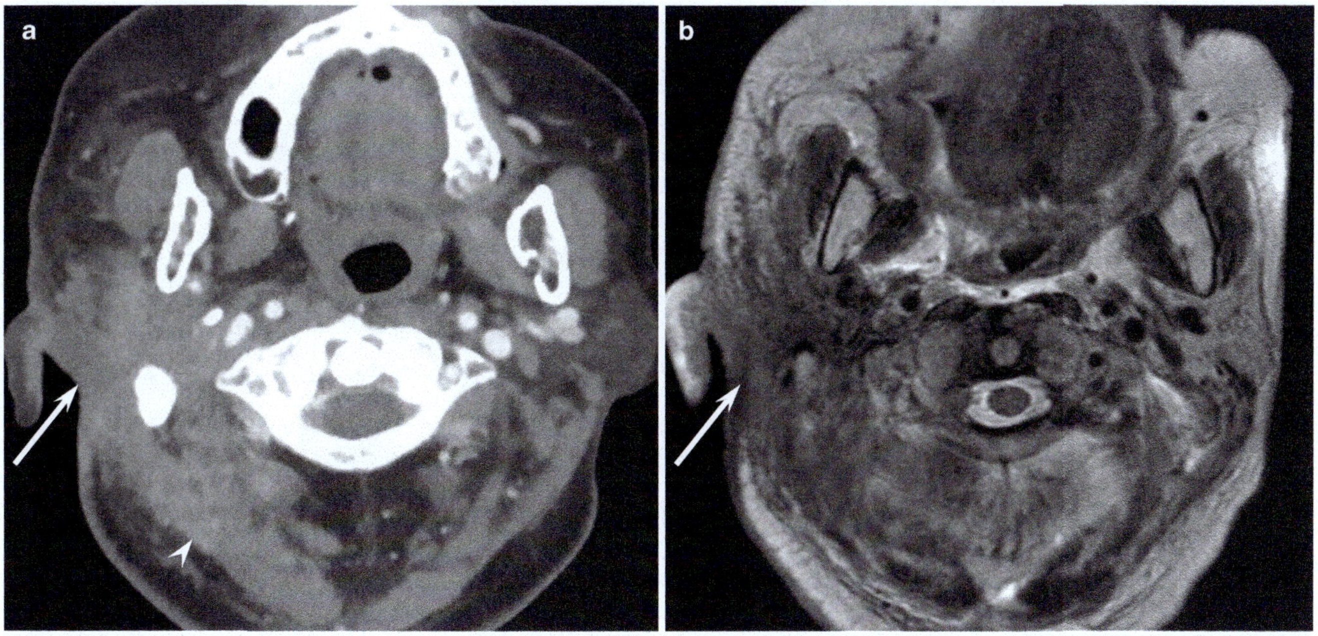

Fig. 8.11 A 75-year-old woman with adenocarcinoma NOS of the right parotid gland. (**a**) Contrast-enhanced CT image shows an ill-defined, heterogeneously enhanced lesion (arrow) with invasion of the surrounding muscle (arrow head). (**b**) T2-weighted image shows an ill-defined, heterogeneously hypointense lesion (arrow)

growth, pain, facial nerve palsy, and nodal metastasis in a significant proportion of cases at presentation [20]. Poor prognosis is caused by a high incidence of local recurrence, cervical nodal involvement, and distant metastasis. The 5-year overall survival rate is estimated to be between 41 and 55%.

Grossly, SDC is generally a firm, ill-defined mass infiltrating the surrounding tissue. Fibrosis within hemorrhagic areas, necrosis, cystic degeneration, and intratumoral calcification may all be observed within tumors. Microscopically, SDC is reminiscent of high-grade ductal carcinoma of the breast composed of large ducts with comedonecrosis and pleomorphic, epithelioid cells with a cribriform growth pattern. Although most cases seem to arise from a preexisting pleomorphic adenoma, de novo cases undoubtedly occur. Perineural spread is a hallmark of SDC, occurring in more than half of patients. Lymphovascular invasion with intravascular tumor emboli is another common histological feature.

Due to its high-grade and aggressive nature, SDC has ill-defined boundaries with infiltration into the surrounding fat space (Figs. 8.12 and 8.13) [30]. On T2-weighted images, solid components usually show low to intermediate signal intensity, and areas of marked hypointensity may be seen, reflecting the histological feature of a marked desmoplastic reaction associated with an infiltrating tumor [30, 31]. As necrosis commonly appears in the form of various degrees of non-enhancing areas, enhancement patterns are usually heterogeneous (Fig. 8.13) [31]. CT imaging can reveal various sizes of intratumoral calcification in 50% of cases (Fig. 8.12) [31].

8.13 Epithelial-Myoepithelial Carcinoma

Epithelial-myoepithelial carcinoma (EMC) is defined as a low-grade salivary gland cancer with expansive borders and lacking a true capsule. EMC is an uncommon neoplasm, accounting for <5% of all salivary gland malignancies. The peak occurrence is in the sixth and seventh decades. There is a slight female predilection, with a female-to-male ratio of 3:2. EMC arises most commonly in the parotid gland, but has also been described in the submandibular gland and minor salivary glands, including in the oral mucosa and the upper and lower respiratory tracts [32]. EMCs in the parotid gland usually present with painless, slow-growing, multinodular masses which may be present for several years prior to diagnosis, whereas those in minor salivary glands can present as ulcerated submucosal masses with ill-defined margins [32]. The 5-year overall survival rate is 80%. EMCs are typically low-grade tumors; thus, regional and distant metastases are uncommon. However, local recurrence after resection is more common.

Grossly, EMC appears as a multinodular, unencapsulated, and mainly solid mass, although cystic change is noted in 30% of cases. Tumor margins are usually well-delineated but may be infiltrative. Microscopically, EMC is a prototypically biphasic tumor, composed of eosinophilic luminal ductal cells and typically clear, polygonal, abluminal myoepithelial cells. Given the partial encapsulation and a rounded border, limited sampling may resemble the appearance of a benign tumor. Several variants have been described, most notably oncocytic, apocrine, and high-grade transformed.

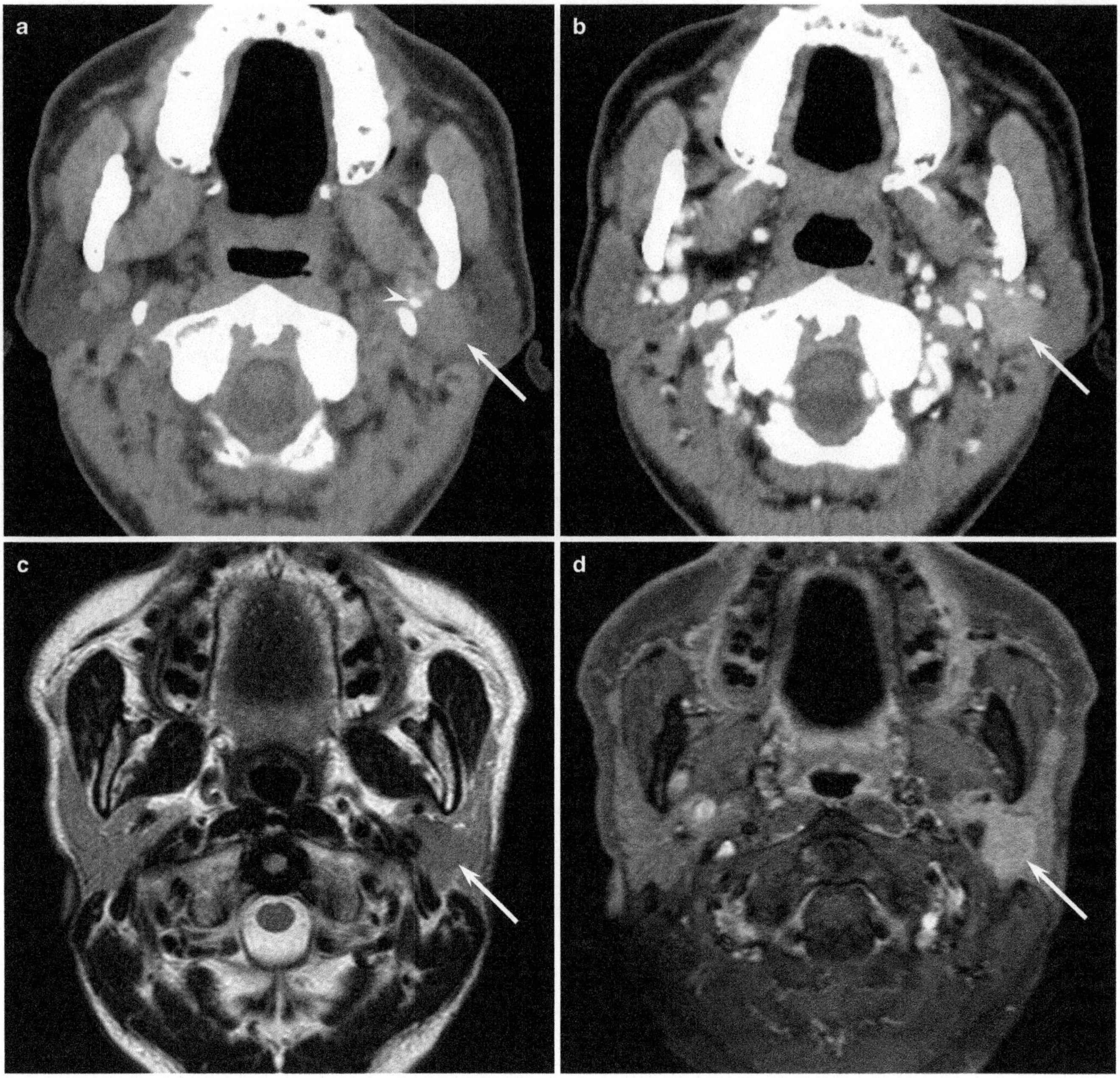

Fig. 8.12 A 71-year-old man with salivary duct carcinoma of the left parotid gland. (**a**) Unenhanced CT image shows an ill-defined lesion (arrow) with calcification (arrow head). (**b**) Contrast-enhanced CT image shows a homogeneously enhanced lesion (arrow). (**c**) T2-weighted image shows a homogeneously isointense lesion (arrow). (**d**) Fat-suppressed gadolinium-enhanced T1-weighted image shows a homogeneously enhanced lesion (arrow)

Although no case series reporting EMC imaging findings can be found, EMCs usually appear as well-circumscribed masses due to their low-grade nature (Fig. 8.14). Solid components on T2-weighted images show intermediate to high signal intensity, and the enhancement pattern is usually heterogeneous [33, 34]. On T1-weighted images, hyperintense areas corresponding to hemorrhagic areas may be seen [34].

8.14 Carcinoma ex Pleomorphic Adenoma

Carcinoma ex pleomorphic adenoma (CXPA) represents an infiltrative and destructive malignancy, arising in pleomorphic adenoma. It constitutes approximately 12% of all malignant salivary gland neoplasms. CXPA arises from long-standing or recurrent pleomorphic adenoma, with incidence increasing from 1.5% at 5 years to 10% at 15 years. It

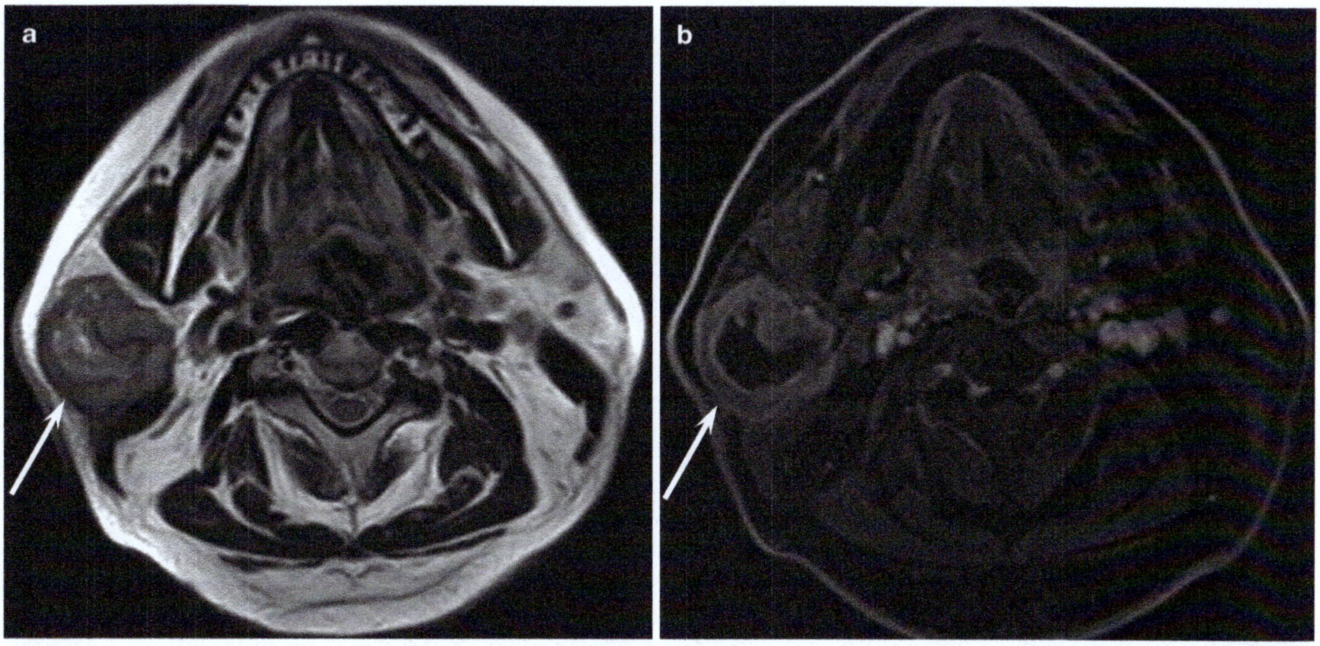

Fig. 8.13 A 62-year-old man with salivary duct carcinoma of the right parotid gland. (**a**) T2-weighted image shows an ill-defined, heterogeneously iso- to hyperintense lesion (arrow). (**b**) Fat-suppressed gadolinium-enhanced T1-weighted image shows a heterogeneously enhanced lesion (arrow) with central unenhanced area

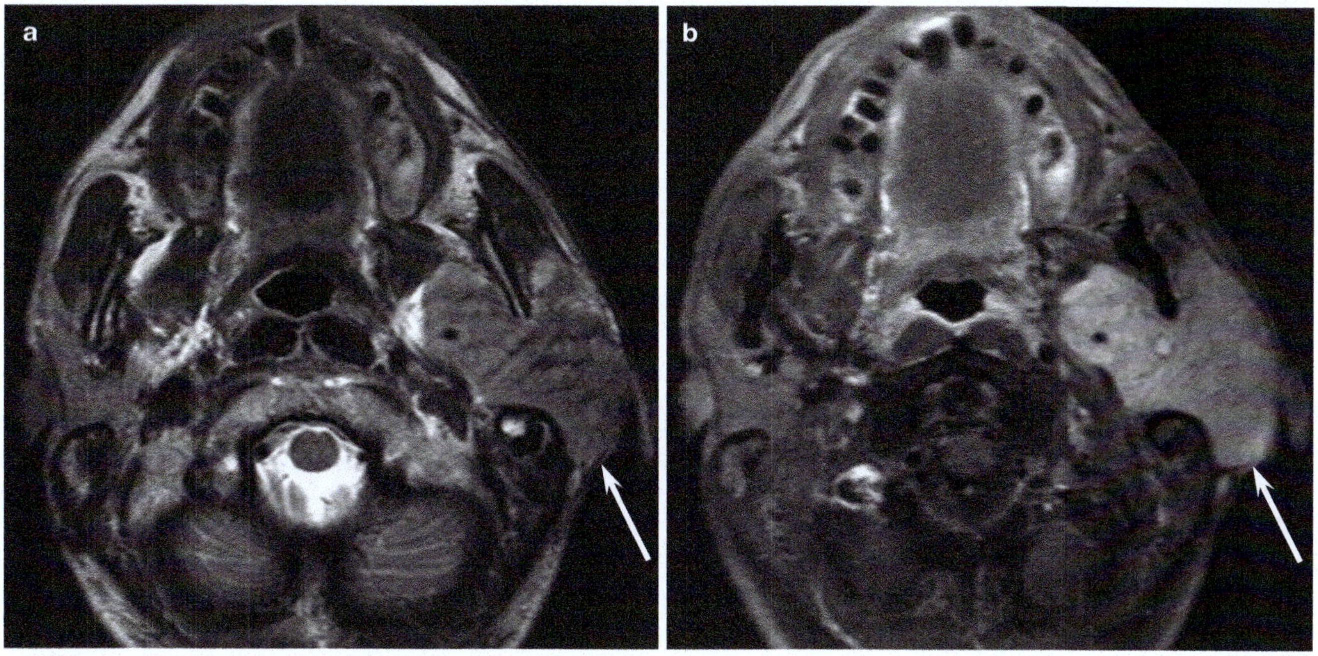

Fig. 8.14 A 41-year-old man with epithelial-myoepithelial carcinoma of the left parotid gland. (**a**) T2-weighted image shows an ill-defined, heterogeneously iso- to hyperintense lesion (arrow). (**b**) Fat-suppressed gadolinium-enhanced T1-weighted image shows a homogeneously enhanced lesion (arrow)

is found predominantly in the sixth to eighth decades and is slightly more common in females, with a female-to-male ratio of 3:2. CXPA predominantly affects the parotid gland, but has also been known to manifest in the submandibular gland and minor salivary glands in the oral cavity, particularly in the hard and soft palates [35]. Although clinical presentation is usually of an asymptomatic, firm mass and often similar to pleomorphic adenoma, features of frank malignancy are usually manifested as sudden rapid growth, fixation, ulceration, facial nerve palsy, and regional

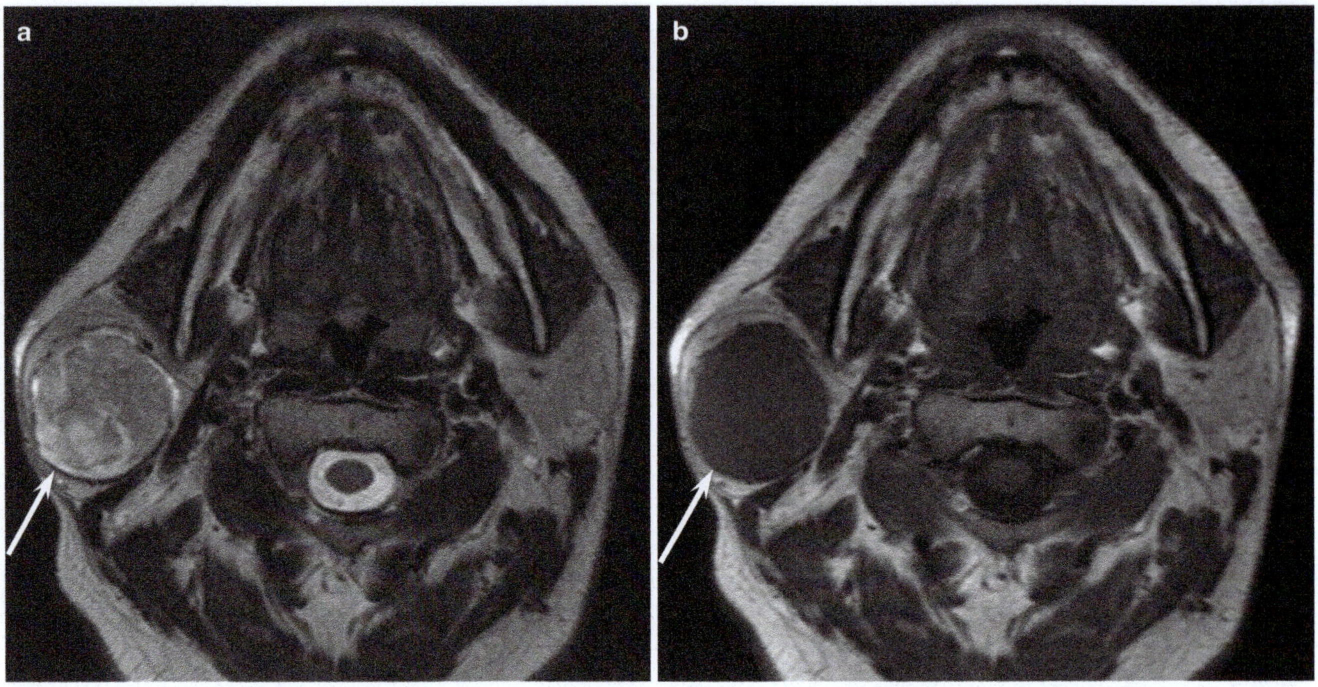

Fig. 8.15 A 46-year-old man with carcinoma ex pleomorphic adenoma of the right parotid gland. (**a**) T2-weighted image shows a well-demarcated, heterogeneously hyperintense lesion (arrow). (**b**) T1-weighted image shows a homogeneously hypointense lesion (arrow) with well-delineated tumor borders

lymphadenopathy with a preexisting, long-standing mass. CXPA prognosis can be predicted based on noninvasive, minimally invasive, or invasive classification. The 5-year overall survival rates vary significantly, ranging from 30 to 70%, due to various phases of transformation, histological subtypes, and tumor extension. Up to 70% of patients will develop local recurrence and/or distant metastases.

Gross appearance varies, but poorly circumscribed, infiltrative tumor margins are often observed. The components of the underlying pleomorphic adenoma are grossly visible in most cases, usually as a sclerotic, calcified nodule. Microscopically, CXPA is composed of a mixture of pleomorphic adenoma and carcinoma. Based on the extension of the carcinomatous components outside the fibrous capsule, CXPA can be subdivided into noninvasive, minimally invasive, and invasive CXPA. The most common histological subtype of malignant components of CXPA is ANOS; however, AdCC, MEC, or SDC may also occur.

The combination of invasive and encapsulated components is a characteristic imaging feature of CXPA [36]. Invasive components have ill-defined margins, central necrosis, occasional extraparotid extension, and low to intermediate signal intensities on T2-weighted images [36]. These are consistent with high-grade malignancies, whereas encapsulated components are demonstrated as hyperintense masses with hypointense rims on T2-weighted images, which are common findings of pleomorphic adenoma [36]. According to proportions of malignant components, CXPA may have several appearances: (1) large pleomorphic adenoma, with no evidence of malignancy (Fig. 8.15), (2) pleomorphic adenoma with a focally aggressive appearance, and (3) entirely aggressive, with no remaining evidence of a pleomorphic adenoma (Fig. 8.16). DWI with ADC measurement may allow differentiation between malignant components and pleomorphic adenoma within CXPA [37].

8.15 Poorly Differentiated Carcinoma

According to the 4th edition of the WHO classification of head and neck tumors, poorly differentiated carcinoma (PDC) of salivary glands, characterized by higher clinical stage and poorer prognosis, includes undifferentiated carcinoma, large cell neuroendocrine carcinoma (LCNEC), and small cell neuroendocrine carcinoma (SmCC). These diagnoses can only be made following the exclusion of metastasis and other primary salivary gland tumors. Among patients with SmCC of salivary glands, the median age is 64 years. and there is a female predilection, with a female-to-male ratio of 2.4:1 [38]. Most tumors occur in the parotid gland, followed by the submandibular gland. Most patients present with painless masses which develop rapidly over several months; some patients experience facial nerve paralysis. Five-year overall survival rate for patients with SmCC is 37%; incidence of cervical lymph node involvement is over 50%, and that of distant metastasis is less than 45% [38].

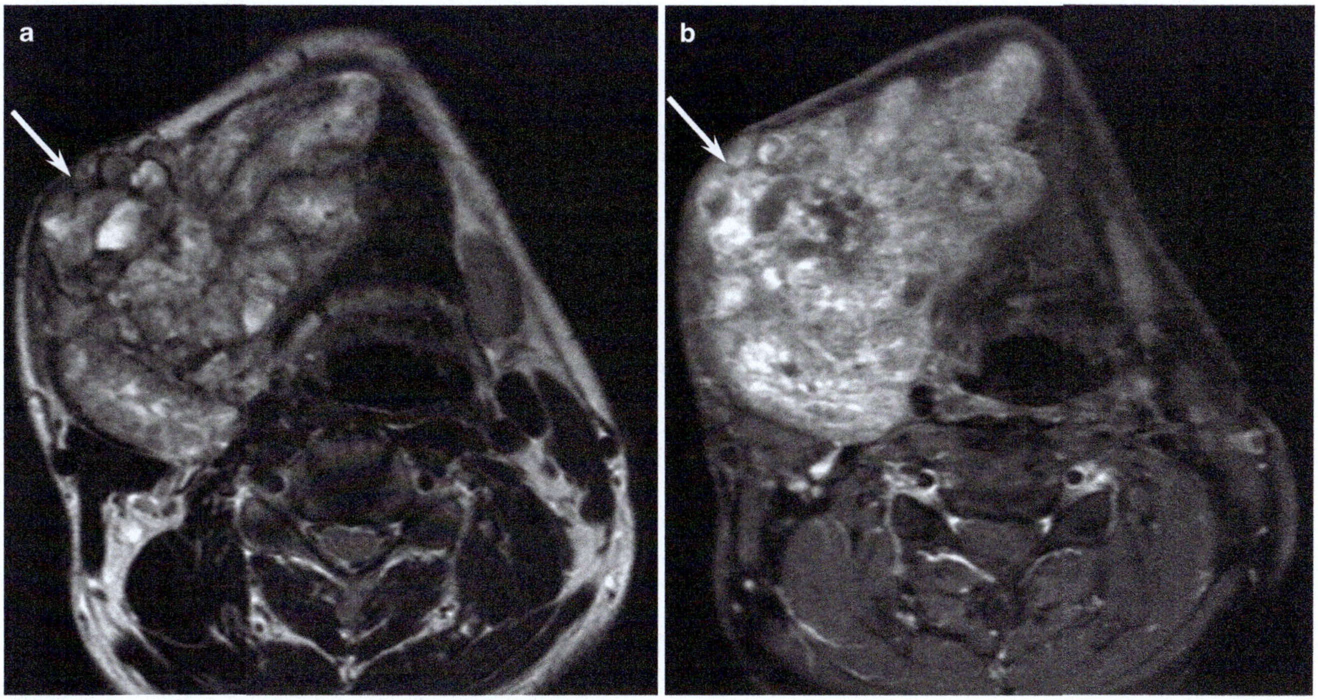

Fig. 8.16 A 58-year-old man with carcinoma ex pleomorphic adenoma of the right submandibular gland. (**a**) T2-weighted image shows a considerably heterogeneous lesion (arrow). (**b**) Fat-suppressed gadolinium-enhanced T1-weighted image shows a heterogeneously enhanced lesion (arrow) with ill-delineated tumor borders

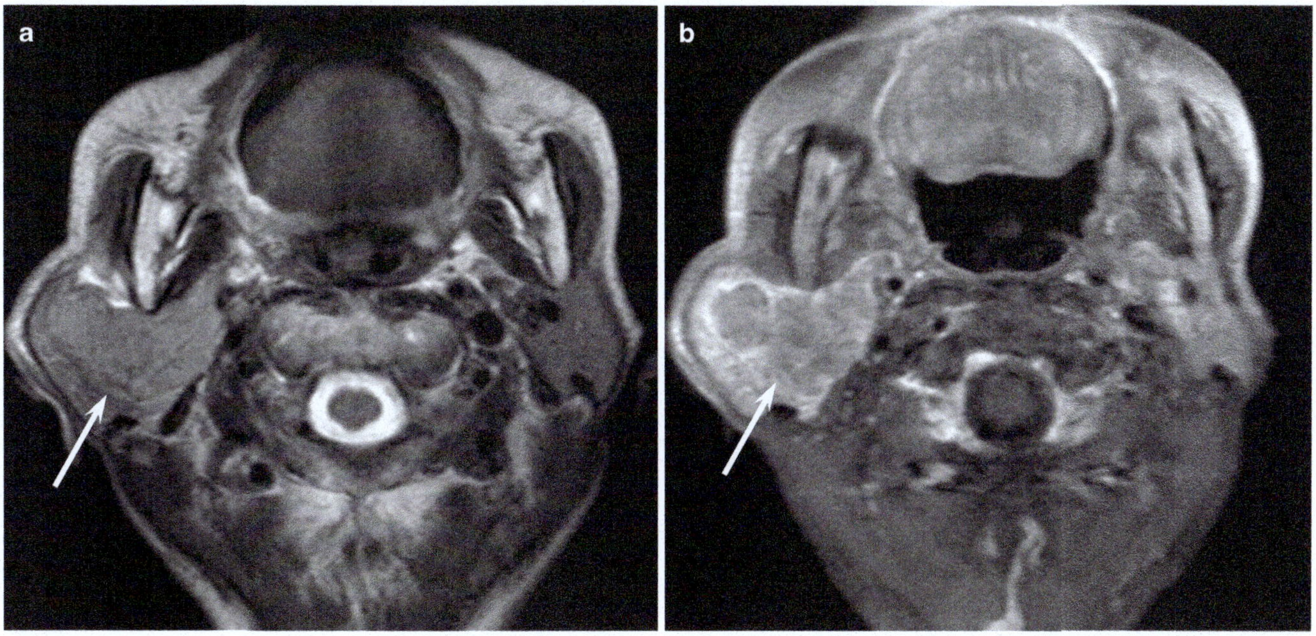

Fig. 8.17 A 84-year-old woman with small cell carcinoma of the right parotid gland. (**a**) T2-weighted image shows an ill-defined, homogeneously isointense lesion (arrow). (**b**) Fat-suppressed gadolinium-enhanced T1-weighted image shows a heterogeneously enhanced lesion (arrow) with ill-delineated tumor borders

Grossly, poorly defined firm masses can be observed. Microscopically, both LCNEC and SmCC are high-grade carcinomas, characterized by organoid cellular growth with minimal differentiation, high mitotic rates, and necrosis. Ill-defined margins accompanied by invasion into surrounding tissues are usually observed in high-grade neuroendocrine carcinoma.

Imaging features of PDC are nonspecific and consistent with those of high-grade malignancy with high tumor cellularity (Fig. 8.17). Relatively large tumors show invasive and destructive growth patterns, reflecting the aggressive nature of the tumor. As the tumor grows, extensive necrosis or hemorrhage can be seen within the tumor.

8.16 Summary

Although MRI can reveal pathological conditions, radiological differentiation of salivary gland tumors is difficult, especially between benign tumors and low-grade malignant tumors. However, radiologists may suggest high-grade malignancies associated with a poor prognosis when MRI demonstrates ill-defined margins with necrosis, hemorrhage, or invasion into surrounding tissue. In salivary gland cancers, MRI also plays an important role in the assessment of tumor extension for predicting prognosis.

References

1. Everson JW, Auclair P, Gnepp DR, Ei-Naggar AK. Tumours of the salivary glands: indroduction. In: Barnes L, Eveson JW, Reichart P, Sidransky D, editors. Pathology and genetics head and neck tumors. Lyon: IARC; 2005. p. 212–5.
2. Wong DS. Signs and symptoms of malignant parotid tumours: an objective assessment. J R Coll Surg Edinb. 2001;46(2):91–5.
3. Witt RL. Major salivary gland cancer. Surg Oncol Clin N Am. 2004;13(1):113–27.
4. WHO Classification of Tumours of the Salivary Glands. In: El-Naggar AK, JKC C, Grandis JR, Takata T, Slootweg PJ, editors. WHO classification of head and neck tumours. Lyon: IARC; 2017. p. 160.
5. Lydiatt WM, Mukherji SK, O'Sullivan B, Patel SG, Shah JP. Major salivary glands. In: Amin M, Edge S, Greene FL, Byrd D, Brookland R, editors. AJCC cancer staging manual. 8th ed. New York: Springer Nature; 2017. p. 95–101.
6. Yabuuchi H, Fukuya T, Tajima T, Hachitanda Y, Tomita K, Koga M. Salivary gland tumors: diagnostic value of gadolinium-enhanced dynamic MR imaging with histopathologic correlation. Radiology. 2003;226(2):345–54.
7. Motoori K, Yamamoto S, Ueda T, et al. Inter- and intratumoral variability in magnetic resonance imaging of pleomorphic adenoma: an attempt to interpret the variable magnetic resonance findings. J Comput Assist Tomogr. 2004;28(2):233–46.
8. Ikeda M, Motoori K, Hanazawa T, et al. Warthin tumor of the parotid gland: diagnostic value of MR imaging with histopathologic correlation. Am J Neuroradiol. 2004;25(7):1256–62.
9. Wang J, Takashima S, Takayama F, et al. Head and neck lesions: characterization with diffusion-weighted echo-planar MR imaging. Radiology. 2001;220(3):621–30.
10. Kato H, Kawaguchi M, Ando T, Mizuta K, Aoki M, Matsuo M. Pleomorphic adenoma of salivary glands: common and uncommon CT and MR imaging features. Jpn J Radiol. 2018;36(8):463–71.
11. Luna MA. Salivary mucoepidermoid carcinoma: revisited. Adv Anat Pathol. 2006;13(6):293–307.
12. Seethala RR, Stenman G. Update from the 4th edition of the World Health Organization classification of head and neck tumours: tumors of the salivary gland. Head Neck Pathol. 2017;11(1):55–67.
13. Okahara M, Kiyosue H, Hori Y, Matsumoto A, Mori H, Yokoyama S. Parotid tumors: MR imaging with pathological correlation. Eur Radiol. 2003;13(Suppl 4):L25–33.
14. Kashiwagi N, Dote K, Kawano K, et al. MRI findings of mucoepidermoid carcinoma of the parotid gland: correlation with pathological features. Br J Radiol. 2012;85(1014):709–13.
15. Spiro RH. Salivary neoplasms: overview of a 35-year experience with 2,807 patients. Head Neck Surg. 1986;8(3):177–84.
16. Szanto PA, Luna MA, Tortoledo ME, White RA. Histologic grading of adenoid cystic carcinoma of the salivary glands. Cancer. 1984;54(6):1062–9.
17. Sigal R, Monnet O, de Baere T, et al. Adenoid cystic carcinoma of the head and neck: evaluation with MR imaging and clinical-pathologic correlation in 27 patients. Radiology. 1992;184(1):95–101.
18. Caldemeyer KS, Mathews VP, Righi PD, Smith RR. Imaging features and clinical significance of perineural spread or extension of head and neck tumors. Radiographics. 1998;18(1):97–110; quiz 147.
19. Al-Zaher N, Obeid A, Al-Salam S, Al-Kayyali BS. Acinic cell carcinoma of the salivary glands: a literature review. Hematol Oncol Stem Cell Ther. 2009;2(1):259–64.
20. Lewis AG, Tong T, Maghami E. Diagnosis and management of malignant salivary gland tumors of the parotid gland. Otolaryngol Clin North Am. 2016;49(2):343–80.
21. Khalele BA. Systematic review of mammary analog secretory carcinoma of salivary glands at 7 years after description. Head Neck. 2017;39(6):1243–8.
22. Chiosea SI, Griffith C, Assaad A, Seethala RR. The profile of acinic cell carcinoma after recognition of mammary analog secretory carcinoma. Am J Surg Pathol. 2012;36(3):343–50.
23. Kashiwagi N, Nakatsuka SI, Murakami T, et al. MR imaging features of mammary analogue secretory carcinoma and acinic cell carcinoma of the salivary gland: a preliminary report. Dentomaxillofac Radiol. 2018;47(5):20170218.
24. Evans HL, Batsakis JG. Polymorphous low-grade adenocarcinoma of minor salivary glands. A study of 14 cases of a distinctive neoplasm. Cancer. 1984;53(4):935–42.
25. Vander Poorten V, Triantafyllou A, Skalova A, et al. Polymorphous adenocarcinoma of the salivary glands: reappraisal and update. Eur Arch Otorhinolaryngol. 2018;275(7):1681–95.
26. Haba R, Kobayashi S, Miki H, et al. Polymorphous low-grade adenocarcinoma of submandibular gland origin. Acta Pathol Jpn. 1993;43(12):774–8.
27. Gonzalez-Garcia R, Rodriguez-Campo FJ, Munoz-Guerra MF, Nam-Cha SH, Sastre-Perez J, Naval-Gias L. Polymorphous low-grade adenocarcinoma of the palate: report of cases. Auris Nasus Larynx. 2005;32(3):275–80.
28. Li J, Wang BY, Nelson M, et al. Salivary adenocarcinoma, not otherwise specified: a collection of orphans. Arch Pathol Lab Med. 2004;128(12):1385–94.
29. Gilbert MR, Sharma A, Schmitt NC, et al. A 20-year review of 75 cases of salivary duct carcinoma. JAMA Otolaryngol Head Neck Surg. 2016;142(5):489–95.
30. Kashiwagi N, Takashima S, Tomita Y, et al. Salivary duct carcinoma of the parotid gland: clinical and MR features in six patients. Br J Radiol. 2009;82(982):800–4.
31. Weon YC, Park SW, Kim HJ, et al. Salivary duct carcinomas: clinical and CT and MR imaging features in 20 patients. Neuroradiology. 2012;54(6):631–40.
32. Dimitrijevic MV, Tomanovic NR, Jesic SD, Arsovic NA, Mircic AL, Krstic AM. Epithelial-myoepithelial carcinoma—review of clinicopathological and immunohistochemical features. Arch Iran Med. 2015;18(4):218–22.
33. Silvers AR, Som PM, Brandwein M. Epithelial-myoepithelial carcinoma of the parotid gland. Am J Neuroradiol. 1996;17(3):560–2.
34. Takumi K, Fukukura Y, Kamiyama T, et al. Epithelial-myoepithelial carcinoma of the parotid gland: correlation of dynamic magnetic resonance imaging, (18)F-fluorodeoxyglucose-positron

emission tomography, and pathological findings. Jpn J Radiol. 2010;28(8):618–22.
35. Antony J, Gopalan V, Smith RA, Lam AK. Carcinoma ex pleomorphic adenoma: a comprehensive review of clinical, pathological and molecular data. Head Neck Pathol. 2012;6(1):1–9.
36. Kashiwagi N, Murakami T, Chikugo T, et al. Carcinoma ex pleomorphic adenoma of the parotid gland. Acta Radiol. 2012;53(3):303–6.
37. Kato H, Kanematsu M, Mizuta K, Ito Y, Hirose Y. Carcinoma ex pleomorphic adenoma of the parotid gland: radiologic-pathologic correlation with MR imaging including diffusion-weighted imaging. AJNR Am J Neuroradiol. 2008;29(5):865–7.
38. Servato JP, da Silva SJ, de Faria PR, Cardoso SV, Loyola AM. Small cell carcinoma of the salivary gland: a systematic literature review and two case reports. Int J Oral Maxillofac Surg. 2013;42(1):89–98.

9 Diagnostic Imaging of Perineural Spread

Anthony A. Mancuso

Abstract

Perineural invasion is one of the patterns of often clinically occult spread of head and neck cancer that can take malignancies far from the site of tumor origin and well beyond the limits of even the most skilled clinician's physical examination. Because of that, perineural spread substantially affects treatment planning and prognosis. These patterns were legacy knowledge observed and described by surgeons, radiotherapists, and pathologists long before the advent of modern imaging with CT and MRI. This manifestation of disease spread has now become routinely "visible" in the treatment planning phase of medical decision making in the last four decades. This chapter will explore factors related to pretreatment diagnostic and surveillance imaging with computed tomography (CT) and magnetic resonance imaging (MRI), which have contributed to an extraordinary, now decades long, outcome improvement in this difficult oncologic treatment scenario.

Keywords

Perineural · Cancer · CT · MRI · Diagnosis · Imaging

Perineural spread of head and neck cancer substantially affects treatment planning and prognosis. The clinical environment with regard to these impacts has changed vastly since first introduced to me by two pioneers in the management of this disease in the 1970s and 1980s. Paul Ward, Chairman of Otolaryngology and Head and Neck at UCLA, used to say, "Whenever I am operating on a patient with adenoid cystic carcinoma, I always know I am cutting across tumor." This represented a profound and realistic understanding of the reality confronting him and his predecessors with regard to the dilemma of perineural spread in the earlier days, of the modern era, and of head and neck cancer treatment. Rod Million, Chairman of Radiation Oncology at the University of Florida College of Medicine, in the 1980s used to routinely offer, at our weekly multidisciplinary Head and Neck Tumor Board, that (paraphrasing) … "perineural involvement is a nearly incurable safe haven for cancers" … when considering likelihood of ultimate disease control. These two "truths" of the past continue to remain partially true; however, there has been much progress in managing this spread pattern aspect of head and neck cancer, considerably lessening its negative impact on ultimate control rates alluded to by Dr. Million.

This chapter will explore factors related to pretreatment diagnostic and surveillance imaging with computed tomography (CT) and magnetic resonance imaging (MRI), which have contributed to an extraordinary, now decades long, outcome improvement in this difficult oncologic treatment scenario. Other pivotal factors contributing to better outcomes are the emergence of targeted, aggressive, radiation therapy techniques and advanced craniofacial/skull base surgery (now primarily endoscopic and much less morbid than in that past time) both substantially aided by diagnostic imaging and imaging guidance of these extraordinary surgical technical/skill advances. The improved outcomes are further facilitated by ever evolving chemotherapy and targeted immunotherapy options.

9.1 The Basics: Growth Along Nerves and Vessels (Perineural and Perivascular Spread)

The most basic contribution of modern diagnostic imaging in head and neck cancer imaging, beginning in the late 1970s with CT and continuing with ever improving capabilities

A. A. Mancuso (✉)
Department of Diagnostic Radiology, University of Florida College of Medicine and UF Health—Shands Hospital, Gainesville, FL, USA
e-mail: mancua@radiology.ufl.edu

H. Ojiri (ed.), *Diagnostic Imaging in Head and Neck Cancer*, https://doi.org/10.1007/978-981-15-3188-0_9

with MRI imaging in the 1980s, is the ability of these advanced imaging modalities to find disease spreading beyond the limits of the physical examination. This capability includes the currently most advanced endoscopic and physiologic testing procedures so that this spread, beneath intact mucosa, is not visible to the most skilled endoscopist. Such diagnostic imaging sometimes even leads to the initial diagnosis of a completely mucosally or otherwise in-apparent primary cancer presenting with a cranial neuropathy (Fig. 9.1). Because of this capability of modern imaging techniques, critical management options often depend primarily on imaging findings. Those imaging findings sometimes call for confirmation by the advantage of *imaging-guided* percutaneous biopsy, when alternative pathways of care, influenced by imaging findings, might critically impact treatment morbidity and/or outcome risk. Perineural invasion is one of these patterns of clinically occult disease spread that can take malignancies far from the site of tumor origin and well beyond the limits of even the most skilled clinician's physical examination (Fig. 9.2).

These infiltrative growth patterns, beyond visible mucosal disease, may follow neurovascular bundles. This is little different from actual "perineural" invasion (PNI) often used as a representative term for this mode of disease extension. Just as submucosal tumor spreads along muscle bundles, perineural/perineurovascular growth can lead to tumor extension quite remote from the site of primary origin (Fig. 9.2). The

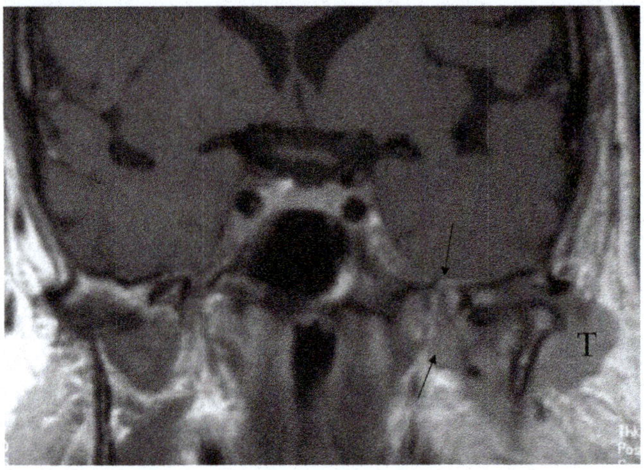

Fig. 9.1 A patient with over a year of chronic, progressive facial pain with a working diagnosis of trigeminal neuralgia. The patient also eventually developed facial weakness. Recent prior outside imaging with both CT and MRI interpreted as negative. The otherwise occult (non-palpable) primary cancer in the left parotid gland (T) spread along the auriculotemporal nerve within the masticator space to access the mandibular division of the trigeminal nerve to spread as far proximally as the foramen ovale/trigeminal ganglion (arrows)

nerves/neurovascular bundles involved can be thought of as spokes extending peripherally from the hub of the primary site. The actual nerves/vessels involved depend largely on that primary site of origin.

For example, mucosal origin head and neck cancers may spread along the carotid sheath (Fig. 9.3), distal maxillary and palatine (Fig. 9.4) neurovascular bundles, and the branches of maxillary division of the trigeminal nerve. A final common pathway of several of these patterns is to the central skull base at the pterygopalatine fossa and, eventually, to the trigeminal ganglion with continued proximal intracranial spread along the trigeminal nerve (Fig. 9.4) possible. Alternatively, mucosal or, occasionally, other origin cancers may access V3 by way of the lingual and inferior alveolar nerve and reach the trigeminal ganglion by way of the foramen ovale (Fig. 9.2). Distal involvement ultimately follows these conduits both centrally and farther distally, both affecting treatment planning. Spread along the carotid sheath eventually invades the jugular fossa and/or carotid canal (Fig. 9.3) and those of the trigeminal branches to the trigeminal cistern nerve rootlets and beyond. Alternatively, perineural spread in parotid cancers and cutaneous malignancies follow branches of the cranial nerves V (most commonly the auriculotemporal nerve) and VII from their most distal ramifications (deep to and within the superficial aponeurotic system of the face) to as far proximally as the brainstem (Fig. 9.1). Moreover, there are situations where these nerves may communicate with one another as happens between the facial and trigeminal nerve by way of the greater superficial petrosal nerve along the petrous ridge and the facial and auriculotemporal nerve deep in the substance of the parotid gland (Fig. 9.5). Multiple cranial neuropathies herald intracranial disease either in the paracavernous region or orbital apex or disseminated meningeal disease or neurotrophic lymphoma.

9.2 Imaging Structural Manifestations

Spread of tumor within or around nerves is sometimes described as growth in "perineural lymphatics." In fact, experimental and autopsy studies demonstrate that the only lymphatic spaces related to peripheral nerves are in the epineurium. The epineurium is a layer of loose areolar tissue surrounding nerve fascicles that contains the vasa vasorum and lymphatics. The perineurium and endoneurium contain no lymphatics. Since tumor may be found in the epi-, peri-, and endoneurium, the term "perineural spread" or "perineural invasion/involvement" (PNI) related to imaging studies should be used generically to describe spread along cranial

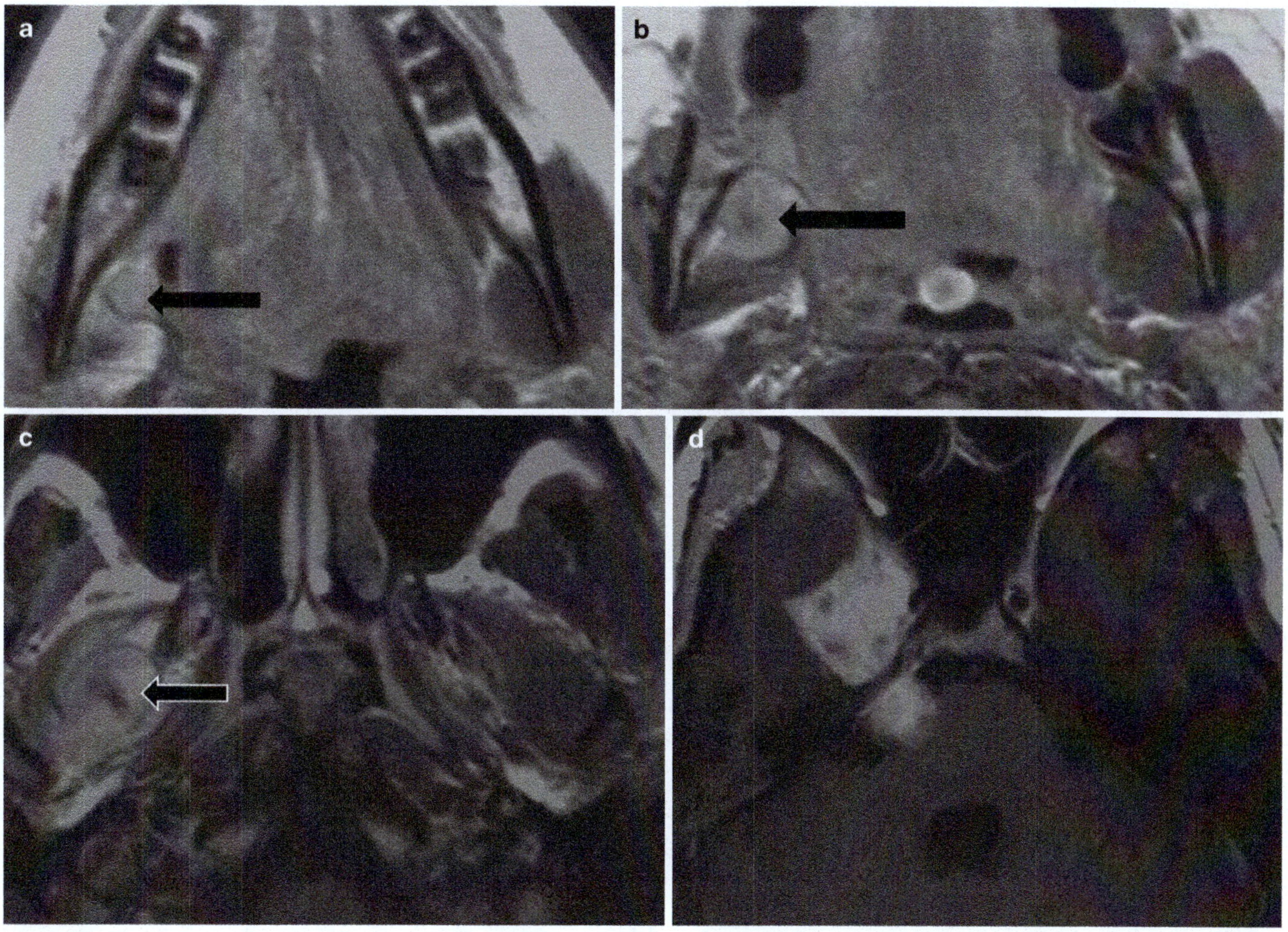

Fig. 9.2 A 12-year-old male presented with a fullness in the right floor of the mouth. (**a**) The infiltrating mass in the floor of the mouth spreads to the adjacent lingual nerve (black arrow). Note that the medial pterygoid muscle on the right is partially atrophic compared to the left side. (**b**) Continued, clinically occult spread along the lingual nerve on the right (black arrow). (**c**) Perineural spread to the third division of the trigeminal nerve within the masticator space and atrophy of the surrounding pterygoid muscle group as a secondary change (black arrow). (**d**) The perineural spread became transcranial along the third division of the trigeminal nerve and then following the trigeminal nerve beneath the petroclival ligament to its root entry zone. Note: The biopsy of the floor of the mouth mass revealed rhabdomyosarcoma. None of the perineural spread was suspected, and these imaging findings markedly altered the original plan for gross total resection as a primary treatment consideration

and peripheral nerves, realizing that the tumor may be in any of the layers within and outside the nerve. Disseminated intracranial disease may be with the cranial nerve (truly neurotrophic) and/or leptomeningeal as a corollary pattern.

On CT and MR, perineural spread is often manifest by obliteration of the tissue (fat) planes around the neurovascular structures in question. Prime examples of fat planes of interest more centrally (at the skull base) are those below the stylomastoid foramen (Fig. 9.5c) and within the pterygomaxillary fossa (Fig. 9.4). More peripherally, loss of tissue (fat) containing planes around the distal infraorbital nerves deep to the superficial musculoaponeurotic system (SMAS) of the face is a reliable indicator of more distal pathologic perineural spread of cancer (Fig. 9.6).

Enlargement and/or abnormal enhancement of the nerves (Figs. 9.1, 9.2, 9.3, 9.4 and 9.5), erosion of the bone forming their exit foramen (Figs. 9.3 and 9.4), and abnormal meningeal enhancement (Fig. 9.7) are other important primary and secondary signs of perineural spread of a benign or, in our case, malignant tumor. These findings may appear "subtle" unless anticipated based on knowledge of the natural history and tendency of these disease patterns as summarized here (Fig. 9.8). These patterns are legacy knowledge observed and described by surgeons, radiotherapists, and pathologists long before the advent of modern imaging with CT and MRI. This manifestation of disease spread has now become routinely "visible" in the treatment planning phase of medical decision making in the last four decades. Careful comparison to the

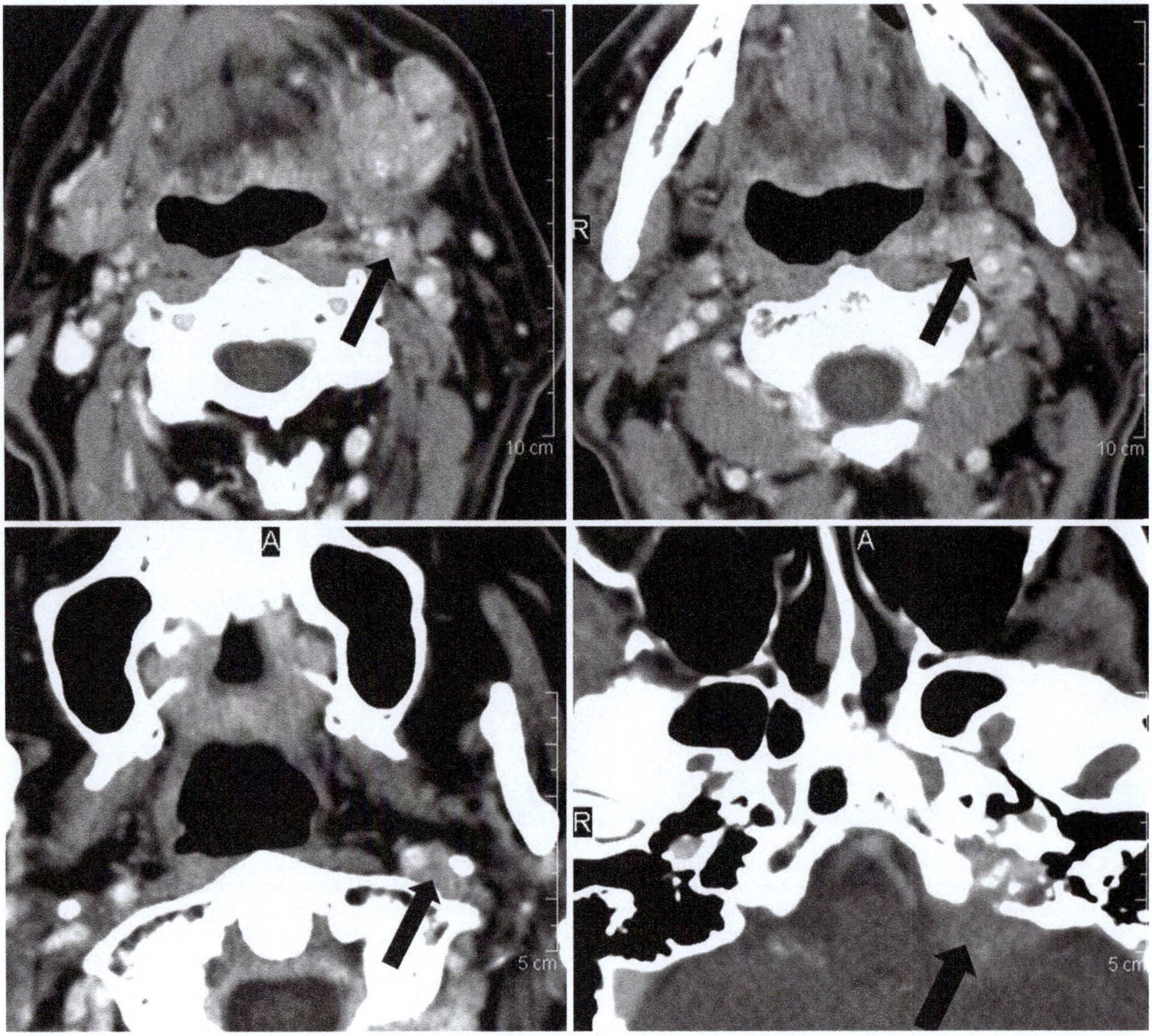

Fig. 9.3 A patient with adenocarcinoma of the left submandibular gland with related level IB lymphadenopathy. Cancer spreads from the primary along the external carotid artery by way of sympathetic nerves (black arrow—upper left); (upper right—black arrow) spread of tumor encases the carotid sheath and continues along the carotid sheath (lower left—black arrow) to finally invade the skull base by way of the jugular fossa with intracranial intradural spread (lower right—black arrow). Note: None of the perineural extension was anticipated the time of the original clinical diagnosis. These imaging findings significantly altered the treatment plan and substantially worsened prognosis

same structures on the uninvolved side is important for detecting subtle change. An awareness of the possibility of such spread in a particular tumor type and/or given primary site and the patient's signs and symptoms combined with anatomic knowledge sufficient for a complete search are all factors important to accurate diagnosis.

Contrast-enhanced MRI (CEMR) is capable of showing perineural spread better than contrast-enhanced computer tomography (CECT) in many patients, especially near and within skull base. A critical factor in the superior rendering of CEMR is that most of the cranial nerves, and their major divisions, are surrounded by a plexus of vessels as they pass through their related bony canals and exit foramina. The resulting perineural enhancement, which is often asymmetric, is a normal variation (Fig. 9.8) that should not be mistaken as a reliable predictor of PNI. The diagnosis of perineural tumor spread on MR and/or CT can be identified as enhancement of the normal size nerve itself or such enhancement combined with nerve enlargement. Enhancement of a nerve can also be due to inflammation and for that reason is a nonspecific imaging finding outside of the diagnostic context of known presence or suspected recurrence of anatomically appropriate primary carcinoma, sarcoma, or lymphoma.

Nerve dysfunction does not necessarily imply invasion. Adjacent tumor can compress nerves while not directly invading them. An interesting example is compression of the lower cranial nerves by enlarged retropharyngeal nodes in nasopharyngeal carcinoma. Compressive nerve deficits may resolve following radiotherapy, whereas nerves

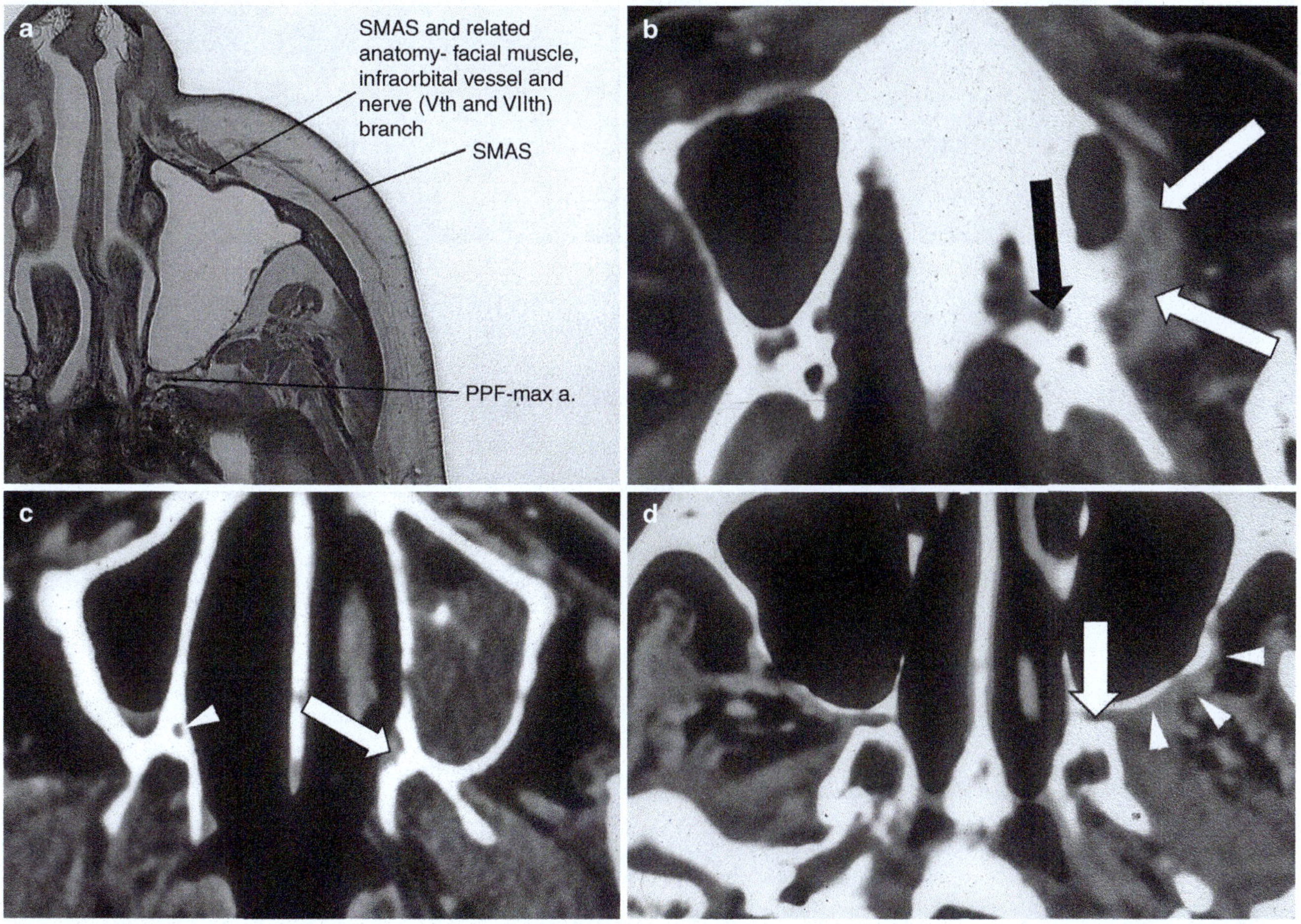

Fig. 9.4 A patient with cancer of the maxillary sinus infrastructure at its junction with the posterior hard palate. (**a**) Anatomic whole organ section, in this case showing the relationship of the posterior superior alveolar vessels and eventual termination of the greater and lesser palatine neurovascular bundles in the pterygopalatine fossa. It also illustrates the relationship between the SMAS layer and distal branches of the maxillary division of the trigeminal nerve; a relationship to be noted in conjunction with illustrative cases that follow. (**b**) Buccal space invasion (white arrows) creates access to the posterior superior alveolar neurovascular bundles. The greater and lesser palatine neurovascular bundles are similarly accessed at opening of the eroded, enlarged greater and lesser palatine distal neural canal (black arrow). (**c**) Shows continued spread along the greater and lesser palatine neural canal on the left side (white arrow) compared to the normal appearance (white arrowhead) on the uninvolved side confirming the CT evidence of involvement of the that neurovascular channel. (**d**) Continued cephalad spread occurs along the posterior superior alveolar neurovascular bundle (arrowheads) as well as the palatine neurovascular bundles reaches the pterygopalatine fossa (arrow). (**e**) Continued cephalad spread in the retroantral fat pad and pterygopalatine fossa to the infraorbital fissure on the left side (arrow) manifest as obliteration of the fat in that area compared to the normal right side (arrowhead). (**f**) CT erosion of the foramen rotundum manifests mainly as thinning of its border (smaller white arrow) with the sphenoid sinus (larger white arrow arrow) compared to the mesial cortex of the foramen rotundum (arrowhead) on the normal side. (**g**) CEMR was done to determine the proximal extent of spread. This coronal post-contrast T1-weighted image confirms spread to the trigeminal ganglion (arrowhead) and second division of the trigeminal nerve (arrow) confirming the CT evidence of involvement of the foramen rotundum and second division of the trigeminal nerve when compared to these structures on the normal side (black arrows)

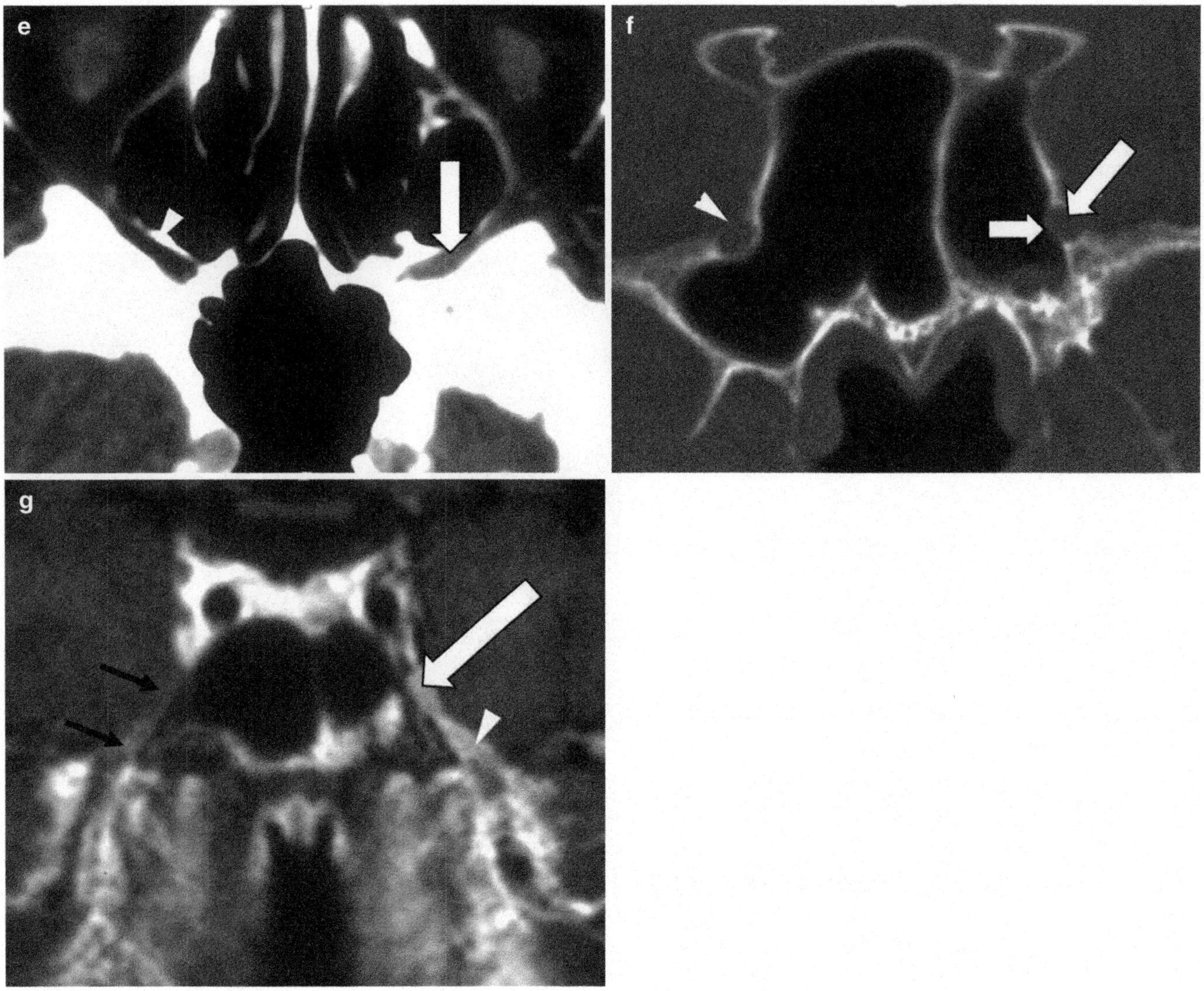

Fig. 9.4 (continued)

invaded by tumor may not recover function so readily following radiotherapy, and in fact, such disease is difficult to control with radiotherapy. Compression by benign tumors is probably more likely to resolve than that caused by a malignant tumor. Atrophy of the end organs/structures such as muscles of the masticator space or of facial expression within SMAS and related long-term paralysis will usually not recover.

9.3 Two General Clinical Scenarios

9.3.1 Skin Cancer

Skin cancer presents typically as a slow-growing mass of the skin or just beneath the skin surface. Paresthesias and formications, a crawling feeling under the skin, suggest perineural spread. This can be an initial presenting complaint but is far more common as a symptom of cranial neuropathy in the recurrent disease setting. A more overt cranial neuropathy may be evident. Clinical diagnosis of recurrent skin cancer in this setting may be delayed because the treating physicians do not associate the history of skin cancer with signs of trigeminal or facial nerve dysfunction. Moreover, the patient may not offer the history of a treated skin cancer or may not even be aware that a treated skin lesion was cancer (Fig. 9.9). Such cases often come to imaging with a clinical suspicion of "trigeminal neuralgia" or atypical facial pain. Failure to recognize the typical patterns of perineural recurrence in this setting is not uncommon and, unfortunately, can lead to substantial delay in confirmation of recurrence. Such

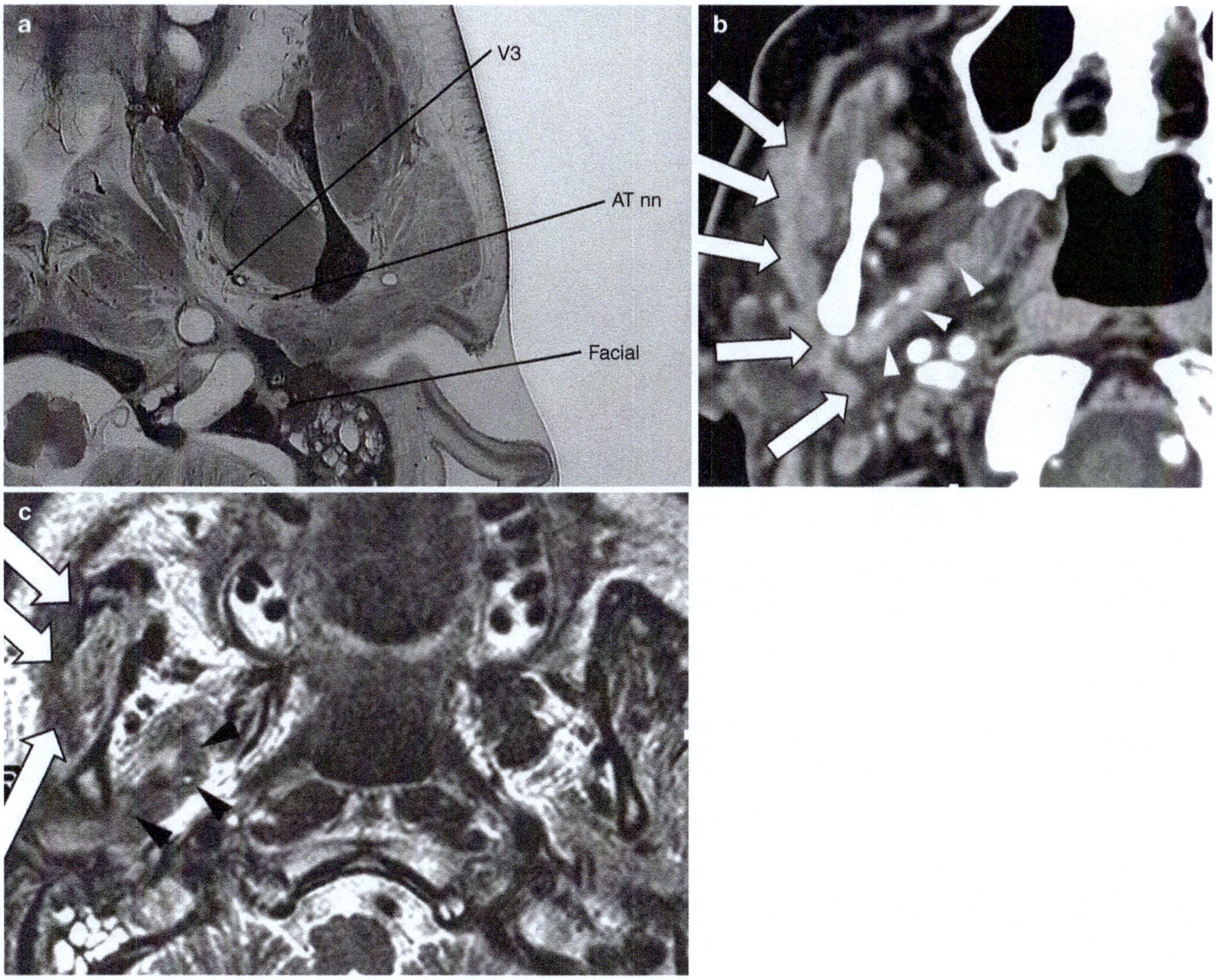

Fig. 9.5 Adult patient reports that presenting with what was called "Bell's palsy"; however, in reality the symptoms were chronic and progressive loss of facial nerve function. Careful history also showed evidence of progressive right-sided facial pain. Prior outside CT and MR studies read over several months interpreted as normal. (**a**) Anatomic whole organ section demonstrating pertinent anatomic relationships between the auriculotemporal nerve (ATn), third (mandibular) division of the trigeminal nerve (V3), and the facial nerve, at this level, within the fat pad below the stylomastoid foramen (facial). (**b**) CECT chosen infiltrating mass within the parotid gland along the expected course of the facial nerve which tracks around the posterior aspect of the mandibular on the along the expected course of the auriculotemporal nerve (arrows) to involve the third division of the trigeminal nerve (arrowheads). This spread pattern should be correlated with the anatomy shown in **a**. (**c**) T2-weighted MRI image showing the extent of the facial nerve and auriculotemporal/V3 spread as correlated to **b** (arrows and arrowheads). The equivalency of signal in the infiltrating tumor to that of muscle is unusual for epithelial malignancies, and this was eventually proven to be a primary neurofibrosarcoma of the facial nerve

delay allows the disease to extend more proximally and increase in volume, both factors considerably increasing the morbidity of radiotherapy and adjunctive treatments and clearly worsening the chances of ultimate control of disease.

Other factors may also contribute to advanced disease at the time of initial imaging. Patient neglect can also lead to advanced lesions with perineural spread at presentation. Less well-differentiated squamous cell cancers and melanoma may also demonstrate a biologic predisposition to being "neurotrophic."

In skin cancer, a systematic search of the most peripheral ramifications of the trigeminal and facial nerve to the brain stem is required. More specific conduits relate to the site of origin of the primary. The common pathways include the following:

1. Forehead—V1 branches to supraorbital notch, orbital apex (Fig. 9.10).
2. Midface—V2 branches to infraorbital canal to pterygopalatine fossa to foramen rotundum (Figs. 9.4, 9.6, and 9.8).

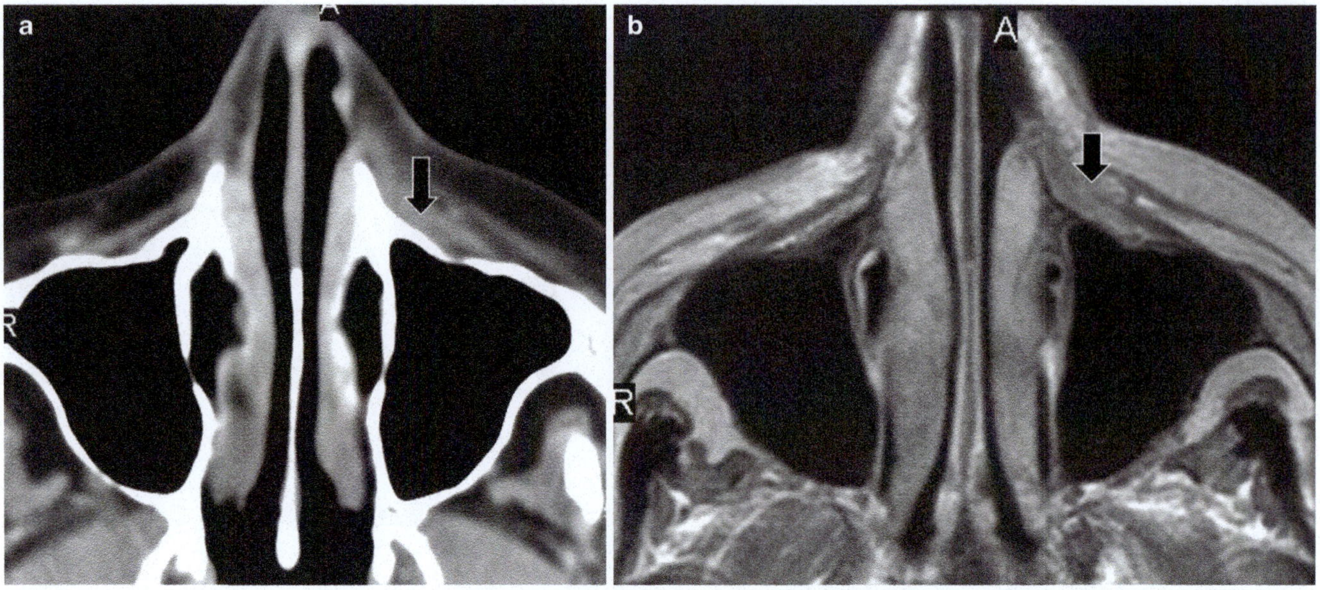

Fig. 9.6 A patient with prior history of treated skin cancer on the left cheek. Patient had slowly progressive facial pain and formications in the distribution of the maxillary division of the left trigeminal nerve present for 2 years. The working clinical diagnosis was trigeminal neuralgia. Repeated outside CT and MR studies shown here were read as normal over that timeframe. (**a**) CT study shows infiltration of the fat pad between the anterior wall of the maxillary sinus and SMAS on the left side compared to the right (arrow). (**b**) A subsequent MRI study, also interpreted as negative, shows similar infiltration of that fat pad (arrow) with mesial extension of the abnormal enhancement to surround the distal infraorbital neurovascular structures. Note: These images should be compared with the normal appearance of these anatomic relationships shown in Fig. 9.4a

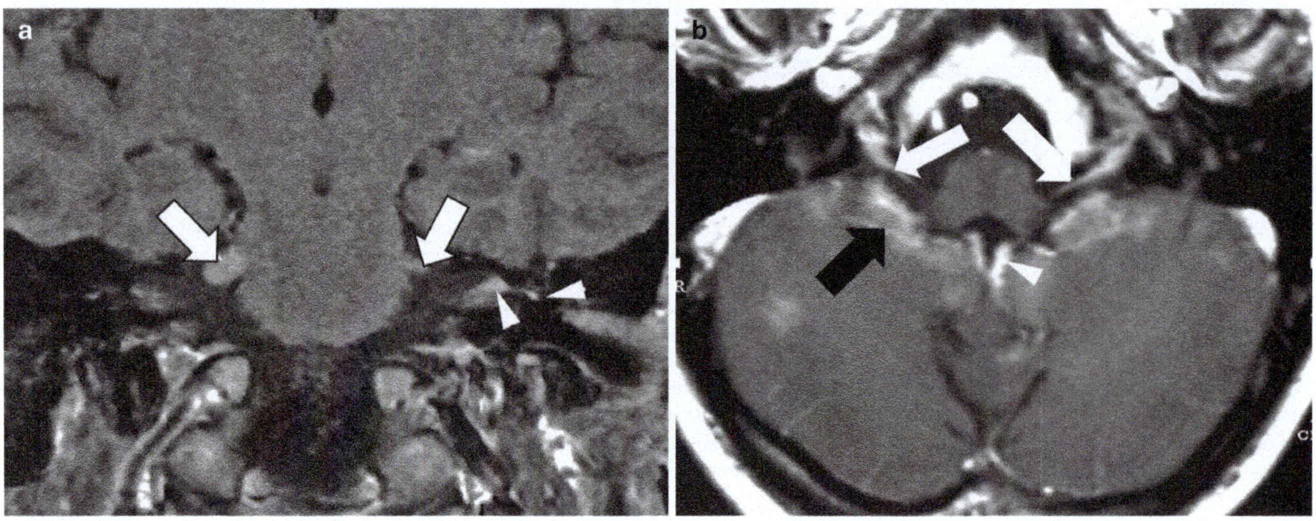

Fig. 9.7 Two patterns of intracranial expression of spread along cranial nerves in two different patients with disseminated lymphoma. (**a**) Neurotrophic lymphoma infiltrates the trigeminal nerves bilaterally (arrows) and involves the seventh and eighth nerves within the left internal auditory canal (arrowheads). (**b**) Leptomeningeal disseminated lymphoma surrounds lower cranial nerves entering the jugular fossa (white arrows), spreads along the ependymal of the fourth ventricle (white arrowhead), and spreads along the pia-arachnoid to involve the cerebellum (black arrow)

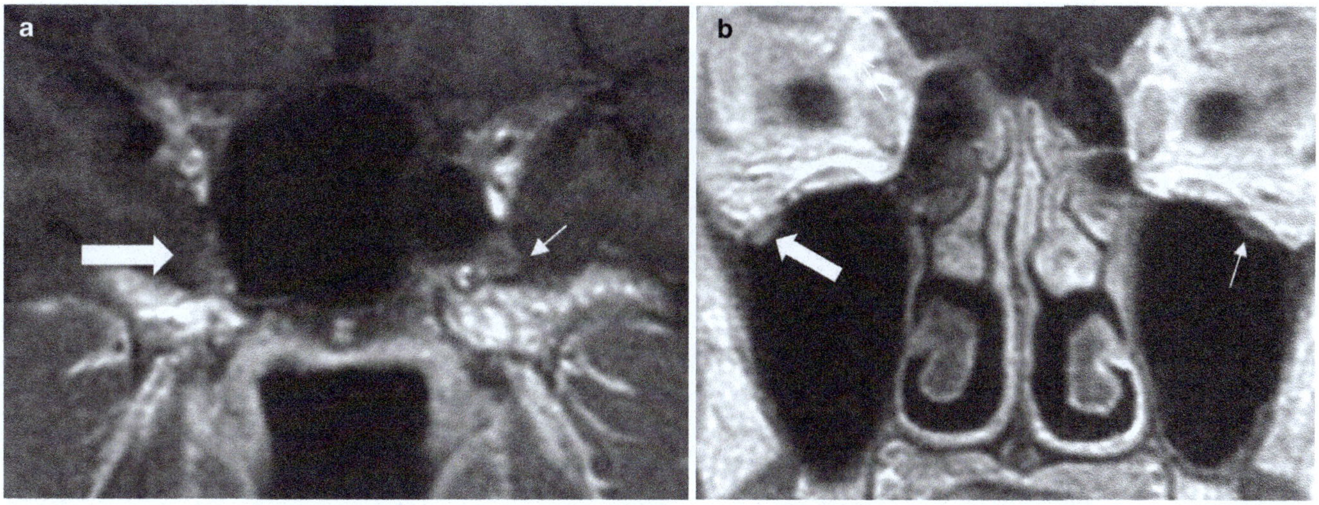

Fig. 9.8 A patient with skin cancer and minor symptoms suggestive of maxillary division trigeminal neuropathy on the right. (**a**) The infraorbital nerve is relatively subtly enlarged and enhances abnormally (large white arrow) compared to the opposite side (small white arrow). (**b**) There is subtle abnormality of the maxillary division of the trigeminal nerve on the right side manifest as irregular enhancement and in distinctness (large white arrow) especially when compared to the normal configuration of the maxillary division on the left with a central non-enhancing nerve surrounded by a normal vascular plexus (small white arrow). Note: This case emphasizes the importance of observation of relatively subtle findings by way of understanding normal anatomic variance and comparing side to side especially in patients with high risk and symptoms even when those symptoms are relatively subtle. Also, it shows the capacity for potential "skip" abnormalities that may be detected by imaging and assure more accurate planning of tumor volume and dosing schedules avoid recurrence related to under dosing of proximal spread of perineural disease

3. Periauricular—V3 in masticator space by way of the auriculotemporal nerve to foramen ovale and facial nerve proximally to stylomastoid foramen course through the facial canal segments to the IAC and peripherally along the trunk and facial nerve branches in the parotid and eventually to and along SMAS (Figs. 9.1, 9.2, 9.5 and 9.9).

The final common pathway for the trigeminal patterns is to the paracavernous region, trigeminal cistern nerve rootlets, and then the trigeminal nerve itself to the pons. Facial nerve spread does not typically go beyond the IAC. Leptomeningeal and dural dissemination is unusual (Fig. 9.9).

9.3.2 Mucosal Origin Cancers and/or Those with Known Neurotrophic Tendencies

A very prevalent failure pattern in mucosal origin head and neck cancers observed by treating clinicians and pathologists in the "pre-advanced imaging" past has been along the cranial nerves. An additional logical observation reported by them was that the involved cranial nerve, at the sites of recurrence, was the main nerves innervating the original primary tumor as well as the major adjacent communicating nerves. This experience, thereby, identified predictable pretreatment disease spread patterns along the cranial nerves innervating the primary mucosal site. In aggregate, this legacy knowledge emphasized the now common awareness that these patterns must to be taken into account when defining clinical target volumes (CTV) for RT treatment planning.

For example, all adenoid cystic carcinomas should be presumed to have a predictable perineural spread risk based on the primary site and site of origin (Fig. 9.1). However, any other adenocarcinoma, all squamous cell mucosal origin cancers, and mucosa-associated lymphoma can follow this particular tendency for path of spread so that assessment of at-risk areas of perineural spread is dominantly dependent on the primary site of origin. In the recurrent setting, when there has been a vascularized free flap reconstruction, one must also consider the possibility of similar patterns of recurrence along the free flap vascular pedicle. In this era of routine posttreatment surveillance, imaging strategies and interpretation must be inclusive of planning and awareness that both the standard, generally predicable, patterns of perineural recurrence and patterns related to the flap construct are possible and might impact potential salvage therapy options.

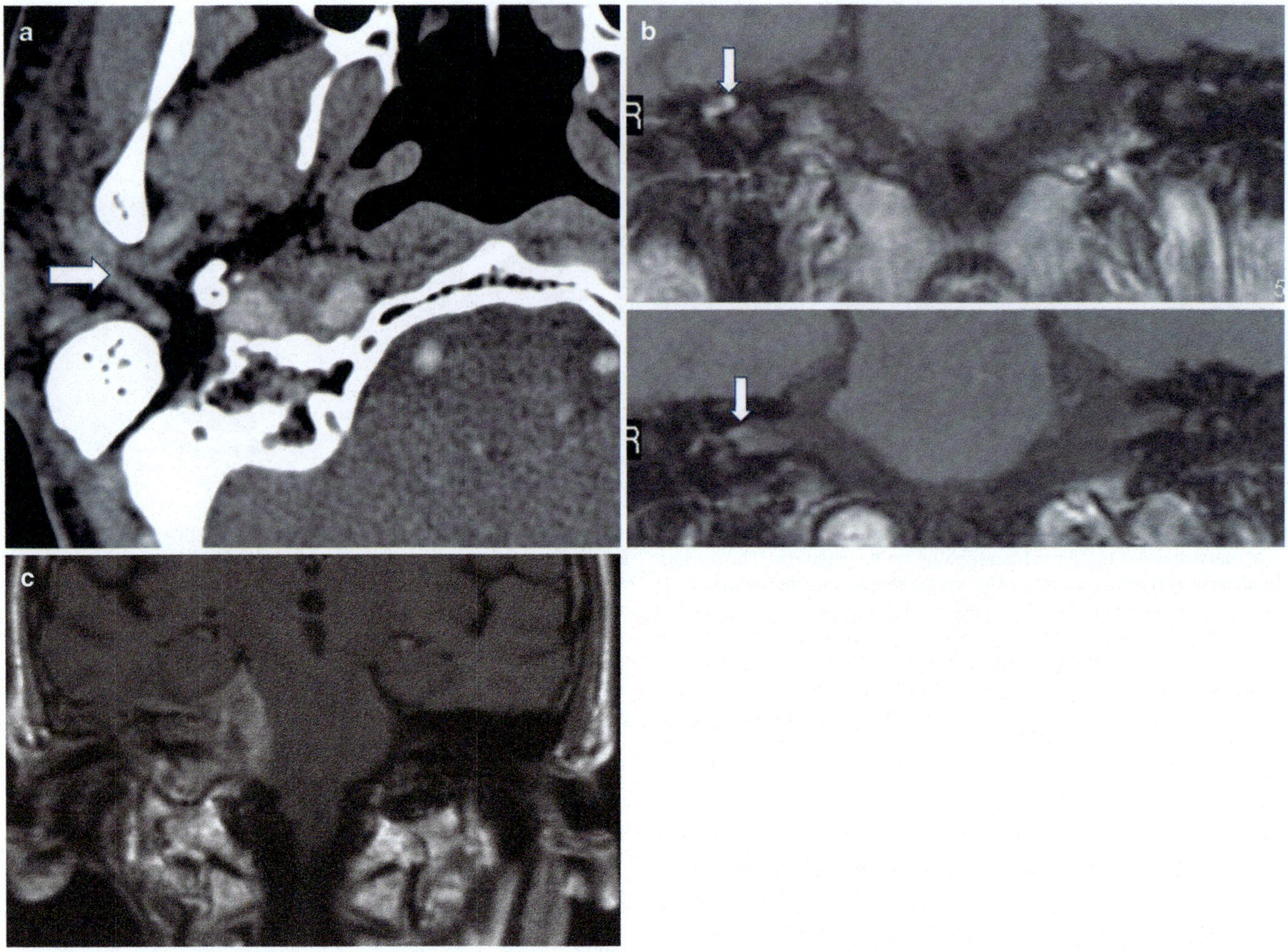

Fig. 9.9 A patient with prior history of treated skin cancer on the right periauricular region. "Bell's palsy" was the working diagnosis over several years in spite of chronic and progressive loss of facial nerve function. The first two studies shown in **a** and **b** were read as normal originally. (**a**) There is abnormal thickening of the facial nerve where it enters the parotid gland (white arrow). This abnormal thickening extends from the fat pad below the stylomastoid foramen into the substance of the parotid gland with subtle evidence of involvement of the adjacent auriculotemporal nerve. Study was interpreted as normal. (**b**) A CEMR was performed about 1 year later for persistent symptoms. The abnormal enhancement of the facial nerve at the first genu and in the fundus of the internal auditory canal (white arrows) was interpreted as normal even though it was very substantially different from the opposite side in a patient with progressive facial nerve weakness. (**c**) A CEMR was performed another year later for persistent, progressive symptoms. That study showed extensive progression to widely involve the temporal bone, adjacent dura, and perineural spread from the IAC to the surface of the brainstem

The diagnostic imager must then design a protocol for each tumor site of origin as well as for surveillance imaging that will cover the pathways of the neurovascular bundles known to pass near or through the area of involvement. This may include something as obvious as a detailed study of the course of the facial nerve through the temporal bone in parotid cancers and, perhaps less obviously, a detailed study of the course of the greater and lesser palatine nerves to the pterygopalatine fossa in hard and soft palate cancers. Properly focused imaging studies can profoundly influence treatment plans in patients with perineural cancer spread and produce improved outcomes. Inattention to such focused imaging will negatively impact outcome. Specific comprehensive protocols for each site are available in other resources.

9.4 Imaging Modalities

Both CT and MRI can detect perineural spread (Figs. 9.1, 9.2, 9.3, 9.4, 9.5, 9.6, 9.7, 9.8, 9.9 and 9.10). Findings may be subtle on either exam. CT can be used for screening, but MRI is more definitive as the disease becomes more proximal to the central nervous system. This makes MRI often the most definitive exam for establishing the full extent of imaging detectable disease. MRI also most confidently confirms, when the MRI study is negative, that the perineural disease, confirmed in a relevant tissue sample, is only microscopic and properly classified as subclinical. A "subclinical" designation of perineural disease also requires the patient to be asymptomatic for a cranial neuropathy. This is an important

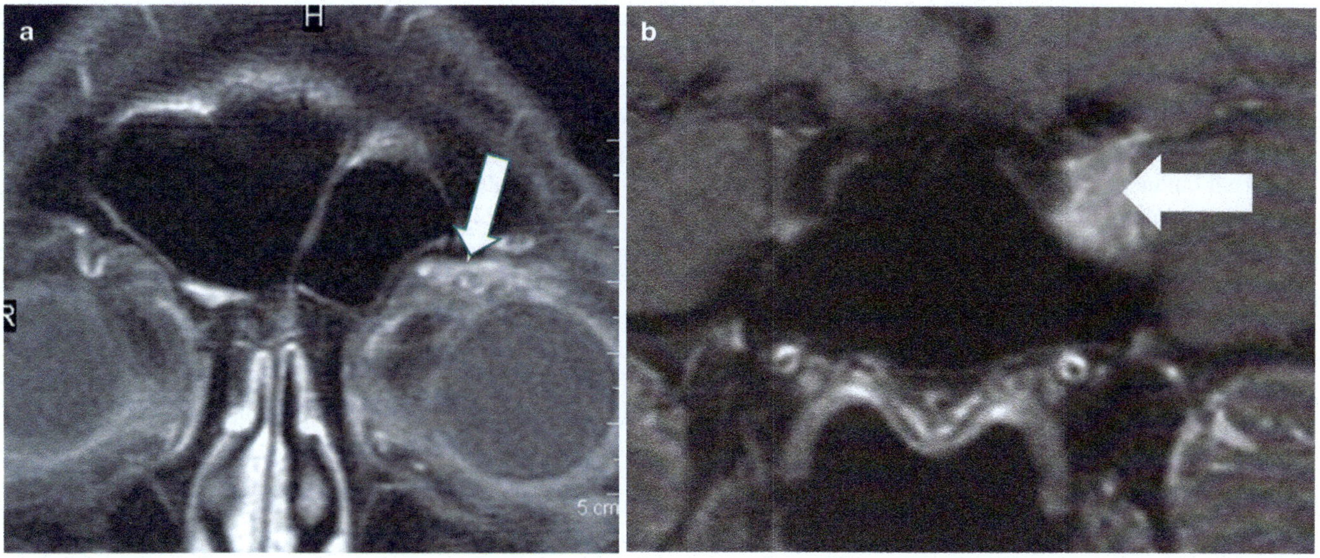

Fig. 9.10 A patient with previously removed left forehead skin cancer and abnormal sensation in the distribution of the ophthalmic division of the trigeminal nerve. (**a**) Fat-suppressed, contrast-enhanced T1-weighted MR coronal image shows infiltration of the fat pad around the supraorbital neurovascular bundle (white arrow). (**b**) Fat-suppressed, contrast-enhanced T1-weighted MR coronal image at the orbital apex shows infiltration of the orbital apex junction with the anterior aspect of the cavernous and para-cavernous region (white arrow)

consideration both with regard to treatment planning and prognosis. Subclinical disease has a substantially better prognosis and often will require less risky and less morbid treatment plans. If tumor fails to enlarge the nerve and/or causes it to enhance abnormally, microscopic spread remains possible with its lesser prognostic and treatment planning implications.

Enlargement and enhancement of inflamed nerves such as is present in viral neuropathies can mimic tumor involvement so that the clinical context of a presenting cranial neuropathy is all important. Infrequently, cancers will initially present even as an acute or subacute cranial neuropathy as might some recurrences. The nonspecificity of positive findings for perineural structural abnormality being present must always be kept in mind as well as in context.

False-positive readings of perineural disease are also to be avoided. A rich vascular plexus accompanies the cranial nerves as they near and course through their exit foramina and often beyond. Such normal perineural enhancement must not be misdiagnosed as an abnormality possibly due to perineural tumor.

9.5 General Treatment Implications

PNI may be incidental or clinical. Incidental PNI is defined as occurring in asymptomatic patients with microscopic invasion of the nerve detected only by histopathology. Clinical PNI includes patients with cranial neuropathy (usually CN V or VII) on physical examination and/or imaging evidence of tumor involvement along the tract of a nerve. Diagnostic imaging, with focused CEMR and CECT, is used to detect and define the extent of PNI. Imaging positive PNI is unusual in a totally symptomatic patient. The presence of PNI also increases the risk of metastases to the regional lymph nodes.

Patients with incidental PNI are most often treated with wide local excision of the primary lesion before the diagnosis is established histologically, and they then typically receive postoperative radiotherapy (RT). Patients with completely resectable clinical PNI typically undergo surgery followed by postoperative RT to reduce the risk of local-regional recurrence. Patients with incompletely resectable clinical PNI cancers are treated with definitive RT. It is the last two circumstances that imaging findings are often treatment choice determinant. The RT clinical target volume (CTV) must cover demonstrable disease of the involved nerve to the base of skull and cavernous sinus. Anticipated subclinical (imaging undetectable) disease beyond that point must also be taken into account. Concurrent chemotherapy may be added, and clinically negative regional lymph nodes should also be electively treated to avoid the substantial risk of subclinical nodal disease.

CEMR, often complementing an initial diagnostic CECT, is generally accepted as essential to the workup of a patient with suspected clinical PNI. MRI is used to detect and define the most proximal extent of PNI since it is often associated with "skip" lesions along the nerve. Such "skip" behavior significantly increases the risk of a recurrence after resection even if negative margins are obtained on surgical pathology. CT may show distal spread more graphically since it can be performed with 1 mm thick sections and in that way as a more definitive spatial resolution with regard to distal pathways of spread. This spatial resolution advantages further enhanced by the distal course of these nerves being typically surrounded by fat and providing suitable contrast resolution.

For all cutaneous squamous cell and basal cell carcinomas, a combination of CT and MRI examination might be necessary to assess the full proximal and distal extent of perineural disease patients with signs and symptoms suggesting perineural spread with a cutaneous lesion located in the corresponding CN distribution. Such an approach may also be necessary in cutaneous lesions when there is histopathological evidence of PNI. A similar combined approach is frequently necessary for mucosal and other common malignancies such as parotid cancer, with a similar risk profile for PNI, as well as for surveillance protocols. MRI is used in the surveillance setting to determine the proximal extent of known treated PNI when there is a reasonable salvage option for treatment of recurrence.

Symptomatic but imaging-negative PNI has a relatively good prognosis after receiving definitive RT alone or combined with surgery. Imaging-positive minimal or moderate volume, peripheral disease has a better local control rate than higher volume more central spread. However, there is a similar survival rate when relatively peripheral, lower volume PNI is compared to patients with more central higher volume disease on pretreatment imaging studies.

10 PET in the Diagnosis of Head and Neck Cancer

Tetsuro Sekine

Abstract

In current clinical practice, the standard approach for initial assessment of head and neck cancer (HNC) is clinical examination followed by neck ultrasound, computed tomography (CT), and magnetic resonance imaging (MRI). Compared with these modalities, fluorodeoxyglucose (FDG)-positron emission tomography (PET) may provide unique information about metabolic characteristics. The abnormal elevation of FDG uptake has been shown to be specifically induced in tumor cells because of its low rate of dephosphorylation. Based on this theory, FDG-PET can be used to detect malignant lesions, differentiate benign from malignant lymph nodes (LNs), detect the primary site of unknown primary tumors, plan radiation therapy, and detect tumor recurrence after treatment. In addition, whole-body PET acquisition can be utilized to provide information about the existence of concurrent or distant carcinoma. Another advantage of PET is the capability of robust semi-quantification of metabolic changes by calculating standardized uptake values (SUV). This information can be used to predict prognosis or assess response to therapy. This chapter aims to highlight the use, benefits, and limitations of PET in HNC.

Keywords

PET/CT · PET/MR · Metabolic tumor volume · Texture analysis · Therapy assessment · Unknown primary tumor · Human papillomavirus · Tumor heterogeneity · TNM staging · Prognostic value

T. Sekine (✉)
Department of Radiology, Nippon Medical School, Bunkyoku, Tokyo, Japan

10.1 FDG-PET Image Acquisition

10.1.1 Patient Preparation

To enhance sensitivity of tumor detection, it is necessary to reduce tracer uptake in normal tissue. For that purpose, adequate patient preparation is required [1]. The most important preparation is fasting with no oral or intravenous fluids containing sugar or dextrose at least 4–6 h before FDG PET. After injecting FDG, the increased blood glucose directly competes between binding sites and enzymes [2]. In addition, increased insulin secondary to elevated blood glucose increases the translocation of glucose transporters, thereby inducing FDG accumulation to organs with a high density of insulin receptors (e.g., skeletal muscles) [1]. Although it is a common misunderstanding, diabetes is not an absolute contraindication to an FDG-PET study. Fasting hyperglycemia does not hamper the clinical value of FDG-PET, although the clinical recommendation for upper plasma glucose level may be 200 mg/dL [3]. Nevertheless, the timing of oral or injected insulin and that of FDG injection should be tailored [3, 4]. Another recommendation is to avoid exercise 24–48 h before the scan to minimize FDG uptake in skeletal muscle. In the context of head and neck PET evaluation, avoiding chewing gum 24 h before FDG injection is also recommended to reduce the uptake in masticatory muscle [5]. The patients should be kept warm 30–60 min before the injection. Particularly in young patients, cold exposure may stimulate brown adipose tissue located around cervical and supraclavicular regions [6].

10.1.2 Scanning Protocols

Among institutions, there still exists some variability in scanning protocols for PET/CT in HNC. The standard PET/CT acquisition consists of whole-body PET with "low-dose" CT scanning for attenuation correction and anatomical orientation. Several attempts have been made to tailor a

H. Ojiri (ed.), *Diagnostic Imaging in Head and Neck Cancer*, https://doi.org/10.1007/978-981-15-3188-0_10

dedicated protocol for head and neck PET [7, 8]. The optimization of the protocol depends on the characteristics of each scanner, but it generally applies a high-resolution matrix (e.g., 256 × 256), dedicates the reconstruction parameter to a small field of view (FOV; e.g., iteration, subset, and point spread function), selects a longer acquisition window for improved signal-to-noise ratio (SNR), uses an arm position that is not elevated but along the body, and applies delayed acquisition [9]. A recent study combining these optimizations reveals that the diagnostic accuracy of dedicated head and neck PET was significantly superior to standard whole-body PET in terms of general lesion detectability (almost twice as many malignancies were detected by dedicated PET scan) and small LN detectability (dedicated PET scan could detect LNs larger than 7 mm). In contrast, whole-body PET can detect LNs larger than 13 mm [10]. As for the CT part, contrast-enhanced diagnostic-quality CT (ceCT) can be integrated into PET scanning [8, 11]. While, in general, the clinical utility of adding ceCT to PET may be limited, the simultaneous acquisition of both modalities can be adequately run for the assessment of equivocal lesions, particularly in necrotic LN metastases [12, 13]. Suenaga et al. evaluated the diagnostic accuracy of PET/CT and PET/ceCT in 170 patients previously treated for HNC. They concluded that the added value of ceCT for PET/CT is minimal [14]. Therefore, National Comprehensive Cancer Network (NCCN) guidelines stated that ceCT may not be necessary as part of posttreatment PET/CT; if PET/CT results are positive, then cross-sectional imaging with contrast enhancement is recommended [15]. Although care should be taken for the error of attenuation correction derived from ceCT, its effect is clinically insignificant [16, 17]. In addition, some additional techniques have been proposed [18]. Weissman et al. first developed the puffed-cheek technique for CT [19], which Chang et al. further validated for PET/CT [20]. Following the success of PET/MR with an SiPM detector (digital PET), commercial PET/CT with SiPM detector (digital PET) of highly improved sensitivity has currently become available as a commercial scanner [21–23]. The increased sensitivity is expected to impact on diagnostic accuracy.

10.1.3 PET/MR

In the recent years, integrated PET/MR machines have been developed by several commercial vendors and introduced in the clinical world [24]. One obvious advantage of the PET/MR system is lower radiation dose by forgoing CT exposure. However, this advantage is of limited value in most patients with HNC who receive radiotherapy. Another advantage is that the higher soft-tissue contrast than the one offered by CT may help to better assess the complex anatomy in head and neck regions. Although this advantage has been proven to be less prominent than expected in the studies that compared diagnostic accuracy between PET/CT and PET/MR, the fused images definitely support better understanding of the correlation between morphological and metabolic changes in most situations [25]. For more detail about T and N staging by PET/MR, please refer to the corresponding chapter.

One of the common drawbacks of the PET/MR system is the low detectability of lung nodules. Although Raad et al. reported that FDG-negative lung nodules were shown to be benign in more than 98%, further evaluation in larger cohort with HNC should be performed [26]. It also remains to be fully determined whether there exists a synergy effect of functional imaging between two modalities (e.g., FDG-PET and diffusion-weighted magnetic resonance imaging) (Fig. 10.1). Although the evidence remains inconclusive, the combination of these two channels of information may be useful for the clinical evaluation of detailed pathophysiologic features or complicated lesions such as those found in post-radiation therapy [27–30]. In summary, to date, the cost-benefit of this expensive machine is still controversial [31]. Synergic combination of PET and MRI information and appropriate scan workflows should be further developed [32, 33].

10.2 FDG-PET Image Evaluation

10.2.1 Quantification and Visual Inspection of FDG Uptake

Generally, the tumor uptake of FDG reflects tumor's aggressiveness with various cellular characteristics, such as histological grading and proliferative activity [34–36]. Therefore, to present detailed tumor characteristics, the semi-quantitative value of FDG uptake known as the standardized uptake value (SUV) is used in clinical practice. SUV can be calculated as the normalized concentration of radioactivity in a lesion. In addition, the SUV normalized by lean body mass (SUL) may also be calculated [37]. More specifically, SUVmax, the highest value of SUV in the target tumor volume of interest, is widely used in clinical practice because it is easy to measure and objective among readers and software. The variability of metabolic activity has been validated. Hong et al. performed pretreatment FDG-PET scans separated by 1 week for stages III–IV HNC patients [38]. Their results showed that the calculated repeatability coefficients for primary SUV max and nodal SUVmax were 18% and 10%, respectively. This is in line with the PET response criteria in solid tumors (PERCIST), which define a partial metabolic response as equal or more than a 30% decrease in SUV after treatment [39, 40]. The same group also reported a repeatability coefficient of mean apparent diffusion

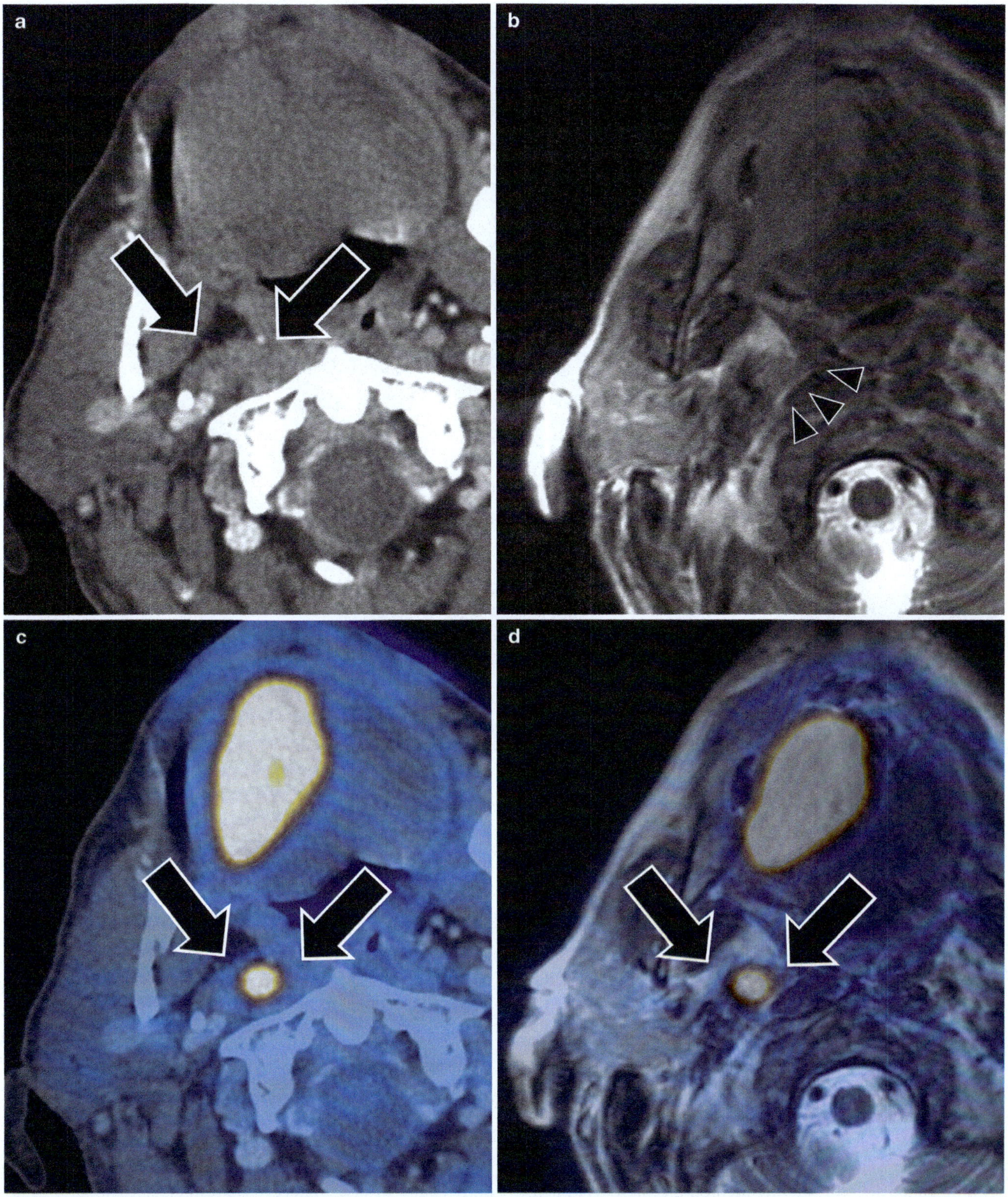

Fig. 10.1 The lymph node metastases adjacent to the prevertebral muscle were clearly depicted on PET/CT (**c**, *thick arrows*) and PET/MR (**d**, *thick arrows*). On contrast-enhanced CT, it was difficult to completely rule out prevertebral muscle infiltration (**a**, *thick arrows*), which eliminated the option of surgical resection. Fat was detected between the tumor and prevertebral fascia on T2WI (**b**, *arrow heads*). This finding had high negative predictive value for evaluation of prevertebral space involvement on MRI. High intensity on echo-planar imaging (*EPI*)-diffusion-weighted magnetic resonance *imaging* (DWI) also reflected tumor cells (**e**, *thick arrows*). However, misregistration on fused T2WI/DWI images was obvious at tumor margin and cerebellum because of the distortion on DWI in the anterior-posterior direction (**f**, *dashed arrows*). This figure is referred to "Sekine T. PET+MR versus PET/CT in the initial staging of head and neck cancer, using a trimodality PET/CT+MR system. Clin Imaging. 2017;42:232–239." (Permission obtained from Elsevier)

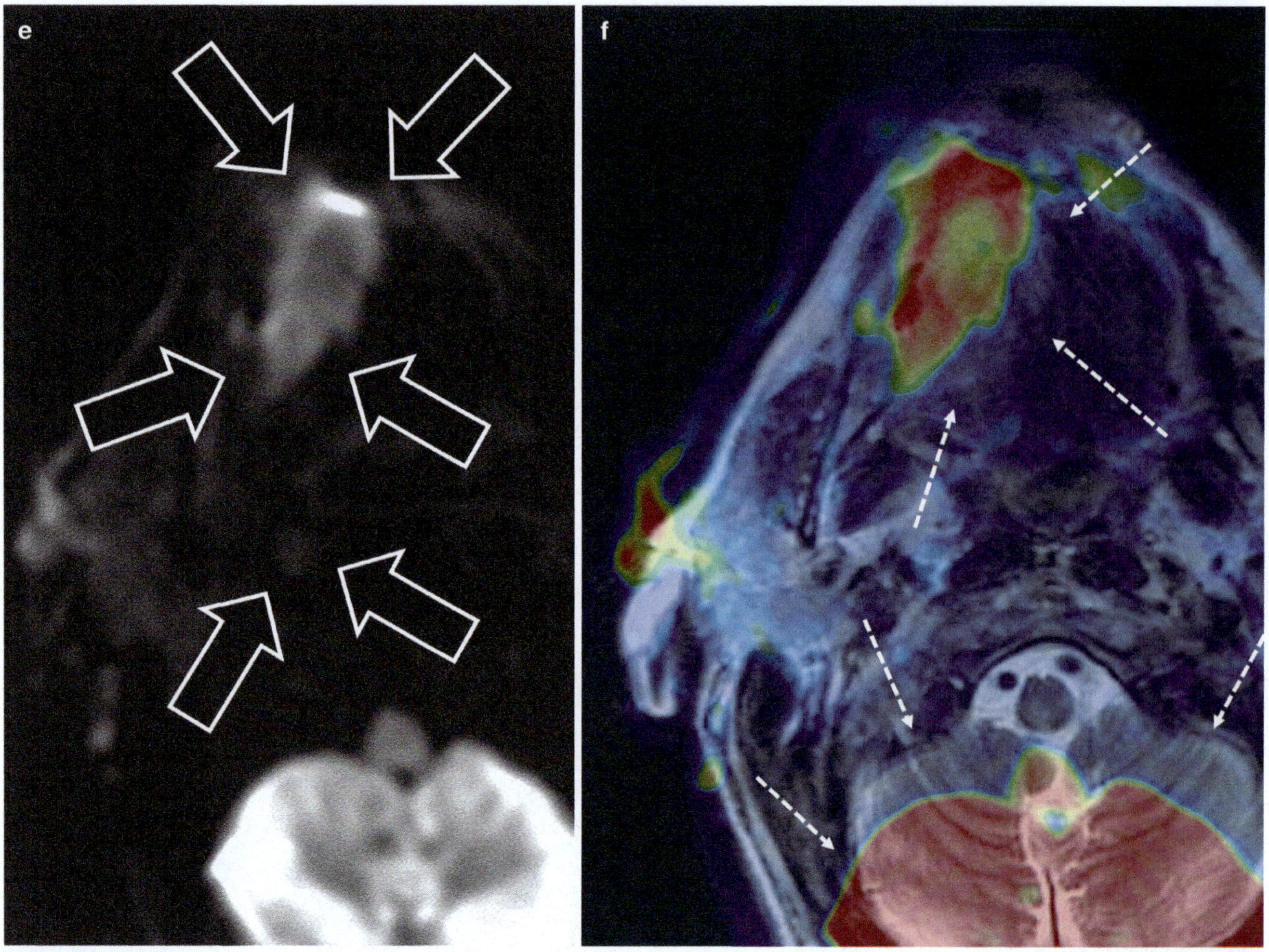

Fig. 10.1 (continued)

coefficient (ADC) of 15% [41]. Another reason for caution regarding the measurement of SUV is that the value highly depends on the sensitivity of the scanner and reconstruction method. To compensate for the variability, quantitative PET harmonization by applying the optimal Gaussian filtering has been recommended [42].

The SUV can be used as an imaging biomarker to predict the prognosis of HNC, especially during the initial staging [43, 44]. Currently, in addition to SUVmax, there has been increasing interest in the use of volumetric SUV parameters, such as MTV or TLG [43, 45]. Although the clear threshold of tumor burden has not been established, fixed thresholds, such as SUV over 2.5, 41% or 50% of the maximum pixel value, or mean liver SUL + 2 or 3 standard deviations, are recommended [3, 40, 46]. To incorporate these volumetric parameters into the clinical interpretation of PET/CT, the practical software to contour the tumor burden should be widely distributed. Ideally, the harmonization function should be also launched to compensate for the difference between PET/CT scanners or reconstruction software updates.

Unlike the clear-cut pretreatment evaluation, posttreatment evaluation using PET/CT is sometimes ambiguous, with the finding of equivocal to false-positive lesions due to secondary therapeutic changes [47–49] (Figs. 10.2 and 10.3). To minimize interobserver variability for these lesions, interpretation criteria for therapy response, such as the Hopkins Criteria, have been proposed and validated (Table 10.1) [50, 51], the performance of which seems at least comparable to the SUV quantification metrics [52]. Similarly, a structured reporting template with standardized criteria for the use of ceCT with/without PET/CT for HNC patient surveillance that links categories to further management recommendations was recently proposed [12, 53, 54]. NI-RADS was developed following the success of other Imaging Reporting and Data System cancer surveillance templates (e.g., BI-RADS for breast cancer, PI-RADS for prostate cancer, and LI-RADS for liver cancer), which have already been incorporated in clinical management [55–57] (Table 10.2). Establishment of such standardized criteria for HNC may also help improve communication between radiologists,

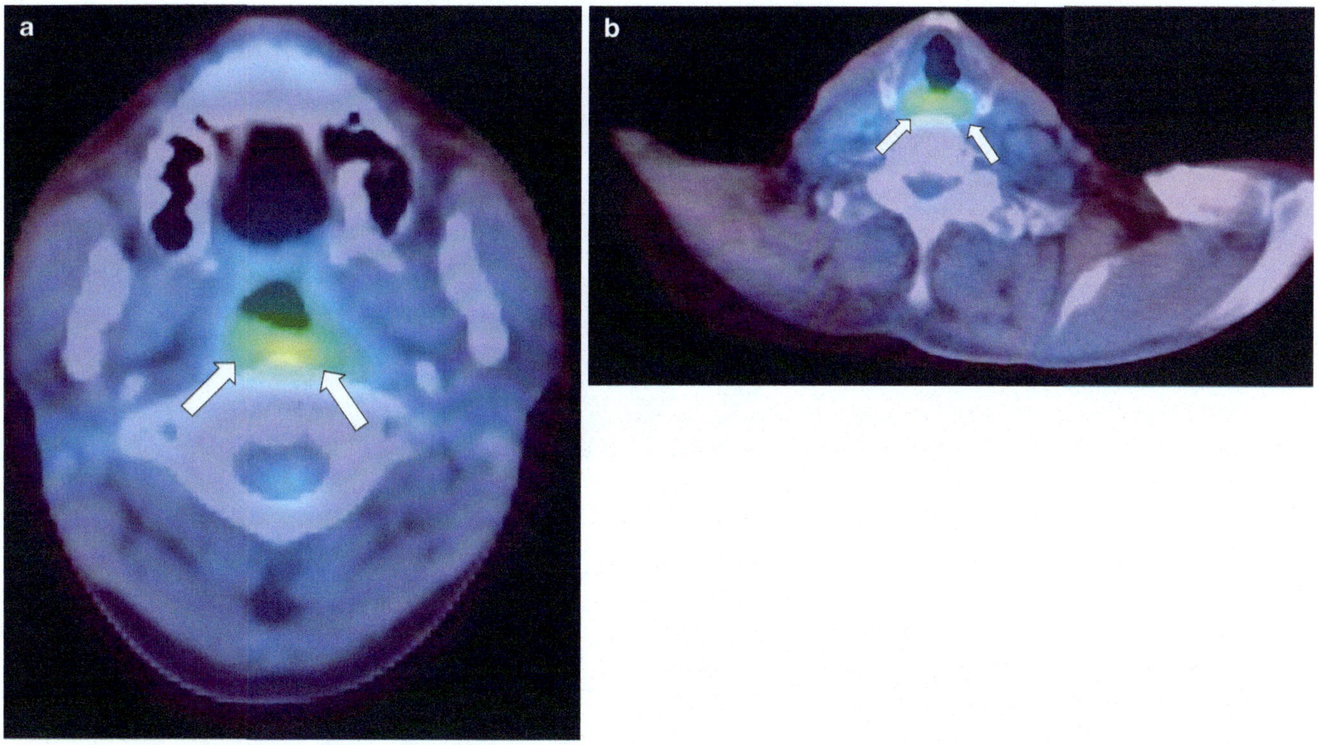

Fig. 10.2 A 43-year-old man with nasopharyngeal carcinoma. The fused PET images scanned 3 months after the completion of radiation therapy presented moderate FDG uptake on the primary lesion (SUVmax 4.38) (**a**, *arrows*). Direct inspection by endoscopy identified the uptake as posttreatment changes. Another 72-year-old man with hypopharyngeal carcinoma displayed inflammatory FDG uptake (SUVmax 4.08) 13 months after the completion of radiation therapy (**b**, *arrows*). As prolonged inflammatory changes with FDG accumulation are not rare up to 3 months or more after the completion of radiation therapy, posttreatment PET images should be interpreted with caution. Assessment of images should be based on the clinical course and other clinical/imaging findings

referring clinicians, and/or patients. These standardized criteria do not use the quantification value of SUV, relying instead on visual qualification (e.g., comparing the radiotracer uptake in the target site with that in a reference region, such as the internal jugular vein or liver) because SUV may be affected by various biological factors, the scanner and scan protocol, and the image reconstruction method [1, 37].

10.2.2 Tumor Heterogeneity

It has been found that tumor heterogeneity is associated with treatment resistance, resulting in worse outcomes in various malignant cancers, including HNC [58–61]. Although there are distinct phenomena underlying genetic (at the nm order) and imaging heterogeneity (mm order), the association between the two is generally accepted [62]. For example, hypoxia or hypoperfusion is linked not only to genetic heterogeneity but also to tracer uptake heterogeneity on FDG-PET [63]. One common finding on PET imaging that reflects tumor heterogeneity is whether the FDG uptake takes a sphere-shaped or a ring-shaped appearance (Fig. 10.4). Koyasu et al. analyzed 108 patients with HNC with the aim to reveal the prognostic value of PET/CT parameters, including SUVmax, MTV, TLG, and uptake pattern (sphere shaped or ring shaped) [64]. The results showed that the hazard ratio of uptake pattern was higher than SUVmax, MTV, or TLG using the univariate cox proportional hazard model (9.58 [4.28–21.45] vs. 2.45 [1.12–5.38], 5.81 [2.33–14.52], or 5.54 [2.22–13.81] for disease-free survival, and 18.92 [7.36–48.62] vs. 5.66 [1.87–17.10], 8.89 [2.58–30.58], or 8.38 [2.44–28.88] for disease-specific survival, respectively). Similar results were also obtained by Apostolova et al. [65]. As expected, quantitative assessment can reduce interobserver variability compared to that associated with visual assessment of tumor uptake heterogeneity [66]. For this purpose, texture analysis has been proposed and validated [67–71]. A few studies with favorable results already exist, which used texture analysis for HNC [72–74]. Although it is difficult to incorporate this complex approach into clinical reading, radiologists should be aware that FDG uptake heterogeneity is associated with worse outcome.

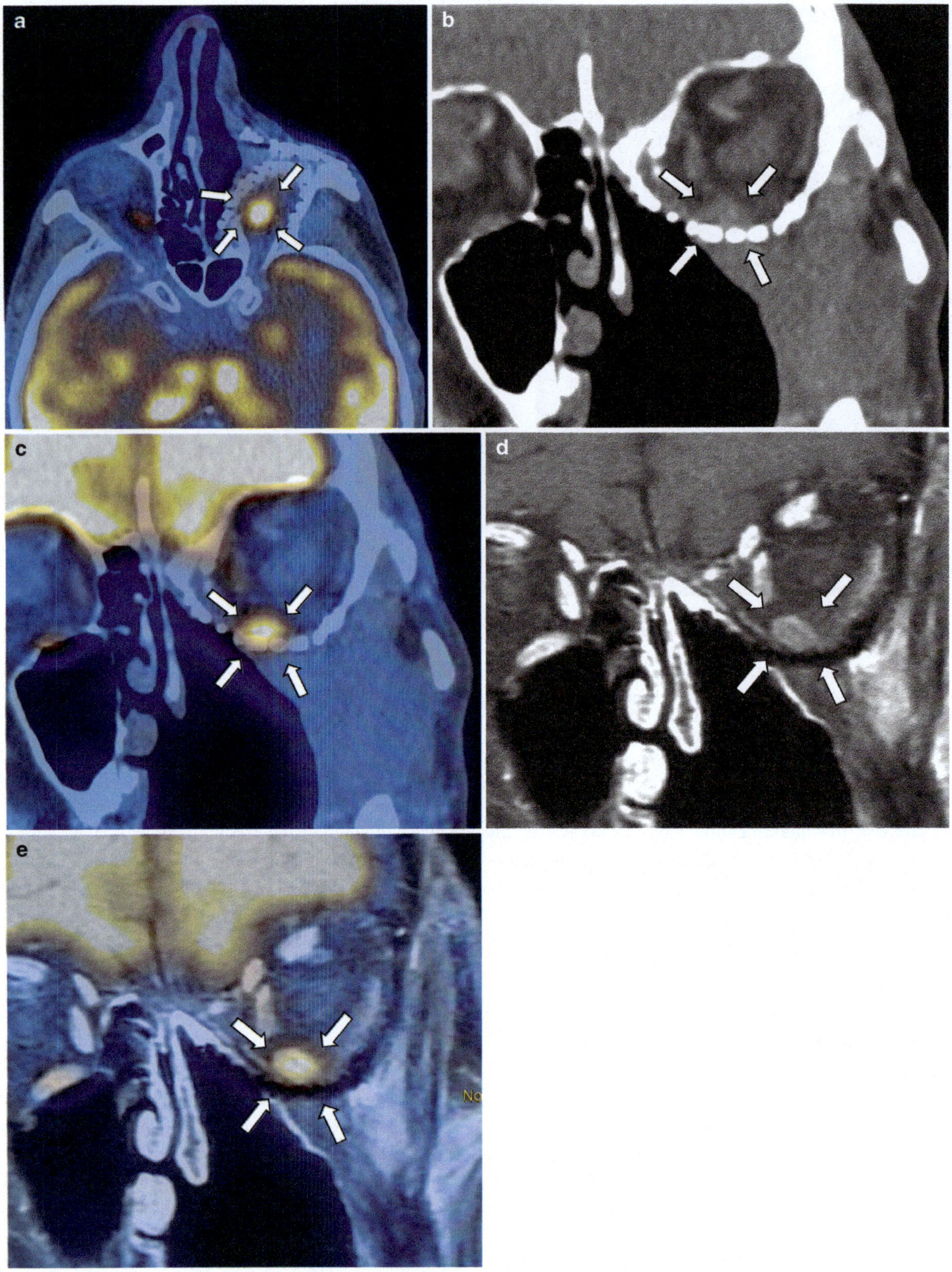

Fig. 10.3 An 82-year-old man after surgery and CRT for hard palate adenocarcinoma. Follow-up imaging after radiotherapy and reconstruction of the floor of the left orbit, which was infiltrated by the tumor. An FDG-avid mass was seen in the left orbit above the reconstructed floor with surrounding stranding of the intraconal and extraconal adipose tissue on axial FDG-PET/CT images (**a**, *arrows*), coronal CT images (**b**, *arrow*), and coronal FDG-PET/CT images (**c**, *arrow*). Contrast-enhanced fat-suppressed coronal MR images (**d**, *arrow*) and FDG PET/MR images (**e**, *arrow*) led to the diagnosis of myositis of the inferior rectus muscle and no evidence of recurrence. This figure is referred to "Sekine T. Emerging topics in PET/CT and PET/MR. Toukeibu Gan. 2018;44:347–352." (Permission obtained from Japan Academic Association for Copyright Clearance)

Table 10.1 Hopkins criteria[a]

Score	18F-FDG uptake pattern	Response category
1	18F-FDG uptake at the primary site and nodes less than IJV	Complete metabolic response
2	Focal 18F-FDG uptake at the primary site and nodes greater than IJV but less than liver	Likely complete metabolic response
3	Diffuse 18F-FDG uptake at the primary site or nodes is greater than IJV or liver	Likely postradiation inflammation
4	Focal 18F-FDG uptake at the primary site or nodes greater than liver	Likely residual tumor
5	Focal and intense 18F-FDG uptake at the primary site or nodes	Residual tumor

Scores 1, 2, and 3, which represent complete metabolic response, likely complete metabolic response, and likely postradiation inflammation, respectively, were considered negative for tumor. Scores 4 and 5, which represent likely residual tumor and residual tumor, respectively, were considered positive for tumor. New lesion would be considered as progressive disease

[a]This table is referred to "Marcus C, Ciarallo A, Tahari AK, Mena E, Koch W, Wahl RL, Kiess AP, Kang H, Subramaniam RM. Head and neck PET/CT: therapy response interpretation criteria (Hopkins Criteria)-interreader reliability, accuracy, and survival outcomes. J Nucl Med. 2014;55:1411–1416"

Table 10.2 NI-RADS category[d]

Category	Primary site	Neck	Imaging findings: Primary site	Imaging findings: Neck	Management
Incomplete	0	0	• New baseline study without any prior imaging available **AND** knowledge that prior imaging exists and will become available as comparison		Assign score in addendum after prior imaging examinations become available
No evidence of recurrence	1	1	• Expected post treatment changes • Non-mass-like distortion of soft tissues • Low-density post-treatment mucosal edema • Diffuse linear mucosal enhancement or FDG • If residual nodal tissue, no FDG uptake		Routine surveillance
Low suspicion	2a	2	• Focal mucosal enhancement or FDG uptake on initial post treatment scan	• Mild/mod FDG in residual nodal tissue • Enlarging or new lymph node without definitive abnormal morphologic features[a] • Any discordance between PET and CECT: enlarging lymph nodeor discrete neck mass but little to no FDG uptake or focal uptake with no CT correlate[b]	2a: Direct visual inspection
	2b		• Deep, ill-defined soft tissue, with only mild/ mod FDG if PET available • Any discordance between PET and CECT: discrete CECT abnormality but little to no FDG uptake or focal FDG uptake but no CT correlate[b]		2b or neck 2: Short interval follow-up (3 months) or PET if scoring on CECT alone
High suspicion	3	3	• Discrete nodule or mass at the primary site with intense focal FDG uptake if PET available • Residual nodal tissue with intense FDG • New enlarged lymph node or enlarging lymph node with abnormal morphologic features[c] on CECT only or focal intense FDG uptake if PET available		Image guided or clinical biopsy if clinically indicated
Definitive recurrence	4	4	• Pathologically proven or definite radiologic and clinical progression		Clinical management

[a]Focal mucosal abnormalities have a high likelihood of being treatment related, especially on the initial posttreatment PET/CECT, so that in most cases, it is prudent to assign a "2a" and let surgeons or oncologists directly inspect. If a more mass-like or nodular mucosal abnormality develops later in the time course of surveillance, it may warrant a "3"

[b]This guideline for PET and CECT discordance only applies if the original tumor was FDG avid

[c]Morphologically abnormal features which are definitive= new necrosis or gross extra nodal extension (ENE) as evidenced by invasion of adjacent structures

[d]This table is referred to "NI-RADS category description" in American College of Radiology HP. At NI-RADS page, ACR states that Neck Imaging Reporting and Data System (NI-RADS) by American College of Radiology is licensed under a Creative Commons Attribution-NonCommercial-NoDerivatives 4.0 International License. https://www.acr.org/Clinical-Resources/Reporting-and-Data-Systems/NI-RADs

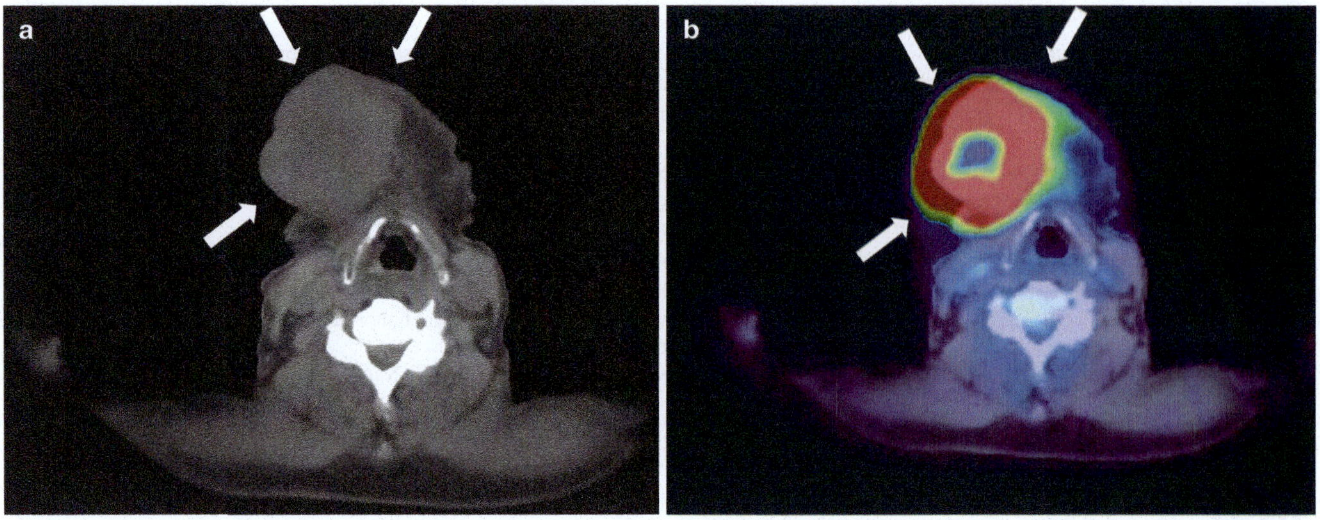

Fig. 10.4 A 72-year-old man with squamous cell carcinoma on the mandibular bone (**a**, *arrows*). Ring-shaped tracer accumulation can be seen on the primary site (**b**, *arrows*). The measured SUVmax was extremely high (24.6). Soon after the scan, chemoradiation therapy was started. However, 5 months after the scan, the patient died due to disease progression despite intensive therapy

10.3 TNM Staging by PET

10.3.1 Initial Treatment Strategy

An early multicenter prospective study recruiting 71 patients conducted by Scott et al. concluded that stand-alone PET study resulted in a change in initial management plans in 33.8% of patients compared to conventional staging procedures including ceCT [75]. Similar results have been obtained in several later studies. Lonneux et al. performed a multicenter prospective study in 233 patients with newly diagnosed and untreated HNC. Their results show that the PET results changed the TNM classification of the disease and altered the management in 13.7% of patients [76]. In the latest multicenter analysis conducted to date, Lowe et al. recruited 287 participants who were clinically diagnosed as N0 (T2N0-T4N0) and underwent neck dissection [77]. The NPV of PET/CT was 0.868 (95% confidence interval [CI], 0.803–0.925) with visual assessment and 0.942 (95% CI, 0.930–0.953) on applying strict SUV threshold (cutoff 1.8). The surgical treatment plan was changed in 51 out of 237 participants (22%) after PET/CT examination. These results suggest that, even in low-to-moderate initial staging, PET/CT could be useful for clinical management decisions [15].

10.3.2 T Staging

In an early study, Dammann et al. revealed that tumor detectability of primary site by stand-alone PET systems was similar to MRI [78]. In patients with severe metallic artifact, tracer accumulation can facilitate tumor delineation compared to conventional CT (Figs. 10.5 and 10.6) [79, 80]. Consistently with these findings, PET/CT can also play a complemental role for assessment of bone invasion in combination with MRI [81, 82] because MRI has high sensitivity but moderate specificity due to inflammatory changes. One common disadvantage of PET is poor spatial resolution, which may limit the detection of small or superficial primary tumors [83].

PET allows biological tumor delineation because FDG uptake directly reflects biological tumor activity. This characteristic can be utilized to improve the planning of radiotherapy. Several studies revealed that radiotherapy planning based on FDG-PET images can improve interobserver variability and reduce target gross tumor volume compared to the planning based on CT images [84, 85].

The utility of PET/MR for T staging or resectability has been demonstrated in several studies with relatively small sample sizes [86–88]. PET/MR emerged as the modality of choice to delineate the tumor margin, particularly in the regions where the quality of CT images suffers due to artifacts, such as dental implants (Figs. 10.5, 10.6 and 10.7) [89]. In addition, information on tumor resectability, such as perineural spreading, can be obtained through a combination of PET and MRI (Figs. 10.8, 10.9 and 10.10) [87]. Physiologic or inflammatory FDG uptake in normal tissue (e.g., palatine tonsils, vocal cords, and teeth) on PET/CT can also confound image interpretation [90, 91] (Fig. 10.11), while MR components of PET/MR add useful information in these regions.

10.3.3 N Staging

Involvement of LNs is common in patients with HNC. Especially in patients with clinical N0, the main treatment dilemma is whether to treat the neck or to adopt a wait-

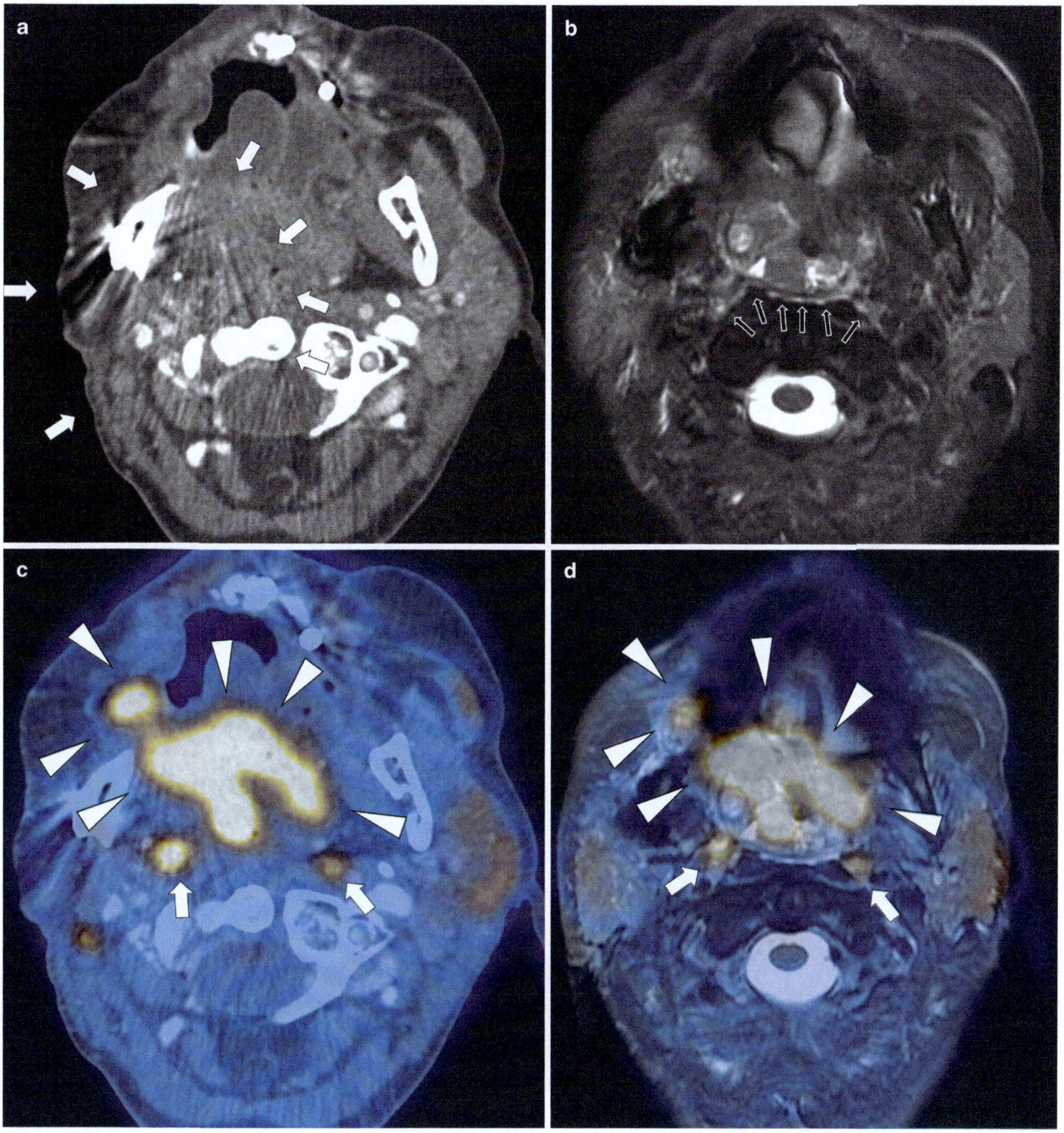

Fig. 10.5 A 59-year-old woman with recurrent squamous cell carcinoma of the floor of the mouth. The severe artifacts from dental implants on CT limited the interpretation of tumor extension (**a**, *arrows*). PET overlay added information about tumor activity (**c**, *arrowheads*); however, the anatomical information was still limited on these images. In contrast, on T2WI, an almost continuously defined thin hyperintense line between the tumor and the prevertebral muscles was seen (**b**, *thin arrows*). With this finding having a high negative predictive value for the absence of prevertebral invasion, the lesion was correctly diagnosed as resectable on PET/MR, which was further confirmed by clinical examination. However, the radical operation was not performed because the patient had multiple lymph node metastases (*arrows* on **c** and **d**). PET/MR images simultaneously provided information on tumor extension and delineation of the interface with anatomical structures (**d**, *arrowheads*). This figure is referred to "Sekine T. Local resectability assessment of head and neck cancer: Positron emission tomography/MRI versus positron emission tomography/CT. Head Neck. 2017;39:1550–1558." (Permission obtained from Wiley)

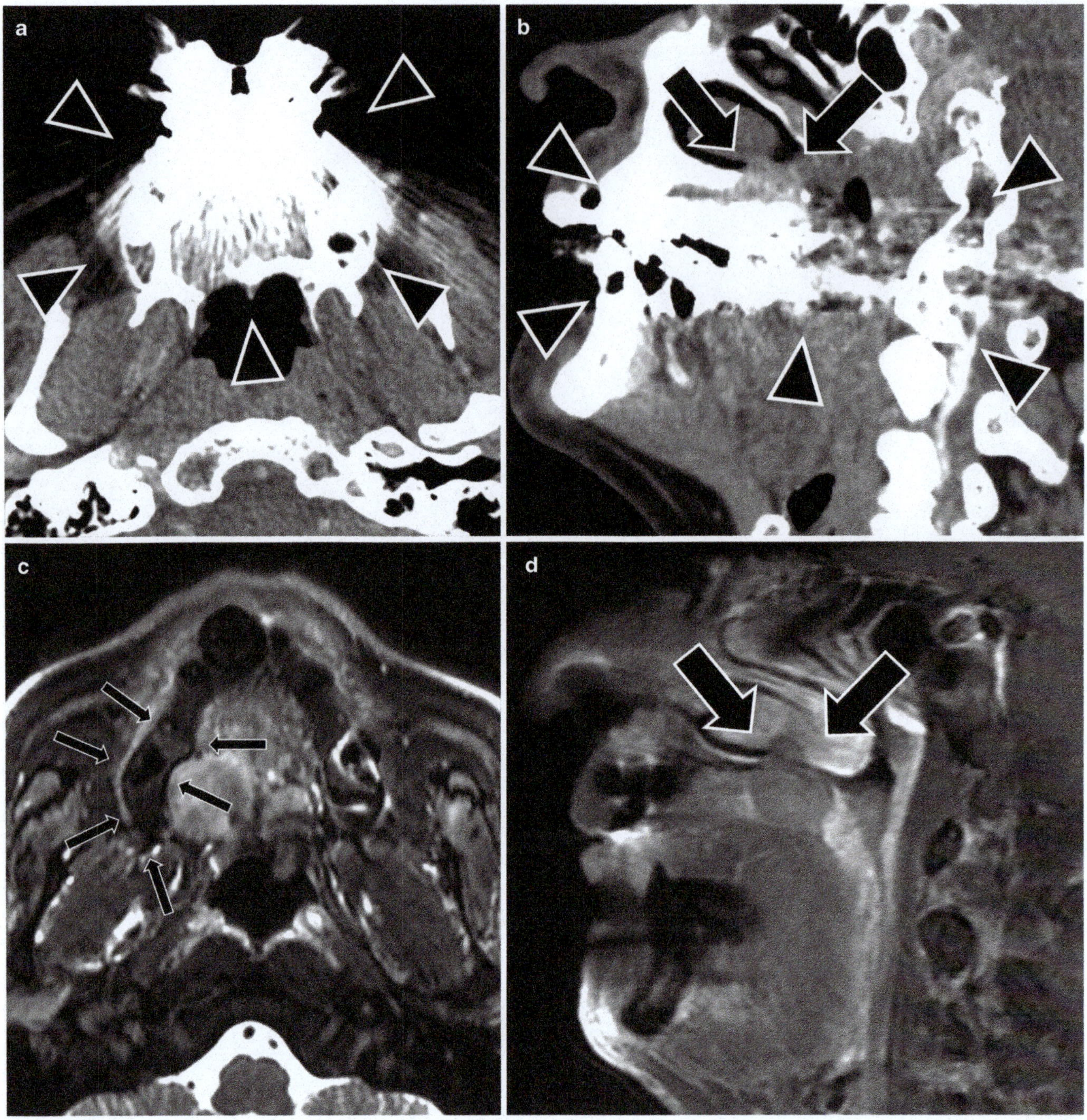

Fig. 10.6 A 67-year-old man with mucoepidermoid carcinoma of the hard palate. The tumor infiltrated the nasal cavity and invaded the inferior nasal concha (**b**, **d**, **f**, and **h**, *thick arrows*), while the alveolar part of the mandible was spared (**c**, *thin arrows*). The margin of the tumor was hard to detect on CT (**a**, **b**) and PET/CT (**e**, **f**) because of artifacts from implants (**a** and **b**, arrowheads) and low soft-tissue contrast. In contrast, the margin was easily recognized on fat-sat T2WI and contrast-enhanced T1WI (**c**, **d**), and fused PET/MR images (**g**, **h**). Consistent with the imaging findings, the patient was finally diagnosed as stage T4a, and surgery was performed. The precise detection of local extension impacted surgical procedure. A subtle FDG uptake on the left side of hard palate was clinically proven as a physiological accumulation (**e** and **g**, dashed arrows). This figure is referred to "Sekine T. PET+MR versus PET/CT in the initial staging of head and neck cancer, using a trimodality PET/CT+MR system. Clin Imaging. 2017;42:232–239." (Permission obtained from Elsevier)

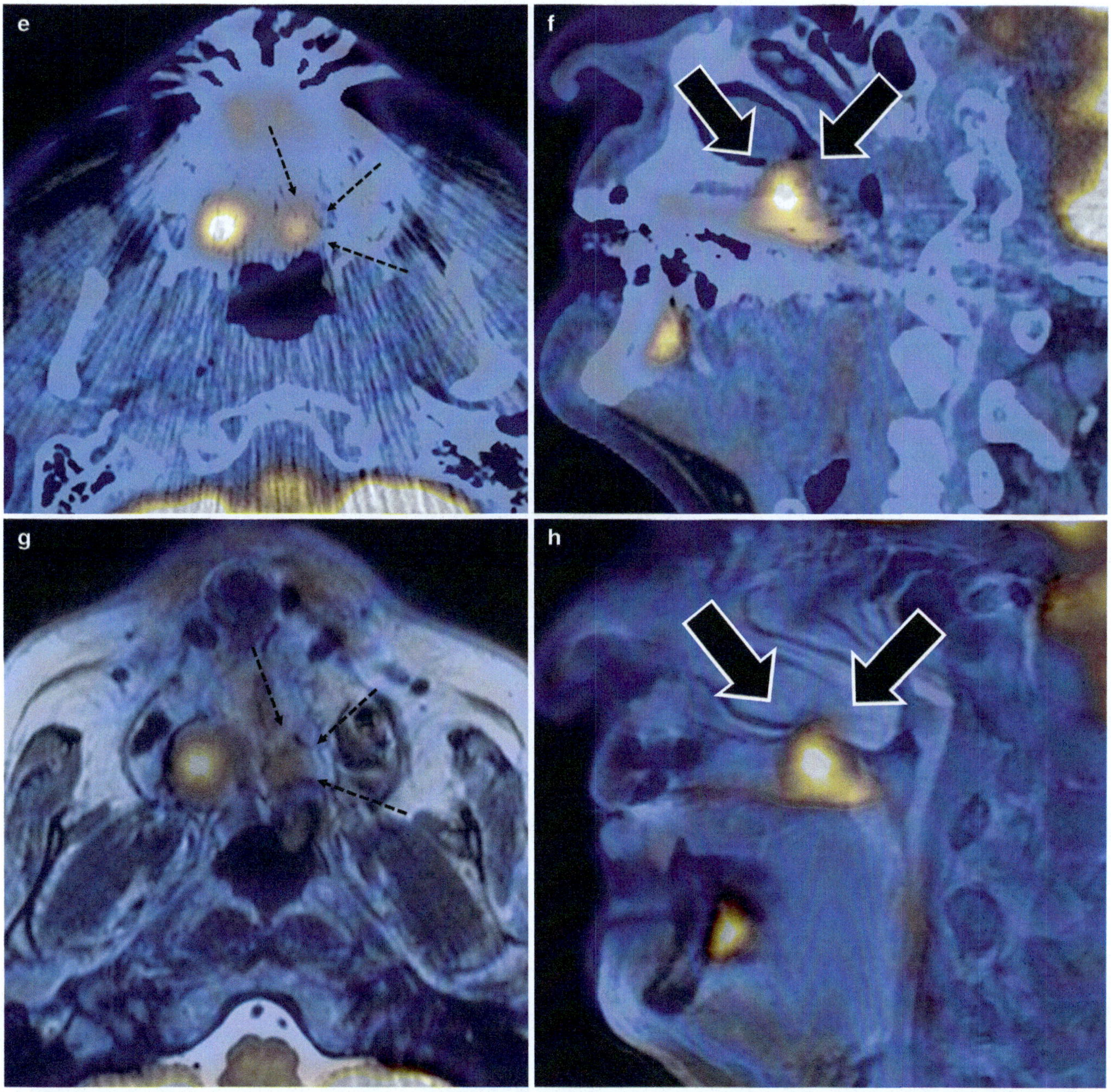

Fig. 10.6 (continued)

and-watch policy. CT and MRI for detection of nodal metastasis have been routinely performed. However, PET has higher sensitivity and specificity for metastatic nodal disease compared with CT and MRI (Fig. 10.12). An earlier meta-analysis across 32 studies (1236 patients in total, with 311 clinical N0 patients) conducted by Kyzas et al. revealed that the PET sensitivity and specificity were 79% (72–85%) and 86% (83–89%) for the detected nodal lesions [92]. In this study, the diagnostic accuracy of PET was found to be superior to other modalities, such as CT, MRI, and ultrasound but with overlapping confidence intervals. In the subgroup of cN0, the results of PET/CT were not satisfactory (sensitivity and specificity, 0.50 (0.37–0.63) and 0.87 (0.76–0.93), respectively). Some possible reasons for the relatively low diagnostic accuracy have been suggested, such as the close anatomic proximity of the LNs to salivary glands and other structures with FDG uptake, smaller size of occult metastases below the spatial resolution of PET/CT, and high glucose level. Liao et al. also performed a meta-analysis focusing on diagnostic accuracy for nodal metastasis in patients with cN0 [93]. They concluded that PET had low-to-moderate sensitivity (0.66 (0.47–0.80)) and was not superior to other modalities, such as CT, MRI, and ultrasound. Another earlier simulation study, however, showed that PET

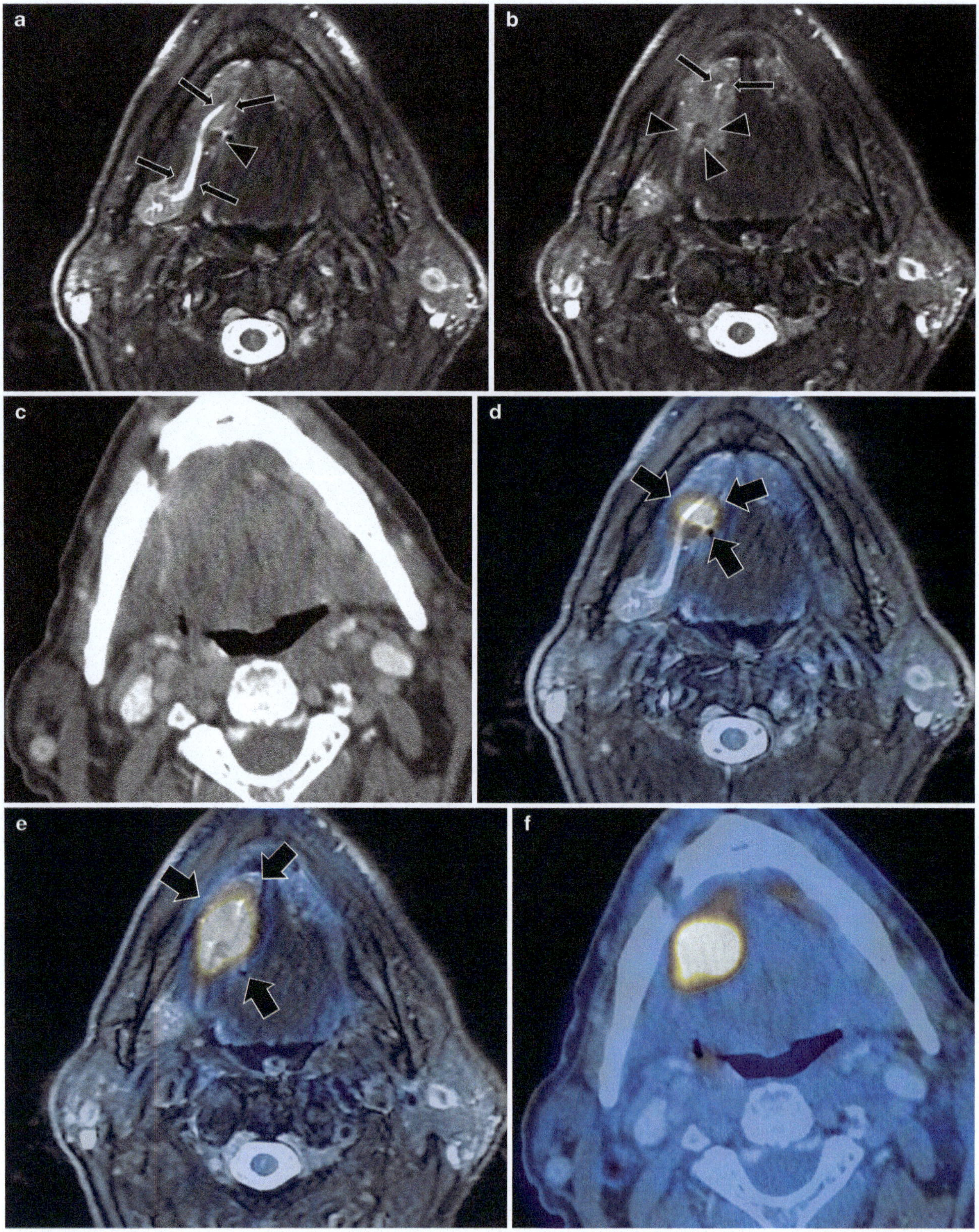

Fig. 10.7 A 69-year-old woman with squamous cell carcinoma of the tongue. A pronounced dilatation of Wharton's duct was observed on fat-saturated T2WI (**a** and **b**, *thin arrows*). This dilatation was due to obstruction by the tumor, which was easily recognized on fused PET/MR images (**d** and **e**, *thick arrows*). This tumor obstruction reflected invasion of the floor of the mouth. The tumor additionally invaded the right hyoglossus muscle (**a** and **b**, *arrowheads*). Consistent with the imaging findings, the patient was finally diagnosed with T4a. The local extent of the tumor was less obvious on contrast-enhanced CT images (**c**) and PET/CT images (**f**). This figure is referred to "Sekine T. PET+MR versus PET/CT in the initial staging of head and neck cancer, using a trimodality PET/CT+MR system. Clin Imaging. 2017;42:232–239." (Permission obtained from Elsevier)

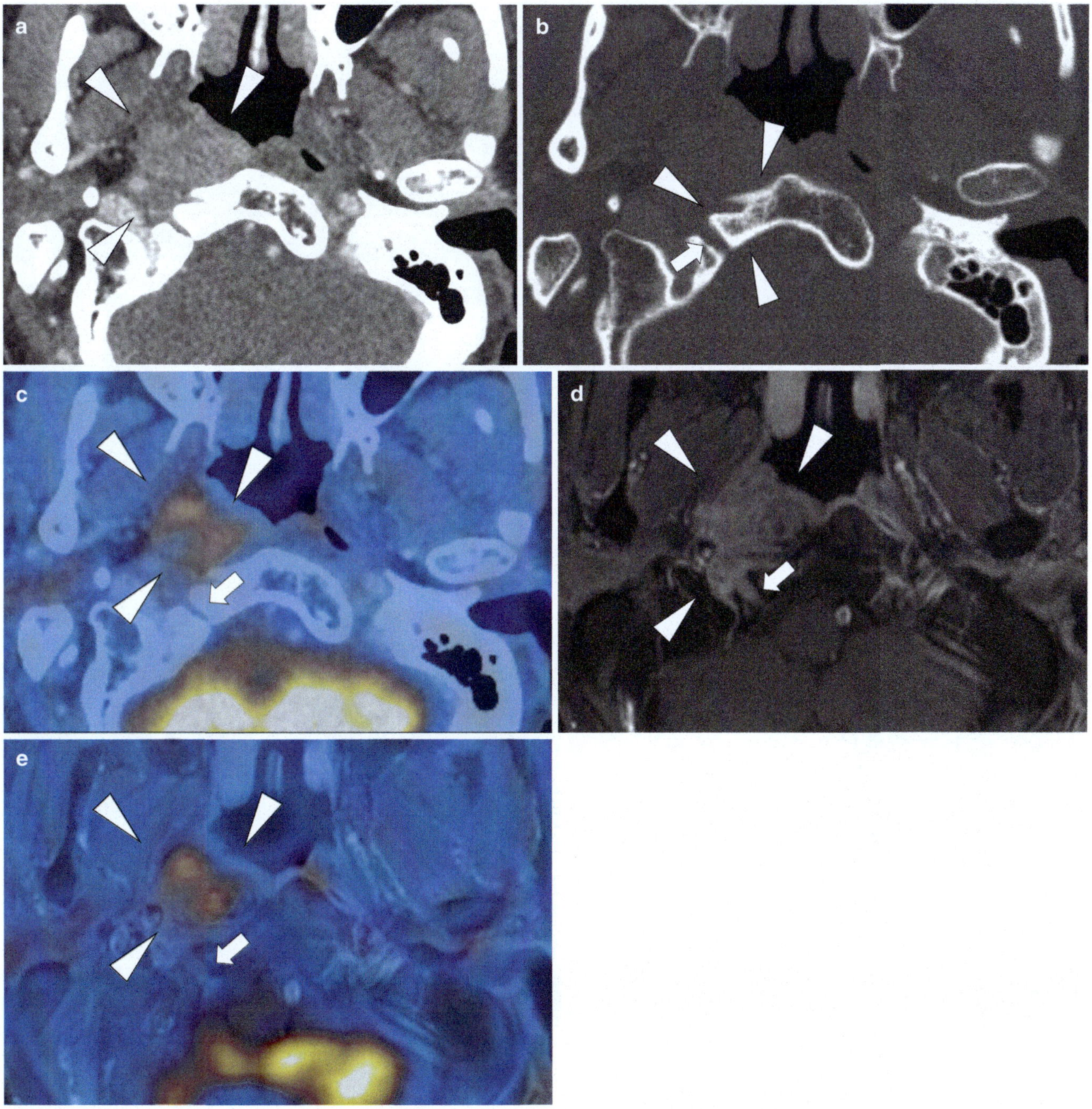

Fig. 10.8 A 54-year-old man after three cycles of cisplatin-based chemotherapy for a poorly differentiated nasopharyngeal carcinoma. Contrast-enhanced CT images in soft tissue window (**a**) and bone window (**b**) showed a mass in the nasopharynx on the right side (**a**, *arrowheads*) with parapharyngeal infiltration. Sclerosis was seen in the clivus adjacent to the mass (**b**, *arrowheads*). The hypoglossal canal was not widened (**b**, *arrow*). Fused PET/CT image (**c**) demonstrated moderate FDG uptake of the mass (*arrowheads*), but no increased FDG uptake within the hypoglossal canal (*arrow*). Contrast-enhanced T1-weighted image (**d**) and fused PET/MR image (**e**) depicted contrast enhancement in the right-sided hypoglossal canal (*arrows* on **d** and **e**, respectively), compatible with perineural spread, which was in continuity with the FDG-avid mass (*arrowheads* on **d** and **e**, respectively). Perineural spread was missed on PET/CT, but evident on PET/MR. This figure is referred to "Sekine T. Local resectability assessment of head and neck cancer: Positron emission tomography/MRI versus positron emission tomography/CT. Head Neck. 2017;39:1550–1558." (Permission obtained from Wiley)

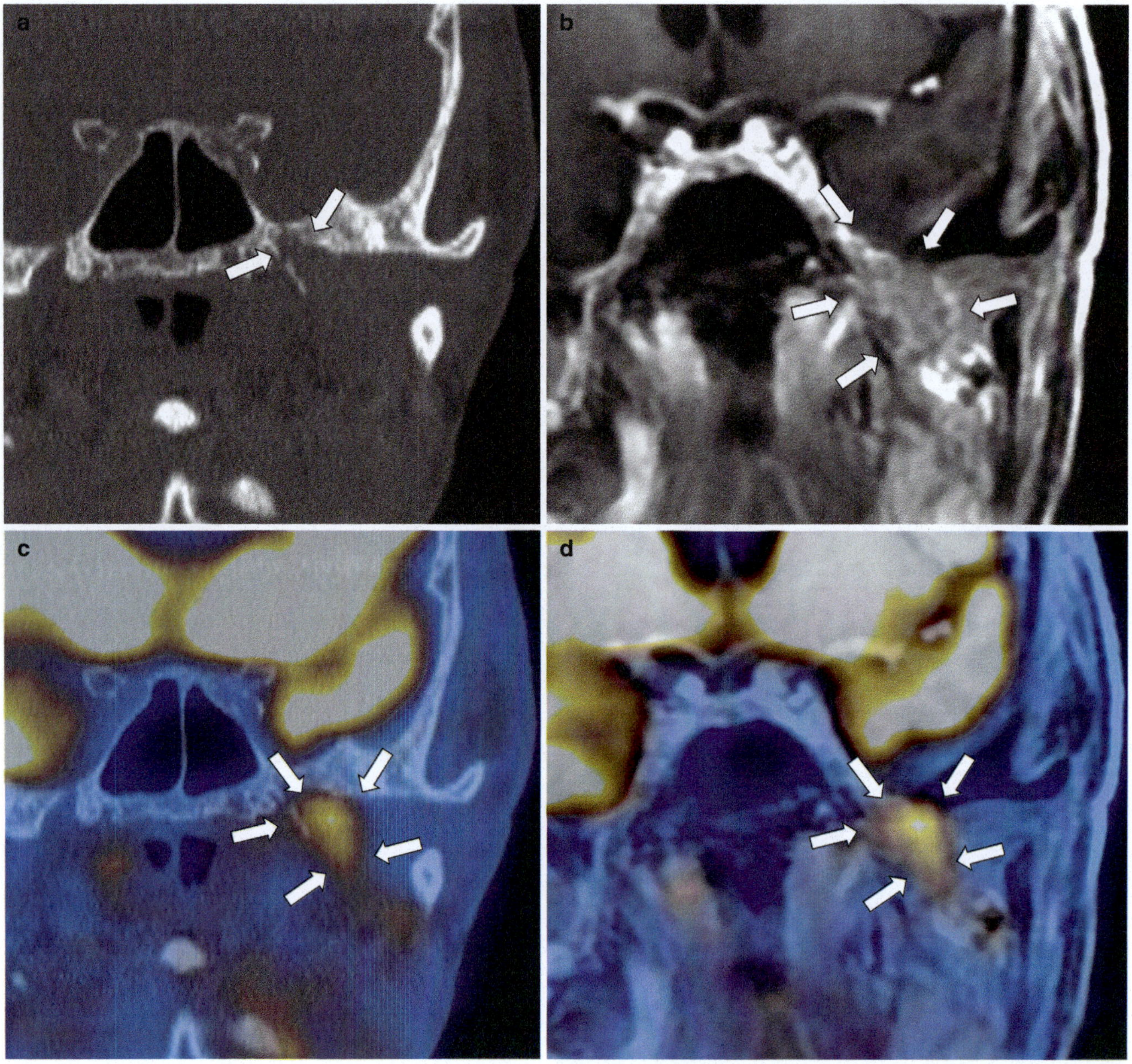

Fig. 10.9 A 76-year-old man after surgery and radiotherapy for mucoepidermoid cancer of the left parotid gland. Contrast-enhanced T1WI allowed a better conspicuity of the perineural spread along the V3 component of the trigeminal nerve through the foramen ovale (**b**, *arrows*). The spread could be seen indirectly as the dilatation of the foramen ovale on CT (**a**, *arrows*). On fused PET images, the lesion was partially seen as FDG uptake along the nerve (**c** and **d**, *arrows*)

was cost-effective in patients with N0, though the sensitivity and specificity of PET were determined too high (86.9% and 94.8%, respectively) [94]. The latest multicenter prospective study from 23 American College of Radiology Imaging Network-qualified institutions analyzed 270 neck sides from 212 participants clinically diagnosed as cN0 [77]. Based on pathological findings, lymph node metastasis was confirmed to be negative in 195 necks in 212 patients. The authors emphasized the presence of a high NPV (0.87 (0.75–0.99)) and the strict criteria with a relatively modern PET system improved sensitivity (74.7%) but decreased specificity (64.1%). Extracapsular spread is an indicator of poor prognosis, which has been newly defined as N3b in the latest AJCC staging system [95, 96]. Although few groups reported that higher SUV uptake may be indicated to contribute the differentiation of extracapsular spread similarly to CT or MRI, standardized criteria have yet to be proven by prospective study [96–99]. Evidence on the clinical performance of PET/MR for N staging is still limited. Most studies revealed that PET/MR has a comparable diagnostic accuracy to that

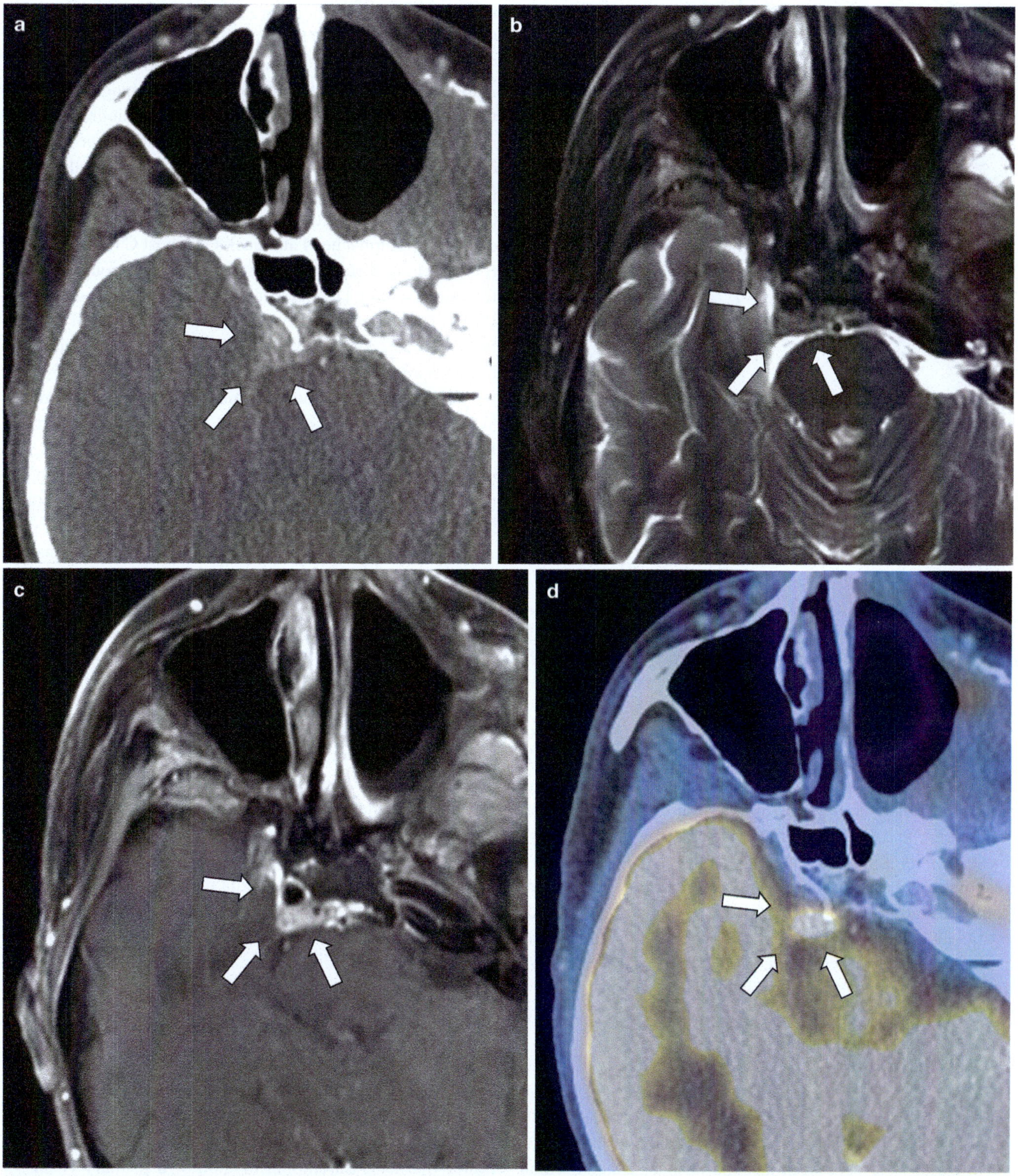

Fig. 10.10 An 82-year-old man after surgery and CRT of an adenocarcinoma of the hard palate. The slightly enhancing lesion around the right cavernous sinus was observed on CT (**a**, *arrows*). The lesion was diagnosed as perineural spread and carotid artery invasion, both on PET/CT and PET/MR. In this lesion, FDG uptake was observed, but distinction from normal brain FDG accumulation was difficult (**d** and **e**, *arrows*). This might be a pitfall of PET images. The tissue contrast of this lesion was clearer on T2WI and ce-T1WI (*arrows* on **b**, **c** and **d**, respectively). This figure is referred to "Sekine T. Local resectability assessment of head and neck cancer: Positron emission tomography/MRI versus positron emission tomography/CT. Head Neck. 2017;39:1550–1558." (Permission obtained from Wiley)

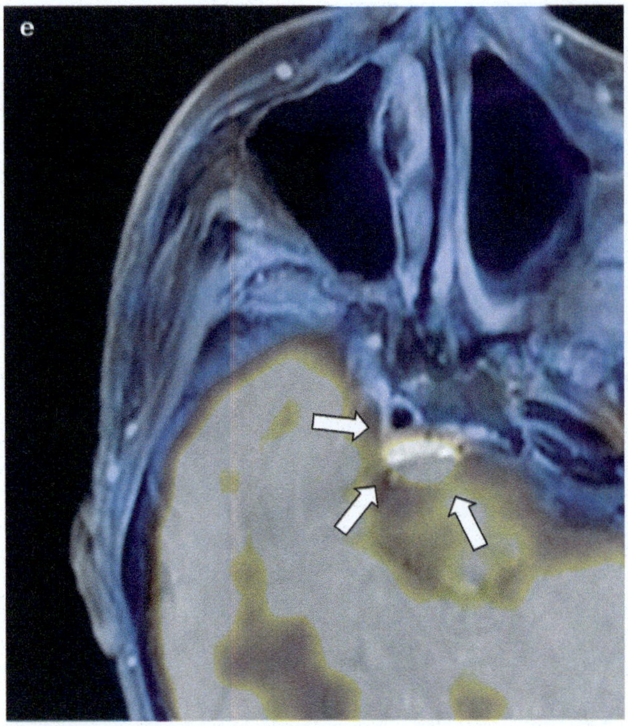

Fig. 10.10 (continued)

of PET/CT, although the image quality was inferior in PET/MR owing to motion artifacts caused by swallowing and carotid pulsation [88, 89, 100] (Fig. 10.13).

Familiarity with the drainage pattern of each nodal site from the primary tumor can improve interpretation in FDG-PET as well as other modalities [101]. During N staging, attention should be paid to midline tumor, nasopharyngeal carcinoma, and epiglottic and oral cavity tumors, because these tumors frequently have bilaterally drainage pattern resulting in the contralateral side of metastasis. There are some limitations associated with PET evaluation. Small or cystic nodal metastases can be overlooked by PET due to the partial volume effect (Figs. 10.14, 10.15, and 10.16). Inflammatory changes can also lead to tracer uptake.

10.3.4 M Staging

Although the reported incidence varies (3.8%–12.0%) among studies, HNSCC has a low-to-moderate prevalence for metastasis or concurrent second primary cancer, which become determining factors in clinical decision-making [102–106]. The lung (70–85%) is the most common site of metastasis, followed by the bone (15–39%) and liver (10–30%) [105]. Consequently, chest radiography and CT screening are still most commonly used. However, compared with these conventional modalities, PET has a high diagnostic accuracy for the detection of metastasis for initial staging (sensitivity and specificity of chest radiography are 41% and 92%, of chest CT are 74% and 63%, and of PET are 92% and 93%, respectively) (Figs. 10.17 and 10.18) [107]. Additionally, compared with dedicated imaging workup using multimodal imaging such as chest radiography, head and neck MRI, and chest CT, PET/CT can detect a significantly higher number of metastases at the initial staging [108]. Kim et al. performed a prospective study with a large cohort of 740 consecutive patients, in which they compared chest radiography, head and neck CT, chest CT, and PET/CT for screening distant metastases and synchronous cancer at the initial staging [109]. In line with several previous studies, PET/CT was found to be superior to conventional modalities. Of note, a significant difference in the detection rate between conventional modalities and PET/CT was observed only in stage III–IV patients, and not in stage I–II patients. While this supports a previous NCCN recommendation that PET/CT should be considered for stage III–IV patients, this recommendation was already revised at the time of publication, and PET/CT is now generally considered for all stages [15, 110].

To reveal the diagnostic accuracy of PET for metastasis not only at the initial staging but also during follow-up, Xu et al. performed a meta-analysis of 12 studies between 2006 and 2010 that included a total of 824 patients for initial stating and 452 for restaging [111]. Of the 1279 eligible patients, 174 (13.7%) had distant metastases or second primary cancers. The pooled sensitivity and specificity were 0.888 (0.827–0.928) and 0.951 (0.936–0.963), respectively. In a more recent study, Gao et al. included 756 patients from 10 studies between 2006 and 2012, all of which performed PET/CT and not stand-alone PET [112]. Their results showed high diagnostic accuracy, with a sensitivity and specificity of 0.92 (0.83–0.96) and 0.93 (0.80–0.98), respectively. Approximately half of the misdiagnoses (false-positives and false-negatives) were caused by the misinterpretation of lung lesions. Thus, FDG-PET is the most accurate single whole-body imaging modality for the detection of distant metastasis and synchronous cancer.

10.3.5 Unknown Primary Tumor

Occult tumors may manifest with metastases to LNs or to organs, with paraneoplastic symptoms or increased serum tumor markers. Carcinoma of unknown primary (CUP) is defined as a metastatic malignancy whose primary site cannot be detected at the time of diagnosis [113]. CUP ranks among the top ten cancer diagnoses worldwide, accounting for 3–5% of all malignant tumors [113, 114]. Prognosis of patients is generally dismal [113, 115, 116]. Recently, cervical CUP was defined as a distinct category by the American Joint Committee on Cancer (AJCC) [117, 118]. In this clas-

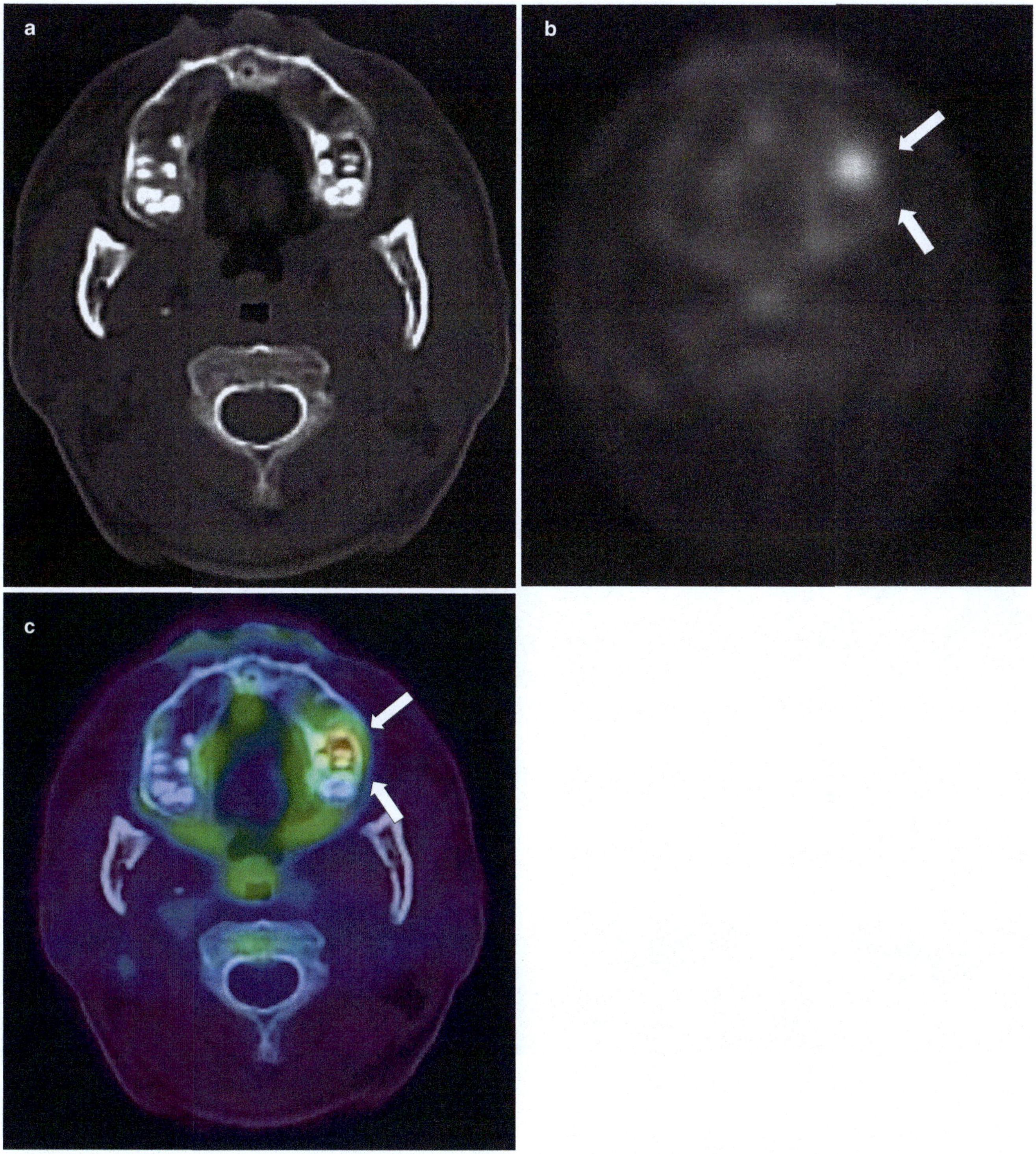

Fig. 10.11 A 50-year-old man with nasopharyngeal carcinoma. CT in bone window, PET and fused images are presented (**a**, **b** and **c**). PET/CT showed nodular FDG uptake around tooth apices on the left side caused by dental infection (**b** and **c**, *arrows*)

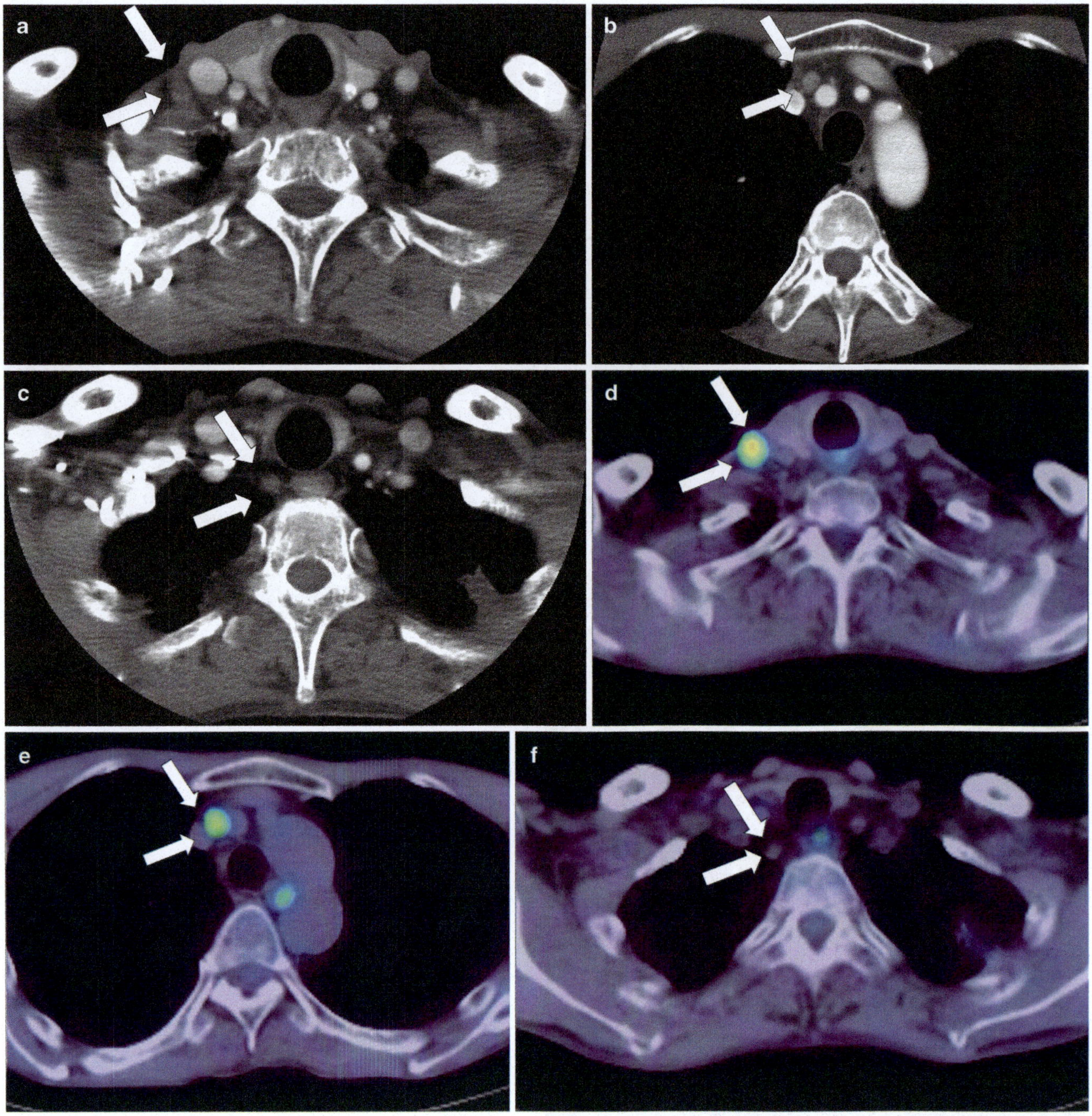

Fig. 10.12 A 56-year-old man with hypopharynx squamous cell carcinoma. Contrast-enhanced CT showed three cervical adenopathies (**a**, **b**, and **c**, *arrows*). Out of three lymph nodes, two had significant FDG uptake (**d** and **e**, *arrows*), while no uptake was observed in the other lymph node. This third lymph node was confirmed to be benign during follow-up (**f**, *arrows*)

sification, if there is evidence of either Epstein–Barr virus (EBV) or HPV histologically, the nasopharyngeal or oropharyngeal classification can be applied. In order to treat CUP patients appropriately, knowledge regarding the presumed primary site and coexisting metastatic lesions is important (Figs. 10.17 and 10.18). Treatment options vary considerably depending on the primary site and extent of metastatic spread [115]. Therefore, whole-body imaging examinations are considered to be the first choice in the evaluation of patients with suspected occult malignancies. In CUP patients, the most prevalent site of occult primaries is the head and neck region [119], where PET/CT is more sensitive than contrast-enhanced CT or MR imaging [120], and PET/CT is considered to have an actual benefit in the management of CUP [121, 122]. Zhu et al. reported a meta-analysis covering 7 studies with a total of 246 patients with

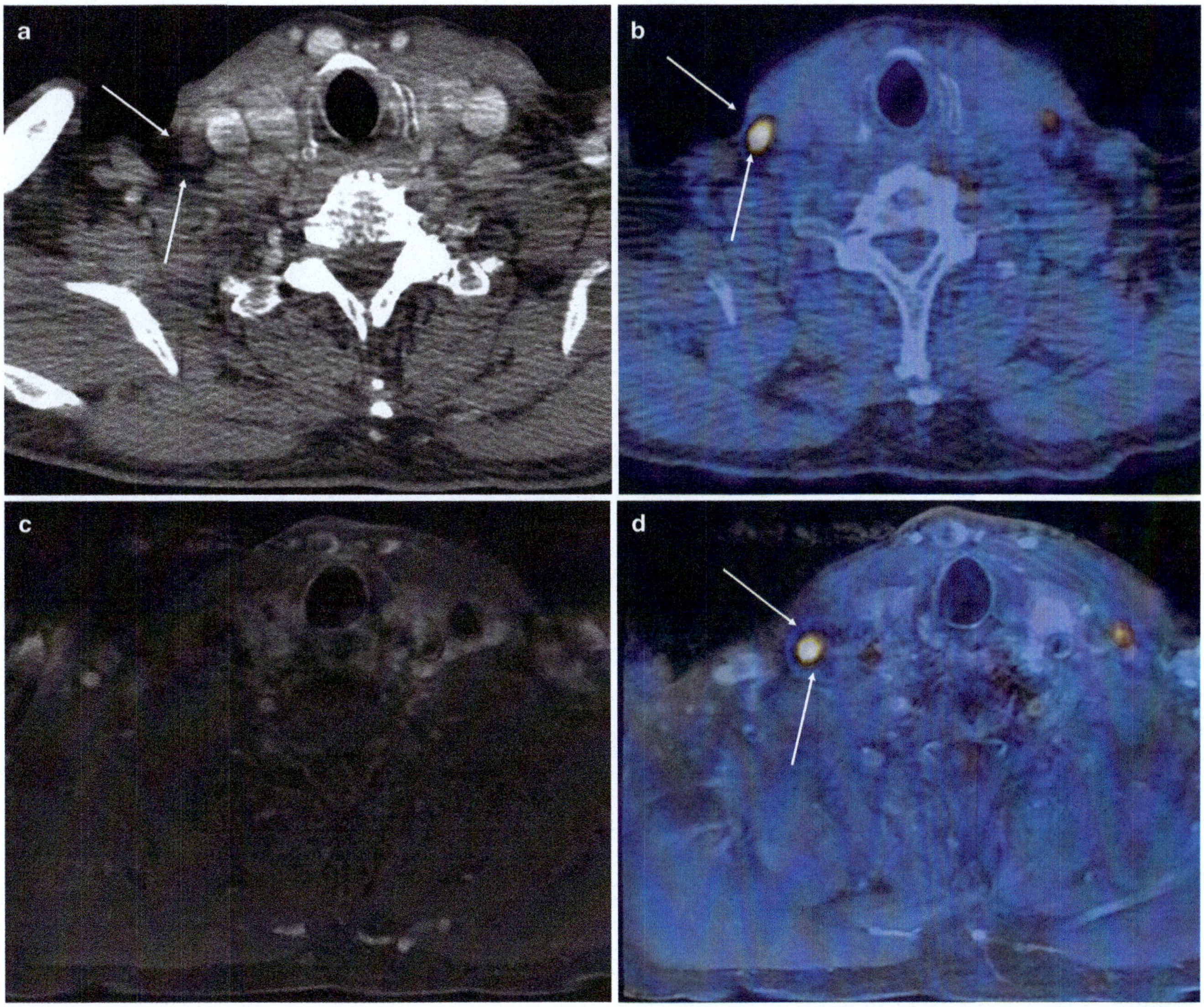

Fig. 10.13 The lymph node metastases were clearly depicted on contrast-enhanced CT (**a**, *arrows*) and PET/CT (**b**, *arrows*). However, it was difficult to point out this lymph node on fat-sat contrast-enhanced T1WI (**c**) because of artifacts due to the motion and pulsation of arteries. PET-fusion added valuable information on this lesion (**d**, *arrows*)

cervical nodal metastases of CUP. The pooled tumor detection rate, sensitivity, and specificity of PET/CT were 0.44 (0.31–0.58), 0.97 (0.63–0.99), and 0.68 (0.49–0.83), respectively. They concluded that while PET/CT had sufficient sensitivity to rule out the presence of primary tumor, it did not adequately detect the primary tumor [123]. Another recent prospective study, which focused on CUP with cervical metastases, was conducted by Lee et al. [120]. They prospectively included 56 patients with initially undetected tumors after endoscopic or physical examination. Altogether, primary tumors were pathologically detected at 32 sites in 31 patients. The results showed that PET/CT is more sensitive for detection of primary tumors than the combination of contrast-enhanced CT and MRI (sensitivity and specificity for PET/CT 69% (51–82%) and 88% (70–96%), respectively vs. 41% (22–61%) and 59% (33–82%) for ceCT MRI). Recent studies revealed that integrated PET/MR has equivalent to superior performance for CUP evaluation compared to that of PET/CT [124, 125]. Due to the significantly lower dose of ionizing radiation, PET/MR may provide benefit for patients who need repeated imaging workup for therapy monitoring and long-term surveillance. NCCN guidelines for CUP (not only cervical CUP but whole-body CUP) concluded that PET/CT may be warranted in some situations, particularly when considering local or regional therapy; however, it is not recommended for routine screening [126]. Meanwhile, NCCN guidelines for HNC recommended that PET/CT scan for head and neck CUP should only be performed if the other tests do not reveal a primary tumor [15].

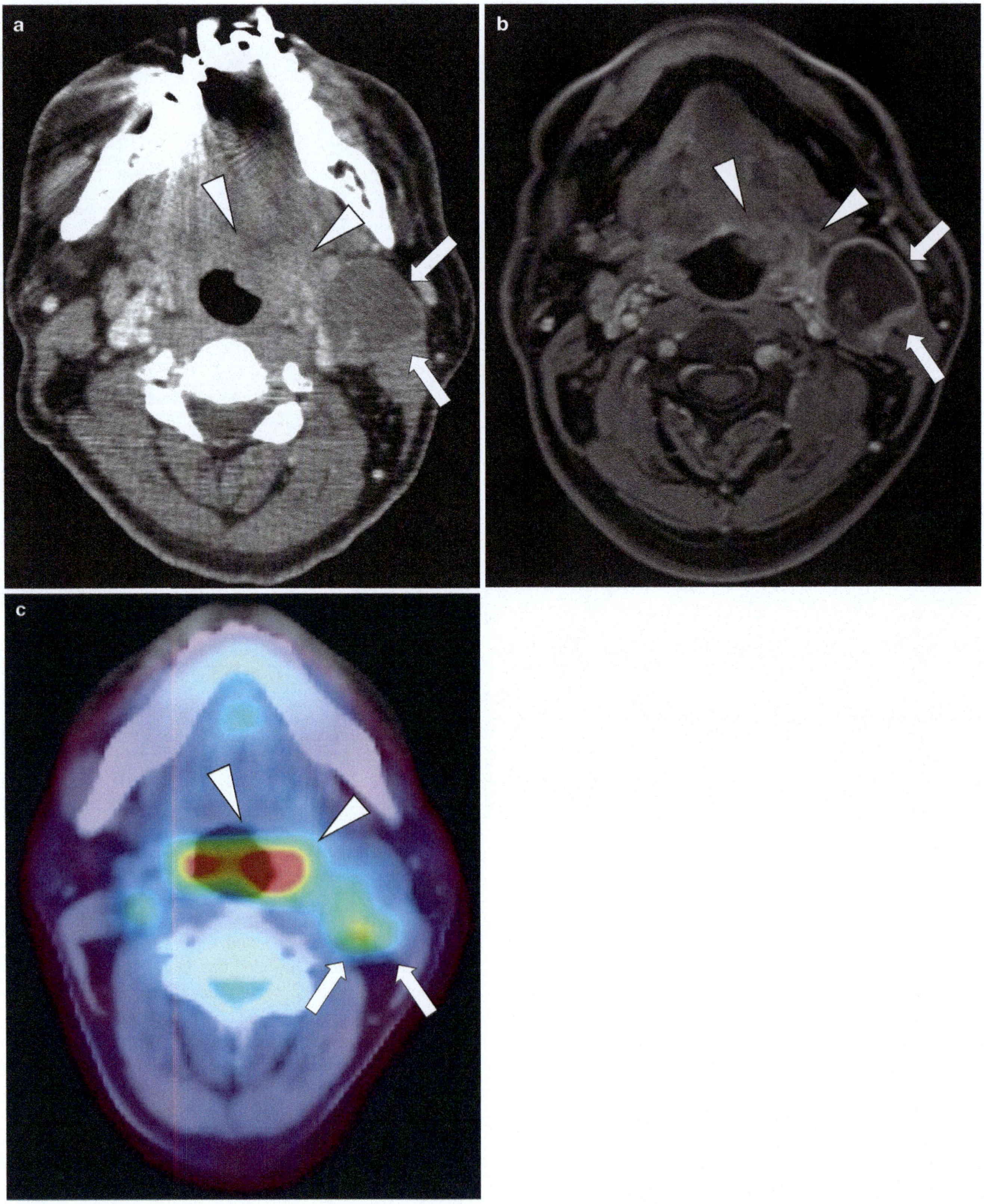

Fig. 10.14 A 49-year-old man with HPV-associated oropharyngeal carcinoma (**a**, **b**, and **c**, *arrowheads*). Contrast-enhanced CT and contrast-enhanced MR presented the necrotic lymph node metastasis on the left side (**a** and **b**, *arrows*). In contrast, fused PET-CT showed only a subtle uptake at the lymph node periphery (**c**, *arrows*)

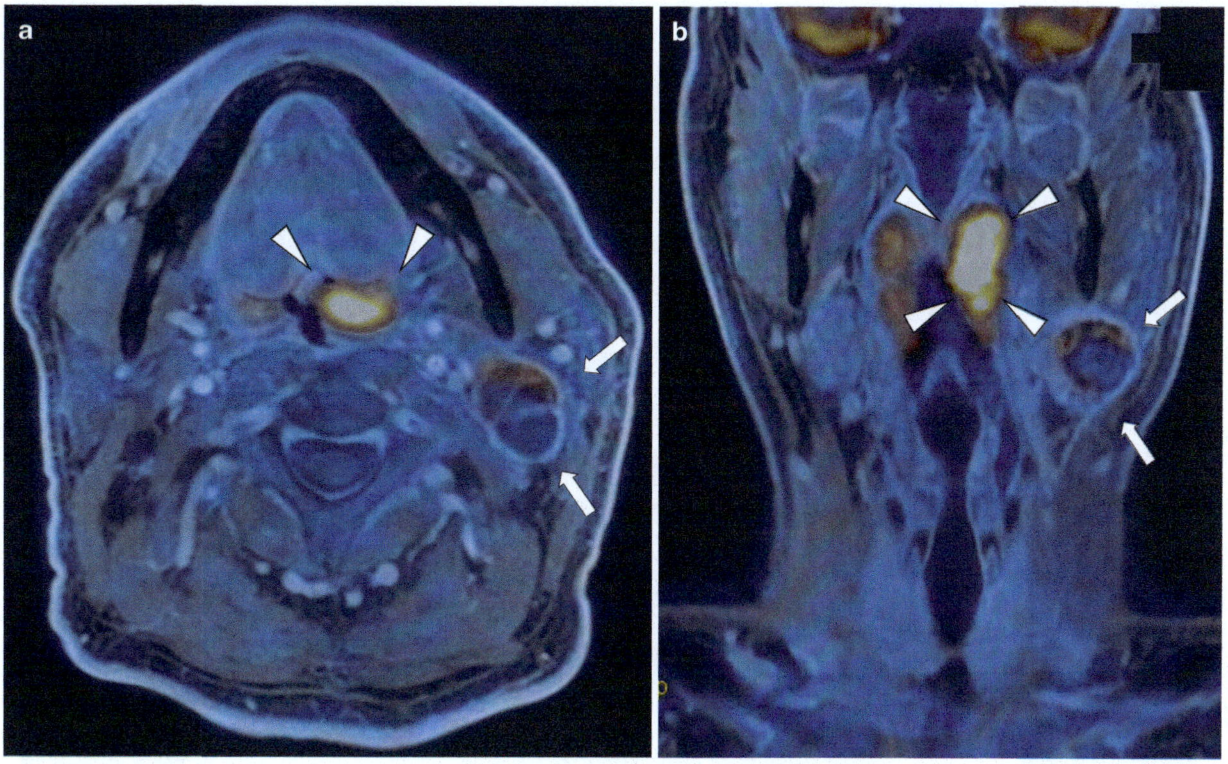

Fig. 10.15 HPV-associated oropharyngeal carcinoma (**a** and **b**, *arrowheads*). Fused PET/MR showed almost no avid necrotic lymph node (*arrows*). (Courtesy of Dr. Hüllner Martin at the Department of Nuclear Medicine, University Hospital Zurich, Switzerland)

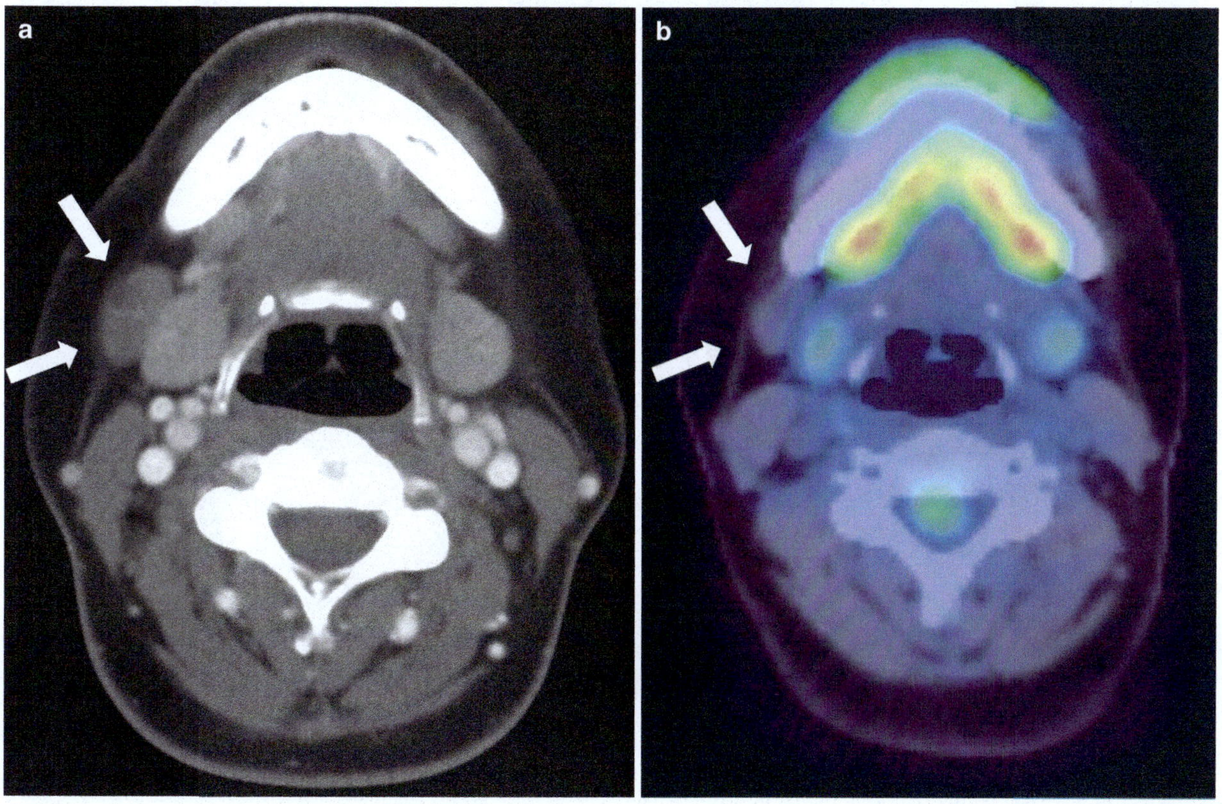

Fig. 10.16 A 41-year-old woman with mucoepidermoid tumor in buccal mucosa. The contrast-enhanced CT after surgical treatment detected a slightly contrast-enhanced lymph node adjacent to the submaxillary gland (**a**, *arrows*). There was no tracer uptake in this lesion on FDG-PET/CT (**b**, *arrows*). As the lymph node was growing during follow-up, surgical resection was performed and the metastasis of mucoepidermoid tumor was pathologically confirmed. Low concentration of tumor cells, which is sometimes observed in mucoepidermoid tumor, was associated with low FDG uptake in this lesion

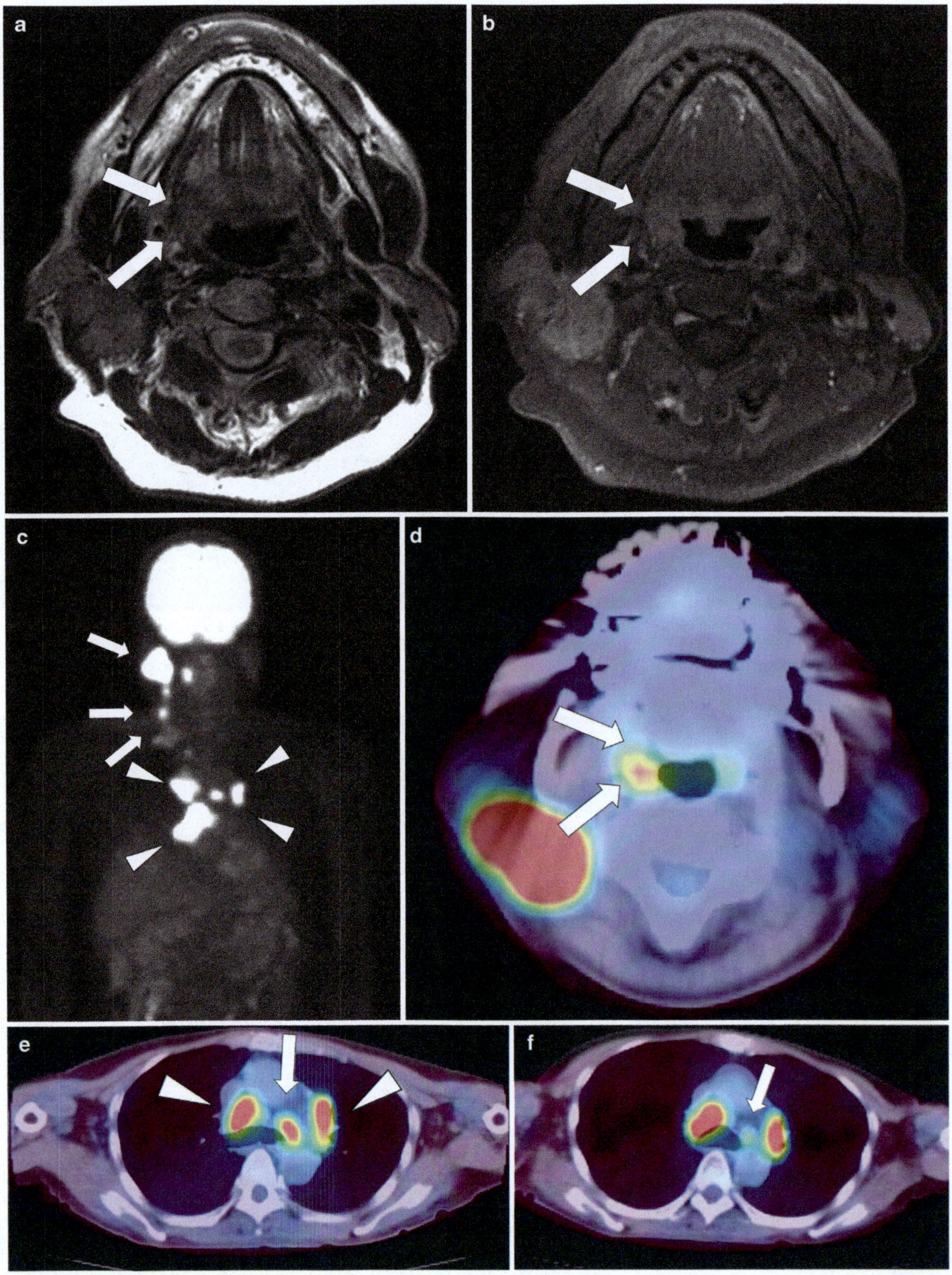

Fig. 10.17 A 69-year-old man with HPV-associated tonsil carcinoma. T2WI and contrast-enhanced T1WI showed no or only subtle morphological changes in the tonsil on the right side (**a** and **b**, *arrows*). The maximum intensity projection (MIP) images of FDG-PET demonstrated existence of multiple lymph node metastases (**c**, *arrows*), though the primary site had moderate SUV uptake (SUVmax 6.48) (**d**, *arrows*). The coexisting sarcoidosis made it difficult to assess whether lymph node metastasis was present in the thoracic area (*arrowheads* of **c** and *arrows* of **e**). The follow-up PET/CT after chemoradiation clearly depicted the metabolic response only in the metastatic lymph node (**e** and **f**, *arrows*)

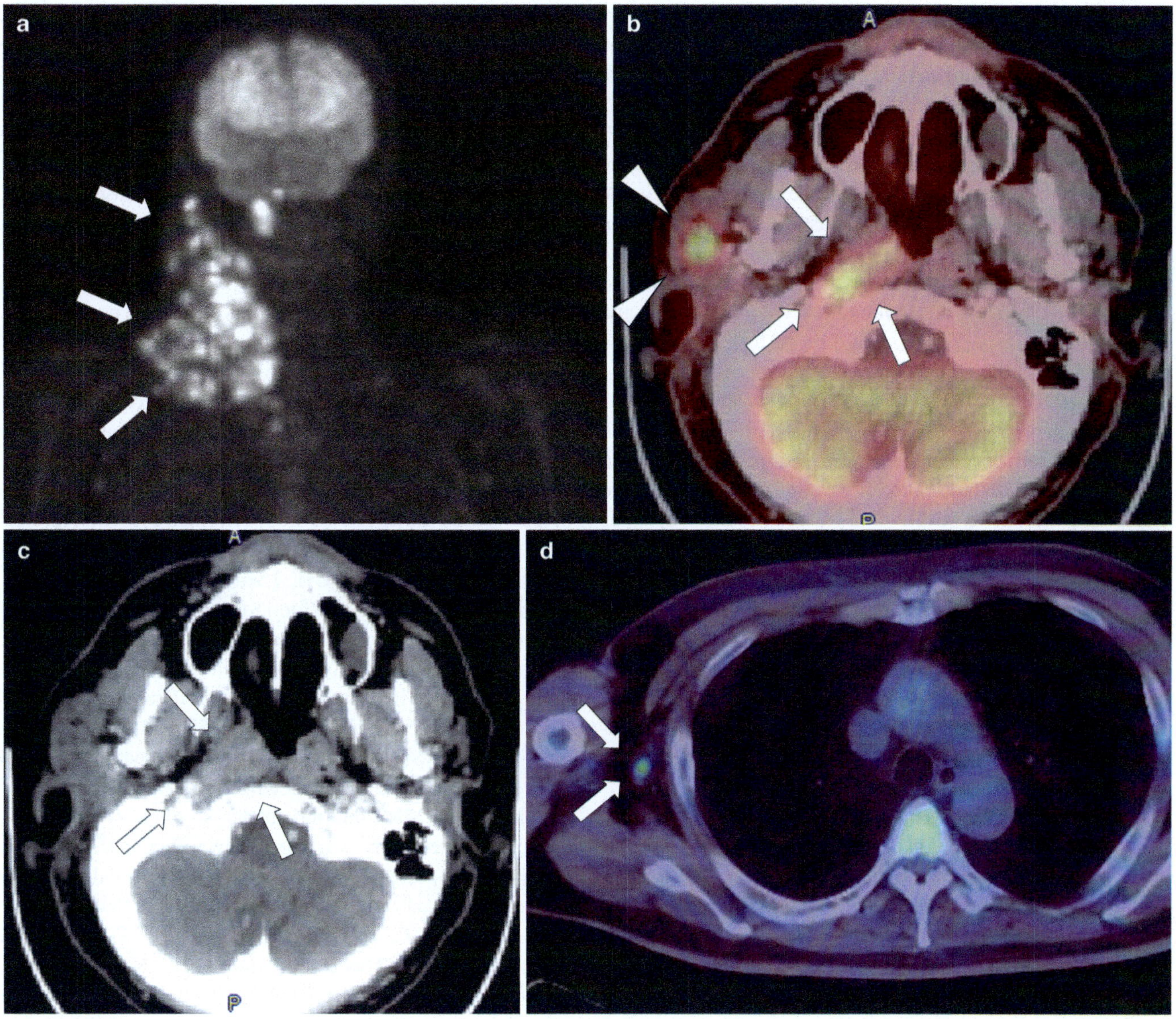

Fig. 10.18 A 54-year-old man with unilateral cervical lymphadenopathy. The biopsy confirmed lymph node metastasis of squamous cell carcinoma with EBV infection. The initial workup consisting of clinical examination, CT, and MRI did not find any primary site. Subsequently, PET was performed. The maximum intensity projection (MIP) images showed multiple FDG uptakes in lymph nodes on the right side (**a**, *arrows*). Fused PET/CT images demonstrated focal uptake in the nasopharynx (**b**, *arrows*). Meanwhile, contrast-enhanced CT showed only subtle morphological changes in this lesion (**c**, *arrows*). The lymph node metastasis was clearly depicted on fused PET/CT images (**b**, *arrowheads*). After the scan, the diagnosis was changed from T0 (unknown primary tumor with EBV infection) to T1 based on the 8th AJCC classification. Simultaneously, the axillary lymph node was also detected (**d**, *arrows*). As a result, the M staging was upstaged from M0 to M1

10.4 Patients with HPV Positive Oropharyngeal Cancer

It has been clarified that HPV-associated HNC is a distinct category of patients with a favorable prognosis [127–129]. The 8th edition of *Union for International Cancer Control (UICC)* TNM staging separately categorized HPV-positive oropharyngeal cancer as a low-risk stratification. In this category, LN staging was generally downstaged (e.g., N2a and N2b were converted to N1) because patients with HPV-positive HNC more likely present with advanced N stage despite favorable outcomes [128]. One of the common imaging findings in this group is cystic LN metastasis [130]. This kind of LN may be missed or misdiagnosed by PET with low-dose CT due to subtle FDG uptake [131], and in such cases, PET/ceCT or PET/MR can be useful for detection (Figs. 10.14 and 10.15) [13, 132]. HPV status also impacts on the ratio and timing of distant metastasis [133, 134]. The HPV-positive HNC generally has low prevalence of distant metastasis. However, when present, distant metastasis sometimes manifests a disseminating phenotype or affects multiple organs, which is rarely seen in HPV-negative patients [135, 136]. As another atypical clinical behavior, metastasis can also occur later after completion of radiation therapy (between 3 and 5 years) [135–137]. Tailored surveillance protocols and clinical interpretations should be considered based on the natural course of this patient group.

In terms of the quantification of FDG uptake, HPV-positive HNC may have different characteristics from HPV-negative HNC. Although there are some discrepancies in the literature, a trend of lower FDG uptake at the primary site and higher FDG uptake at LN metastasis was observed in HPV-positive patients [138–140]. This feature may indicate that the evaluation of prognosis by using an SUV value (e.g., SUV max, SUV peak, metabolic tumor volume [MTV], and total lesion glycosis [TLG]) should be performed under the consideration of the HPV status.

The role of posttreatment PET/CT assessment of patients with HPV-associated HNC was evaluated by Awan et al. [141]. They retrospectively included 108 patients (68 with HPV-positive status and 40 with HPV-negative status) who underwent definitive CRT. The median follow-up was 2.38 years. In terms of PET/CT assessment for the regional recurrence of HPV-positive patients, NPV was higher, but PPV was lower compared to that of patients with an HPV-negative status (100% and 50%, respectively, vs. 88.5% and 72.7%). Despite the good outcome of patients with an HPV-positive status, the negative posttreatment PET/CT scan status in this group acts as an independent predictor of recurrence-free survival (see Sect. 10.5.4 for more detailed studies). Several clinical trials of RT-dose de-escalation for HPV-associated HNC have been run [142]. In NRG-HN002, an ongoing randomized phase II trial for patients with HPV-positive status, the predictive value of posttreatment PET/CT evaluation for locoregional control, and progression-free survival will be evaluated as a secondary objective, potentially revealing the different role of PET/CT in this condition [143].

10.5 Implication for Patient Management

10.5.1 Scan Timing for Therapy Assessment

The timing of performing PET/CT is important. Posttreatment inflammation can yield false-positive results (Figs. 10.2 and 10.3). Ong et al. evaluated diagnostic performance for the assessment of tumor recurrence after concurrent chemoradiation therapy (CRT) in 65 patients with advanced HNC [144]. Although the sample size was small (7 heminecks had positive findings), the results showed that PET/CT scans at 8–12 weeks after treatment have low specificity (33%) and low positive predictive value (PPV, 14%) compared to the scans after 12 weeks (with specificity and PPV reaching 94% and 67%, respectively). Subsequent meta-analyses confirmed that a minimum of 12 weeks after radiation is the optimal duration to avoid false-positive lesions on PET/CT [48, 145–148]. A recent study that evaluated the probability of a correct PET/CT result as a function of the time after the end of CRT concluded that the probability reached a plateau after 11 weeks [149]. Therefore, the European Association of Nuclear Medicine (EANM) guidelines recommend that the optimal interval is at least 10 days for chemotherapy and 3 months after radiotherapy [3]. NCCN guidelines also recommend that the first PET/CT scan for follow-up should be performed at a minimum of 12 weeks after treatment to reduce the rate of false-positives. In the meantime, other modalities may be more useful for the assessment of treatment response [150–152]. Although early response assessment with FDG-PET during CRT has been performed for research purposes, it is still rarely performed in clinical settings [38, 152–154].

The use of PET surveillance in patients without clinical findings suspicious of recurrence is controversial [15, 49]. Abgral et al. prospectively enrolled 91 HNC patients (including 5 patients with initial stage I, 18 with stage II, 19 with stage III, and 49 with stage IV) without any clinical evidence of recurrence [155]. PET/CT was performed 11.6 ± 4.4 months after the end of treatment. Thirty patients (none with initial stage I, 6 with initial stage II, 7 with initial stage III, and 17 with initial stage IV) were found to have proven recurrence and 61 patients to have no recurrence, using histopathology findings or 6-month follow-up as reference diagnostic. The findings revealed high sensitivity and moderate specificity of PET for HNC recurrence (100% and 85%, respectively). In a meta-analysis, Sheikhbahaei et al. performed a subgroup analysis between the groups with and without clinical or imaging (CT or MRI) findings suspicious of recurrence [146]. The pooled sensitivity was subtly lower, but specificity was higher in the patients with negative suspicious findings of recurrence compared to the group with positive findings (0.89 [0.78–0.95] and 0.92 [0.86–0.95] vs. 0.94 [0.90–0.96] and 0.78 [0.69–0.85]). The results should be cautiously interpreted because of their vulnerability to the risk of selection bias. The improved specificity in the patients without clinical findings may be caused by the increase of true-positives in the lesions considered negative by CT or MRI, not the increase of true-negatives. In contrast, the improved sensitivity in patients with clinical findings may be due to the increase in true-negatives in the lesions considered positive by CT or MRI.

Among all instances of recurrence of HNC post-definitive treatment, 65.4–79% recurrences occur within 1 year and 88.5–95% recurrences occur within 2 years [156, 157]. Therefore, several studies have sought to determine whether early PET/CT surveillance (e.g., 3 months after treatment) is sufficient to detect later recurrence. Ho et al. performed a 10-year retrospective analysis of patients with HNC [158], in which they included 284 patients who underwent PET/CT 3 months after treatment. Among those with negative 3-month imaging, 175 had PET/CT 12 months later. Of those with negative findings both at 3- and 12-month PET/CT scans, 77 had 24-month PET/CT examination. The results show that 12-month PET/CT detected only 2% of locoregional recurrence and 24-month PET/CT did no locoregional recurrence.

In terms of distant metastasis, 12- and 24-month PET/CT detected 6% and 4% of distant metastasis, respectively, after a negative 3-month PET/CT. However, PET/CT-detected recurrence between 3 and 24 months did not contribute to improving disease-free survival or median survival compared to clinically detected recurrence over the same duration. Spector et al. also revealed a similar finding that PET-based detection of distant metastasis did not improve life expectancy compared to other imaging (chest X-ray or CT)-based detection [159]. McDermott et al. sought to clarify how many PET/CT surveillance scans were efficient [160] by recruiting 512 patients who underwent consecutive PET/CT scans for surveillance purposes. Restaging PET/CT scans were excluded. The surveillance scans were performed 2, 5, 8, and 14 months after therapy. The results showed that the negative predictive value (NPV) of the first surveillance was high but insufficient (91%). However, two consecutive PET/CT scans with negative findings scored sufficiently high NPV (98%), suggesting that further PET/CT surveillance is wasteful. Another study recruiting 88 patients also showed that 95% of asymptomatic recurrences were detected within 24 months after treatment, indicating PET/CT surveillance beyond 24 months may not be cost-effective [157]. Based on the aforementioned studies, routine PET/CT surveillance should be discouraged, and NCCN guidelines do not recommend repeated PET/CT for asymptomatic patients who have completed initial treatment and had one negative baseline scan [15, 49, 161]. However, in the real world, most physicians perform routine surveillance PET/CT [161]. There are several conceivable causes for this discrepancy. Physicians may not be aware of the lack of supportive survival data, they may remain optimistic about improved outcomes based on their personal experience, they may respond to patients' expectations, or they believe the importance of reassurance provided by a negative scan [161, 162].

Finally, several current studies have revealed that HNC cases positive for human papillomavirus (HPV) display different posttreatment changes in terms of FDG accumulation. Therefore, tailored PET/CT surveillance protocols with different timings may be needed (See Sect. 10.4).

10.5.2 Prognostic Value of Baseline FDG-PET

There have been several studies confirming that FDG avidity on pretherapy FDG-PET can be used to stratify survival outcomes in patients with HNC [163, 164]. Recently, to evaluate the performance of PET-based prognostic prediction, Pak et al. conducted a systematic review including 1180 patients from 30 studies [165]. They revealed that patients with higher volumetric parameters, MTV and TLG, had a higher risk for both recurrence (hazard ratio, 3.06 [2.33–4.01] and 3.10 [2.27–4.24]) and death (hazard ratio, 3.51 [2.62–4.72] and 3.14 [2.24–4.40]). They also conducted a subanalysis comparing the prognosis-predicting performance of SUV_{max}, MTV, and TLG. Although it was not a direct comparison between the metrics, the hazard ratio of SUV_{max} was lower than that of the volumetric metrics (1.83 [1.39–2.42] for recurrence and 2.36 (1.48–3.77) for death). This result was confirmed by other meta-analysis studies as well [166, 167]. In one of these two studies, the authors revealed that the prognostic value of SUV_{max} for event-free survival and overall survival was significantly different between nasopharyngeal carcinoma (NPC) and non-nasopharyngeal carcinoma (non-NPC) (2.36 [1.41–3.97] vs. 1.67 [1.29–2.18] for event-free survival and 2.41 [1.24–4.65] vs. 1.07 [1.01–1.13] for overall survival) [167]. In the other study, the authors highlighted that MTV was superior to the 7th AJCC TNM staging for predicting disease-free survival and overall survival [166]. This superiority may be partially derived from the fact that the 7th AJCC TNM staging did not consider HPV status, which affects not only the prognosis but also the accumulation pattern of PET. Over the last decade, a vast number of studies have investigated the prognostic value of PET incorporating the HPV status [73, 168–171]. Although the results are contradictory among studies, there is indication that PET parameters tend to predict prognosis for non-HPV HNC, but not for HPV-related HNC [168, 169, 172].

10.5.3 Prognostic Value of Intratreatment or Posttreatment FDG-PET

Metabolic information, as provided by intratreatment (interim) PET or posttreatment PET, can predict the treatment response of initial therapy (Fig. 10.19). Sheikhbahaei et al. performed a meta-analysis which focused on predicting prognosis through intratherapy or posttherapy PET [173]. From 26 studies, 600 patients were included for the evaluation of overall survival and 479 for event-free survival. The results revealed that positive findings on intratreatment or posttreatment PET presented an increased risk with a hazard ratio of 3.55 (2.55–5.37) for overall survival and 4.73 (2.61–8.56) for progression or recurrence. The risk-ratio analysis also proved that a positive PET finding was associated with an increased risk of death not only within 2 years of follow-up (6.19 [3.04–12.62]) but also within 3–5 years of follow-up (2.42 [1.76–3.32]). In a subgroup analysis, the effect of the timing of PET evaluation on the prediction of prognosis was estimated (interim versus posttreatment, or before versus after 12 weeks from completion of treatment). Posttreatment evaluation tended to be superior to interim evaluation. Likewise, PET evaluation 12 weeks after the completion of radiation had a higher predictive value than that at 12 weeks prior, although the difference was not significant. More specifically, another systematic review focusing on the prognostic value of interim PET by Garibaldi et al. [153] included 533 patients from 23 studies. The authors concluded that posttreatment PET had greater prognostic power than interim PET, but the possibility to adjust the treatment strategy based on interim PET as an

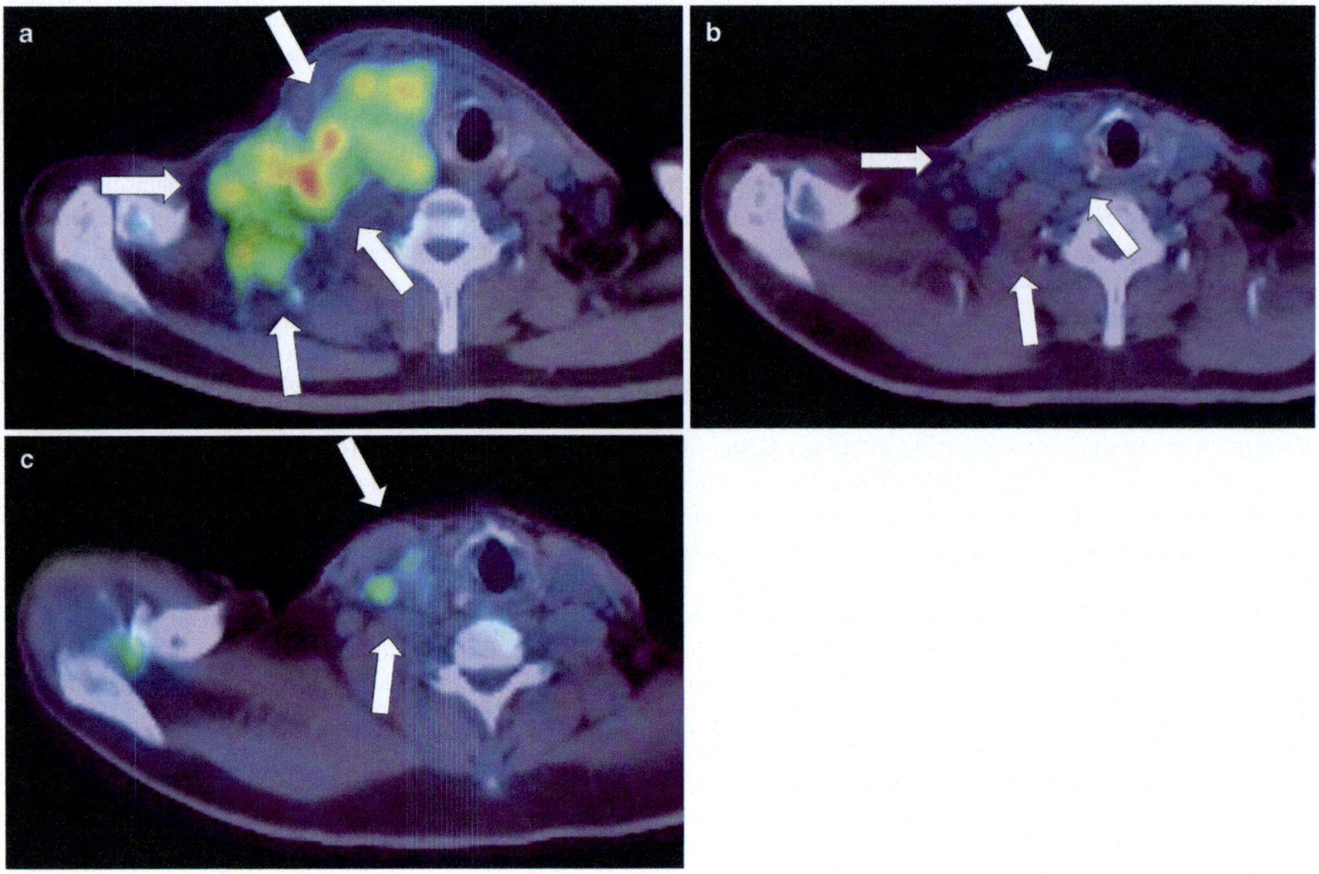

Fig. 10.19 A 54-year-old man with unilateral cervical lymphadenopathy (**a**, *arrows*) (same patient as in Fig. 10.18). After the initial workup including PET/CT, first-line chemoradiation therapy was performed. Two months after the induction of first-line therapy, intertreatment PET/CT was performed for the evaluation of treatment response. The SUV uptake of the tumor site decreased significantly (**b**, *arrows*). Based on these findings, the same regimen of chemoradiation therapy was continued. Four months after intertreatment PET, PET/CT was performed again. The images demonstrate FDG-avid lymph-node recurrence, indicating the failure of the first-line treatment (**c**, *arrows*). Immediately after the scan, the second-line chemotherapy was inducted

early assessment had much greater clinical relevance. More recently, another systematic review by Martens et al. [152] including 17 studies revealed that SUV_{max} can be used as a predictive value, with a pooled hazard ratio of 2.32 (1.39–3.87) for locoregional failure and 2.59 (1.64–4.12) for overall survival. TLG can also be used as a predictive value, with a pooled hazard ratio of 5.68 (2.86–11.31) for locoregional control and 3.04 (1.70–5.42) for overall survival. Nonetheless, the research designs in these reviews were widely heterogeneous (e.g., scan timing, treatment strategy, and methodology of assessment). The ongoing prospective multicenter study, TEmPoRAL (Positron Emission Tomography (PET) During Radiochemotherapy to Treat Otorhinolaryngological Cancer, ClinicalTrials.gov NCT02469922), has been designed to enroll more than 100 patients undergoing interim PET once or twice and use a standardized evaluation. The prognostic value of pretreatment, interim, and posttreatment PET for locoregional relapse will be evaluated after trial completion (due in November 2020).

10.5.4 PET/CT Evaluation for Residual Nodal Disease After CRT

Radiation, or chemoradiation, has become the initial treatment of choice for patients with HNC. After primary treatment of patients with advanced nodal disease (N2 or N3), image-guided decision-making for further surgery (i.e., neck dissection) is generally recommended [15]. A high NPV of posttreatment PET/CT can be utilized to safely avoid unnecessary neck dissection. Mehanna et al. published the results of the prospective, randomized, and controlled PET-NECK trial, which recruited 564 patients from 37 centers in the United Kingdom who underwent primary CRT [174]. In the trial, half of the patients were assigned to the planned-surgery group and the remaining to the PET/CT-guided surveillance group. There was no statistical difference in survival between the two groups, even after adjustment for HPV status during the follow-up phase (with a minimum duration of 24 months and median of 36 months). The surgical complications of delayed neck dissection in the surveillance group were not more frequent than those in the planned-surgery group. In the surveillance group, approximately 80% of patients were considered safe for neck dissection, resulting in saving 2190 U.S. Dollars per patient [175]. The authors, however, indicated that PET/CT-guided surveillance offers further room for improvement in clinical management, as the persistence of post-CRT nodal FDG accumulation in HPV-positive patients may cause false-positive results. Helsen et al. evaluated the diagnostic accuracy of the current PET/CT system in detecting nodal disease within 6 months after treatment by including 1293 patients from 20 studies [176]. The pooled estimated sensitivity and specificity were 85% (76–91%) and 93% (89–96%), respectively. They revealed that the diagnostic performance was lower in patients with HPV-positive status than in those with HPV-negative status (sensitivity and specificity, 75% vs. 89% and 87% vs. 95%, respectively). HPV-positive lesions are considered more sensitive to radiation than HPV-negative lesions [177]. Therefore, delayed regrowth of the persistent tumor cells after radiation may cause false-negative results at the first PET surveillance [176]. In terms of lower specificity, intratumoral T-cell-based antitumor immune response may lead to prolonged secondary inflammatory changes in the treated LNs [127, 176]. In a study evaluating the temporal change of LN metastasis following treatment, LN size regression was more prolonged in patients with HPV-positive status than in patients without HPV-positive status [178]. Interestingly, the LN regression curve was not separate between both groups until 12 weeks. Therefore, to overcome the low specificity for LN detection in HPV-positive patients, Liu et al. performed repeat PET/CT at 16 weeks to assess the persistence of findings with tumor uptake on 12-week PET/CT in a study that retrospectively included 342 consecutive patients with HPV-associated HNC [47]. Out of 342 patients, 41 showed incomplete response by PET/CT examination at 12 weeks. In this setting, NPV was high, but PPV was low (98% and 12%, respectively). If the patients with stable FDG avidity between 12 and 16 weeks were assigned into the local failure group, repeat PET/CT excluded 32 patients (78%) from unnecessary surgery despite a low PPV (50%). Notably, the PET-NECK trial already confirmed the benefit of 12-week PET/CT surveillance in patients with HPV-positive status despite the drawback of PET assessment described above [174]. In some patient groups (elderly, poor performance status, comorbidity), chemotherapy is not suitable, and only radiotherapy is performed. The high NPV of PET/CT for residual nodal detection was also confirmed in patients who underwent definitive radiotherapy without chemotherapy [179].

10.5.5 Surveillance Following Definitive Treatment of HNC

Early detection of recurrent disease or second primary tumors is of paramount importance for early salvage treatment, which potentially results in survival benefit [180]. Although conventional imaging modalities such as CT and MRI are mainly used for this purpose, their detectability is affected by morphological changes caused by surgery or radiotherapy [181] (Fig. 10.20). As PET is capable of captur-

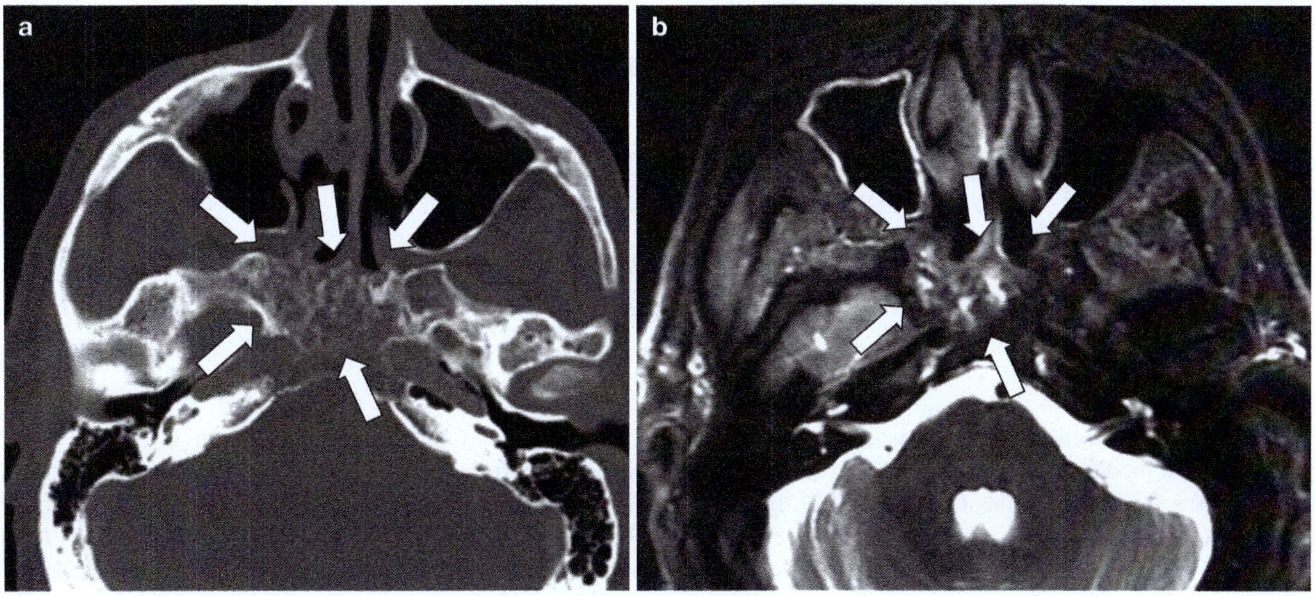

Fig. 10.20 A 72-year-old man after surgery and 21 months after CRT for epipharynx SCC. The skull base bone was heterogeneous on CT, fat-sat T2WI and contrast-enhanced T1WI (**a**, **b**, and **c**, *arrows*). These findings were potentially indicative of recurrent SCC and skull base invasion. Meanwhile, fused PET images showed that there was no FDG uptake in the lesion (**d** and **e**). As a result, tumor recurrence was definitely ruled out. This figure is referred to "Sekine T. Emerging topics in PET/CT and PET/MR. Toukeibu Gan. 2018;44:347–352." (Permission obtained from Japan Academic Association for Copyright Clearance)

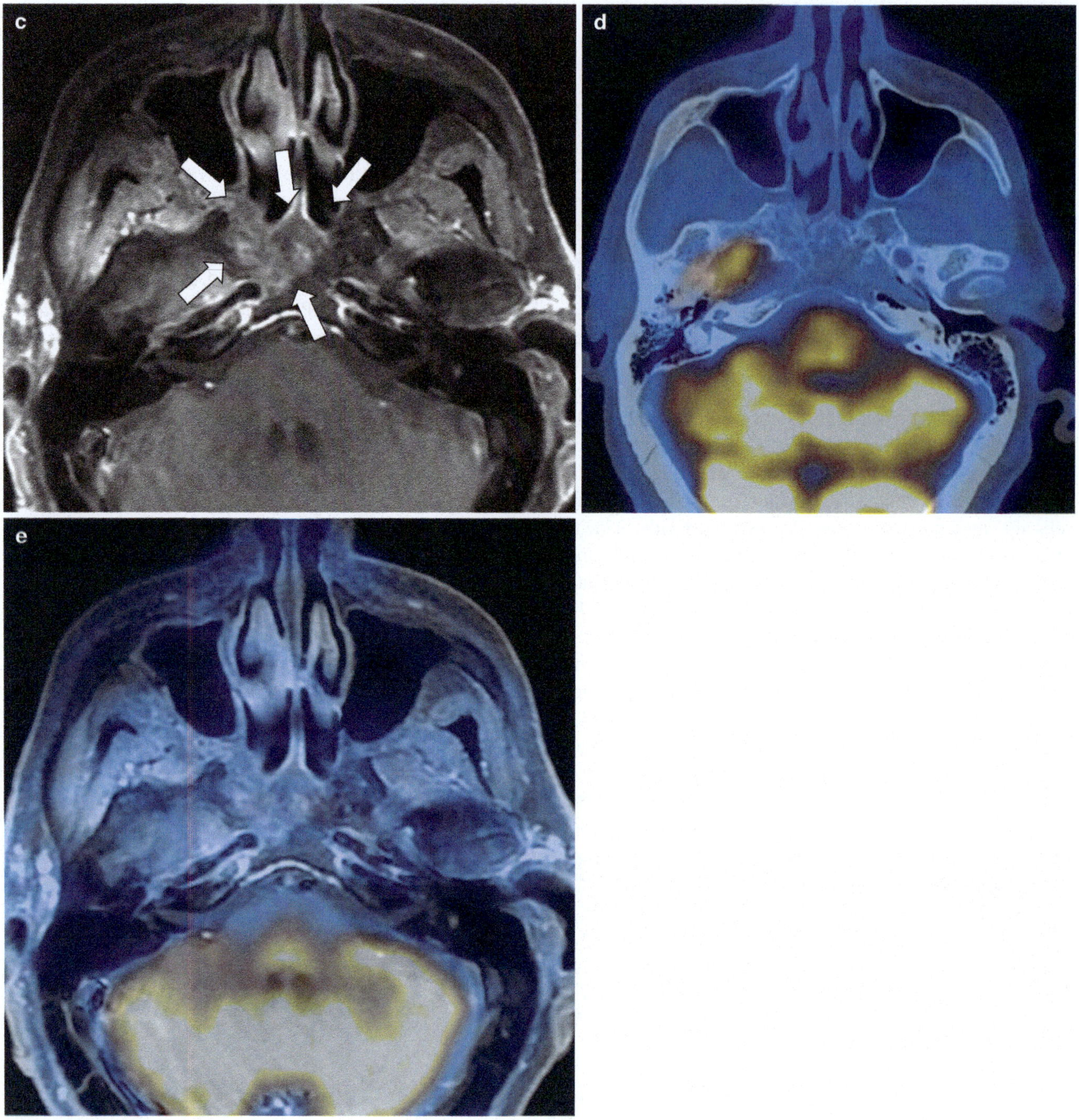

Fig. 10.20 (continued)

ing tumor metabolic changes, it is considered as one of the most accurate modalities available for differentiating recurrent diseases from posttreatment changes [182]. In a meta-analysis, Gupta et al. recruited 2335 patients from 51 studies between 1990 and 2010 [48]. Stand-alone PET scans were also included. In the patient group scanned for more than 12 weeks posttreatment, the pooled sensitivity and specificity for the primary site were 91.9% [82.7–97.1%] and 86.9% [82.8–90.4%], and those for the neck nodes were 90.4% [79.6–96.6%] and 94.3% [91.6–96.3%], respectively. A recent meta-analysis conducted by Wong et al. recruited 2627 patients from 24 studies between 2010 and 2016, reflecting current PET/CT technology and recent advances in HNC management [148]. The sensitivity and specificity of PET/CT detectability for local failure were 85% [79–90%] and 92% [90–94%], respectively. The diagnostic accuracy was significantly improved in PET/CT after 3 months compared to that before 3 months (with a sensitivity and specificity of 87% and 93% vs. 60% and 84%, respectively). These results are in line with those of other earlier meta-analyses [48, 145–147]. The clinical performance of PET/MR for surveillance was also evaluated by Queiroz et al., who prospectively included 87 patients who underwent both PET/ceCT and PET/ceMR for restaging/follow-up of HNC [89]. Their results showed that both PET/CT and PET/MR had superior diagnostic accuracy to ceCT or ceMR, but the diagnostic accuracy between PET/CT and PET/MR did not differ (sensitivity and specificity of 63.9% and 96.3% for ceCT, 62.9% and 96.7% for ceMR, 85.7% and 92.7% for PET/ceCT, and 85.7% and 93.9% for PET/ceMR, respectively). The authors presented two main advantages of PET/MR over PET/CT for the evaluation of oropharynx regions. First, PET/MR can eliminate implanted metal artifacts better than that by PET/CT (Figs. 10.5 and 10.6). Second, PET/MR can perform a detailed evaluation of the perineural spread (Figs. 10.8, 10.9 and 10.10). These advantages were also confirmed by other studies [87, 88]. Meanwhile, inferior image quality of PET/MR in hypopharynx/larynx regions was observed due to the motion artifact with swallowing or carotid pulsation (Fig. 10.13). Additionally, it was occasionally difficult to distinguish postradiotherapy osteo/cartilage necrosis after radiation therapy from the tumor recurrence. There was a significant overlap in the SUV_{max} between these two groups. Although CT and MRI do provide additional information, pathological confirmation is essential in complicated cases [27, 87, 183] (Fig. 10.21).

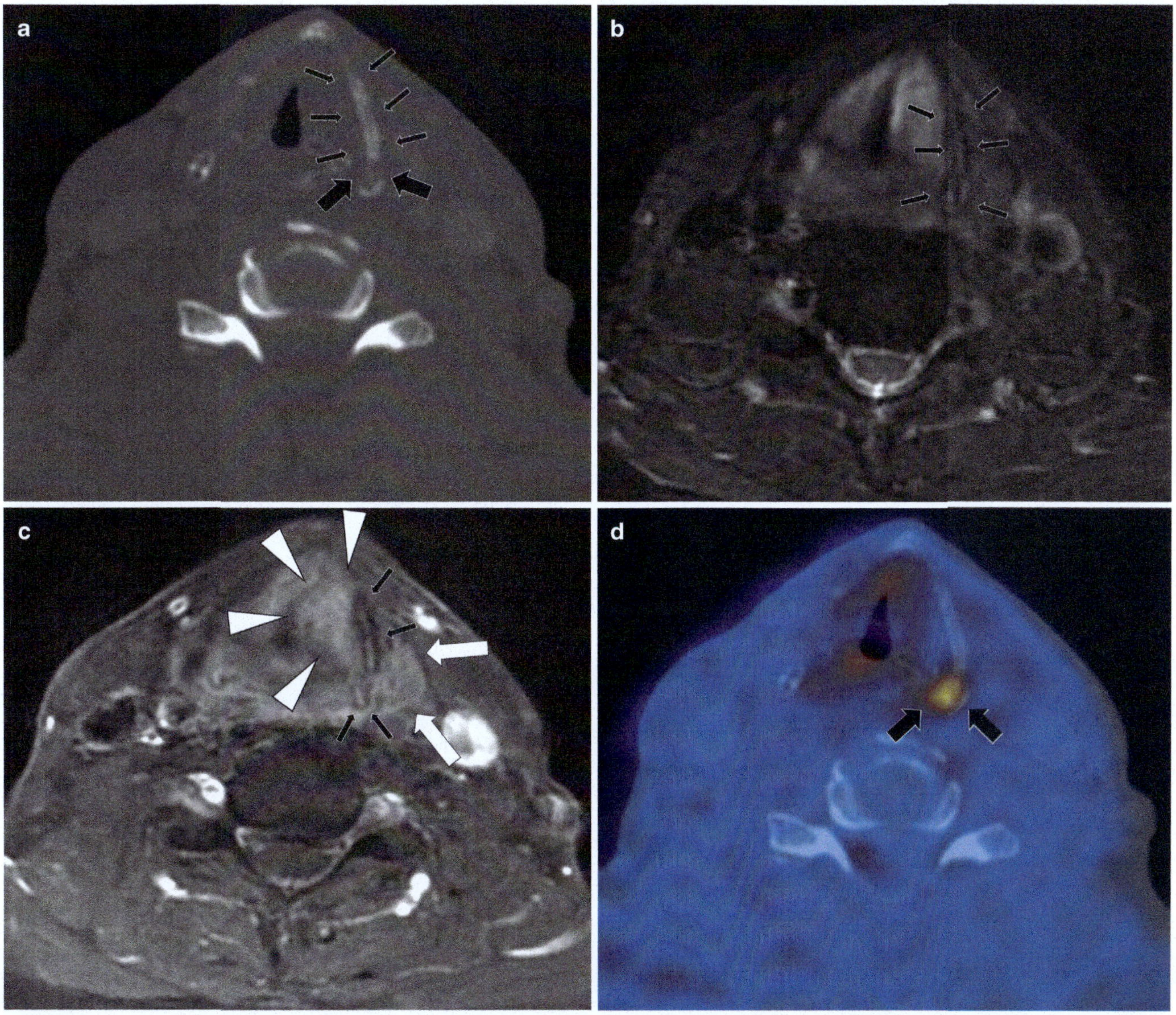

Fig. 10.21 A 62-year-old man with supraglottic laryngeal SCC. Images were obtained 7 years after radiation therapy. CT showed an irregular calcification (**a**, *thin arrows*) and erosion (**a**, *thick arrows*) of the left thyroid cartilage lamina. Hyperintensity was noted on fat-sat T2WI (**b**, *arrows*) and on contrast-enhanced T1WI (**c**, *thin arrows*). Corresponding to the bone erosion on CT (**a**, *thick arrows*), fused PET images demonstrated focal uptake in the thyroid cartilage (**d** and **e**, *arrows*). This finding indicated potentially recurrent SCC with cartilage invasion. Pronounced soft tissue swelling might be an imaging sign of radiation necrosis (**c**, *arrowheads*). However, one would expect FDG positivity with tumor recurrence. There was no air deposit around this lesion. Biopsy of this lesion confirmed radiation necrosis without evidence of malignant cells. This figure is referred to "Sekine T. Local resectability assessment of head and neck cancer: Positron emission tomography/MRI versus positron emission tomography/CT. Head Neck. 2017;39:1550–1558." (Permission obtained from Wiley)

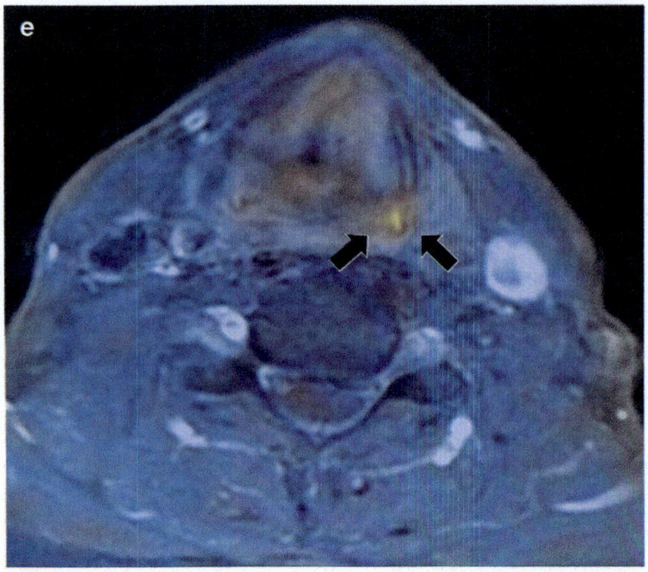

Fig. 10.21 (continued)

10.6 Summary

FDG-PET is useful in HNC for initial evaluation, prognosis prediction, therapy response assessment to avoid unnecessary planned neck dissection, and surveillance. The newly developed PET/MR may enhance this advantage, though its evidence is currently limited. Presently, interim PET or routine surveillance is not encouraged in asymptomatic patients. Future research is needed in the field of standardized interpretation (especially in patients after the competition of chemoradiation), tumor heterogeneity evaluation by PET, and the utility of PET in HPV-associated HNC.

References

1. Surasi DS, Bhambhvani P, Baldwin JA, Almodovar SE, O'Malley JP. (1)(8)F-FDG PET and PET/CT patient preparation: a review of the literature. J Nucl Med Technol. 2014;42:5–13.
2. Wahl RL, Henry CA, Ethier SP. Serum glucose: effects on tumor and normal tissue accumulation of 2-[F-18]-fluoro-2-deoxy-D-glucose in rodents with mammary carcinoma. Radiology. 1992;183:643–7.
3. Boellaard R, Delgado-Bolton R, Oyen WJ, et al. FDG PET/CT: EANM procedure guidelines for tumour imaging: version 2.0. Eur J Nucl Med Mol Imaging. 2015;42:328–54.
4. Delbeke D, Coleman RE, Guiberteau MJ, et al. Procedure guideline for tumor imaging with 18F-FDG PET/CT 1.0. J Nucl Med. 2006;47:885–95.
5. Kathula SK, Mantil J. Chewing gum causing a very high FDG uptake of the tongue on PET scan. Clin Nucl Med. 2007;32:122–3.
6. Cohade C, Osman M, Pannu HK, Wahl RL. Uptake in supraclavicular area fat ("USA-Fat"): description on 18F-FDG PET/CT. J Nucl Med. 2003;44:170–6.
7. Yamamoto Y, Wong TZ, Turkington TG, Hawk TC, Coleman RE. Head and neck cancer: dedicated FDG PET/CT protocol for detection—phantom and initial clinical studies. Radiology. 2007;244:263–72.
8. Wong TZ, Paulson EK, Nelson RC, Patz EF Jr, Coleman RE. Practical approach to diagnostic CT combined with PET. Am J Roentgenol. 2007;188:622–9.
9. Rodrigues RS, Bozza FA, Christian PE, et al. Comparison of whole-body PET/CT, dedicated high-resolution head and neck PET/CT, and contrast-enhanced CT in preoperative staging of clinically M0 squamous cell carcinoma of the head and neck. J Nucl Med. 2009;50:1205–13.
10. Ciappuccini R, Aide N, Blanchard D, et al. Incremental value of a dedicated head and neck acquisition during 18F-FDG PET/CT in patients with differentiated thyroid cancer. PLoS One. 2016;11:e0162482.
11. Subramaniam RM, Agarwal A, Colucci A, Ferraro R, Paidpally V, Mercier G. Impact of concurrent diagnostic level CT with PET/CT on the utilization of stand-alone CT and MRI in the management of head and neck cancer patients. Clin Nucl Med. 2013;38:790–4.
12. Aiken AH, Farley A, Baugnon KL, et al. Implementation of a Novel Surveillance Template for Head and Neck Cancer: Neck Imaging Reporting and Data System (NI-RADS). J Am Coll Radiol. 2016;13:743–746 e741.
13. Haerle SK, Strobel K, Ahmad N, Soltermann A, Schmid DT, Stoeckli SJ. Contrast-enhanced (1)(8)F-FDG-PET/CT for the assessment of necrotic lymph node metastases. Head Neck. 2011;33:324–9.
14. Suenaga Y, Kitajima K, Ishihara T, et al. FDG-PET/contrast-enhanced CT as a post-treatment tool in head and neck squamous cell carcinoma: comparison with FDG-PET/non-contrast-enhanced CT and contrast-enhanced CT. Eur Radiol. 2016;26:1018–30.
15. Network NCC. NCCN clinical practice guidelines in oncology: head and neck cancers. Version 2.2019. 2019.
16. Mawlawi O, Erasmus JJ, Munden RF, et al. Quantifying the effect of IV contrast media on integrated PET/CT: clinical evaluation. Am J Roentgenol. 2006;186:308–19.
17. Nakamoto Y, Chin BB, Kraitchman DL, Lawler LP, Marshall LT, Wahl RL. Effects of nonionic intravenous contrast agents at PET/CT imaging: phantom and canine studies. Radiology. 2003;227:817–24.
18. Kumar R, Mukherjee A, Mittal BR. Special techniques in PET/computed tomography imaging for evaluation of head and neck cancer. PET Clin. 2016;11:13–20.
19. Weissman JL, Carrau RL. "Puffed-cheek" CT improves evaluation of the oral cavity. Am J Neuroradiol. 2001;22:741–4.
20. Chang CY, Yang BH, Lin KH, Liu RS, Wang SJ, Shih WJ. Feasibility and incremental benefit of puffed-cheek 18F-FDG PET/CT on oral cancer patients. Clin Nucl Med. 2013;38:e374–8.
21. Sonni I, Baratto L, Park S, et al. Initial experience with a SiPM-based PET/CT scanner: influence of acquisition time on image quality. EJNMMI Phys. 2018;5:9.
22. Sekine T, Delso G, Zeimpekis KG, et al. Reduction of (18)F-FDG dose in clinical PET/MR imaging by using silicon photomultiplier detectors. Radiology. 2018;286:249–59.
23. Wright CL, Washington IR, Bhatt AD, Knopp MV. Emerging opportunities for digital PET/CT to advance locoregional therapy in head and neck cancer. Semin Radiat Oncol. 2019;29:93–101.
24. Delso G, Furst S, Jakoby B, et al. Performance measurements of the Siemens mMR integrated whole-body PET/MR scanner. J Nucl Med. 2011;52:1914–22.
25. Spick C, Herrmann K, Czernin J. 18F-FDG PET/CT and PET/MRI perform equally well in cancer: evidence from studies on more than 2,300 patients. J Nucl Med. 2016;57:420–30.
26. Raad RA, Friedman KP, Heacock L, Ponzo F, Melsaether A, Chandarana H. Outcome of small lung nodules missed on hybrid

PET/MRI in patients with primary malignancy. J Magn Reson Imaging. 2016;43(2):504–11.
27. Becker M, Varoquaux AD, Combescure C, et al. Local recurrence of squamous cell carcinoma of the head and neck after radio(chemo)therapy: diagnostic performance of FDG-PET/MRI with diffusion-weighted sequences. Eur Radiol. 2018;28(2):651–63.
28. Queiroz MA, Hullner M, Kuhn F, et al. Use of diffusion-weighted imaging (DWI) in PET/MRI for head and neck cancer evaluation. Eur J Nucl Med Mol Imaging. 2014;41:2212–21.
29. Kim YI, Cheon GJ, Kang SY, et al. Prognostic value of simultaneous (18)F-FDG PET/MRI using a combination of metabolo-volumetric parameters and apparent diffusion coefficient in treated head and neck cancer. EJNMMI Res. 2018;8:2.
30. Rasmussen JH, Nørgaard M, Hansen AE, et al. Feasibility of multiparametric imaging with PET/MR in head and neck squamous cell carcinoma. J Nucl Med. 2017;58:69–74.
31. Kuwert T, Ritt P. PET/MRI and PET/CT: is there room for both at the top of the food chain? Eur J Nucl Med Mol Imaging. 2016;43:209–11.
32. Queiroz MA, Huellner MW. PET/MR in cancers of the head and neck. Semin Nucl Med. 2015;45:248–65.
33. Kuhn FP, Hullner M, Mader CE, et al. Contrast-enhanced PET/MR imaging versus contrast-enhanced PET/CT in head and neck cancer: how much MR information is needed? J Nucl Med. 2014;55:551–8.
34. Haberkorn U, Strauss LG, Reisser C, et al. Glucose uptake, perfusion, and cell proliferation in head and neck tumors: relation of positron emission tomography to flow cytometry. J Nucl Med. 1991;32:1548–55.
35. Na KJ, Choi H. Tumor metabolic features identified by (18) F-FDG PET correlate with gene networks of immune cell microenvironment in head and neck cancer. J Nucl Med. 2018;59:31–7.
36. Gronroos TJ, Lehtio K, Soderstrom KO, et al. Hypoxia, blood flow and metabolism in squamous-cell carcinoma of the head and neck: correlations between multiple immunohistochemical parameters and PET. BMC Cancer. 2014;14:876.
37. Adams MC, Turkington TG, Wilson JM, Wong TZ. A systematic review of the factors affecting accuracy of SUV measurements. Am J Roentgenol. 2010;195:310–20.
38. Hoang JK, Das SK, Choudhury KR, Yoo DS, Brizel DM. Using FDG-PET to measure early treatment response in head and neck squamous cell carcinoma: quantifying intrinsic variability in order to understand treatment-induced change. Am J Neuroradiol. 2013;34:1428–33.
39. Wahl RL, Jacene H, Kasamon Y, Lodge MA. From RECIST to PERCIST: evolving considerations for PET response criteria in solid tumors. J Nucl Med. 2009;50(Suppl 1):122S–50S.
40. JH O, Lodge MA, Wahl RL. Practical PERCIST: a simplified guide to PET response criteria in solid tumors 1.0. Radiology. 2016;280:576–84.
41. Hoang JK, Choudhury KR, Chang J, Craciunescu OI, Yoo DS, Brizel DM. Diffusion-weighted imaging for head and neck squamous cell carcinoma: quantifying repeatability to understand early treatment-induced change. Am J Roentgenol. 2014;203:1104–8.
42. Aide N, Lasnon C, Veit-Haibach P, Sera T, Sattler B, Boellaard R. EANM/EARL harmonization strategies in PET quantification: from daily practice to multicentre oncological studies. Eur J Nucl Med Mol Imaging. 2017;44:17–31.
43. Paidpally V, Chirindel A, Lam S, Agrawal N, Quon H, Subramaniam RM. FDG-PET/CT imaging biomarkers in head and neck squamous cell carcinoma. Imaging Med. 2012;4:633–47.
44. Differding S, Hanin FX, Gregoire V. PET imaging biomarkers in head and neck cancer. Eur J Nucl Med Mol Imaging. 2015;42:613–22.
45. Ziai P, Hayeri MR, Salei A, et al. Role of optimal quantification of FDG PET imaging in the clinical practice of radiology. Radiographics. 2016;36:481–96.
46. Im HJ, Bradshaw T, Solaiyappan M, Cho SY. Current methods to define metabolic tumor volume in positron emission tomography: which one is better? Nucl Med Mol Imaging. 2018;52:5–15.
47. Liu HY, Milne R, Lock G, et al. Utility of a repeat PET/CT scan in HPV-associated oropharyngeal cancer following incomplete nodal response from (chemo)radiotherapy. Oral Oncol. 2019;88:153–9.
48. Gupta T, Master Z, Kannan S, et al. Diagnostic performance of post-treatment FDG PET or FDG PET/CT imaging in head and neck cancer: a systematic review and meta-analysis. Eur J Nucl Med Mol Imaging. 2011;38:2083–95.
49. Goel R, Moore W, Sumer B, Khan S, Sher D, Subramaniam RM. Clinical practice in PET/CT for the management of head and neck squamous cell cancer. Am J Roentgenol. 2017;209:289–303.
50. Marcus C, Ciarallo A, Tahari AK, et al. Head and neck PET/CT: therapy response interpretation criteria (Hopkins Criteria)-interreader reliability, accuracy, and survival outcomes. J Nucl Med. 2014;55:1411–6.
51. Kendi AT, Brandon D, Switchenko J, et al. Head and neck PET/CT therapy response interpretation criteria (Hopkins criteria)—external validation study. Am J Nucl Med Mol Imaging. 2017;7:174–80.
52. Sjovall J, Bitzen U, Kjellen E, Nilsson P, Wahlberg P, Brun E. Qualitative interpretation of PET scans using a Likert scale to assess neck node response to radiotherapy in head and neck cancer. Eur J Nucl Med Mol Imaging. 2016;43:609–16.
53. Krieger DA, Hudgins PA, Nayak GK, et al. Initial performance of NI-RADS to predict residual or recurrent head and neck squamous cell carcinoma. Am J Neuroradiol. 2017;38:1193–9.
54. Wangaryattawanich P, Branstetter BF, Hughes M, Clump DA 2nd, Heron DE, Rath TJ. Negative predictive value of NI-RADS Category 2 in the first posttreatment FDG-PET/CT in head and neck squamous cell carcinoma. Am J Neuroradiol. 2018;39:1884–8.
55. Weinreb JC, Barentsz JO, Choyke PL, et al. PI-RADS prostate imaging—Reporting and Data System: 2015, Version 2. Eur Urol. 2016;69:16–40.
56. Radiology ACo. Breast imaging reporting and data system. BI-RADS. 2003.
57. Mitchell DG, Bruix J, Sherman M, Sirlin CB. LI-RADS (Liver Imaging Reporting and Data System): summary, discussion, and consensus of the LI-RADS Management Working Group and future directions. Hepatology. 2015;61:1056–65.
58. Burrell RA, McGranahan N, Bartek J, Swanton C. The causes and consequences of genetic heterogeneity in cancer evolution. Nature. 2013;501:338–45.
59. Mroz EA, Tward AD, Hammon RJ, Ren Y, Rocco JW. Intra-tumor genetic heterogeneity and mortality in head and neck cancer: analysis of data from the Cancer Genome Atlas. PLoS Med. 2015;12:e1001786.
60. Mroz EA, Tward AD, Pickering CR, Myers JN, Ferris RL, Rocco JW. High intratumor genetic heterogeneity is related to worse outcome in patients with head and neck squamous cell carcinoma. Cancer. 2013;119:3034–42.
61. Gerlinger M, Rowan AJ, Horswell S, et al. Intratumor heterogeneity and branched evolution revealed by multiregion sequencing. N Engl J Med. 2012;366:883–92.
62. Karlo CA, Di Paolo PL, Chaim J, et al. Radiogenomics of clear cell renal cell carcinoma: associations between CT imaging features and mutations. Radiology. 2014;270:464–71.
63. Zhao S, Kuge Y, Mochizuki T, et al. Biologic correlates of intratumoral heterogeneity in 18F-FDG distribution with regional expression of glucose transporters and hexokinase-II in experimental tumor. J Nucl Med. 2005;46:675–82.

64. Koyasu S, Nakamoto Y, Kikuchi M, et al. Prognostic value of pretreatment 18F-FDG PET/CT parameters including visual evaluation in patients with head and neck squamous cell carcinoma. Am J Roentgenol. 2014;202:851–8.
65. Apostolova I, Steffen IG, Wedel F, et al. Asphericity of pretherapeutic tumour FDG uptake provides independent prognostic value in head-and-neck cancer. Eur Radiol. 2014;24:2077–87.
66. Tixier F, Hatt M, Valla C, et al. Visual versus quantitative assessment of intratumor 18F-FDG PET uptake heterogeneity: prognostic value in non-small cell lung cancer. J Nucl Med. 2014;55:1235–41.
67. Brooks FJ, Grigsby PW. The effect of small tumor volumes on studies of intratumoral heterogeneity of tracer uptake. J Nucl Med. 2014;55:37–42.
68. Tixier F, Hatt M, Le Rest CC, Le Pogam A, Corcos L, Visvikis D. Reproducibility of tumor uptake heterogeneity characterization through textural feature analysis in 18F-FDG PET. J Nucl Med. 2012;53:693–700.
69. Hatt M, Majdoub M, Vallieres M, et al. 18F-FDG PET uptake characterization through texture analysis: investigating the complementary nature of heterogeneity and functional tumor volume in a multi-cancer site patient cohort. J Nucl Med. 2015;56:38–44.
70. Chicklore S, Goh V, Siddique M, Roy A, Marsden PK, Cook GJ. Quantifying tumour heterogeneity in 18F-FDG PET/CT imaging by texture analysis. Eur J Nucl Med Mol Imaging. 2013;40:133–40.
71. Hatt M, Tixier F, Pierce L, Kinahan PE, Le Rest CC, Visvikis D. Characterization of PET/CT images using texture analysis: the past, the present... any future? Eur J Nucl Med Mol Imaging. 2017;44:151–65.
72. Cheng NM, Fang YH, Lee LY, et al. Zone-size nonuniformity of 18F-FDG PET regional textural features predicts survival in patients with oropharyngeal cancer. Eur J Nucl Med Mol Imaging. 2015;42:419–28.
73. Mena E, Taghipour M, Sheikhbahaei S, et al. Value of intratumoral metabolic heterogeneity and quantitative 18F-FDG PET/CT parameters to predict prognosis in patients with HPV-positive primary oropharyngeal squamous cell carcinoma. Clin Nucl Med. 2017;42:e227–34.
74. Cheng NM, Fang YH, Chang JT, et al. Textural features of pretreatment 18F-FDG PET/CT images: prognostic significance in patients with advanced T-stage oropharyngeal squamous cell carcinoma. J Nucl Med. 2013;54:1703–9.
75. Scott AM, Gunawardana DH, Bartholomeusz D, Ramshaw JE, Lin P. PET changes management and improves prognostic stratification in patients with head and neck cancer: results of a multicenter prospective study. J Nucl Med. 2008;49:1593–600.
76. Lonneux M, Hamoir M, Reychler H, et al. Positron emission tomography with [18F]fluorodeoxyglucose improves staging and patient management in patients with head and neck squamous cell carcinoma: a multicenter prospective study. J Clin Oncol. 2010;28:1190–5.
77. Lowe VJ, Duan F, Subramaniam RM, et al. Multicenter trial of [(18)F]fluorodeoxyglucose positron emission tomography/computed tomography staging of head and neck cancer and negative predictive value and surgical impact in the N0 neck: results from ACRIN 6685. J Clin Oncol. 2019;37:1704–12.
78. Dammann F, Horger M, Mueller-Berg M, et al. Rational diagnosis of squamous cell carcinoma of the head and neck region: comparative evaluation of CT, MRI, and 18FDG PET. Am J Roentgenol. 2005;184:1326–31.
79. Baek CH, Chung MK, Son YI, et al. Tumor volume assessment by 18F-FDG PET/CT in patients with oral cavity cancer with dental artifacts on CT or MR images. J Nucl Med. 2008;49:1422–8.
80. Hong HR, Jin S, Koo HJ, et al. Clinical values of (18) F-FDG PET/CT in oral cavity cancer with dental artifacts on CT or MRI. J Surg Oncol. 2014;110:696–701.
81. Abd El-Hafez YG, Chen CC, Ng SH, et al. Comparison of PET/CT and MRI for the detection of bone marrow invasion in patients with squamous cell carcinoma of the oral cavity. Oral Oncol. 2011;47:288–95.
82. Babin E, Desmonts C, Hamon M, Benateau H, Hitier M. PET/CT for assessing mandibular invasion by intraoral squamous cell carcinomas. Clin Otolaryngol. 2008;33:47–51.
83. Ng SH, Chan SC, Yen TC, et al. Staging of untreated nasopharyngeal carcinoma with PET/CT: comparison with conventional imaging work-up. Eur J Nucl Med Mol Imaging. 2009;36:12–22.
84. Leclerc M, Lartigau E, Lacornerie T, Daisne JF, Kramar A, Gregoire V. Primary tumor delineation based on (18)FDG PET for locally advanced head and neck cancer treated by chemoradiotherapy. Radiother Oncol. 2015;116:87–93.
85. Anderson CM, Sun W, Buatti JM, et al. Interobserver and intermodality variability in GTV delineation on simulation CT, FDG-PET, and MR images of head and neck cancer. Jacobs J Radiat Oncol. 2014;1:006.
86. Huang SH, Chien CY, Lin WC, et al. A comparative study of fused FDG PET/MRI, PET/CT, MRI, and CT imaging for assessing surrounding tissue invasion of advanced buccal squamous cell carcinoma. Clin Nucl Med. 2011;36:518–25.
87. Sekine T, Barbosa FG, Delso G, et al. Local resectability assessment of head and neck cancer: positron emission tomography/MRI versus positron emission tomography/CT. Head Neck. 2017;39:1550–8.
88. Sekine T, Barbosa F, Kuhn FP, et al. PET+ MR versus PET/CT in the initial staging of head and neck cancer, using a trimodality PET/CT+ MR system. Clin Imaging. 2017;42:232–9.
89. Queiroz MA, Hullner M, Kuhn F, et al. PET/MRI and PET/CT in follow-up of head and neck cancer patients. Eur J Nucl Med Mol Imaging. 2014;41:1066–75.
90. Blodgett TM, Fukui MB, Snyderman CH, et al. Combined PET-CT in the head and neck. Radiographics. 2005;25:897–912.
91. Cho YS, Moon SH, Choi JY, Choe YS, Kim BT, Lee KH. Clinical significance of incidental 18F-FDG uptake in the pyriform sinus detected by PET/CT. Clin Nucl Med. 2016;41:e82–6.
92. Kyzas PA, Evangelou E, Denaxa-Kyza D, Ioannidis JP. 18F-fluorodeoxyglucose positron emission tomography to evaluate cervical node metastases in patients with head and neck squamous cell carcinoma: a meta-analysis. J Natl Cancer Inst. 2008;100:712–20.
93. Liao LJ, Lo WC, Hsu WL, Wang CT, Lai MS. Detection of cervical lymph node metastasis in head and neck cancer patients with clinically N0 neck-a meta-analysis comparing different imaging modalities. BMC Cancer. 2012;12:236.
94. Hollenbeak CS, Lowe VJ, Stack BC Jr. The cost-effectiveness of fluorodeoxyglucose 18-F positron emission tomography in the N0 neck. Cancer. 2001;92:2341–8.
95. Sahovaler A, Krishnan RJ, Yeh DH, et al. Outcomes of cutaneous squamous cell carcinoma in the head and neck region with regional lymph node metastasis: a systematic review and meta-analysis. JAMA Otolaryngol Head Neck Surg. 2019;145:352–60.
96. Mermod M, Tolstonog G, Simon C, Monnier Y. Extracapsular spread in head and neck squamous cell carcinoma: a systematic review and meta-analysis. Oral Oncol. 2016;62:60–71.
97. Su Z, Duan Z, Pan W, et al. Predicting extracapsular spread of head and neck cancers using different imaging techniques: a systematic review and meta-analysis. Int J Oral Maxillofac Surg. 2016;45:413–21.
98. Chun BJ, Yoo Ie R, Joo YH, et al. Efficacy of 18F-fluorodeoxyglucose positron emission tomography/CT imaging for extracapsular spread of laryngeal squamous cell carcinoma. Head Neck. 2016;38:290–3.
99. Kubicek GJ, Champ C, Fogh S, et al. FDG-PET staging and importance of lymph node SUV in head and neck cancer. Head Neck Oncol. 2010;2:19.

100. Platzek I, Beuthien-Baumann B, Schneider M, et al. FDG PET/MR for lymph node staging in head and neck cancer. Eur J Radiol. 2014;83:1163–8.
101. Hoang JK, Vanka J, Ludwig BJ, Glastonbury CM. Evaluation of cervical lymph nodes in head and neck cancer with CT and MRI: tips, traps, and a systematic approach. Am J Roentgenol. 2013;200:W17–25.
102. Kowalski LP, Carvalho AL, Martins Priante AV, Magrin J. Predictive factors for distant metastasis from oral and oropharyngeal squamous cell carcinoma. Oral Oncol. 2005;41:534–41.
103. Jackel MC, Rausch H. Distant metastasis of squamous epithelial carcinomas of the upper aerodigestive tract. The effect of clinical tumor parameters and course of illness. HNO. 1999;47:38–44.
104. Merino OR, Lindberg RD, Fletcher GH. An analysis of distant metastases from squamous cell carcinoma of the upper respiratory and digestive tracts. Cancer. 1977;40:145–51.
105. Takes RP, Rinaldo A, Silver CE, et al. Distant metastases from head and neck squamous cell carcinoma. Part I. Basic aspects. Oral Oncol. 2012;48:775–9.
106. de Bree R, Deurloo EE, Snow GB, Leemans CR. Screening for distant metastases in patients with head and neck cancer. Laryngoscope. 2000;110:397–401.
107. Krabbe CA, Pruim J, van der Laan BF, Rodiger LA, Roodenburg JL. FDG-PET and detection of distant metastases and simultaneous tumors in head and neck squamous cell carcinoma: a comparison with chest radiography and chest CT. Oral Oncol. 2009;45:234–40.
108. Rohde M, Nielsen AL, Johansen J, et al. Head-to-head comparison of chest X-ray/head and neck MRI, chest CT/head and neck MRI, and (18)F-FDG PET/CT for detection of distant metastases and synchronous cancer in oral, pharyngeal, and laryngeal cancer. J Nucl Med. 2017;58:1919–24.
109. Kim Y, Roh JL, Kim JS, et al. Chest radiography or chest CT plus head and neck CT versus (18)F-FDG PET/CT for detection of distant metastasis and synchronous cancer in patients with head and neck cancer. Oral Oncol. 2019;88:109–14.
110. Network NCC. NCCN Clinical practice guidelines in oncology: head and neck cancers. Version 2.2017. 2017.
111. Xu GZ, Guan DJ, He ZY. (18)FDG-PET/CT for detecting distant metastases and second primary cancers in patients with head and neck cancer. A meta-analysis. Oral Oncol. 2011;47:560–5.
112. Gao S, Li S, Yang X, Tang Q. 18FDG PET-CT for distant metastases in patients with recurrent head and neck cancer after definitive treatment. A meta-analysis. Oral Oncol. 2014;50:163–7.
113. Pavlidis N. Forty years experience of treating cancer of unknown primary. Acta Oncol. 2007;46:592–601.
114. Kwee TC, Basu S, Cheng G, Alavi A. FDG PET/CT in carcinoma of unknown primary. Eur J Nucl Med Mol Imaging. 2010;37:635–44.
115. Riihimaki M, Thomsen H, Hemminki A, Sundquist K, Hemminki K. Comparison of survival of patients with metastases from known versus unknown primaries: survival in metastatic cancer. BMC Cancer. 2013;13:36.
116. van de Wouw AJ, Jansen RL, Speel EJ, Hillen HF. The unknown biology of the unknown primary tumour: a literature review. Ann Oncol. 2003;14:191–6.
117. Patel S, Lydiatt W, Ridge J. Cervical lymph nodes and unknown primary tumors of the head and neck. In: AJCC cancer staging manual. 8th ed. Cham: Springer Nature; 2017. p. 67–78.
118. O'Sullivan B. Head and neck tumours. UICC TNM classification of malignant tumours. 8th ed. Chichester: Wiley; 2017. p. 17–54.
119. Kwee TC, Kwee RM. Combined FDG-PET/CT for the detection of unknown primary tumors: systematic review and meta-analysis. Eur Radiol. 2009;19:731–44.
120. Lee JR, Kim JS, Roh J-L, et al. Detection of occult primary tumors in patients with cervical metastases of unknown primary tumors: comparison of 18F FDG PET/CT with contrast-enhanced CT or CT/MR imaging—prospective study. Radiology. 2015;274:764–71.
121. Pawaskar AS, Basu S. Role of 2-fluoro-2-deoxyglucose PET/computed tomography in carcinoma of unknown primary. PET Clin. 2015;10:297–310.
122. Varadhachary GR. Carcinoma of unknown primary: focused evaluation. J Natl Compr Canc Netw. 2011;9:1406–12.
123. Zhu L, Wang N. 18F-fluorodeoxyglucose positron emission tomography-computed tomography as a diagnostic tool in patients with cervical nodal metastases of unknown primary site: a meta-analysis. Surg Oncol. 2013;22:190–4.
124. Sekine T, Barbosa FG, Sah BR, et al. PET/MR outperforms PET/CT in suspected occult tumors. Clin Nucl Med. 2017;42:e88–95.
125. Ruhlmann V, Ruhlmann M, Bellendorf A, et al. Hybrid imaging for detection of carcinoma of unknown primary: a preliminary comparison trial of whole-body PET/MRI versus PET/CT. Eur J Radiol. 2016;85:1941–7.
126. Network NCC. NCCN Clinical practice guidelines in oncology: Occult Primary (cancer of Unknown Primary [CUP]). Version 2.2019. 2019.
127. Mirghani H, Amen F, Tao Y, Deutsch E, Levy A. Increased radiosensitivity of HPV-positive head and neck cancers: molecular basis and therapeutic perspectives. Cancer Treat Rev. 2015;41:844–52.
128. Fakhry C, Westra WH, Li S, et al. Improved survival of patients with human papillomavirus-positive head and neck squamous cell carcinoma in a prospective clinical trial. J Natl Cancer Inst. 2008;100:261–9.
129. Gillison ML, D'Souza G, Westra W, et al. Distinct risk factor profiles for human papillomavirus type 16-positive and human papillomavirus type 16-negative head and neck cancers. J Natl Cancer Inst. 2008;100:407–20.
130. Goldenberg D, Begum S, Westra WH, et al. Cystic lymph node metastasis in patients with head and neck cancer: an HPV-associated phenomenon. Head Neck. 2008;30:898–903.
131. Abadi P, Johansen A, Godballe C, Gerke O, Hoilund-Carlsen PF, Thomassen A. (18)F-FDG PET/CT to differentiate malignant necrotic lymph node from benign cystic lesions in the neck. Ann Nucl Med. 2017;31:101–8.
132. Subramaniam RM, Alluri KC, Tahari AK, Aygun N, Quon H. PET/CT imaging and human papilloma virus-positive oropharyngeal squamous cell cancer: evolving clinical imaging paradigm. J Nucl Med. 2014;55:431–8.
133. Xu CC, Biron VL, Puttagunta L, Seikaly H. HPV status and second primary tumours in oropharyngeal squamous cell carcinoma. J Otolaryngol Head Neck Surg. 2013;42:36.
134. Martel M, Alemany L, Taberna M, et al. The role of HPV on the risk of second primary neoplasia in patients with oropharyngeal carcinoma. Oral Oncol. 2017;64:37–43.
135. Huang SH, Perez-Ordonez B, Liu FF, et al. Atypical clinical behavior of p16-confirmed HPV-related oropharyngeal squamous cell carcinoma treated with radical radiotherapy. Int J Radiat Oncol Biol Phys. 2012;82:276–83.
136. Huang SH, Perez-Ordonez B, Weinreb I, et al. Natural course of distant metastases following radiotherapy or chemoradiotherapy in HPV-related oropharyngeal cancer. Oral Oncol. 2013;49:79–85.
137. O'Sullivan B, Huang SH, Perez-Ordonez B, et al. Outcomes of HPV-related oropharyngeal cancer patients treated by radiotherapy alone using altered fractionation. Radiother Oncol. 2012;103:49–56.
138. Tahari AK, Alluri KC, Quon H, Koch W, Wahl RL, Subramaniam RM. FDG PET/CT imaging of oropharyngeal squamous cell carcinoma: characteristics of human papillomavirus-positive and -negative tumors. Clin Nucl Med. 2014;39:225–31.
139. Joo YH, Yoo Ie R, Cho KJ, Park JO, Nam IC, Kim MS. Preoperative 18F-FDG PET/CT and high-risk HPV in patients with oropharyngeal squamous cell carcinoma. Head Neck. 2014;36:323–7.

140. Kendi AT, Magliocca K, Corey A, et al. Do 18F-FDG PET/CT parameters in oropharyngeal and oral cavity squamous cell carcinomas indicate HPV status? Clin Nucl Med. 2015;40:e196–200.
141. Awan MJ, Lavertu P, Zender C, et al. Post-treatment PET/CT and p16 status for predicting treatment outcomes in locally advanced head and neck cancer after definitive radiation. Eur J Nucl Med Mol Imaging. 2017;44:988–97.
142. Yom SS, Gillison ML, Trotti AM. Dose de-escalation in human papillomavirus-associated oropharyngeal cancer: first tracks on powder. Int J Radiat Oncol Biol Phys. 2015;93:986–8.
143. Oncology N. NRG-HN002: a randomized phase II trial for patients with p16 positive, non-smoking associated, locoregionally advanced oropharyngeal cancer, NCT02254278. 2015. https://clinicaltrials.gov/ct2/show/NCT02254278.
144. Ong SC, Schoder H, Lee NY, et al. Clinical utility of 18F-FDG PET/CT in assessing the neck after concurrent chemoradiotherapy for locoregional advanced head and neck cancer. J Nucl Med. 2008;49:532–40.
145. Isles MG, McConkey C, Mehanna HM. A systematic review and meta-analysis of the role of positron emission tomography in the follow up of head and neck squamous cell carcinoma following radiotherapy or chemoradiotherapy. Clin Otolaryngol. 2008;33:210–22.
146. Sheikhbahaei S, Taghipour M, Ahmad R, et al. Diagnostic accuracy of follow-up FDG PET or PET/CT in patients with head and neck cancer after definitive treatment: a systematic review and meta-analysis. Am J Roentgenol. 2015;205:629–39.
147. Kao J, Vu HL, Genden EM, et al. The diagnostic and prognostic utility of positron emission tomography/computed tomography-based follow-up after radiotherapy for head and neck cancer. Cancer. 2009;115:4586–94.
148. Wong ET, Dmytriw AA, Yu E, et al. (18) F-FDG PET/CT for locoregional surveillance following definitive treatment of head and neck cancer: a meta-analysis of reported studies. Head Neck. 2019;41:551–61.
149. Helsen N, Roothans D, Van Den Heuvel B, et al. 18F-FDG-PET/CT for the detection of disease in patients with head and neck cancer treated with radiotherapy. PLoS One. 2017;12:e0182350.
150. Kim S, Loevner L, Quon H, et al. Diffusion-weighted magnetic resonance imaging for predicting and detecting early response to chemoradiation therapy of squamous cell carcinomas of the head and neck. Clin Cancer Res. 2009;15:986–94.
151. Wong KH, Panek R, Welsh L, et al. The predictive value of early assessment after 1 cycle of induction chemotherapy with 18F-FDG PET/CT and diffusion-weighted MRI for response to radical chemoradiotherapy in head and neck squamous cell carcinoma. J Nucl Med. 2016;57:1843–50.
152. Martens RM, Noij DP, Ali M, et al. Functional imaging early during (chemo)radiotherapy for response prediction in head and neck squamous cell carcinoma; a systematic review. Oral Oncol. 2019;88:75–83.
153. Garibaldi C, Ronchi S, Cremonesi M, et al. Interim (18)F-FDG PET/CT during chemoradiation therapy in the management of head and neck cancer patients: a systematic review. Int J Radiat Oncol Biol Phys. 2017;98:555–73.
154. Min M, Lin P, Lee MT, et al. Prognostic role of metabolic parameters of (18)F-FDG PET-CT scan performed during radiation therapy in locally advanced head and neck squamous cell carcinoma. Eur J Nucl Med Mol Imaging. 2015;42:1984–94.
155. Abgral R, Querellou S, Potard G, et al. Does 18F-FDG PET/CT improve the detection of posttreatment recurrence of head and neck squamous cell carcinoma in patients negative for disease on clinical follow-up? J Nucl Med. 2009;50:24–9.
156. Leemans CR, Tiwari R, Nauta JJ, van der Waal I, Snow GB. Recurrence at the primary site in head and neck cancer and the significance of neck lymph node metastases as a prognostic factor. Cancer. 1994;73:187–90.
157. Beswick DM, Gooding WE, Johnson JT, Branstetter BF. Temporal patterns of head and neck squamous cell carcinoma recurrence with positron-emission tomography/computed tomography monitoring. Laryngoscope. 2012;122:1512–7.
158. Ho AS, Tsao GJ, Chen FW, et al. Impact of positron emission tomography/computed tomography surveillance at 12 and 24 months for detecting head and neck cancer recurrence. Cancer. 2013;119:1349–56.
159. Spector ME, Chinn SB, Rosko AJ, et al. Diagnostic modalities for distant metastasis in head and neck squamous cell carcinoma: are we changing life expectancy? Laryngoscope. 2012;122:1507–11.
160. McDermott M, Hughes M, Rath T, et al. Negative predictive value of surveillance PET/CT in head and neck squamous cell cancer. Am J Neuroradiol. 2013;34:1632–6.
161. Roman BR, Patel SG, Wang MB, et al. Guideline familiarity predicts variation in self-reported use of routine surveillance PET/CT by physicians who treat head and neck cancer. J Natl Compr Canc Netw. 2015;13:69–77.
162. Cabana MD, Rand CS, Powe NR, et al. Why don't physicians follow clinical practice guidelines? A framework for improvement. JAMA. 1999;282:1458–65.
163. Zhang B, Li X, Lu X. Standardized uptake value is of prognostic value for outcome in head and neck squamous cell carcinoma. Acta Otolaryngol. 2010;130:756–62.
164. Xie P, Li M, Zhao H, Sun X, Fu Z, Yu J. 18F-FDG PET or PET-CT to evaluate prognosis for head and neck cancer: a meta-analysis. J Cancer Res Clin Oncol. 2011;137:1085–93.
165. Pak K, Cheon GJ, Nam HY, et al. Prognostic value of metabolic tumor volume and total lesion glycolysis in head and neck cancer: a systematic review and meta-analysis. J Nucl Med. 2014;55:884–90.
166. Castelli J, De Bari B, Depeursinge A, et al. Overview of the predictive value of quantitative 18 FDG PET in head and neck cancer treated with chemoradiotherapy. Crit Rev Oncol Hematol. 2016;108:40–51.
167. Wang L, Bai J, Duan P. Prognostic value of 18F-FDG PET/CT functional parameters in patients with head and neck cancer: a meta-analysis. Nucl Med Commun. 2019;40:361–9.
168. Gouw ZAR, La Fontaine MD, van Kranen S, et al. The prognostic value of baseline 18F-FDG PET/CT in human papillomavirus-positive versus human papillomavirus-negative patients with oropharyngeal cancer. Clin Nucl Med. 2019;44:e323–8.
169. Moan JM, Amdal CD, Malinen E, Svestad JG, Bogsrud TV, Dale E. The prognostic role of 18F-fluorodeoxyglucose PET in head and neck cancer depends on HPV status. Radiother Oncol. 2019;140:54–61.
170. Floberg JM, DeWees TA, Chin RI, et al. Pretreatment metabolic tumor volume as a prognostic factor in HPV-associated oropharyngeal cancer in the context of AJCC 8th edition staging. Head Neck. 2018;40:2280–7.
171. Chotchutipan T, Rosen BS, Hawkins PG, et al. Volumetric (18) F-FDG-PET parameters as predictors of locoregional failure in low-risk HPV-related oropharyngeal cancer after definitive chemoradiation therapy. Head Neck. 2019;41:366–73.
172. Castelli J, Depeursinge A, Devillers A, et al. PET-based prognostic survival model after radiotherapy for head and neck cancer. Eur J Nucl Med Mol Imaging. 2019;46:638–49.
173. Sheikhbahaei S, Ahn SJ, Moriarty E, Kang H, Fakhry C, Subramaniam RM. Intratherapy or posttherapy FDG PET or FDG PET/CT for patients with head and neck cancer: a systematic review and meta-analysis of prognostic studies. Am J Roentgenol. 2015;205:1102–13.
174. Mehanna H, Wong WL, McConkey CC, et al. PET-CT surveillance versus neck dissection in advanced head and neck cancer. N Engl J Med. 2016;374:1444–54.
175. Mehanna H, McConkey CC, Rahman JK, et al. PET-NECK: a multicentre randomised Phase III non-inferiority trial comparing a positron emission tomography-computerised tomography-guided watch-and-wait policy with planned neck dissection in the management of locally advanced (N2/N3) nodal metastases in patients

with squamous cell head and neck cancer. Health Technol Assess. 2017;21:1–122.
176. Helsen N, Van den Wyngaert T, Carp L, Stroobants S. FDG-PET/CT for treatment response assessment in head and neck squamous cell carcinoma: a systematic review and meta-analysis of diagnostic performance. Eur J Nucl Med Mol Imaging. 2018;45:1063–71.
177. Ang KK, Harris J, Wheeler R, et al. Human papillomavirus and survival of patients with oropharyngeal cancer. N Engl J Med. 2010;363:24–35.
178. Huang SH, O'Sullivan B, Xu W, et al. Temporal nodal regression and regional control after primary radiation therapy for N2-N3 head-and-neck cancer stratified by HPV status. Int J Radiat Oncol Biol Phys. 2013;87:1078–85.
179. Arunsingh M, Vaidyanathan S, Dyker KE, Sen M, Scarsbrook AF, Prestwich RJD. Accuracy of response assessment positron emission tomography-computed tomography following definitive radiotherapy without chemotherapy for head and neck squamous cell carcinoma. Clin Oncol (R Coll Radiol). 2019;31:212–8.
180. Wong LY, Wei WI, Lam LK, Yuen AP. Salvage of recurrent head and neck squamous cell carcinoma after primary curative surgery. Head Neck. 2003;25:953–9.
181. Lell M, Baum U, Greess H, et al. Head and neck tumors: imaging recurrent tumor and post-therapeutic changes with CT and MRI. Eur J Radiol. 2000;33:239–47.
182. Srinivasan A, Mohan S, Mukherji SK. Biologic imaging of head and neck cancer: the present and the future. Am J Neuroradiol. 2012;33:586–94.
183. Alhilali L, Reynolds AR, Fakhran S. Osteoradionecrosis after radiation therapy for head and neck cancer: differentiation from recurrent disease with CT and PET/CT imaging. Am J Neuroradiol. 2014;35:1405–11.

The manufacturer's authorised representative in the EU is Springer Nature Customer Service Centre GmbH, Europaplatz 3, 69115 Heidelberg, Germany. If you have any concerns regarding our products, please contact ProductSafety@springernature.com

Printed and bound by CPI Group (UK) Ltd, Croydon, CR0 4YY
30/09/2026
02225269-0001